Management *of* PAIN & ANXIETY *in the* Dental Office

Management *of* PAIN & ANXIETY

in the Dental Office

RAYMOND A. DIONNE, DDS, PhD***

Bethesda, Maryland

JAMES C. PHERO, DMD

Professor of Clinical Anesthesia, Clinical Pediatrics, and Clinical Surgery
University of Cincinnati College of Medicine;
Faculty, UC Physicians Pain Center
Cincinnati, Ohio

DANIEL E. BECKER, DDS

Professor, Allied Health Sciences
Sinclair Community College;
Associate Director of Medical Education, General Practice Dental Residency,
Miami Valley Hospital
Dayton, Ohio

*Dr. Dionne is a Senior Investigator at the National Institute of Dental and Craniofacial Research, NIH. His participation as an editor for this book was performed outside the scope of his employment as a US Government employee. His contributions represent his personal opinion and not necessarily those of the US Government.

SAUNDERS
An Imprint of Elsevier

SAUNDERS
An Imprint of Elsevier

The Curtis Center
Independence Square West
Philadelphia, Pennsylvania 19106

NOTICE

Pharmacology is an ever-changing field. Standard safety precautions must be followed, but as new research and clinical experience broaden our knowledge, changes in treatment and drug therapy may become necessary or appropriate. Readers are advised to check the most current product information provided by the manufacturer of each drug to be administered to verify the recommended dose, the method and duration of administration, and contraindications. It is the responsibility of the treating physician, relying on experience and knowledge of the patient, to determine dosages and the best treatment for each individual patient. Neither the publisher nor the editor assumes any liability for any injury and/or damage to persons or property arising from this publication.

Stack
ISBN-13: 978-0-7216-7278-6
ISBN-10: 0-7216-7278-7

Acquisitions Editor: Penny Rudolph
Developmental Editor: Jaime Pendill
Project Manager: Linda McKinley
Designer: Julia Dummitt

MANAGEMENT OF PAIN AND ANXIETY IN THE DENTAL OFFICE

Printed in the United States of America

Last digit is print number: 9   8   7   6   5   4   3   2

CONTRIBUTORS

C. Richard Bennett, DDS, PhD
Professor and Chairman, Department of
Anesthesiology; Professor, Department of
Pharmacology, University of Pittsburgh School of
Dental Medicine, Pittsburgh, Pennsylvania

Jeffrey D. Bennett, DMD
Associate Professor, Department of Oral and
Maxillofacial Surgery, University of Connecticut
School of Dental Medicine, Farmington,
Connecticut

Charles W. Berthold, DDS, MS
Gratis Faculty Member, Department of
Pharmacology and Department of General
Dentistry, Louisiana State University Health
Science Center, New Orleans, Louisiana

Bruce E. Bradley, DDS, PhD
Associate Professor, Department of Oral and
Maxillofacial Surgery, University of Michigan
School of Dentistry, Ann Arbor, Michigan

Glenn T. Clark, MS, DDS
Professor and Chair, Department of Oral Medicine
and Oral Pain, University of California–Los Angeles
School of Dentistry, Los Angeles, California

Stephen A. Cooper, DMD, PhD
Board of Overseers, Department of Oral Surgery,
University of Pennsylvania, Philadelphia,
Pennsylvania; Senior Vice President, Medical and
Clinical Affairs, Whitehall-Robins Healthcare,
Department of Scientific Affairs, Whitehall-Robins
Healthcare, Madison, New Jersey

Jane M. Fall-Dickson, RN, PhD, AOCN
Clinical Research Fellow, National Institute of
Dental and Craniofacial Research, National
Institutes of Health, Bethesda, Maryland

Raymond S. Garrison, DDS, MS
Professor and Chairman, Department of Dentistry,
Wake Forest University School of Medicine,
Winston-Salem, North Carolina

Joseph A. Giovannitti, Jr., DMD
Private Practice, Dallas, Texas

Daniel A. Haas, DDS, PhD, FRCD (C)
Professor and Associate Dean; Head of Department
of Clinical Sciences; Head of Discipline of
Anaesthesia, Faculty of Dentistry, University of
Toronto, Toronto, Ontario, Canada

Kenneth M. Hargreaves, DDS, PhD
Professor and Chair, Department of Endodontics,
University of Texas Health Science Center at San
Antonio, San Antonio, Texas

Kate M. Hathaway, PhD
Associate Professor and Licensed Psychologist,
Department of TMD and Orofacial Pain, University
of Minnesota School of Dentistry, Minneapolis,
Minnesota

J. Mel Hawkins, DDS, BScD(AN), FADSA, DADBA
Director, Intravenous Sedation Continuing
Education, Department of Anaesthesia, Faculty of
Dentistry, University of Toronto, Toronto, Ontario,
Canada

Mark N. Hochman, DDS
Clinical Associate Professor, Departments of
Orthodontics and Implant Dentistry, New York
University College of Dentistry, New York, New
York; Scientific Consultant, Milestone Scientific,
Inc, Livingston, New Jersey; Private Practice, New
York, New York

Stephen R. Holliday, DDS
Associate Professor, Department of Allied Health
Sciences, Sinclair Community College; Associate
Director of Medical Education, General Practice
Dental Residency, Miami Valley Hospital, Dayton,
Ohio

Milton I. Houpt, DDS, PhD
Professor, Chairman and Director of Postdoctoral
Program, Department of Pediatric Dentistry,
UMDNJ–New Jersey Dental School, Newark,
New Jersey

Yoshiki Imamura, DDS, PhD
Associate Professor, Department of Dental
Anesthesiology, Kyushu Dental College; Head,
Department of Orofacial Pain and Neurofunction
Clinic, Kyushu Dental College Hospital,
Kitakyushu, Fukuoka, Japan

Yuzuru Kaneko, DDS, PhD
Professor in Chief, Department of Anesthesiology, Tokyo Dental College, Tokyo, Japan

David P. Kretzschmar, DDS, MS
Assistant Professor, Department of Oral and Maxillofacial Surgery, Wake Forest University School of Medicine, Winston-Salem, North Carolina

John P. Lawrence, MD
Assistant Professor of Clinical Anesthesia, University of Cincinnati College of Medicine, Cincinnati, Ohio

John W. Leyman, DDS
Associate Professor, Department of Dental Anesthesiology, Loma Linda University School of Dentistry, Loma Linda, California

Leonard J. Lind, MD, FCCM
Clinical Professor, Department of Anesthesia, University of Cincinnati College of Medicine, Cincinnati, Ohio; Anesthesiologist and Medical Director, PACU and SDS, Department of Anesthesia, University Hospital, Cincinnati, Ohio

Hideo Matsuura, DDS, PhD, IJBDA
Professor Emeritus, Faculty of Dentistry, Department of Dental Anesthesiology, Osaka University, Suita City, Osaka Prefecture, Japan

John Gerard Meechan, BSc, BDS, FDSRCPS, PhD
Senior Lecturer and Honorary Consultant, Department of Oral Surgery, Newcastle Dental School, England

Stephen B. Milam, DDS, PhD
Professor and Chairman; Hugh B. Tilson Endowed Chair, Department of Oral and Maxillofacial Surgery, University of Texas Health Science Center at San Antonio, San Antonio, Texas

Peter Milgrom, DDS
Professor, Department of Public Health Sciences; Director, Dental Fears Research Clinic; Adjunct Professor of Health Services, University of Washington, Seattle, Washington

Jenny Z. Mitchell, MD
Assistant Professor of Clinical Anesthesia, University of Cincinnati College of Medicine, Cincinnati, Ohio

Paul A. Moore, DMD, PhD, MPH
Professor, Department of Dental Public Health, University of Pittsburgh School of Dental Medicine; Adjunct Professor, Department of Pharmacology, University of Pittsburgh School of Pharmacy; Adjunct Professor, Department of Epidemiology, University of Pittsburgh Graduate School of Public Health, Pittsburgh, Pennsylvania

John K. Neubert, DDS, PhD
Clinical Research Fellow, Pain and Neurosensory Mechanisms Branch, National Institute of Dental and Craniofacial Research, National Institutes of Health, Bethesda, Maryland

Jeffrey P. Okeson, DMD
Professor and Director, Orofacial Pain Center, Department of Oral Health Science, University of Kentucky College of Dentistry, Lexington, Kentucky

George E. Parsons, PhD
Private Practice, Cincinnati, Ohio

James A. Roelofse, MBChB, MMED, PhD
Professor, Department of Maxillofacial Surgery and Anesthesiology, University of Stellenbosch, South Africa

Morton B. Rosenberg, DMD
Professor, Department of Oral and Maxillofacial Surgery; Head, Division of Anesthesia and Pain Control; Associate Professor, Department of Anesthesia, Tufts University School of Medicine, Boston, Massachusetts

Lauren E. Ta, DDS, MS
Clinical Research Fellow, Pain and Neurosurgery Mechanisms Branch, National Institute of Dental and Craniofacial Research, Bethesda, Maryland

Larry D. Trapp, DDS
Associate Professor, Department of Dental Anesthesiology, Loma Linda University School of Dentistry, Loma Linda, California

John A. Yagiela, DDS, PhD
Professor and Chair, Division of Diagnostic and Surgical Services, University of California–Los Angeles School of Dentistry; Professor, Department of Anesthesiology, University of California–Los Angeles School of Medicine, Los Angeles, California

Pain was defined in 1906 in *The Devil's Dictionary as* "an uncomfortable frame of mind that may have a physical basis in something that is being done to the body, or may be purely mental . . ." It would not stretch the definition to suggest the mental portion can also be manifested in anxiety.

The understanding of "pain" as an entity has evolved over the past five decades, first by scientists and practitioners, dentists, and other health care providers and in the past decade by society in general. Significantly, in the past decade, that understanding has been transmitted to treatment of pain in its various body sites and its symptomatic manifestations to the point that the public expectations are focused on treatment rather than "suffering in silence."

Drs. Dionne, Phero, and Becker have devoted a significant amount of time in their illustrious careers to the understanding and management of pain and anxiety in the dental office. The initial text on this subject edited by Drs. Dionne and Phero was published in 1991. The 2002 text bears only a slight resemblance to its precursor. Just as the scientific knowledge and psychosocial and therapeutic aspects of pain have expanded, the same has been true in the area of pain and anxiety in dental practice.

Management of Pain and Anxiety in the Dental Office encapsulates this growth of information by using 37 authors from the United States and 7 other nations. This text covers all aspects of orofacial pain, both acute and chronic, as well as the spectrum of conscious sedation through general anesthesia. Many new topics not covered in the previous text are covered in this text, including up-to-date expansions of the basic science topics necessary to any thorough presentation of pain management. The authors have targeted this text primarily "to meet the reference and didactic needs of the doctoral and postgraduate dentist." I have no doubt, however, that all practitioners of pain management who encounter patients with orofacial pain will find information in this text that will be of great value to their practice.

Phillip O. Bridenbaugh, MD
Professor and Chairman,
Department of Anesthesia
University of Cincinnati Medical Center
Cincinnati, Ohio

Pain has always been a barrier to dentistry, serving as the inspiration for pioneering efforts by dentists to control pain. The discovery of anesthesia based on the observations of a dentist, Horace Wells, is considered one of medicine's greatest achievements. Outpatient anesthesia and conscious sedation owes much to the contributions of dentists such as Morgan Allison, Edward Driscoll, Neils Jorgensen, Leonard Monheim, and Sylvia Shane. The use of nitrous oxide as a sedation technique was popularized by a practicing dentist, Harry Langa.

Dentistry has also contributed significantly over the past 25 years in the continuing quest to ameliorate acute pain with the development of the oral surgery model by Stephen Cooper as the most widely used method for testing new analgesic drugs and mechanisms of analgesia in humans. The enigma of chronic orofacial pain and the growing recognition of the need to base therapy on scientifically validated approaches, often characterized as evidence-based medicine, now represent new challenges to the dental profession in the control of pain. This text attempts to address these challenges by providing clinical advice and treatment recommendations for the control of both acute and chronic pain based on the best scientific evidence and balancing benefit-to-risk considerations for the patient.

The text is divided into five parts. Part I contains four chapters that provide the basic principles underlying the control of pain and patient apprehension in the dental setting. Part II reviews the pharmacology of the drug classes most commonly used to achieve pain control in outpatients. Part III describes the management of patients across the range of pharmacologic techniques used in dental practice. Part IV discusses the unique considerations associated with the management of patients with special requirements. Part V devotes five chapters to the most problematic area of pain management, the diagnosis and management of chronic pain. The emphasis throughout the book is not only that the drugs and management modalities should be scientifically validated but also that safety is a paramount consideration in treating patients for mostly elective procedures, both from an ethical imperative and in the current medicolegal environment.

We wish to thank the large number of contributors and our publisher for tolerating our many missed deadlines and editorial shortcomings. We also appreciate the encouragement and the often needed "push" by Jaime Pendill and Penny Rudolph of Elsevier/Saunders and the editorial expertise applied by Carol Weis of Top Graphics.

This edition is dedicated to Ronald Dubner, DDS, PhD, in recognition of his contributions to the study of pain and its application to dentistry over the past four decades. He has contributed significantly to our understanding of pain and its control, trained a generation of pain researchers and defined a tradition of excellence for pain research by dentists, for dentistry, and for the benefit of our patients.

Raymond A. Dionne
James C. Phero
Daniel E. Becker

CONTENTS

Management
of
PAIN & ANXIETY
in the
Dental Office

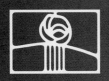

PRINCIPLES OF PAIN
AND ANXIETY CONTROL

CHAPTER 1

Overcoming Pain and Anxiety in Dentistry

RAYMOND A. DIONNE

YUZURU KANEKO

CHAPTER OUTLINE

Pain and dentistry are often synonymous in the minds of patients, especially those with poor dentition due to multiple extractions, periodontal disease requiring surgery, or symptomatic teeth requiring endodontic therapy. Many dental procedures can cause pain, even with the benefit of local anesthesia. Surgical procedures may result in significant postoperative pain, edema, and even limited mouth opening for 2 to 3 days postoperatively. Dental therapy can evoke perioperative anxiety, especially in pediatric patients, those with special needs, phobic patients, or those undergoing procedures usually associated with dread, such as "root canals" or removal of impacted third molars.

Although behavioral approaches and clinical expertise result in successful outcomes in many situations, pharmacologic approaches are frequently used to alleviate patient apprehension, attenuate postoperative pain, and provide symptomatic treatment of chronic orofacial pain. The safe and effective application of drug therapy is based on knowledge of the drug's pharmacology, appreciation for its interaction with normal physiology, and recognition of adverse effects and their management (Box 1-1).

This text addresses the management of acute and chronic pain and dental patient apprehension based on accepted pharmacologic therapies and special applications for dental outpatients. The emphasis is on critical review of the primary literature to substantiate the safety and efficacy for indications that have not been subjected to formal approval through the normal regulatory process for new drugs.

The most problematic area of orofacial pain, the *temporomandibular disorders* (TMDs), are usually self-limited and resolve over time with symptomatic, reversible treatments. A small fraction of patients with chronic orofacial pain are resistant to treatment and often seek or receive professional advice to pursue more aggressive therapy. Irreversible treatments are generally discouraged because they are usually ineffective and may result in iatrogenic injury. The dearth of clinical trials on which to base therapeutic recommendations for TMDs produces a dilemma: the severity and the chronicity of the pain prompt treatment, but few standard therapies have been validated. In areas where the literature on clinical trials attempting to validate treatments is limited, this text provides conservative therapeutic recommendations for chronic orofacial pain by extrapolation from similar indications in other patient populations.

Our overall objective is to provide scientifically based recommendations for treatment of pain and anxiety in dental outpatients, with *patient safety* as the paramount consideration. The foundation knowledge is presented first, the relevant drug classes reviewed, and the various therapeutic modalities for acute pain and management of perioperative patient anxiety presented. The last four chapters focus on the diagnosis and treatment of chronic orofacial pain with the same approach, although with limited support from the scanty scientific literature. The overall goals are to improve pain therapeutics, provide a basis for safer methods of anxiety management, and suggest conservative approaches to the management of TMDs.

Pain and Dentistry

Fear of pain associated with dentistry persists despite the decreasing incidence of dental disease and continuing improvements in the control of pain. The most common method for blocking pain during dental procedures—the intraoral administration of local anesthetic—is aversive in its own right due to the pain associated with its administration and the perceived threat of needle puncture. This assertion is supported by a survey finding that individuals who reported themselves as highly fearful of dentistry worry about receiving oral injections.[1] Another survey of the general population demonstrated an association between high dental anxiety and missed or delayed dental appointments.[2] These observations support previous findings that avoidance of dental care due to fear of dentistry represents a significant barrier to oral health[3,4] (Box 1-2). Fear of dental pain is magnified in pediatric patients, emotionally and physically disabled patients, and those who have

---

BOX 1-1

Therapeutic Recommendation

Although pharmacologic methods for controlling pain and apprehension are in common use, only analgesic therapy for acute pain is based on careful regulatory review. For sedation, anesthesia, and chronic pain treatment, dentists should only employ drug modalities that are based on careful review of the scientific literature documenting both safety and efficacy.

BOX 1-2

Therapeutic Recommendation

Effective control of pain and apprehension associated with dentistry is a preventive strategy that every dentist should incorporate into his or her practices and likely results in improved oral health by minimizing avoidance of dental care.

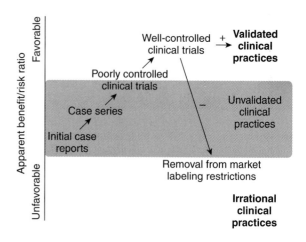

Fig. 1-1 Natural history of therapeutic modalities for pain management. Favorable reports based on case series or poorly controlled clinical trials are often superseded by well-controlled trials that demonstrate whether a treatment is a validated clinical practice, an invalidated clinical practice, or should be removed from the market or its use otherwise restricted. (From Dionne RA: *Oral Surg Oral Med Oral Pathol Oral Radiol Endod* 83:135, 1997.)

become fearful as a result of previous unpleasant dental or medical procedures. As a consequence, some dental outpatients require anxiolytic modalities.

For low levels of apprehension, behavioral methods and judicious use of topical and local anesthesia often suffice. Pharmacologic adjuncts, such as nitrous oxide or an orally administered sedative, are usually needed for moderate levels of patient anxiety that prevents or interferes with the planned procedure. Truly phobic patients, patients with special needs who are not able to accept treatment, and patients undergoing extremely painful procedures (e.g., removal of impacted third molars) often require parenteral sedation or general anesthesia. The relative efficacy and safety of these modalities vary greatly depending on the clinician's level of training as well as the drug, dose, and route of administration. As a result of these considerations, most dentists other than oral surgeons still rely on oral sedation as the primary method for managing anxiety in outpatients.

Natural History of Pain Therapeutics

The natural history of therapeutic interventions for the management of pain covers a wide range (Fig. 1-1). Novel treatments first described on the basis of initial case reports, case series, or poorly controlled clinical trials usually appear to have therapeutic benefit, or the results would not be publicized. After evaluation of a putative therapy in well-controlled clinical trials, several alternative interpretations are possible. If several trials indicate that the treatment is effective and has minimum toxicity, it is considered to be a validated therapeutic practice. An example of this outcome is the use of nonsteroidal antiinflammatory drugs (NSAIDs) for the control of acute orofacial pain. If the treatment is found not to be effective or toxicity becomes evident, the drug is removed from

the market (e.g., zomepirac [Zomax] in the 1970s), or labeling restrictions are imposed (e.g., oral ketorolac [Toradol] more recently).

Most therapies that are used for chronic orofacial pain do not fall under the jurisdiction of the U.S. Food and Drug Administration (FDA) as either drugs or devices and are not subjected to rigorous examination before being used in humans. Other review processes, such as the U.S. Pharmacopeial Convention, use expert panels to review non-FDA-approved uses for marketed drugs but do not address devices or clinical practices. As a consequence, most drugs, devices, and therapeutic strategies that are used for chronic orofacial pain, and to a lesser extent for conscious sedation, fall into the category of nonvalidated clinical practices. This does not imply that these treatment modalities do not have some therapeutic value. Rather, they have not been subjected to well-controlled trials that allow the biomedical community to determine if the modality is a validated clinical practice with efficacy that exceeds the potential for toxicity, or perhaps to determine that their use represents an irrational clinical practice that should be discontinued. The hazard of using a seemingly effective therapy in humans without appropriate validation of safety is illustrated by the use of Proplast implants for the treatment of TMDs.

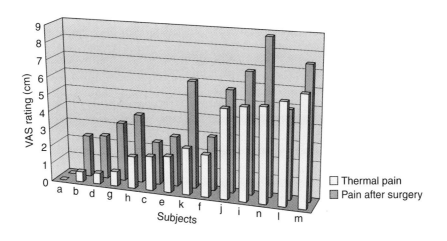

Fig. 1-2 Wide variation in clinical pain report among subjects undergoing a single extraction of a full-boney impacted third molar.

The principles of managing dental pain and anxiety rest on the same principles that apply to the use of all therapeutic modalities: (1) demonstrated efficacy for the indication, (2) acceptable incidence and severity of adverse reactions for the condition being treated, and (3) safety when used in large numbers of patients for prolonged periods.

Mechanistic Complexity of Pain

The complexity and multiplicity of pain mechanisms and the difficulty in separating nociceptive processing from normal physiologic processes represent a significant barrier to pain therapy. It is now recognized that gender and genetic factors also contribute to individual variation in pain perception, processing, and appreciation. Use of analgesic drugs in fixed doses that have been validated in a relatively homogenous patient sample may not result in effective therapy when used in a patient population with wide genetic diversity in pain processing and drug metabolism. For example, a fourfold variation was seen in postsurgical pain levels for patients undergoing a near-identical procedure: the removal of a single impacted third molar, after offset of a limited dose of local anesthetic (Fig. 1-2). This variation is likely caused by individual differences in pain processing, since application of a fixed thermal stimuli to the skin of the same cranial nerve dermatome also resulted in similar variation across the sample. The similarity in individual responses to both experimental and clini-

cal pain supports the concept of a molecular genetic basis to variations in pain across patients.

Genetic factors may also influence the clinical efficacy of medications used for pain and anxiety control. Codeine, for example, is metabolized to a number of metabolites with potential opiate activity, including morphine.[5] In subjects characterized as either good or poor drug metabolizers based on prior challenge with a test compound (sparteine), a wide variation in blood levels of morphine were demonstrated. Good metabolizers produced detectable levels of morphine, whereas poor metabolizers produced negligible morphine after codeine administration; codeine levels were similar between the two groups. The efficacy of the codeine for experimental pain was significantly related to the circulating morphine levels but unrelated to the codeine levels in the blood, suggesting that the morphine metabolite, not the parent drug, was responsible for the analgesic effect. If this observation in a limited number of subjects with experimental pain can be extrapolated to clinical pain, genetic factors related to drug metabolism may also impact on analgesic efficacy when treating pain clinically.

Although the peripheral effects of clinically useful drugs such as aspirin and NSAIDs are generally attributed to suppression of the enzyme cyclooxygenase in the periphery, many other cytokines are capable of producing pain at a site of tissue injury. The inability to demonstrate an analgesic mechanism for acetaminophen, peripheral sites of action for opioids, or central sites of action for NSAIDs suggests a mechanistic complexity to pain processes, both peripherally and centrally. The search continues, however, for the development of drugs with selective effects on a single neurotransmitter or inflammatory mediator in hopes of producing effective analgesia with minimal effects on other systems. Disappointment over the results of early clinical trials across a series of prototypic neurokinin antagonists[6] suggest the limitations of selective blockade of just one of many possible pathways for signaling pain, especially if accompanied by inflammation. Similarly, selective blockade of the neurokinin-2 receptor does not produce any detectable analgesia.[7] If blockade of the two receptors for a potent pain-producing substance, substance P, does not result in detectable analgesia across a series of studies, selective blockade of other mediators of pain may also prove inadequate.

Current methods for assessing new analgesic drugs arose from the pioneering work of Henry Beecher and colleagues in the 1950s, evolved in the 1960s through the extensive work of Houde, Wallenstein, and Rogers, and became standardized in the 1970s. Although these methods have been largely unchanged for more than 25 years, since the introduction of the oral surgery model,[8] rapid expansion in the neurosciences and biotechnology now holds promise for many new investigational treatments for pain. The ability to test novel mechanisms and prototypic drugs rapidly and efficiently is largely limited by use of clinical models, experimental designs, and pain measurement methods from an earlier scientific era. Persistence in continuing to evaluate potentially important analgesic mechanisms and novel treatments may be hampered by regulatory and pharmaceutical reluctance to evolve in parallel with the rapidly expanding scientific basis for understanding pain and its relief. In addition, the high cost and relatively slow pace of clinical analgesic trials increase the cost of drug development, delay financial return on the large investment in drug development, and limit introduction of treatments for relatively small clinical indications. More importantly, the incidence of chronic pain in the U.S. population, the limitations of currently available analgesic drugs, and the high impact of untreated pain suggest a need for better pain management.

This text presents strategies for enhancing analgesic therapy with existing drugs and combinations in the absence of FDA-approved indications where the evidence supports this use and when safety has been established through other clinical uses.

Pain Prevention

Interfering with nociceptive input into the central nervous system (CNS), especially in the perioperative period, also interferes with processes that contribute to the development of greater pain at later times, a process characterized as *central sensitization*.[9] The consequence of sensitization is that innocuous sensations may be interpreted as painful because of these CNS changes, termed *central hyperalgesia*, and are thought to persist long after the initiating stimulus has ended. This phenomenon and the related process of sensitization of peripheral nociceptors are probably additive and contribute to both the intensity and the duration of pain postoperatively. Recognition of the possible clinical importance of the development of central sensitization has led to attempts to block its development and thus minimize postoperative pain and lower analgesic demand during recovery. The ability to lower analgesic use is particularly desirable in ambulatory patients, who are much more sensitive to the adverse effects of opioid drugs, including nausea and vomiting. Decreasing pain and adverse drug effects not only makes the postoperative period less unpleasant, but it also enhances return to normal function and likely lowers apprehension about future clinical procedures.

How can these results be applied to the management of pain in the dental environment? The use of a long-acting local anesthetic (e.g., bupivacaine, etidocaine) before a painful procedure (e.g., removal of impacted third molar) results in less pain during the first 4 hours after surgery (Fig. 1-3, *A*) and should attenuate pain intensity over the next 48 hours (Fig. 1-3, *B*). The administration of an NSAID before pain onset will suppress the release of inflammatory mediators, especially prostaglandins, which contribute to the sensitization of peripheral nociceptors. Patients will experience a much slower onset and less intense postoperative pain after NSAID pretreatment, thereby lessening the development of central sensitization as well. The combination of NSAID pretreatment before pain onset and the use of a long-acting local anesthetic greatly reduces pain after oral surgery, such that many patients report little pain for 6 to 7 hours postoperatively.[10,11] Additional benefits with NSAID pretreatment include less postoperative edema and lessening of limitation in mouth opening, both considered to be cardinal signs of acute inflammation.[12]

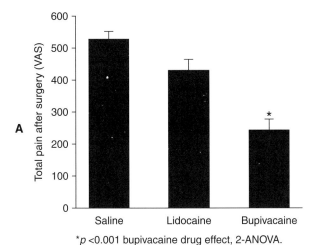

A

*p <0.001 bupivacaine drug effect, 2-ANOVA.

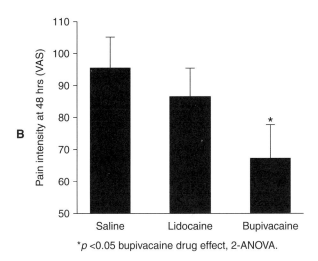

B

*p <0.05 bupivacaine drug effect, 2-ANOVA.

Fig. 1-3 Reduction in postoperative pain in the immediate postoperative period **(A)** resulting in a reduction in pain at 48 hours **(B)**, presumably by blocking the development of central sensitization leading to hyperalgesia at later time points. (Modified from Gordon S et al: *J Dent Res* 76:153,1997.)

Controversy on Safety of Anesthesia and Sedation

A television documentary in the mid-1980s focused public concern over the safety of dental anesthesia and sedation, with resultant changes in virtually all state dental practice acts and implementation of professional guidelines for the use of anesthesia and sedation in the dental office. Levels of training increased, requirements for monitoring and office inspections were implemented, and even the use of some drug classes (e.g., barbiturates) came under regulatory scrutiny. Although no objective data has ever been published, clinical impression suggests that patient safety has improved for the use of general anesthesia and parenteral sedation in the dental office. The paucity of dentists trained in anesthesia and sedation, the regulatory limits to the use of parenteral sedation, and the limited therapeutic options when referring anxious patients to an oral surgeon (i.e., extractions) force general dentists to manage most patients in need of sedation with an oral drug.

The choice of which drug, combination of drugs, and dose for oral sedation is complex and largely based on tradition rather than data from well-controlled studies.[13] The morbidity and mortality attributed to pediatric sedation by another television show in the 1990s *(60 Minutes II)* illustrates that selection of a sedative drug regimen should be weighted heavily in favor of patient safety. Among the drug classes used for oral premedication in dentistry (barbiturates, chloral hydrate, opioids, antihistamines, and phenothiazines), benzodiazepines are the most selective for anxiety relief with the greatest margin of safety. Diazepam (Valium) largely replaced the barbiturates for oral sedation, but it is metabolized to active metabolites that produce residual sedation long after the procedure. Oral diazepam produces significant anxiety relief in adults, but its effect cannot be readily differentiated from placebo in children, suggesting the need for a more effective benzodiazepine for oral pediatric sedation.

Balancing Efficacy and Safety

Selection of the sedation modality, the drugs, and the dose range to balance clinical efficacy and patient safety involves complex decisions that depend on not only knowledge of the drugs being used but also the level of training of the clinician and the expectations of the patient. The choice of sedative modality is based largely on the patient's level of apprehension, the perceived need for amnesia, and duration and difficulty of the procedure. The overriding consideration is patient safety, however, since virtually any significant morbidity or mortality is considered unacceptable in an otherwise healthy outpatient undergoing an elective dental procedure.

The safety of anxiolytic drug use for dental patients depends primarily on the drug, dose, and route of administration. This is illustrated for diazepam (Valium), one of the most common sedative drugs in dentistry (Table 1-1). Oral administration of diazepam 10 mg results in a minimally to moderately sedated patient, usually with no changes in vital signs other than those associated with relaxation from an anxious state, and it requires no specialized training beyond the doctoral level. Intravenous administration of the same dose will usually result in a very relaxed patient with some transient changes in vital signs but introduces the potential for greater morbidity than oral administration of the same dose. Because of many earlier reports of serious morbidity and mortality in the dental office associated with parenteral sedation, dentists are now required to obtain advanced training beyond the doctoral level and to monitor vital signs frequently. If a greater dose of diazepam is given by the same route of administration, a state of deep sedation may be produced, medicolegally considered synonymous with general anesthesia. This requires advanced training of 1 to 2 years beyond the doctoral level, continuous monitoring by a second individual who is not the operator, and even higher levels of professional liability coverage.

This example illustrates that the safety of drugs used for sedation in dental patients depends greatly on (1) the drug, (2) the route of administration, and (3) the total dose administered. These three parameters largely predict the resultant pharmacologic effects and the frequency and severity of adverse reactions, thereby indicating the level of training required to sedate patients safely before outpatient dental procedures.

The selection of drugs, doses, and the route of administration has historically been left to the discretion of individual educators and clinicians. The resultant diversity of drugs and combinations in current clinical use is indicated by a survey that identified 82 distinct drug combinations used for intravenous sedation by 264 respondents.[14] The scientific basis for the use of such a broad spectrum of drugs and combinations has not been established. Very few drugs have an FDA-approved indication for sedation in outpatients. Although the FDA does not regulate the practice of medicine or dentistry, they do determine whether a specific use of a drug meets regulatory standards for safety and efficacy (see following discussion). Few well-controlled clinical trials have evaluated the use of sedative drugs in dental patients. Many published studies are inadequate due to methodologic flaws, such as a failure to include a placebo or standard treatment for comparison, the use of observer end points (the appearance of sedation) rather than patient self-report (anxiety relief), small sample sizes resulting in a failure to differentiate between treatments due to variability, and the use of drug combinations without first demonstrating independent and additive effects for each of the components. Expert opinions or clinical observations in the absence of an adequate body of well-controlled studies are insufficient for differentiating the subjective effects of drugs from placebo responses, observer and patient bias, individual variability, and chance occurrences. Moreover, even

TABLE 1-1   📖

Diazepam Dose and Administration in Dental Patients

Diazepam Dose	Route of Administration	Level of Consciousness	Monitoring	Training
10 mg	Oral	Slightly to moderately sedated	Responsiveness to verbal commands	DDS
10 mg	Intravenous	Moderately sedated	Blood pressure Respiration rate Oxygen saturation	Sedation permit; varies by state
20 mg	Intravenous	Moderately to heavily sedated	Blood pressure Respiration rate Oxygen saturation	Anesthesia permit; varies by state

extensive clinical observations may be insufficient to detect serious morbidity or mortality that occurs with low frequency. As a consequence, therapeutic recommendations for the use of sedative drugs in dental patients are often nonvalidated clinical practices based on unsubstantiated assertions.

Selecting a drug or combination for use as a sedative in dental patients should be weighed heavily in favor of patient safety over efficacy. A wide spectrum of safety exists between general anesthesia and deep sedation at one extreme and oral sedation or nitrous oxide at the other end (Fig. 1-4). General anesthesia and deep sedation are effective in virtually all patients but carry significant risk of morbidity and mortality requiring extensive postdoctoral training, continuous monitoring, and a separate anesthetist to give the drug and monitor the patient. *Parenteral sedation* still carries the risk of transient morbidity if dose, patient responsiveness, and the experience of the administrator are not carefully balanced. *Nitrous oxide* requires minimal additional training beyond the doctoral level, is efficacious in less anxious pa-

tients, but requires scrupulous scavenging of waste gases to avoid contamination of the operatory with subsequent chronic exposure to dental personnel. *Oral sedation*, in contrast, can be as efficacious as parenteral premedication, requires little monitoring when appropriate doses are used, and is unlikely to result in serious morbidity.

Dentists without advanced training in parenteral sedation should limit their use of sedative drugs to oral administration and nitrous oxide. Clinicians with appropriate training in parenteral sedation can usually treat all but the most phobic patients with oral sedation or intravenous sedation with a benzodiazepine. The addition of other drug classes, such as opioids and barbiturates, usually provides little additional benefit to the patient but does increase the potential for respiratory depression, inadvertent loss of consciousness, and other adverse drug reactions. The chapters that address anesthesia and sedation assume that dentists treating patients with sedative drugs follow professional and regulatory guidelines for training in the drug modality selected.

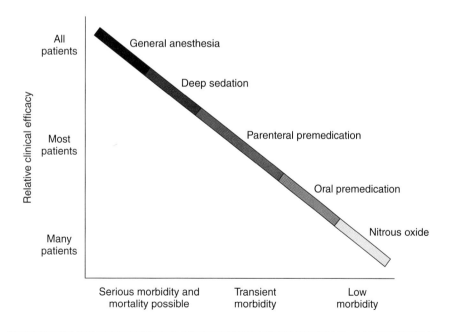

Fig. 1-4 Relationship between the clinical efficacy of drugs used for anxiety relief and patient safety. Increasing clinical efficacy is directly related to greater potential for morbidity, while the use of modalities such as nitrous oxide and oral premedication are effective in many patients with only a low risk of morbidity. (From Dionne RA: *Oral Maxillofac Surg Clin North Am* 4:990, 1992.)

Management of Chronic Orofacial Pain

The management of chronic orofacial pain has a long history of therapeutic misadventures, charismatic-based treatment philosophies, controversies over the correct nomenclature, and a lack of scientific documentation for most clinical practices. The dental profession has struggled to develop a systematic approach to nomenclature, treatment, and clinical research through numerous conferences, workshops, and attempts at consensus. Despite these efforts, there is still no generally accepted agreement on the etiology of chronic orofacial pain, its natural history, the role of occlusion, the need for aggressive treatment, and the effectiveness, safety, and indications for most current practices. These differences are often fostered by a lack of appreciation of the difference between clinical observations, which may form the basis for therapeutic innovation, and the need to verify the safety and efficacy of treatments in studies that control for factors that can mimic clinical success. Tricyclic antidepressants are an example of a treatment for chronic pain that arose from the clinical observations of astute clinicians but was subjected to scientific validation by well-controlled clinical trials.

Drug classes for TMDs range from short-term treatment with NSAIDs and muscle relaxants for pain of presumed muscular origin to chronic administration of antidepressants for less well-characterized pain. In general, claims of efficacy based on clinical observations are often superseded by equivocal findings of efficacy or belated recognition of adverse effects and toxicity with long-term administration. The principles of pain management for TMDs rest on the same principles that apply to the use of all drugs: demonstrated efficacy for the indication, an acceptable incidence of adverse reactions for the condition being treated, and safety when used in large numbers of patients for prolonged periods.

History of Anesthesia and Sedation

The primary role of dentists in the discovery of anesthesia is not surprising because few surgical procedures were performed in the early part of the nineteenth century. Physicians and surgeons infrequently produced pain deliberately, so the problem of pain was probably a low priority. This was not the case with early dental practitioners, who were treating patients with pain every day and thus had daily incentive for discovering the means to relieve pain.

General Anesthesia

The history of modern anesthesia began in 1844 with the use of nitrous oxide and in 1846 with the use of ether. "Nitrous air" was first produced by the British scientist Joseph Priestley in 1776. In 1800, Humphrey Davy found that the gas he called "laughing gas" had anesthetic and sedative effects.[15] At the time, laughing gas was used as pneumatic therapy to treat patients with tuberculosis and was exploited for fun and pleasure. The use of nitrous oxide spread to the United States, where it was accidentally discovered to have special qualities.

On December 10, 1844, Gardner Quincy Colton, a chemist, was demonstrating the properties of nitrous oxide during a traveling show in Hartford, Connecticut.[16] Samuel Cooley, a member of the audience and a local drugstore clerk, came on stage and inhaled the gas, then began to dance and dash around, injuring his legs. A 29-year-old dentist named Horace Wells noticed that despite an apparently serious wound, Cooley did not exhibit signs of pain. Wells recognized that the gas had an analgesic or anesthetic effect that might be useful to reduce the pain of surgical treatment and tooth extraction. Wells asked Colton to bring the nitrous oxide equipment to his office the next day. Wells inhaled the gas until he lost consciousness. As part of an experiment to test Wells' theory, Dr. John M. Riggs, a friend of Wells, removed one of his upper wisdom teeth. Later, expressing his concern surrounding this first therapeutic use of nitrous oxide, Riggs explained that he felt as though he were entering an unknown world. Wells exclaimed, "It is the greatest discovery ever made. I did not feel it so much as the prick of a pin."[17]

In a surgery room at the Massachusetts General Hospital, before a group of medical students and physicians, including the famous surgeon Professor John Collins Warren, Wells unsuccessfully demonstrated his nitrous oxide anesthesia. After a medical student inhaled the gas, Wells attempted to extract his tooth; the student moved and groaned. Although patients often exhibit these signs under light anesthesia even though they are not in pain, at the time, these facts were not known to the audience, who accused Wells of fraud.

On October 16, 1886, in the same operating theater where Wells failed to demonstrate the anesthetic effect of nitrous oxide, William Morton, a dentist and a Harvard Medical School student, successfully anesthetized a patient with ether.[18] During the ether demonstration, Professor Warren removed a submandibular lymph node from the patient. Professor

Warren stood before the audience to claim, "Gentlemen, this is no humbug." Surgical anesthesia emerged from the darkness at this moment.

Wells' failure to demonstrate anesthesia in his patient meant that for nearly 20 years, nitrous oxide was not used as an anesthetic agent.[19] Interestingly, both Wells' failure and Morton's success can be attributed to what we now know about the pharmacokinetics of these agents. Nitrous oxide has a weak anesthetic action, and inhalation of nitrous oxide from a bag can cause hypoxia. Ether, on the other hand, is volatile, and the gas has a strong anesthetic action. When ether is administered, it is mixed with air. This procedure does not induce hypoxia in the etherized patient. An advantage of nitrous oxide was only fast induction. From the viewpoint of anesthetic power and safety, ether was clearly superior to nitrous oxide at the time of their discovery. The properties of nitrous oxide meant that Wells failed to be named as the discoverer of general anesthesia. Ironically, Wells was also discredited as a dentist.[20] Although Morton received the honor of discovering general anesthesia, he was frustrated in his attempts to profit from this discovery by a man named Charles T. Jackson, a physician, geologist, and chemist. Jackson insisted that he had suggested to Morton that ether could be used as anesthetic.

It was later discovered that two other physicians may have been overlooked. Dr. Crawford Long of Atlanta used ether with mesmerism during the amputation of a leg 2 years before Morton's demonstration. A physician named Clark used ether as an anesthetic during a tooth extraction months before Long's demonstration. Neither publicized his observations, in contrast to Wells and Morton, who recognized the value of anesthesia and attempted to proclaim its benefits.

Local Anesthesia

Cocaine. The first article that appeared in a dental journal describing local anesthesia concluded that cocaine was not effective as a local anesthetic in dentistry, as follows:[21]

> Cocaine Hydrochlorate—As this substance is attracting considerable attention as a local anesthetic for the eye, it may occur to dentists to try it for sensitive dentine. As I do not find it of any special value for this purpose, it may be worthwhile to mention the fact, as it is very experimenting with so costly and comparatively useless a substance for this purpose.

On September 15, 1884, Josef Brettauer read a paper at an ophthalmologic congress in Heidelberg written by Carl Koller, an ophthalmologist at the University of Vienna. Koller's paper described the anesthetic effect of cocaine. The topical effect was demonstrated by applying it to the ocular surface of a patient. Local anesthesia was the second important discovery in the history of anesthesia. News of Koller's discovery immediately spread worldwide.

Four years earlier, in 1880, the local anesthetic action of cocaine was noted in frogs by the Estonian B. von Anrep, who recommended the application of cocaine to the human. Moleno Y. Maiz, a Peruvian physician, recognized the anesthetic actions of cocaine as early as 1860 and asked, "Could we use it as a local anesthetic?" Sigmund Freud, later famous as a psychiatrist, found that cocaine reduced his gingival pain during his studies of the effects of cocaine on psychiatric patients. Freud noted the anesthetic effect of cocaine in a paper that alerted Koller. Koller performed animal experiments and confirmed the anesthetic effect of cocaine in patients just 4 days before presenting his paper at the meeting in Heidelberg.

On January 20, 1885, Raymond presented a report at the meeting of the New York Dental Association on the local injection of cocaine during the treatment of six patients. William Stewart Halsted had performed the injections in Raymond's report. Halsted obtained excellent effects with a block anesthesia at the mandibular, infraorbital, and mental foramina. Halsted, only 32 years old at the time, was selected to become a member of the New York Surgical Association and became one of the most successful surgeons of this select group. Halsted began experiments on local injection, serving as his own research subject.[22] Halsted systematically demonstrated the clinical value of local anesthesia in dentistry, and he was the first clinician to demonstrate that the block anesthesia used in the oral and maxillofacial nerves could be applied to other nerve trunks. Unfortunately, Halsted became addicted to cocaine, and within 6 months of his first experiments, he was forced to stop his work and was repeatedly admitted to hospitals for treatment of his cocaine addiction. After a 2-year struggle, Halsted began working as a laboratory technician in the newly established department of pathology at Johns Hopkins Medical School. By 1892 he had fully recovered and joined the staff of the department of surgery. Soon he was appointed professor and subsequently contributed to the development of modern surgery. Halsted's contribution to the development of local anesthesia was neglected for many years because he failed to publish many of his studies. In 1920 the American Dental Association (ADA) recognized Halsted's contributions and honored him 6 months before his death, crediting him as the founder of regional nerve block anesthesia.[23]

When cocaine was used as a local anesthetic, two problems became evident: the weak anesthetic effect of cocaine and acute intoxication. Heinlich Braun, a German surgeon, combined epinephrine extract from the adrenal medulla with cocaine solution in 1897. Epinephrine constricts the blood vessels, decreasing the rate of absorption of cocaine into the blood. Braun determined the appropriate concentration of epinephrine to combine with cocaine by injecting himself subcutaneously. Braun found that the addition of epinephrine produced an extended duration of anesthesia, increased anesthetic efficacy, and prevented intoxication by constricting blood vessels in the region near the injection site. At the time of Braun's discovery, the only way to reduce the rate of absorption of cocaine from an arm or a leg during surgery was to tie the extremity with a tourniquet. For this reason, Braun named his new method "the chemical tourniquet."

Procaine.   Although Schleich and Reclus attempted to improve the safety associated with its use, cocaine is far from the ideal local anesthetic. Cocaine's weak anesthetic effect, its toxicity, and the short duration are all problematic. The search for better local anesthetics began shortly after cocaine's discovery. As early as 1860, Nieman found that cocaine is a benzoic acid ester. Investigations of the relationship between its chemical structure and its pharmacologic effects demonstrated that the anesthetic effect of cocaine is attributed to the benzoic acid moiety.

In 1904, Alfred Einhorn in Munich successfully synthesized a cocaine derivative called *procaine.* Much less toxic than its parent compound, procaine could be safely administered in doses that were 10 times greater than with cocaine. Because of its toxicity, the maximum dose of cocaine was limited to 100 mg. Braun was the first to use procaine clinically.

Lidocaine.   In 1943, Lofgren and Lundqvist, a Swedish chemist, successfully synthesized the first amide local anesthetic, named *lidocaine,* after more than 100 compounds had been investigated. Lidocaine is more potent than procaine, has greater stability, has no irritating action, and is less allergenic. Since 1947, lidocaine has been used extensively throughout the world.

Sedation

Nitrous Oxide.   The use of low concentrations of nitrous oxide for sedation began about 1950. Both Langa of the United States and Lubin of Denmark contributed to the development of the nitrous oxide sedation technique. The euphoria caused by inhalation of nitrous oxide was well known since the middle of the eighteenth century and led to the accidental discovery of general anesthesia. One hundred years later, nitrous oxide was also found to be useful for controlling anxiety during dental procedures.

Intravenous Drugs.   The first intravenous (IV) administration of drugs to control anxiety was performed by Niels Bjorn Jorgensen at Loma Linda University in 1945. A combination of scopolamine, pentobarbital, and meperidine was used for premedication, now characterized as the Jorgensen technique. *Diazepam,* a benzodiazepine, was the first sedative to be used as a single agent for dental patients, by Davidau in France. *Midazolam* is now preferred because it produces less vascular pain and irritation, results in anxiety relief and amnesia, and is more rapidly metabolized than diazepam.

A variety of drugs, including benzodiazepines, barbiturates, opioids, and propofol, are now used by dentists for IV sedation.[14] A major advantage of IV sedation is the ability to titrate the amount of drug administered to produce conscious sedation safely at a dose that balances efficacy and safety for the individual patient. The safety of an IV benzodiazepine for dental outpatients is supported by a recent clinical trial in nearly 1000 patients comparing midazolam to combinations of midazolam with an opioid or an opioid plus a barbiturate.[24] The available data suggest that careful titration of a benzodiazepine, alone or in combination with appropriate doses of an opioid or an opioid and barbiturate, can be very safe when performed by an appropriately trained dentist.[24]

Therapeutic Recommendations

Despite the implementation of modalities to prevent dental diseases (e.g., fluoride, flossing, sealants) and vast improvements in restorative materials, many dental procedures are painful and anxiety provoking. Analgesic and anesthetic drugs will continue to be needed for the foreseeable future to alleviate perioperative pain and anxiety, especially in pediatric patients and patients with special needs. In addition, the management of chronic orofacial pain often requires symptomatic treatment for self-limited conditions, and nonpharmacologic modalities may be addressing the etiology or behavior that is sustaining the chronic pain.

In patients who have failed conservative treatments or have developed iatrogenic complications of surgical treatments, palliative use of drugs to manage pain chronically is preferable to continued surgical procedures. Although the clinical conditions, patient populations, and durations of treatment vary across these indications, patient safety is paramount. The selection of a drug, dose, route of administration, and duration of treatment should be based on the results of controlled clinical trials demonstrating a favorable relationship between efficacy and safety.

The authors and editors of this text provide the scientific basis that underlies individualized therapeutic decisions for clinical practice. Ultimately, continued scientific and therapeutic inquiry will provide enhanced knowledge to address problematic areas of pain therapy and will help to individualize treatments based on each patient's "molecular signature."[25] In the absence of an adequate body of evidence in some therapeutic areas, the adage "first, do no harm" still provides a logical starting point for therapeutic decisions.

References

1. Milgrom P, Coldwell SE, Getz T, et al: Four dimensions of fear of dental injections, *J Am Dent Assoc* 128:756-766, 1997.
2. Dionne RA, Gordon SM, McCullagh LM, et al: Assessment of clinical needs for anesthesia and sedation in the general population, *J Am Dent Assoc* 129:167-173, 1998.
3. Berggren J, Maynert G: Dental fear and avoidance: causes, symptoms, and consequences, *J Am Dent Assoc* 109:247, 1984.
4. Gatchel RJ, Ingersol BD, Bowman L, et al: The prevalence of dental fear and avoidance: a recent study, *J Am Dent Assoc* 107:609, 1983.
5. Findlay JWA, Jones EC, Butz RF, et al: Plasma codeine and morphine combinations after therapeutic doses of codeine-containing analgesics, *Clin Pharmacol Ther* 24:60-68, 1978.
6. Dionne RA: Clinical analgesic trials of NK1 antagonists, *Curr Opin Cent Periph Nerv Syst Drugs* 1:84-87, 1999.
7. Dionne RA, Jaber L, Gilron I, et al: Effect of the NK-2 antagonist SR 48968C on acute pain and inflammation (abstract), *Proc Am Soc Clin Pharmacol Ther* 67:02, 2000.
8. Cooper SA, Beaver WT: A model to evaluate mild analgesics in oral surgery outpatients, *Clin Pharmacol Ther* 20:241-250, 1976.
9. Woolf CJ: Evidence for a central component of post-injury pain hypersensitivity, *Nature* 306:686-688, 1983.
10. Dionne RA, Wirdzek PR, Fox PC, et al: Suppression of postoperative pain by the combination of a non-steroidal anti-inflammatory drug, flurbiprofen, and a long-acting local anesthetic, etidocaine, *J Am Dent Assoc* 108:598-601, 1984.
11. Dionne RA: Suppression of dental pain by the preoperative administration of flurbiprofen, *Am J Med* 80(suppl 3A):41-49, 1986.
12. Troullos ES, Hargreaves KM, Butler DP, et al: Comparison of non-steroidal anti-inflammatory drugs, ibuprofen and flurbiprofen, to methylprednisolone and placebo for acute pain, swelling, and trismus, *J Oral Maxillofac Surg* 48:945-952, 1990.
13. Dionne RA: Oral sedation, *Compendium* 19:868-877, 1998.
14. Dionne RA, Gift HC: Drugs used for parenteral sedation in dental practice, *Anesth Prog* 35:199, 1988.
15. Smith WDA: A history of nitrous oxide and oxygen anesthesia. Part 1. Joseph Priestley to Humphrey Davy, *Br J Anaesth* 37:790-798, 1965.
16. Colton GQ: Experience in the use of nitrous oxide gas, *Br J Dent Sci* 11:253-257, 1868.
17. Archer WH: Life and letter of Horace Wells, discoverer of anesthesia, *J Am Coll Dent* 11(2):81-211, 1944.
18. Green NM: A consideration of factors in discovery of anesthesia and their effects on its development, *Anesthesiology* 33:515-522, 1971.
19. Green NM: Anesthesia and the development of surgery (1846-1896), *Anesth Analg* 58:5-12, 1979.
20. Menczer FM, Mittlemen M, Wildsmith JAW: The story of the man who first used nitrous oxide as an anesthetic has a tragic ending: Horace Wells, *J Am Dent Assoc* 110:773-776, 1985.
21. WHR: Cocaine hydrochlorate, *Dent Cosmos* 26:767, 1884.
22. Olch PD: William S. Halsted and local anesthesia: contribution and complications, *Anesthesiology* 42:479-486, 1975.
23. Clarke JH: History of regional anesthesia. In Jastak JT, Yagiela JA: *Regional anesthesia of the oral cavity,* St Louis, 1981, Mosby.
24. Dionne RA, Yagiela JA, Moore PA, et al: Comparing efficacy and safety of four intravenous sedation regimens in dental outpatients, *J Am Dent Assoc* 132:740-751, 2001.
25. Hunt SP, Mantyh PW: The molecular dynamics of pain control, *Nature Rev Neurosci* 2:83-91, 2001.

CHAPTER 2

Mechanisms of Orofacial Pain and Analgesia

Kenneth M. Hargreaves
Stephen B. Milam

CHAPTER OUTLINE

Dentists should be skilled in the treatment of acute orofacial pain because it often accompanies even meticulous clinical care. Just as successful dental therapy requires knowledge of anatomy, physiology, and the materials used, treating patients in acute pain depends on a foundation of basic and clinical sciences. This understanding requires an appreciation of the inflammatory mediators, neurotransmitters, and relevant nervous system pathways involved in the perception and modification of pain and the clinical pharmacology of therapeutic agents that control pain.

This chapter contributes to this foundation by reviewing peripheral mechanisms involved in detecting painful stimuli, peripheral mechanisms of hyperalgesia, central mechanisms of pain perception and hyperalgesia, and endogenous pain suppression systems. This information is discussed in the context of two common types of acute pain, dentinal pain and inflammatory pain, and chronic pain syndromes.

Peripheral Pain Mechanisms

Cutaneous Pain

The perception of pain is thought to signal the occurrence of tissue damage or the potential for damage.[1] Noxious stimuli, which can produce tissue damage, are detected by the terminal endings of two major classes of *nociceptive* (pain-detecting) afferent nerve fibers. These *nociceptors* are distributed throughout the skin, oral mucosa, and tooth pulp. The *A delta fibers* are relatively fast-conducting, lightly myelinated fibers. They respond primarily to noxious mechanical but generally not to chemical or thermal stimuli. A delta fibers have been proposed to mediate the initial sensation of pain, or *first pain*, which has a sharp or bright perceptual quality.[2,3] The second group of nociceptive fibers are the *C fibers*. These slow-conducting, unmyelinated nerve fibers respond to thermal, mechanical, and chemical stimuli. The C fibers likely mediate *second pain*, which occurs after the initial "sharp pricking" pain and is generally described as having a dull, aching or burning perceptual quality.

Analysis of the fiber population in a human spinal cutaneous nerve indicates that there are approximately three to five times more C fibers than A delta fibers, although presumably not all these fibers are nociceptors.[4] Other classes of cutaneous nociceptors have been described but have not been as well characterized. Most knowledge on the detection of pain comes from studies on cutaneous C and A delta fibers.

Primary afferent nerves fan out as they enter their cutaneous receptive fields. Compared with C fibers, A delta fibers innervating spinal dermatomes generally have a greater number of receptive fields spread over a greater surface area.[5] Although free nerve terminals lack morphologic specialization compared with other forms of cutaneous receptor types (e.g., pacinian corpuscles), they possess biochemical specialization in terms of membrane receptors and stored neuropeptide substances. Interestingly, ultrastructural studies have demonstrated that free nerve endings contain agranular vesicles,[6-8] which may release neuropeptides such as substance P in the modulation of inflammatory responses to tissue damage.

The response of free nerve endings to a suprathreshold stimulus is believed to be similar to other forms of receptor transduction, with the development of a local nonpropagated receptor potential that must exceed some threshold value to trigger a self-propagating action potential. The *action potential*, as a signal for the occurrence of tissue damage, is then conveyed along the primary nociceptive afferent; these fibers represent the peripheral distribution of cranial and upper cervical nerves that terminate in the medullary or spinal dorsal horns.

The detection of noxious stimuli in the orofacial region and the encoding of pain is conveyed primarily by nerves of the trigeminal system. The *trigeminal nerve*, or fifth cranial nerve, is the largest of the cranial nerves; its three branches (ophthalamic, maxillary, mandibular) innervate almost all the face and anterior scalp (Fig. 2-1). The trigeminal nerve also innervates mucous membranes of the mouth, gingiva, the teeth, anterior two thirds of the tongue, nasal cavities, sinuses, meninges, the jaw, and tongue muscles.

Remaining orofacial areas are innervated by other cranial nerves. The *facial* (seventh cranial) *nerve* encodes pain from the skin of the mastoid region and the external auditory meatus; most of the function of this nerve, however, is involved in taste sensation. The *glossopharyngeal* (ninth cranial) *nerve* innervates the back of the tongue, the tonsillar region, tympanic cavity, and antrum, as well as oronasal portions of the pharynx. The *vagus* (tenth cranial) *nerve* innervates the larynx, part of the ear, and the external auditory meatus. With the trigeminal nerve, these nerves provide the peripheral innervation necessary for the detection of cutaneous and dentinal pain.

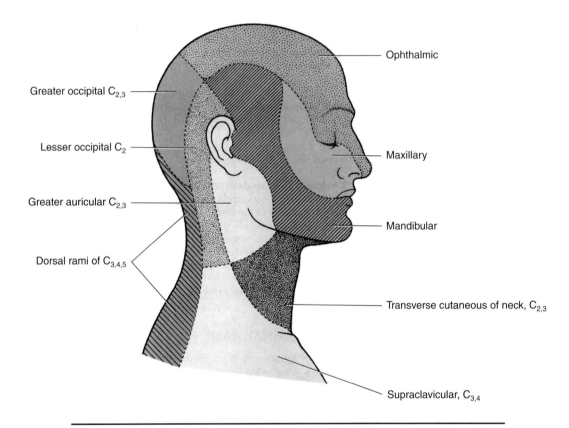

Ophthalmic

Greater occipital $C_{2,3}$

Lesser occipital C_2

Greater auricular $C_{2,3}$

Dorsal rami of $C_{3,4,5}$

Maxillary

Mandibular

Transverse cutaneous of neck, $C_{2,3}$

Supraclavicular, $C_{3,4}$

Fig. 2-1 Cutaneous distribution of peripheral nerves encoding orofacial sensation. Noxious stimuli, resulting in the sensation of pain, are detected by A delta and C fibers located in the trigeminal and upper cervical nerves. (From *Gray's anatomy*, ed 38, New York, 1995, Churchill Livingstone.)

Dentinal Pain

The tooth is heavily endowed with nociceptive nerve fibers. For example, approximately 700 A delta fibers and 1800 C fibers exit through the apical foramen of the adult bicuspid.[9] Stimulation of these pulpal nerve fibers by thermal, mechanical, or chemical stimuli results in a nearly pure sensation of pain. Electrical stimulation with a pulp tester also activates the A delta fibers.

Numerous studies have examined the micro-anatomy of tooth pulp innervation.[8,10,11] Dentinal tubules are well innervated near the pulp horns, with up to 74% of the tubules containing nerve fibers; these fibers can extend 200 μm into the tubule. At the midcrown level of the pulp, fewer tubules are innervated with shorter intratubular distances. In contrast, root dentin is poorly innervated. For all innervated tubules, the nerve fibers are close to odontoblasts, although anatomic connections are not evident.[7] The proximity of these two cell types

suggests that odontoblasts and afferent terminal endings may have biochemical connections (e.g., via expression of receptors) and thereby participate in the sensory transduction of noxious stimuli. This participation may signal dentinal fluid movement to the nerve ending. This cellular relationship may be the physiologic basis for the hydrodynamic theory of dentinal pain.

The *hydrodynamic theory* of dentinal pain has strong experimental support and postulates that movement of fluid through the dentinal tubules results in pain.[12-14] Stimuli, including air blasts, cold, and hypertonic sugars ("sweets"), can produce dentinal tubule fluid movement (Fig. 2-2). Movement of this fluid results in stimulation of nociceptive nerve fibers located on the pulpal side of the dentinal tubules. The fluid movement is thought to serve as a fluid transducer, signaling the presence of stimuli at the outer opening of the dentinal tubules. Removal of dentinal fluid abolishes the ability to detect these

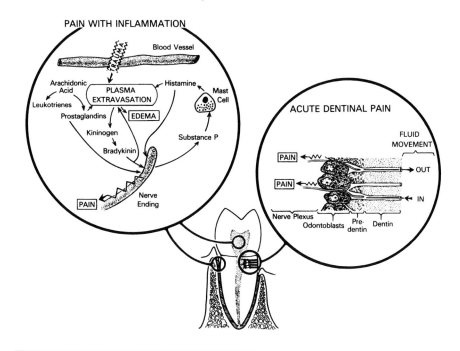

Fig. 2-2 Two mechanisms for peripheral stimulation of nociceptive (pain-detecting) nerve fibers in orofacial region. *Insert,* Pain with inflammation. Trauma activates a cascade resulting in the synthesis or release of prostaglandins, bradykinin, substance P, and histamine (as well as other mediators not shown). Interrelationships among these inflammatory mediators form a positive feedback loop, allowing inflammation to persist long after cessation of the dental procedure. *Insert,* Acute dentinal pain. According to the hydrodynamic theory, stimuli that cause fluid movement in exposed dentinal tubules result in stimulation of nociceptive nerve fibers. (From Hargreaves KM, Troullos E, Dionne R: *Dent Clin North Am* 31:675-694, 1987.)

stimuli; sensitivity returns when the fluid is replenished.[15] It is not known how nerve fibers detect fluid movement. However, the sharp quality of the resulting pain suggests activation of A delta nociceptive fibers.[16] Interestingly, dentinal sensitivity appears to recede with age or after chronic irritation. The increase in secondary or reparative dentin during these processes is thought to diminish fluid flow through the tubules.[17]

After exposure of dentin, either by loss of enamel or by loss of cementum and gingiva, dentinal sensitivity can develop. The buccal surfaces of canines and bicuspids are common sites of dentin exposure, probably because of their susceptibility for toothbrush-induced abrasion.[18] Dentinal sensitivity is characterized as a sharp pain that occurs soon after a provoking stimulus.[17,19] Current therapeutic approaches for blocking dentinal pain are directed at a physical blockade of fluid movement in the tubules. This is accomplished by application of agents such as stron-

tium, fluoride, potassium nitrate, and potassium oxalate. A method using electric current to enhance ion uptake into the tooth, termed *iontophoresis,* has been advocated,[20] but its efficacy has not been established.[21] Application of unfilled resins to exposed dentinal tubules is reported to have a prolonged effect.[22,23]

Inflammatory Pain

Inflammation and pain are common sequelae of dental procedures that produce tissue damage. Knowledge of inflammation and pain is of particular relevance for surgical, endodontic, and restorative treatment. The response to tissue damage constitutes the classic signs of inflammation: pain, edema, local increased temperature, redness, and loss of function (Fig. 2-3). Surgical extraction of impacted third molars produces the signs of inflammation; these findings emphasize the relationships among trauma

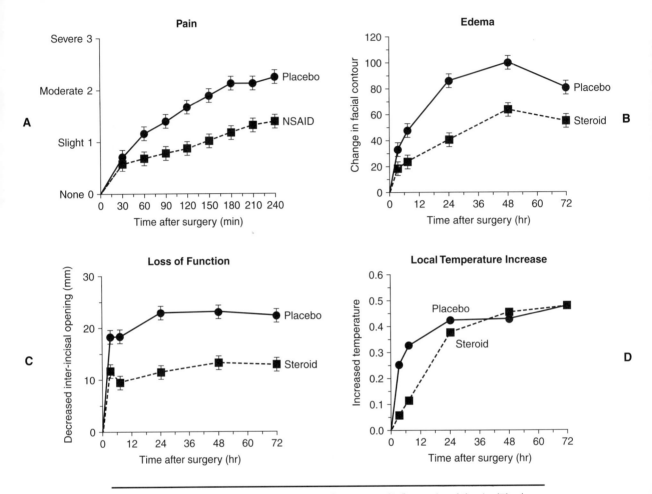

Fig. 2-3 Oral surgery as model of inflammation. Classic signs of inflammation, **(A)** pain, **(B)** edema, **(C)** hyperthermia, erythema (not evaluated), and **(D)** loss of function were assessed in 24 patients undergoing surgical extraction of impacted third molars. Process of inflammation occurs in dental procedures involving tissue damage, and its duration greatly exceeds that of the actual treatment. (Modified from Troullos E et al *J Oral Maxillofac Surg* 48:945, 1990.)

(or infection), inflammation, and posttreatment sequelae. Understanding the process of inflammation can improve care by minimizing the synthesis or release of local inflammatory mediators.

Three lines of evidence are generally required for acceptance of a substance as a local mediator of inflammation: (1) the substance must possess pharmacologic properties that are proinflammatory; (2) measured levels of the substance must be elevated during inflammation; and (3) pharmacologic antagonists to the mediator should possess antiinflammatory properties. Importantly, fulfillment of this last criterion

should have therapeutic benefit by blocking chemically mediated pathophysiologic events.

Products of arachidonic acid metabolism have strong support as inflammatory mediators. *Eicosanoids,* the family name for this class of mediators, are end products of arachidonic acid metabolism and are synthesized as needed. Under conditions of tissue damage, phospholipase A_2 and other enzymes liberate arachidonic acid from phospholipids embedded in cell membranes (see Fig. 2-2). At this point, enzymatic oxidative metabolism can proceed along two divergent pathways to produce several active compounds. The first pathway uses the cyclooxygenase (COX) enzymes, and the second pathway uses the lipoxygenase enzymes.

Prostaglandin levels are elevated in samples collected from inflamed tissue in both humans and animals.[23-25] Prostaglandins are generated in inflamed tissues by arachidonic acid peroxidation, a process that is mediated by enzymes known as *cyclooxygenases*. Two distinct cyclooxygenases are currently known, COX-1 and COX-2. It has been proposed that these enzymes, although similar in action, serve different physiologic functions. Based on analyses of gene structure and expression, COX-1 has characteristics of "housekeeping" genes and is expressed in most tissues. The primary function of *COX-1* is to generate prostaglandins required for normal tissue homeostatic functions. For example, prostanoids are important for gastric mucus and bicarbonate secretion, for renal blood flow regulation, and for normal platelet function.

In contrast, *COX-2* is not typically synthesized in normal tissues. Rather, it is synthesized rapidly in response to a variety of biochemical stimuli, including cytokines (e.g., interleukin-1β, tumor necrosis factor-α, lipopolysaccharide), growth factors (e.g., transforming growth factor-β, epidermal growth factor, platelet-derived growth factor, fibroblast growth factor), and free radicals generated in inflamed tissues.[26,27]

The Lewis strain of rats injected intradermally with Freund's complete adjuvant develop a polyarthritis with characteristics similar to rheumatoid arthritis.[28] COX-2 is rapidly induced in affected joints of these animals.[28,29] Immunostaining of articular tissues from these animals and from patients with rheumatoid arthritis has revealed several cellular sources of upregulated COX-2, including synoviocytes, endothelial cells, chondrocytes, infiltrating mononuclear inflammatory cells, and subchondral osteoblasts. Interestingly, COX-2 immunostaining is only detected in endothelial cells and isolated mononuclear inflammatory cells in articular tissues obtained from nonarthritic traumatized human joints.[28]

Administration of pharmacologic doses of prostaglandins results in increased vascular permeability, activated leukocytic migration, and sensitized nociceptive afferent nerves.[30,31] Several of these factors may be involved in inflammation; for example, prostacyclin is more potent than prostaglandin E_2 (PGE$_2$), although shorter acting, for producing hyperalgesia.[32]

COX-2 expression is suppressed by aspirin-like drugs or nonsteroidal antiinflammatory drugs (NSAIDs), glucocorticoids, and antiinflammatory cytokines (e.g., interleukin-4, interleukin-13).[26,28,29] Selective COX-2 inhibitors have recently been released for clinical use based on the assumptions that (1) prostaglandins mediating inflammation and pain are generated primarily from the action of COX-2, and (2) prostaglandins produced by COX-1 activity are essential for normal organ function (e.g., gastric and renal blood flow, gastric mucus and bicarbonate secretion). Theoretically, selective COX-2 inhibitors should relieve pain and inflammation without affecting prostaglandin-dependent organ functions. However, this theory has recently been challenged.

A second pathway of arachidonic acid metabolism is catalyzed by the enzyme lipoxygenase and results in the formation of the leukotrienes. *Leukotrienes* are the major biologically active products of the 5-lipoxygenation of arachidonic acid. Leukotrienes are relatively short-acting biochemicals. For example, LTB$_4$ has a biologic half-life of 3.5 minutes in the presence of neutrophils.[33] Leukotrienes promote plasma extravasation, particularly in the presence of PGE$_2$. Furthermore, leukotrienes, especially LTB$_4$, are chemotactic for inflammatory cells. LTB$_4$ stimulates these cells to produce free radicals. This effect could contribute to the limited half-life of LTB$_4$ in the presence of these cells, since free radicals can inactivate the leukotriene, particularly in the presence of redox active iron. Therefore evidence indicates that leukotrienes play an important role in the evolution of inflammation.

Thermal hyperalgesia has been observed within 6 hours of an intradermal injection of LTB$_4$ in humans.[34] In these experiments the response threshold to thermal stimulation was reduced approximately 15% by LTB$_4$. LTB$_4$ also induces hyperalgesia in animals. Using a rat model in which hyperalgesia was defined as a relative decrease in tactile pressure required to evoke withdrawal of a paw previously injected with a test substance, Levine et al[35] demonstrated LTB$_4$-induced hyperalgesia. The molar potency of LTB$_4$ for this effect was approximately three times that of bradykinin. Interestingly, bradyknin-induced hyperalgesia was antagonized by preadministration of indomethacin, but LTB$_4$-induced hyperalgesia was unaffected by preadministration of the NSAID. Moreover, LTB$_4$-induced hyperalgesia could be prevented by depletion of polymorphonuclear leukocytes before administration of the leukotriene.[35]

Leukocyte depletion was accomplished in these experiments by repeated intravenous administrations of either hydroxyurea or methotrexate.

Based on these findings, it appears that hyperalgesia induced by LTB_4 is mediated by secondary mechanisms. LTB_4 is a potent chemotactic agent and activator of polymorphonuclear leukocytes. These cells in turn produce a variety of biochemicals that may contribute directly or indirectly to hyperalgesia. However, onset of the hyperalgesic response in this study was rapid, within 20 minutes, and therefore the cell-mediated events responsible for induction of hyperalgesia likely were not dependent on protein synthesis. In support of this concept, Levine et al[36] have provided additional evidence that dihydroxyeicosatetraenoic acid (diHETE) products derived from polymorphonuclear leukocytes elicit hyperalgesia by a specific diHETE receptor-mediated mechanism.

In light of these studies, it is curious to note that LTB_4 appears to reduce spontaneous discharge by primary afferent neurons supplying canine dental pulp. Gazelius et al[37] observed this effect when the leukotriene was applied to freshly exposed pulps of cat teeth. These investigators also found that LTB_4 suppressed excitation of pulpal neurons evoked by exposure to hypertonic saline. In this study the leukotriene preparation required either ethanol or methanol as a solvent. Although the final alcohol concentration did not exceed 3% in the injected solution, it is not clear if the alcohol contaminant contributed to the observed effects. Other investigators have provided contrary results using the same animal model. Madison et al[38] found that LTB_4 treatment (25 mg/ml) significantly enhanced intradental nerve activity evoked by hypertonic saline. These investigators concluded that LTB_4 sensitizes pulpal nociceptors, although the exact mechanism was not explored.

In summary, the effects of leukotrienes on peripheral nerve functions are complex. The evidence indicates that primary afferent neural activities can be modified by leukotrienes; however, many of the effects of leukotrienes on nociception may be indirectly mediated by the actions of inflammatory cells. Agents that block leukotriene synthesis or action possess antiinflammatory activity.[36,39]

Histamine, another inflammatory mediator, is released in tissue after degranulation of mast cells and basophils (see Fig. 2-2). This limited supply reservoir, coupled with a short half-life, suggests that histamine may act only in the early stages of inflammation. In addition, histamine release may vary according to the form of tissue injury; it does not appear to be equally involved in all types of inflammation.[40] Local tissue injection of histamine produces several proinflammatory responses, such as vasodilation, flare, edema, or pain and itching.[41,42] Elevated histamine levels have been reported during inflammation.[43] In addition, histamine receptor antagonists have demonstrated efficacy in blocking many signs of inflammation in clinical studies, including those involving oral surgery patients.[44]

Bradykinin is a peptide liberated by the enzymatic cleavage of kininogen by the enzyme kallikrein (see Fig. 2-2). The precursors for the bradykinin system, prekallikrein and kininogen, circulate as components of blood. Since kallikrein is activated as part of the intrinsic clotting cascade, bradykinin can be locally released at any time, wherever there is damage to blood vessels. The synthetic capability of the bradykinin system is immense; plasma levels of bradykinin can increase more than 10,000-fold under appropriate in vitro conditions. Bradykinin pharmacology reveals a wide spectrum of proinflammatory actions. This peptide activates nociceptive afferent nerves, increases vascular permeability, promotes vasodilation, and induces positive chemotaxis of leukocytes.[30,45] The second criterion for an inflammatory mediator, measurement of elevated levels during inflammation, has been recently demonstrated in patients undergoing oral surgery.[46] Surgical wound levels of immunoreactive bradykinin increase significantly after extraction of impacted third molars (Fig. 2-4). Finally, agents that block either bradykinin synthesis[46] or action[47,48] possess analgesic or antiinflammatory effects.

In general, the various inflammatory mediators have two main effects on the peripheral nociceptive nerve ending. First, they excite and sensitize the peripheral nerve ending.[2,3] Sensitized endings have spontaneous activity, a decreased threshold, and prolonged responses ("afterdischarges") to suprathreshold stimuli. A second effect of inflammatory mediators is to stimulate the release of neuropeptides stored in the peripheral nociceptive nerve ending. The cell body of the primary afferent nerve fiber synthesizes the neuropeptides substance P and calcitonin gene-related peptide (CGRP), as well as other substances, which are transported both to the central nervous system (CNS) and to the periphery.[49] These neuropeptides are highly concentrated in dental pulp nerves,[50,51] and electrical stimulation of the inferior

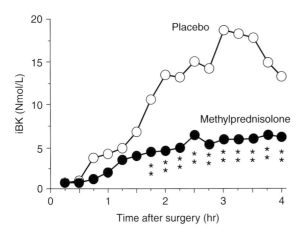

Fig. 2-4 Effect of pretreatment with methylprednisolone on tissue levels of immunoreactive bradykinin *(iBK)* in 36 oral surgery patients. ***p* >0.01. (From Hargreaves KM et al: *Clin Pharmacol Ther* 44:613-621, 1988.)

alveolar nerve releases substantial amounts of substance P from pulpal tissue.[52] In peripheral tissue, substance P and CGRP have proinflammatory properties. They act synergistically with other inflammatory mediators to stimulate histamine release from mast cells and induce plasma extravasation.[53,54] In addition, substance P stimulates monocytes to release substances such as interleukin-1β, tumor necrosis factor, and interleukin-6.[55] More recent studies have implicated neuropeptide release with regulation of wound healing, tissue necrosis, and dentinogenesis. Thus the peripheral nerve not only detects and signals the occurrence of tissue damage but also participates in the development of tissue inflammation and responses to trauma or infection.

In contrast to dentinal pain, pain associated with inflammation has a prolonged time course. This is caused in part by the sustained actions of peripheral mediators, which are thought to interact in the development of a local positive feedback cycle. Tissue trauma or byproducts of infection can activate the synthesis of prostaglandins and the release of bradykinin from its blood-borne precursor, kininogen. Since prostaglandins, bradykinin, and histamine all increase either the permeability or the vasodilation of local blood vessels,[30,53] they act synergistically to increase plasma extravasation (see Fig. 2-2). This accumulation of extravasated fluid into tissue spaces

produces the clinical sign of edema. In addition, plasma extravasation replenishes these short-lived local mediators by providing a fresh supply of kininogen, prostaglandins (released by bradykinin), histamine, and other mediators. The continued synthesis or release of these inflammatory mediators explains the prolonged time course of inflammation, which far exceeds the initial stimulation of the dental procedure (see Fig. 2-3). The clinical time course of postextraction pain and edema emphasizes this prolonged duration of the inflammatory process. Pain often reaches moderate to severe intensity by 3 to 5 hours,[54] and edema peaks by 48 to 72 hours[55] after extraction of impacted third molars. The effects and interactions of these inflammatory mediators produce the signs of inflammation observed after traumatic dental procedures.

Central Pain Mechanisms

Rostral Transmission of Pain

This section describes the neuroanatomic relationships underlying the perception and modification of pain. As previously reviewed, A delta and C fibers from the orofacial region transmit nociceptive signals primarily via trigeminal nerves to the trigeminal nucleus caudalis; noxious information from additional regions is conveyed by other cranial nerves.[56,57] The nucleus caudalis is located in the medulla; its organization and function in processing pain signals are similar to the area on the dorsal aspect of the spinal cord known as the dorsal horn.[56] For this reason, the nucleus caudalis has been termed the *medullary dorsal horn.* For both areas, the dorsal horn is composed of multiple layers much like an onion, with the outermost layer termed *lamina I.*

The medullary and spinal dorsal horns contain four major components related to the processing of noxious stimuli: central terminals of afferent fibers, local circuit neurons, projection neurons, and descending neurons. The first component, *primary nociceptive afferents* (e.g., A delta and C fibers), enter the medullary dorsal horn via the trigeminal tract (Fig. 2-5). Nerves that enter the spinal dorsal horn traverse the lateral aspect of the tract of Lissauer. For both the medullary and the spinal dorsal horns, A delta and C fibers terminate primarily in laminae I, IIa, and V. The primary nociceptive afferents transmit information by the

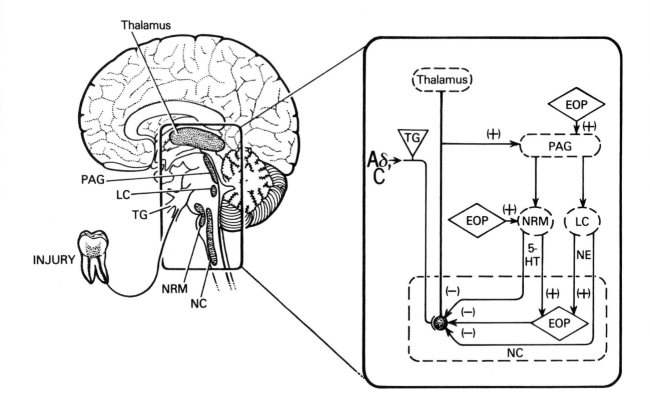

Fig. 2-5 Perception and modulation of orofacial pain. Damage of peripheral tissue activates A delta or C nociceptive fibers, which enter the central nervous system and synapse in the nucleus caudalis *(NC)* of the trigeminal system. The second-order neuron projects to the thalamus; the information is then relayed to the cortex. *Insert,* Endogenous pain suppression system: functional relationship of several neurotransmitters for modulation of nociceptive information at first synapse in NC (actual anatomic relationships are more complex). Peripheral activation of A delta or C fibers stimulates the projection neuron in the NC (filled cell body), which relays stimulus to the thalamus. This signal is also transmitted to the periaqueductal gray *(PAG)*, which receives additional input from other areas not shown. PAG in turn activates the nucleus raphe magnus *(NRM)* and the locus ceruleus *(LC)*. NRM sends fibers to the first synapse in the NC, where it inhibits transmission of nociceptive information through secretion of serotonin *(5-HT)* and other neurotransmitters. Similarly, LC sends fibers to the first synapse, where norepinephrine *(NE)* is released to inhibit transmission. Note that neurons secreting endogenous opioid peptide *(EOP)* are present at all three levels of this system. *TG,* Trigeminal ganglion; +, excitatory action; −, inhibitory action. (From Hargreaves KM, Troullos E, Dionne R: *Dent Clin North Am* 31:675-694, 1987.)

synaptic release of neuropeptides (e.g., substance P, CGRP) and amino acids (e.g., glutamate).

The second component of the dorsal horn, the *local circuit neurons,* consist of two major subtypes, the islet cell and the stalked cell. The islet cell is found throughout lamina II and is thought to be an inhibitory interneuron possibly employing GABA or enkephalin as neurotransmitters.[2,3] The stalked cells are found primarily at the junction between lamina

I and II and have been proposed to be excitatory interneurons conveying nociceptive output from primary afferents to projection neurons located in lamina I. Thus local circuit neurons play a critical role in conveying and probably modulating nociceptive signals from the primary afferents to the projection neurons.

The third component of the dorsal horn is the *projection neurons.* Projection neurons and local circuit

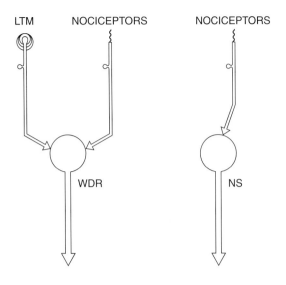

LTM   NOCICEPTORS   NOCICEPTORS

WDR   NS

Fig. 2-6 Two major types of projection neurons: wide dynamic range *(WDR)* and nociceptive specific *(NS)*. These neurons can be distinguished based on the peripheral input. WDR neurons receive input from nociceptors (e.g., A delta and C fibers) and low-threshold mechanoreceptors *(LTM)*. In contrast, NS neurons receive input only from nociceptors. (From Dubner R: *Compend Cont Educ Dent* 7:408-416, 1986.)

neurons can be divided into two major classes, *wide dynamic range* (WDR) and *nociceptive-specific* (NS) neurons (Fig. 2-6). The WDR neurons are activated by weak mechanical stimuli (e.g., hair movement) but respond maximally to intense and potentially tissue-damaging stimuli. In contrast, the NS neurons respond only to intense noxious forms of mechanical, thermal, or chemical stimuli.

Two major projection, or output, systems for pain are the *trigeminothalamic tract* (TTT) and the *spinothalamic tract* (STT) for the medullary and spinal dorsal horns, respectively. These tracts are composed of axonal projections from the WDR and NS neurons. These axons cross to the contralateral side of the medulla or spinal cord and ascend rostrally to the thalamus. From the thalamus, additional neurons convey this information to the cerebral cortex. Axonal collaterals of the TTT and STT terminate in rostral medullary reticular formation and the periaqueductal gray. The projection and local circuit neurons encode information about the location, intensity, duration, and stimulus type of the noxious input.

The fourth component of the dorsal horns is the terminal endings of *descending neurons* (see Fig. 2-5). These neurons form an important component of the endogenous pain modulatory system, which is reviewed in the next section.

Since the cerebral cortex is an important center for integrating all perceptual modalities together with higher functions, such as expectation and recall of previous events, it is not surprising that the cortex is involved in pain perception and response. Evidence suggests that the cerebral cortex is involved with the sensory-discriminative aspect of pain.[58] For example, both WDR and NS neurons have been recorded in monkey cortex. Additional studies suggest that the cortex may activate the endogenous analgesic system and thus represents its most rostral component.

Endogenous Pain Suppression Systems

The perception of pain is not simply a function of the magnitude of the noxious stimulus. Rather, the perception of pain can be altered by drugs that inhibit nociceptive inputs or by drugs and stimuli that activate endogenous analgesic systems. Research conducted in the last decade has determined that pain transmission can be modulated in the first few synapses of the medullary and spinal dorsal horns by an endogenous pain suppression system.[2,59] Although the concept of an "endogenous analgesic system" may appear exotic, it is simply another example of the ability of the CNS to regulate incoming sensory information. For example, several well-characterized systems are known to modulate visual, olfactory, and acoustic sensory input, often at the first few synapses in the CNS.[60]

A model of endogenous pain suppression systems can be considered as a three-tiered system involving the periaqueductal gray, medulla, and spinal cord.[2,59] The insert in Fig. 2-5 schematically depicts this system as it is functionally proposed; the actual neuroanatomic organization is more complex and still incompletely understood. An important component of this analgesic system are the *endogenous opioid peptides* (EOPs), which possess many properties of exogenous opiates (e.g., morphine, codeine). Enkephalin, dynorphin, and β-endorphin are all members of the EOP family. Importantly, EOPs are found at all three levels of the pain suppression system. This fact underlies the analgesic potency of opioids and exogenous opiates, since their administration activates this system at all levels, producing a multiplicative analgesic effect.[61]

In this model the highest, or most rostral, level of the pain suppression system is at a site in the gray matter of the brainstem, known as the *periaqueductal gray* (PAG). The name is descriptive of its location surrounding the aqueduct, which carries cerebrospinal fluid from the third to the fourth ventricle. The PAG plays a critical role in suppression of pain by integrating information from cortical and brainstem regions with incoming nociceptive signals. Local circuit neurons in the PAG contain enkephalin and dynorphin.[62] In addition, nerves originating from the hypothalamus contain β-endorphin and make synaptic contacts in the PAG.[63] At the level of the PAG, these peptides are thought to stimulate descending fibers, which in turn activate the middle level of this system (see Fig 2-5). Indeed, injection of opiates into this region produces a potent, long-lasting analgesia.

The middle level of the pain suppression system includes the nucleus raphe magnus (NRM), nearby medullary reticular nuclei, and the locus ceruleus (LC). Similar to the PAG, the middle level contains enkephalin and dynorphin interneurons. Microinjection of opiates into this region also produces a potent behavioral analgesia in laboratory animals. From this level, fibers project to the medullary (nucleus caudalis) and spinal dorsal horns. Many of these descending fibers contain serotonin (from the NRM) or norepinephrine (from the LC). Extending this observation, several investigators have demonstrated that microinjection of morphine into the PAG results in a significant release of serotonin and norepinephrine in the spinal cord.[2] In addition, the analgesic effects of morphine can be inhibited by administration of antagonists of serotonin and norepinephrine.[64] Other neurotransmitters may also participate in these descending pathways.[2,59]

The medullary and spinal dorsal horns are the lowest, or most caudal, level of the pain suppression system (see Fig 2-5). It is here that descending fibers from the middle level modulate the ultimate activity of the WDR and NS neurons. Pain signals may be suppressed by a direct action of the descending fibers by means of inhibitory synaptic contacts with the projection neurons. Alternatively, pain signals may be suppressed indirectly by descending fibers, which activate inhibitory local circuit neurons (that may contain opioid peptides), or by a combination of the two. Local injection of opiates into the dorsal horn region produces a profound analgesia in both animals and humans in pain. Both opioid peptides and

opiate receptors play a pivotal role in modulating pain transmission at the level of the first few synapses in the CNS.

This endogenous analgesic system can be activated by pain or by stress. Numerous findings indicate that stressful and aversive stimuli are capable of producing analgesia in both humans and animals.[65] One strategy to determine if EOPs are released to suppress pain involves administration of *naloxone*, an opiate receptor antagonist. Although naloxone does not alter the perception of pain when injected under basal conditions,[66] it significantly increases the patient's perception of pain when administered under conditions of stress. Naloxone-induced hyperalgesia is observed during oral surgery; pretreatment with the opiate antagonist results in significantly greater intraoperative pain compared with placebo-treated patients (Fig. 2-7).[67] In addition, naloxone increases pain experienced in the acute postoperative period after oral surgery.[68,69] These findings indicate that the endogenous analgesic system can be activated in patients undergoing stressful dental procedures. In addition, the finding that naloxone more than doubles the amount of intraoperative pain compared with placebo-treated patients indicates the magnitude of pain relief that accompanies activation of this endogenous analgesic system. Other endogenous analgesic systems, such as the endocannabinoids, have also been proposed to modulate acute and chronic pain states.[70]

In addition to a neurally mediated pain suppression system, an endocrine system may also exist. For example, β-endorphin, an EOP, is released from the pituitary gland under conditions of stress of pain. Several studies have demonstrated that oral surgery and acute postoperative pain constitute physiologically relevant stimuli for secretion of immunoreactive β-endorphin.[67,71]

Circulating levels of immunoreactive β-endorphin increase in placebo-treated patients during oral surgery and after loss of local anesthesia; levels are also increased in a compensatory fashion during naloxone-induced hyperalgesia (see Fig. 2-7). The potential role of pituitary β-endorphin in modulating pain has been evaluated under conditions designed to stimulate its release and activate endogenous pain suppression systems.[72,73] These observations may be clinically relevant, since oral surgery patients pretreated with low doses of dexamethasone have lower levels of circulating β-endorphin and significantly greater levels of postoperative pain compared with patients treated

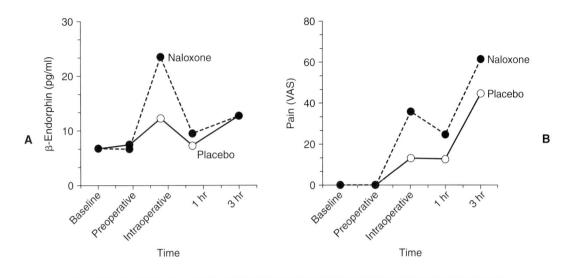

Fig. 2-7 Stress associated with oral surgery is sufficient to increase circulating levels of immunoreactive β-endorphin **(A)** and activate an endogenous opioid–analgesic system **(B).** Twelve patients/group were injected intravenously with either placebo or naloxone (10 mg) and underwent extraction of impacted third molars with 2% lidocaine and 1:100,000 epinephrine. (Modified from Hargreaves KM et al: *Clin Pharmacol Ther* 40:165-171, 1986.)

with placebo.[74] Additional studies have extended these findings by administration of corticotropin-releasing factor (CRF) to postoperative patients. CRF is the endogenous signal for evoking the release of pituitary β-endorphin in response to stressors such as surgery or postoperative pain.[75] Administration of CRF stimulated β-endorphin secretion and significantly reduced postoperative pain in patients after extraction of impacted third molars.[71] The existence of a peripheral site of action for opiate-induced analgesia[76] provides a potential target for circulating opioid peptides.

Hyperalgesia and Allodynia

Acute inflammation due to orofacial infections or dental procedures that produce tissue injury can elicit hyperalgesia. Hyperalgesia is characterized by spontaneous pain, a decreased pain threshold, and an increased magnitude of perceived pain for any given stimulus.[2,3] Hyperalgesia is a common finding in many clinical models of inflammation. Hyperalgesia due to pulpal inflammation may decrease pain threshold to the point where the arterial pressure wave following a heartbeat stimulates pul-

pal nociceptive nerve fibers.[77] This may underlie the "throbbing" pain of pulpitis.[78] Examination of an endodontic pain patient represents the systematic testing for the signs of hyperalgesia: spontaneous pain, reduced pain threshold (e.g., percussion/palpation tests, pain on chewing), and increased pain responsiveness.[79]

Hyperalgesia is caused by both peripheral and central mechanisms. Peripheral mechanisms include the concentration and composition of inflammatory mediators. As reviewed earlier, inflammatory mediators differ in the ability to activate nociceptors, or nociceptors selectively express receptors that are activated by inflammatory mediators. This receptor-mediator interaction requires that the mediator be present at sufficient concentrations. Thus both the composition of mediators in the inflamed tissue and the concentration of each mediator are critical factors in modulating nociceptor function. The result of receptor activation can be depolarization of the nociceptor (sending an action potential back to the CNS) or sensitization (reducing the threshold level to subsequent stimuli). A reduction in the thermal or mechanical thresholds indicates that tissue pressure and temperature are important factors in mediating hyperalgesia. For example, a pulpal nociceptor can have its thermal threshold reduced to body temperature, indicating that this unit will continuously depolarize under these conditions. This may explain the common clinical observation of patients using ice water to reduce spontaneous pain in molars with irreversible pulpitis.[80] The persistence of inflammation can produce phenotypic and morphologic changes in peripheral nociceptors. For example, pulpal inflammation can lead to sprouting of nociceptor terminals in inflamed pulp or periradicular tissue and alterations in neuropeptide content in these fibers.[81,82]

Under certain conditions, non-nociceptors may also contribute to peripheral mechanisms of hyperalgesia. For example, tissue injury can lead to changes whereby sympathetic fibers stimulate C-fiber nociceptors.[83] In addition, certain non-nociceptors (e.g., A beta fibers) may begin to express substance P after tissue injury.[84] Collectively, these findings indicate that several peripheral mechanisms may contribute to the development of hyperalgesia in orofacial pain patients.

In addition to these peripheral changes, evidence indicates that several central mechanisms may mediate the development of hyperalgesia. For example, we and others have shown that central terminals of capsaicin-sensitive nociceptors demonstrate increased basal and evoked release of neuropeptides after tissue inflammation.[85] Interestingly, this enhanced release appears to be mediated by spinal prostaglandins because it is blocked by NSAIDs.[86] Thus inflammation evokes both peripheral and central release of prostaglandins.[25,87] Additional studies have indicated that central sensitization may occur after peripheral injury. *Central sensitization* is characterized as increased excitability of central neurons due to an afferent barrage that includes contribution by C-fiber nociceptors,[88] which is thought to be a major central mechanism of hyperalgesia. Additional phenotypic and morphologic changes may also mediate central hyperalgesia.[80,89]

Multiple peripheral and central mechanisms appear to exist for hyperalgesia. These responses to tissue injury are dynamic, altering over both time and in response to various types of tissue injury. Thus the relative contribution of these mechanisms probably varies among patients and pain etiologies. This conclusion is clinically important because the combination of multiple mechanisms and variable expression of these mechanisms probably contributes to the variability in treatment efficacy and diagnostic accuracy in treating acute and chronic pain patients.

Acute Pain Management

Acute pain typically results from an injurious insult and is self-limiting. The report of pain typically stops before the precipitating injury heals completely. Strategies for acute pain management are based on knowledge of peripheral and central mechanisms of nociception. In general, acute pain management may involve a three-pronged approach: (1) inhibition of biochemical processes signaling tissue injury, (2) blockade of nociceptive impulses along the peripheral nerves, and (3) activation of endogenous analgesic mechanisms in the CNS. These approaches can be employed simultaneously to result in additive analgesia.

Peripherally Acting Drugs

Inflammation represents a complex series of physiologic reactions required for normal healing after physical injury or infection. As previously mentioned, mediators formed during the evolution of the inflammatory process contribute to the genesis of acute pain by stimulation or sensitization of primary afferent neurons by peripheral and central mechanisms.

The biochemical composition of the local environment of inflamed tissue is complex. Protons, cytokines, prostanoids, leukotrienes, neuropeptides, histamine, bradykinin, and free radicals are ingredients of the "inflammatory soup" that defines the biochemical environment of inflamed tissue. Although each of these molecular species may directly or indirectly contribute to inflammatory pain, inflammatory pains probably result from an interplay of neuronal signals generated by the inflammatory soup. In other words, inflammatory pains likely result from synergistic biochemical interactions with primary afferent neurons.

If a particular biochemical in the inflammatory soup is a primary contributor to the genesis of inflammatory pain, drugs that block its actions or synthesis should provide significant analgesia. Agents that block the actions of histamine[44] or substance P[54] and the synthesis of bradykinin[46] or prostaglandins[90] all possess analgesic activity in animal models of inflammation. In addition, combinations of these agents can exert additive effects,[44] which is consistent with the view that the total composition of the inflammatory soup governs the genesis and maintenance of inflammatory pains.

Pharmacologic management of pain can be accomplished either by blocking the nociceptive *input* at the receptor or the nociceptive *impulse* along the peripheral nerve. As previously mentioned, various biochemicals at inflammatory sites affect nociceptive input by direct or indirect mechanisms. For example, prostaglandins, especially PGE[2], sensitize nociceptive nerve endings and thereby potentiate the actions of other inflammatory mediators, such as bradykinin.[91] Sensitization of peripheral nociceptors is minimized in the absence of PGE[2], and pain sensations are thus attenuated. Therefore drugs designed to block prostaglandin synthesis or function should be effective analgesics for some inflammatory pains.

Aspirin-like drugs, which include aspirin, acetaminophen, and NSAIDs, exert their actions in damaged tissue. These drugs inhibit generation of the pain signal and accompanying sensitization at the nerve ending through blockade of prostaglandin synthesis.[92,93] In addition, NSAIDs have been reported to possess moderate efficacy for inhibiting postoperative edema.[94] However, there appears to be a maximal effect, or *ceiling effect*, beyond which additional increments of drug do not produce significantly greater analgesia. This ceiling effect probably reflects the contribution of other inflammatory mediators that are unaffected by aspirin-like drugs.

The physiologic mechanism for the synthesis of prostaglandins is the activation of phospholipase A[2] and cylcooxygenase during the process of tissue damage (e.g., during surgery). This information has an important practical application: pretreating patients with NSAIDs before surgery. The rationale for this therapy is the blockade of enzymes before the initiation of tissue damage. Although the advantages of pretreatment has been most clearly established for ibuprofen,[95] several other drugs, including flurbiprofen, have been demonstrated to reduce pain. Pretreating patients with ibuprofen delays the onset and reduces the magnitude of postoperative pain.[55] This prescription strategy emphasizes how clinicians can improve patient care by knowledge of pain physiology.

Inhibition of prostaglandin synthesis can also be accomplished with administration of *glucocorticoids.* This group of steroids has very potent antiinflammatory activity. Glucocorticoids inhibit all phases of inflammation, such as capillary dilation, migration of leukocytes, and phagocytosis. Steroids have been demonstrated to activate synthesis of a protein inhibitor of phospholipase A[2] called *lipocortin*.[93,96] Blockade of arachidonic acid formation by inhibit-

ing phospholipase A[2] is an early step in the cascade and thus prevents formation of both cyclooxygenase and lipoxygenase end products. In addition, glucocorticoids induce the synthesis of angiotensin-converting enzyme (ACE), a peptidase that degrades bradykinin, and the synthesis of vasotonin, a peptide that promotes vascular stability.[97] These multiple mechanisms for the suppression of inflammatory mediators probably account for the impressive antiinflammatory potency of steroids.

Because of their potent antiinflammatory properties, glucocorticoids would be expected to be analgesic for dental pain. Studies in third molar extraction pain, however, have been equivocal. Although some authors have reported modest levels of analgesia,[98,99] other investigators, using both a placebo control and an active control (NSAID pretreatment), found that the glucocorticoid was not significantly different from placebo.[94,100] Reasons for the poor analgesic activity of steroids are unclear. This antiinflammatory effect with poor analgesia may be caused by glucocorticoids inhibiting both inflammation and an endogenous analgesic system.[74] However, this issue requires further investigation.

Another approach to peripheral pain management is to block the nociceptive impulse as it moves along the nerve axon. Local anesthetics prevent the propagation of an action potential in peripheral nerves by interfering with sodium channel permeability.[101] Nociceptive A delta and C fibers are very susceptible to blockade by local anesthetics. Local anesthetics with increased potency and prolonged duration of action have been developed based on their enhanced physicochemical properties, such as increased lipid solubility and greater protein binding. Thus sustained blockade of A delta and C fibers can result in prolonged suppression of postoperative pain.[102]

Centrally Acting Drugs

Traditional pharmacologic pain management usually involves the administration of opioid analgesics. Parenteral opioid analgesics are the standard of care for severe pain in hospitalized patients. As described, the profound analgesic efficacy of opioid drugs results from their ability to mimic the actions of the family of EOPs. Since EOPs are present at all levels of the endogenous analgesic system, opioid drugs can activate this system to suppress the transmission of nociceptive signals at the medullary and spinal dorsal horns. Unfortunately, the oral efficacy of most opioid drugs is very poor. An additional problem with opioids relates to their propensity for nausea in ambulatory patients.

Since most dental pain situations involve ambulatory outpatients requiring oral analgesics, the usefulness of opioids is limited to an adjunctive role. In general, the combination of an aspirin-like drug with an opioid increases analgesia at the cost of an increased incidence of side effects.

Chronic Pain

Acute Pain Versus Chronic Pain

Acute pain and chronic pain have not been defined in meaningful biologic terms. *Acute* pain is typically defined as pain associated with tissue injury that is self-limiting. Acute pain by definition is self-limiting and usually resolves before healing of the injured site is complete. Two types of acute pain are (1) self-limiting, inflammatory pain and (2) self-limiting, noninflammatory pain.

Traditionally, *chronic pain* has been defined simply as a pain state persisting for longer than 3 to 6 months. However, this definition is arbitrary and does not consider the possibility that chronic pain states differ significantly from acute pain states with respect to the biologic processes involved in their genesis and maintenance. The evolution of a chronic pain state may follow a continuum of biologic events that begins with an acute pain episode and progresses over time to a chronic pain state. If so, the temporal element may be significant in the development of chronic pain.

Alternatively, the biologic pathway to a chronic pain state may diverge from acute pain mechanisms very early after a precipitating event. If this is true, the temporal element would be insignificant. Ultimately, the temporal element often used to delineate chronic pain states from acute pain states may simply distinguish a self-limiting process (i.e., acute pain) from one that is protracted or perpetual (i.e., chronic pain). In other words, the duration of pain may be relatively unimportant. Rather, the significant difference between acute and chronic pain may be a failure in homeostatic mechanisms contributing to the latter state. Factors such as nature of the precipitating event, genetic predisposition (including gender), nutrition, and age may affect critical homeostatic mechanisms that ultimately delineate acute and chronic pain states.

Persistent Versus Recurring Chronic Pain

Chronic pains can be divided into two basic types: (1) persistent and unrelenting and (2) recurring and remitting. Unlike acute pains, chronic pains may persist in the absence of obvious injury. Persistent, non-self-limiting pains are continuous, unrelenting pains that may vary in both intensity and quality over time. For example, individuals who have postherpetic neuralgia are subjected to daily continuous pains that may vary in intensity from mild to severe. Furthermore, pains associated with postherpetic neuralgia may vary in quality. Some patients may describe these pains as constant burning pains that can escalate to stabbing or "electric-shock-like" pains.

Patients may suffer from chronic pains that may remit or become quiescent but recur over time. For example, some individuals have extremely painful vascular headaches that may persist for weeks or months and then suddenly remit. *Cluster headaches* recur in "clusters" of time throughout the patient's life. The patient suffering from cluster headaches may be pain-free for months in a remission period. However, the headaches typically recur and may persist for months after a pain-free period. Cluster headaches are an example of recurring, remitting, non-self-limiting pain.

Many patients suffering from persistent pain are depressed. Many become socially withdrawn, and interpersonal relationships with significant others often deteriorate over time. In addition, some patients with persistent pain may lose employment and face significant economic pressure due to lost income and rising health care expenses. Treating clinicians are often frustrated as well because relatively little scientific information is available to direct reliable diagnostic studies and treatment. As a result, a trial-and-error approach is often taken to the management of these patients, and treatments are often ineffective. Physician-patient relationships often are strained. The physiologic impact of sustained psychological stress on the pathogenesis of persistent pain is poorly understood at present.

Often, persistent pain is present in the absence of overt tissue injury. Unlike sudden-onset pains that can be readily linked to physical insult or injury, some persistent pains may begin spontaneously without overt cause or may continue long after a site of injury has healed. Recent evidence suggests that some persistent pains may be attributed to physical changes induced in the CNS or peripheral nervous system after an initial injury. For example, mechanical allodynia may be ascribed to the sprouting of large-diameter primary afferent neurons (i.e., A delta neurons) into superficial laminae of the spinal cord or brainstem after peripheral nerve injury.[103] A delta primary afferent neurons typically are involved in perceptions of touch and proprioception. Under pathologic conditions, such as nerve injury, C-fiber inputs to superficial laminae of the spinal cord are lost, and A delta fibers sprout into the region previously occupied by them. In addition, evidence indicates that these A delta fibers begin to synthesize neuropeptides that are typically made by C-fiber populations believed to be involved in nociception. This phenotypic switching process is described earlier. In other words, after some types of peripheral nerve injuries in susceptible individuals, A delta fibers populate regions of the spinal cord thought to be involved in nociception. Furthermore, these A delta fibers apparently acquire the capacity to communicate with neurons in the nociceptive pathway by synthesizing signaling molecules (i.e., neuropeptides) involved in interneural signaling. These changes could explain the phenomenon of mechanical allodynia, a condition in which non-noxious mechanical stimuli (e.g., light touch normally perceived via A delta activation) are painful.

New Approaches for Pain Management

Over the last decade, great strides have been made in knowledge of the physiology of pain. However, clinical applications of these findings are still in various stages of development using new classes of analgesics.

One approach with some clinical support is the use of *antihistamines* as adjunctive analgesic agents. Histamine is released during mast cell degranulation. Generalizing from animal studies,[45] antihistamines should demonstrate greater efficacy when given before surgery, but this has yet to be established in the clinic. Several clinical studies have demonstrated that antihistamines serve as effective adjunctive analgesics in the oral surgery model.[44]

Other peripherally acting drugs have been developed but are still under preliminary evaluation, including antagonists to inflammatory mediators such as leukotrienes;[39,104] diHETES[36] and platelet-activating factor[105] may possess activity for some clinical diseases of inflammatory origin. One notable example has received early clinical testing; bradykinin receptor antagonists that possess activity in animals[48] are analgesic in humans experiencing an experimental form of inflammation.[106] An additional approach for drug development comes from the finding that lipocortin, an endogenous peptide, inhibits phospholipase A_2. This endogenous enzyme inhibitor may have clinical implications because analogs of lipocortin have been synthesized that exert antiinflammatory effects in animals.[107]

Another approach for antiinflammatory drug development is the blockade of substances released from the endings of afferent[54,108] and possibly sympathetic efferent nerves.[109] Finally, the demonstration of peripheral analgesic actions of opiates[76] suggests that peripherally acting analogs may exert opiate-like analgesia in the absence of centrally mediated side effects (e.g., nausea, sedation).

It is anticipated that as the biologic processes that underlie the genesis of persistent pain are discovered, improved diagnostics and therapies will emerge. This is already evident in the new "smart" therapies that have been developed to eliminate pain but preserve other neural functions. One such approach involves the delivery of a cytotoxin (saporin) to a specific subset of sensory neurons (i.e., those producing functional NK-1 receptors that bind substance P) involved in nociception.[110] Saporin is conjugated to substance P, creating a hybrid molecule that binds to the NK-1 receptor, which is then internalized by the neuron.[111] Once internalized, the saporin component of the novel hybrid molecule disrupts ribosomal function, resulting in death of the neuron. Since saporin is only effective when internalized through this receptor-mediated process, neighboring neurons (and other cell types) that do not express functional NK-1 receptors are unaffected. Therefore this approach selectively eliminates neuronal subpopulations involved in nociception and preserves other important neural functions (e.g., touch, proprioception, motor function). This approach is a clear example of how an understanding of the molecular mechanisms of nociception can lead to specific, effective therapies for persistent pains.

References

1. International Association for the Study of Pain, Subcommittee on Taxonomy: Pain terms: a list with definitions and notes on usage, *Pain* 6:249-252, 1979.

2. Dubner R, Bennett G: Spinal and trigeminal mechanisms of nociception, *Ann Rev Neurosci* 6:381-418, 1983.

3. Willis W: *The pain system*, New York, 1985, Karger.

4. Ochoa J, Mair W: The normal sural nerve in man. I. Ultrastructure and numbers of fibers and cells, *Acta Neuropathol (Berl)* 13:127-216, 1969.

5. Burgess P, Perl E: Cutaneous mechanoreceptors and nociceptors. In Iggo A, editor: *Handbook of sensory physiology*, vol 2, Heidelberg, 1973, Springer-Verlag.

6. Tervo T, Palkama A: Innervation of the rabbit cornea: a histochemical and electron-microscopic study, *Acta Anat (Basel)* 102:164-175, 1978.

7. Byers M: Dental sensory receptors, *Int Rev Neurobiol* 25:39-94, 1984.

8. Arwill T, Edwall L, Lilja J, et al: Ultrastructure of nerves in the dentinal-pulp border zone after sensory and autonomic nerve transection in the cat, *Acta Odontol Scand* 31:273-281, 1973.

9. Johnson D, Harshbarger J, Rymer H: Quantitative assessment of neural development in human premolars, *Anat Rec* 205:421-429, 1983.

10. Fristad I: Dental innervation: functions and plasticity after peripheral injury, *Acta Odontol Scand* 55:236-254, 1997.

11. Byers MR, Narhi MV: Dental injury models: experimental tools for understanding neuroinflammatory interactions and polymodal nociceptor functions, *Crit Rev Oral Biol Med* 10:4-39, 1999.

12. Brannstrom M, Astrom A: A study on the mechanism of pain elicited from the dentin, *J Dent Res* 43:619-625, 1964.

13. Trowbridge H: Review of dental pain: histology and physiology, *J Endodont* 12:445-452, 1986.

14. Orchardson RJ, Collins W: Dentine sensitivity, *Hyg Forum* 34:6-12, 1984.

15. Lilja J, Nordenvall K, Brannstrom M: Dentin sensitivity, odontoblasts, and nerves under desiccated or infected experimental cavities, *Swed Dent J* 6:93-103, 1982.

16. Narhi M: The characteristics of intradental sensory units and their responses to stimulation, *J Dent Res* 64:564-571, 1985.

17. Dowell P, Addy M, Dummer P: Dentine hypersensitivity: aetiology, differential diagnosis, and management, *Br Dent J* 158:92-96, 1985.

18. Orchardson R, Collins W: Dentine sensitivity, *Hyg Forum* 34:6-12, 1984.

19. Berman L: Dentinal sensitivity and hypersensitivity, *J Periodontol* 56:216-222, 1985.

20. Scott HM: Reduction of sensitivity by electrophoresis, *J Dent Child* 29:225-241, 1962.

21. Brough KM, Anderson DM, Love J, Overman PR: The effectiveness of iontophoresis in reducing dentin hypersensitivity, *J Am Dent Assoc* 111:761-765, 1985.

22. Brannstrom M, Johnson G, Nordenvall K: Transmission and control of dentinal pain: resin impregnation for the desensitization of dentin, *J Am Dent Assoc* 99:612-616, 1979.

23. Dayton R, DeMarco T, DeMarco D: Treatment of hypersensitive root surfaces with dental adhesive materials, *J Periodontol* 45:873-880, 1974.

24. Greaves M, Sondergaard J, McDonald-Gibson W: Recovery of prostaglandins in human cutaneous inflammation, *Br Med J* 2:258-260, 1971.

25. Roszkowski MT, Swift JQ, Hargreaves KM: Effect of ibuprofen and methylprednisolone on surgical wound levels of substance P, eicosanoids, bradykinin, and post-operative pain following removal of impacted third molars, 2001.

26. Simmons P, Salmon J, Moncada S: The release of leukotriene B_4 during experimental inflammation, *Biochem Pharmacol* 32:1353-1359, 1983.

27. Seibert K, Zhang Y, Leahy K, et al: Pharmacological and biochemical demonstration of the role of cyclooxygenase-2 in inflammation and pain, *Proc Natl Acad Sci U S A* 91:12013-12017, 1994.

28. Sano H, Hla T, Maier JAM, et al: In vivo cyclooxygenase expression in synovial tissues of patients with rheumatoid arthritis and osteoarthritis and rats with adjuvant and streptococcal cell-wall arthritis, *J Clin Invest* 89:97-108, 1992.

29. Anderson GD, Hauser SD, McGarity KL, et al: Selective inhibition of cyclooxygenase (COX)-2 reverses inflammation and expression of COX-2 and interleukin-6 in rat adjuvant arthritis, *J Clin Invest* 97:2672-2679, 1996.

30. Basran G, Morley J, Paul W, et al: Evidence in man of synergistic interaction between putative mediators of acute inflammation and asthma, *Lancet* i:935-937, 1982.

31. Goetzl E, Gorman R: Chemotactic and chemokinetic stimulation of human eosinophil and neutrophil polymorphonuclear leukocytes by 12-hydroxy-5,8,10-heptadecatrienoic acid, *J Immunol* 142:526-529, 1978.

32. Ferreira S, Nakamura M, Abreu-Castro M: The hyperalgesic effects of prostacyclin and PGE_2, *Prostaglandins* 16:31-37, 1978.

33. Bray M: The pharmacology and pathophysiology of leukotriene B_4, *Br Med Bull* 39:249-254, 1983.

34. Bisgaard H, Kristensen J: Leukotriene B_4 produces hyperalgesia in humans, *Prostaglandins* 30:791-797, 1985.

35. Levine J, Wau W, Kwiat G, et al: Leukotriene B_4 produces hyperalgesia that is dependent on polymorphonuclear leukocytes, *Science* 225:743-745, 1984.

36. Levine J, Lam D, Taiwo Y, et al: Hyperalgesic properties of arachidonic acid, *Proc Natl Acad Sci U S A* 83:5331-5334, 1986.

37. Gazelius B, Panopoulos P, Odlander B, et al: Inhibition of interdental nerve excitability by leukotriene-B_4 and leukotriene-C_4, *Acta Physiol Scand* 120:141-143, 1984.

38. Madison S, Whitsel EA, Suarezroca H, et al: Sensitizing effects of leukotriene-B_4 on interdental primary afferents, *Pain* 49:99-104, 1992.

39. Barnes N, Piper P, Costello J: The effect of an oral leukotriene antagonist L649,923 on histamine and leukotriene D4–induced bronchoconstriction in normal man. In Samuelsson B, Paoletti R, editors: *Advances in prostaglandin, thromboxane, and leukotriene research*, New York, 1982, Raven.

40. Van Arman C, Begany A, Miller L, et al: Some details of the inflammations caused by yeast and carrageenan, *J Pharmacol Exp Ther* 150:328-334, 1965.

41. Saucedo R, Erill S: Morphine-induced skin wheals: a possible model for the study of histamine release, *Clin Pharmacol Ther* 38:365-370, 1985.

42. Fjellner B, Hagermark O: Potentiation of histamine-induced itch and flare responses in human skin by the enkephalin analogue FK 33-824, beta endorphin, and morphine, *Arch Dermatol Res* 274:29-37, 1982.

43. Frewin D, Cleland L, Jonsson J, et al: Histamine levels in human synovial fluid, *J Rheumatol* 13:13-14, 1986.

44. Rumore M, Schlichting D: Clinical efficacy of antihistamines as analgesics, *Pain* 25:7-22, 1986.

45. Dawson W, Willoughby D: Inflammation: mechanisms and mediators. In Lombardino J, editor: *Non-steroidal antiinflammatory drugs*, New York, 1985, Wiley.

46. Hargreaves KM, Troullos E, Dionne R, et al: Bradykinin is increased during acute and chronic inflammation: therapeutic implications, *Clin Pharmacol Ther* 44:613-621, 1988.

47. Steranka L, Dehass C, Vavrek R, et al: Antinociceptive effects of bradykinin antagonists, *Eur J Pharmacol* 136:261-262, 1987.

48. Costello A, Hargreaves KM: Suppression of carrageenan-induced hyperalgesia, hyperthermia, and edema by a bradykinin antagonist, *Eur J Pharmacol* 171:259-263, 1989.

49. Rosenfeld M, Mermod J, Amara S: Production of a novel neuropeptide encoded by the calcitonin gene via tissue-specific RNA processing, *Nature* 304:129-135, 1983.

50. Olgart L, Gazelius B, Brodin E, et al: Release of substance P–like immunoreactivity from the dental pulp, *Acta Physiol Scand* 101:510-512, 1977.

51. Uddman R, Grunditz T, Sundler F: Calcitonin gene-related peptide: a sensory transmitter in dental pulps? *Scand J Dent Res* 94:219-224, 1986.

52. Olgart L, Hokfelt T, Nilsson G, et al: Localization of substance P–like immunoreactivity in nerves in the tooth pulp, *Pain* 4:153-159, 1977.

53. Morton C, Chahl L: Pharmacology of the neurogenic oedema response to electrical stimulation of the saphenous nerve in the rat, *Arch Pharmacol* 314:271-276, 1980.

54. Lembeck F, Holzer P: Substance P as a neurogenic mediator of antidromic vasodilation and neurogenic plasma extravasation, *Arch Pharmacol* 310:175-183, 1979.

55. Lotz M, Vaughan J, Carson D: Effect of neuropeptides on production of inflammatory cytokines by human monocytes, *Science* 241:1218-1221, 1988.

56. Gobel S, Falls W, Hockfield S: The division of the dorsal and ventral horns of the mammalian caudal medulla into eight layers using anatomical criteria. In Anderson D, Matthews B, editors: *Pain in the trigeminal region*, Amsterdam, 1977, Elsevier.

57. Dubner R, Hayes R, Hoffman D: Neural and behavioral correlates of pain in the trigeminal system. In Bonica J, editor: *Pain*, New York, 1980, Raven.

58. Kenshalo D, Willis W: The role of the cerebral cortex in pain sensation. In Jones EG, Peters A, editors: *The cerebral cortex*, New York, 1989, Plenum.

59. Basbaum A, Fields H: Endogenous pain control systems: brainstem spinal pathways and endorphin circuitry, *Annu Rev Neurosci* 7:309-338, 1984.

60. Carpenter M, Sutin J: *Human neuroanatomy*, ed 8, Baltimore, 1983, Williams & Wilkins.

61. Yeung J, Rudy T: Multiplicative interactions between narcotic agonists expressed at spinal and supraspinal sites of antinociceptive action as revealed by concurrent intrathecal and intracerebroventricular injections of morphine, *J Pharmacol Exp Ther* 215:633-642, 1980.

62. Basbaum A, Jacknow D, Mulcahy J, et al: Studies on the contribution of different endogenous opioid peptides to the control of pain. In Yokota Y, Dubner R, editors: *Current topics in pain research and therapy*, Amsterdam, 1983, Elsevier.

63. Bloom F, Battenberg E, Rossier J, et al: Neurons containing beta-endorphin in rat brain exist separately from those containing enkephalin: immunocytochemical studies, *Proc Natl Acad Sci U S A* 75:1591-1595, 1978.

64. Yaksh T: Direct evidence that spinal serotonin and noradrenaline terminals mediate the spinal antinociceptive effects of morphine in the periaqueductal gray, *Brain Res* 160:180-185, 1979.

65. Terman G, Shavit Y, Lewis J, et al: Intrinsic mechanisms of pain inhibition: activation by stress, *Science* 226:1270-1277, 1984.

66. Grevert P, Goldstein A: Endorphins: naloxone fails to alter experimental pain or mood in humans, *Science* 199:1093-1095, 1978.

67. Hargreaves KM, Dionne R, Goldstein D, et al: Naloxone, fentanyl, and diazepam modify plasma beta-endorphin levels during surgery, *Clin Pharmacol Ther* 40:165-171, 1986.

68. Gracely R, Dubner R, Wolskee P, et al: Placebo and naloxone can alter post-surgical pain by separate mechanisms, *Nature* 306:264-265, 1983.

69. Levine J, Gordon N, Fields H: The mechanism of placebo analgesia, *Lancet* ii:654-657, 1978.

70. Richardson JD, Aanonsen L, Hargreaves KM: Hypoactivity of the spinal cannabinoid system results in an NMDA-dependent hyperalgesia, *J Neurosci* 18:451-457, 1998.

71. Hargreaves KM, Mueller G, Dubner R, et al: Corticotropin releasing factor (CRF) produces analgesia in humans and rats, *Brain Res* 422:154-157, 1987.

72. Amir S, Amit Z: Endogenous opioid ligands may mediate stress-induced changes in the affective properties of pain related behavior in rats, *Life Sci* 23:1143-1152, 1978.

73. Marek P, Panocka I, Hartman G: Dexamethasone reverses adrenalectomy enhancement of footshock-induced analgesia in mice, *Pharmacol Biochem Behav* 18:167-169, 1983.

74. Hargreaves K, Schmidt E, Mueller G, et al: Dexamethasone alters plasma levels of beta-endorphin and post-operative pain, *Clin Pharmacol Ther* 42:601-607, 1987.

75. Vale W, Spiess J, Rivier C, et al: Characterization of a 41-residue ovine hypothalamic peptide that stimulates secretion of corticotropin and beta-endorphin, *Science* 213:1394-1397, 1981.

76. Joris J, Dubner R, Hargreaves KM: Opiate analgesia at peripheral sites: a target for opioids released during stress and inflammation? *Anesth Analg* 66:1277-1281, 1987.

77. Nahri M: Activation of dental pulp nerves of the cat and the dog with hydrostatic pressure, *Proc Fin Dent Soc* 74(suppl 5):1-64, 1978.

78. Narhi M: The characteristics of intradental sensory units and their responses to stimulation, *J Dent Res* 64:564-571, 1985.

79. Hargreaves KM, Swift JQ, Roszkowski MT, et al: Pharmacology of peripheral neuropeptide and inflammatory mediator release, *Oral Surg Oral Med Oral Pathol* 78:503-510, 1994.

80. Hargreaves KM, Hutter JW: Endodontic pharmacology. In Cohen S, Burns R, editors: *Pathways of the pulp*, ed 7, St Louis, 1998, Mosby.

81. Byers M, Taylor P, Khayat B, et al: Effects of injury and inflammation on pulpal and periapical nerves, *J Endodont* 16:78, 1990.

82. Buck S, Reese K, Hargreaves KM: Pulpal exposure alters neuropeptide levels in inflamed dental pulp: evaluation of axonal transport, *J Endodont* 25:718, 1999.

83. Perl E: Causalgia, pathological pain, and adrenergic receptors, *Proc Natl Acad Sci U S A* 96:7664, 1999.

84. Neumann S, Doubell T, Leslie T, et al: Inflammatory pain hypersensitivity mediated by phenotype switch in myelinated primary sensory neurons, *Nature* 384:360, 1996.

85. Garry MG, Hargreaves KM: Enhanced release of immunoreactive CGRP and substance P from spinal dorsal horn slices occurs during carrageenan inflammation, *Brain Res* 582:139-142, 1992.

86. Southall M, Michael R, Vasko M: Intrathecal NSAIDs attenuate inflammation-induced neuropeptide release from rat spinal cord slices, *Pain* 78:39-48, 1998.

87. Dirig D, Yaksh T: Spinal synthesis and release of prostanoids after peripheral injury and inflammation, *Adv Exp Med Biol* 469:401-408, 1999.

88. Woolf C: Windup and central sensitization are not equivalent, *Pain* 66:105, 1996.

89. Sessle B, Iwati K: Central nociceptive pathways. In Lavigne G, Lund J, Sessle B, Dubner R, editors: *Orofacial pain: basic sciences to clinical management*, Chicago, 2000, Quintessence.

90. Gilfoil T, Klavins I, Grumbach L: Effects of acetylsalicylic acid on the edema and hyperesthesia of the experimentally inflamed rat's paw, *J Pharmacol Exp Ther* 142:1-5, 1963.

91. Ferreira SH: Prostaglandins, aspirin-like drugs, and analgesia, *Nature New Biol* 240:200-203, 1972.

92. Ferreira SH, Moncada S, Vane JR: Prostaglandins and the mechanism of analgesia produced by aspirin-like drugs, *Br J Pharmacol* 49:86-97, 1973.

93. Flower RJ, Blackwell GJ: Anti-inflammatory steroids induce biosynthesis of a phospholipase A2 inhibitor which [sic] prevents prostaglandin generation, *Nature* 278:456-459, 1979.

94. Troullos E, Hargreaves KM, Butler D, Dionne R: Comparison of two non-steroidal anti-inflammatory drugs, flurbiprofen and ibuprofen, to methylprednisolone for suppression of post-operative pain and edema, *J Oral Maxillofac Surg*, 48(9):945-952, 1990.

95. Jackson D, Hargreaves KM, Moore P: Prophylactic ibuprofen for the prevention of post-operative pain. *J Am Dent Assoc* 1990.

96. Munck A, Guyre PM, Holbrook NJ: Physiological functions of glucocorticoids in stress and their relation to pharmacological actions, *Endocr Rev* 5:25-44, 1984.

97. DisRosa M, Calignano A, Carnuccio R, et al: Multiple control of inflammation by glucocorticoids, *Agents Actions* 17:284-289, 1985.

98. Skjelbred P, Lokken P: Post-operative pain and inflammatory reaction reduced by injection of a corticosteroid, *Eur J Clin Pharmacol* 21:391-396, 1982.

99. Beirne OR, Hollander B: The effect of methylprednisolone on pain, trismus, and swelling after removal of third molars, *Oral Surg* 61:134-138, 1986.

100. Sisk AL, Bonnington GJ: Evaluation of methylprednisolone and flurbiprofen for inhibition of the postoperative inflammatory response, *Oral Surg* 60:137-145, 1985.

101. Covino BG, Vassallo HG: *Local anesthetics: mechanisms of action and clinical use*, New York, 1976, Grune & Stratton.

102. Sisk AL, Dionne RA, Wirdzek PR: Evaluation of etidocaine hydrochloride for local anesthesia and postoperative pain control in oral surgery, *J Oral Maxillofac Surg* 42:84-88, 1984.

103. Doubell TP, Mannion RJ, Woolf CJ: The dorsal horn: state-dependent sensory processing, plasticity, and the generation of pain. In Wall PD, Melzack R, editors: *Textbook of pain*, New York, 1999, Churchill Livingstone.

104. Fleisch J, Rinkema L, Haisch K, et al: LY171883, 1-(2-hydroxy-3-propyl-4-(1'H-tetrazol-5-yL)butoxyl) phenyl) ethanone, an orally active leukotriene D4 antagonist, *J Pharmacol Exp Ther* 233:148-157, 1985.

105. Braquet P, Shen T, Tougui L, et al: Perspectives in platelet activating research, *Pharmacol Rev* 39:97-146, 1987.

106. Whalley E, Clegg S, Stewart J, et al: The effect of kinin agonists and antagonists on the pain response of the human blister base, *Arch Pharmacol* 335:652-655, 1987.

107. Mierle L, Cordella-Miele E, Facchiano A, et al: Novel anti-inflammatory peptides from the region of highest similarity between uteroglobin and lipocortin. I, *Nature* 335:726-730, 1988.

108. Vaught J: Substance P antagonists and analgesia: a review of the hypothesis, *Life Sci* 43:1419-1431, 1988.

109. Levine J, Coddere T, Helms C, et al: β2-adrenergic mechanisms in experimental arthritis, *Proc Natl Acad Sci U S A* 85:4553-4556, 1988.

110. Hunt SP, O'Brien JA, Palmer JA, et al: Role of substance P in nociception, analgesia, and aggression. In Wood J, editor: *Molecular basis of pain induction*, New York, 2000, Wiley-Liss.

111. Nichols ML, Allen BJ, Rogers SD, et al: Transmission of chronic nociception by spinal neurons expressing the substance P receptor, *Science* 286:1558-1561, 1999.

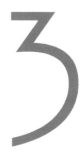

CHAPTER 3

Nonpharmacologic Methods for Managing Pain and Anxiety

PETER MILGROM

CHAPTER OUTLINE

Why Treat Anxious Patients?

People communicate discomfort in a number of ways. Even the most experienced clinician is often unsure how to interpret a patient's response to dental treatment. Is it really pain, or is the patient just jumpy? Is it painful or merely unpleasant? Why is this particular patient so upset? Because the dental treatment environment is so familiar, the dentist often forgets just how uncomfortable it can be to the patient. A clinician may focus on the mechanical aspects of treatment and fail to comprehend fully the nature and extent of a patient's distress. Without appropriate empathy, a dentist may become insensitive and discount what the patient reports. Clearly, however, pain and anxiety are major patient concerns. The dentist may ask certain questions as part of the routine preoperative patient history or during the patient interview (Box 3-1).[1]

Why should the dentist be concerned about anxious patients? There are three obvious reasons. First, building a private general dental practice or having a well-respected public clinic program is a function of having new patients return for regular care and recruiting referrals from current patients. Practices with a satisfied, loyal following are successful. Second, working with patients in acute pain and distress is stressful for the dental practitioner. Minimizing the number of difficult patients reduces the pressure on the dentist and prevents professional burnout. Third, dental auxiliary staff are most happy in well-organized, low-stress environments. A practice that does well with the difficult patient will be a source of pride to staff, and turnover will be low. Assigning responsibilities to dental hygienists and assistants in the preparation and care of the anxious patient increases staff skills and builds loyalty to the practice, which further reduces pressure on the dentist.

Why should the dentist not just refer difficult patients to someone else? The clinician may ask: Who needs them? Who needs this frustration? These are good questions, but the answers are less obvious. Once an anxious patient has approached a dental office, even if in pain, he or she is now ready to tackle the problem. If these patients are handled well, they could be on the road to success in managing their dental anxiety and obtaining good dental care. Such patients become loyal members of a practice, and the dentist serves a public health role in helping the patient. Referring a patient at this stage will likely be unsuccessful, since it is very difficult for many of

these potential patients to summon the courage to come to the initial dentist. If the dentist places barriers in the patient's path, it may take even more courage to approach a second dentist, and many will not succeed. Another reason for not making a referral is that patients with the most complex and interesting dental pathology often avoid dental treatment. If a referral is made at this stage, the dentist is denied the stimulation and professional growth associated with challenging technical problems.

Relationship between Pain and Anxiety

Pain is complex. There is no simple pathway from the teeth and periodontium to the brain. Pain is not simply a function of tissue damage. Many factors, such as emotions, beliefs, past experience, expectations, as well as drugs the patient takes, affect the pain experience. Pain and anxiety are two sides of the same coin. Pain can cause a person to be anxious, and an anxious patient is likely to experience more pain than a patient who is not anxious. Therefore interventions that modulate anxiety reduce pain. For example, many patients express concern about the pain of palatal injections. In fact, patients may anticipate the pain of injections as being so severe that they try to avoid the injection and then experience more discomfort in treatment due to lack of local anesthesia. If the dentist explains that topical agents can reduce the pain of injection, the patient's resistance to the injection and the anticipatory arousal can also be lessened. The agent itself then obtunds the peripheral response.

Circumstances determine how a patient responds. Imagine being caught out in a snowstorm in the mountains when your car breaks down. The cold would be intolerable. However, it would be the same cold experienced when skiing in the snow on a holiday, and the cold while skiing would seldom be described as "intolerable." The temperature (or the cold stimulus) may be the same, but the interpretation of the event is different. Discomfort is exacerbated when people are trapped in a situation beyond their control. The truly anxious person describes dental treatment similarly, which might explain why it is so difficult to treat a patient with irreversible pulpitis. The patient may have been up all night in pain, and such emotionally distraught patients often perceive pressure as pain, making them almost impossible to numb. Using analgesics, allowing the patient to rest, and providing adequate nutrition can transform the situation from failure to success. Attending to both the pain and the anxiety components of the dental treatment experience is required by the empathetic practitioner.

Pediatric Considerations

Appropriate pain control and anxiety control are important considerations in pediatric dentistry. Studies have demonstrated that clinicians often underestimate children's pain. What many children describe as painful may seem merely unpleasant to the dental practitioner.[2] Until recent times it was axiomatic that children felt less pain than adults. Today, we know this is incorrect. Children do not usually sit still in uncomfortable positions for even short periods. Pain is quickly translated into uncooperative behavior aimed at escape. Even if anesthetic agents were foolproof, children in the dental treatment situation might experience distress. Thus how the child is managed psychologically impacts the efficacy of pain control and the clinician's ability to deliver appropriate care.

Dentists give many young children sedative drugs to help manage their distress and help them tolerate dental procedures. Unfortunately, when local anesthesia is not optimal,[3] many cases of conscious sedation fail, and the children face deep sedation or general anesthesia. Recognizing that drugs alone will not help a child is essential to a safe and balanced approach to caring for young people.

Individualizing Treatment

Surveys in the community consistently find that about one in seven patients do not have adequate anesthesia when their teeth are stimulated by the drill, even though they had been given local anesthetic.[4] The dentist should ask a new patient if he or she has ever experienced painful treatment. Usually the patient will readily tell the dentist about the problem. Some may never have experienced pain-free care, and others may have had just a single painful experience. Just asking about the previous experience can help reduce the fearfulness by demonstrating the practitioner's concern. Certain questions may be a helpful starting place in discussing injections and pain (Box 3-2).

In most cases an empathetic response and acceptance of the information will suffice if careful anesthetic technique is used. The practitioner should avoid saying, "That can't happen here." Clinicians should only pledge to do their best to control pain. An antianxiety strategy may not be necessary if the problem is delimited.

Other potential patients may be afraid of the dental treatment or the anesthetic injection itself. Asking patients what happened at their last dental treatment visit can be a good starting point. It is also useful to ask what the patient thinks could be done to make future treatment experience less difficult. Usually such patients can self-diagnose their problem. For example, one patient reported, "The dentist is always in a rush. If only I could have a few minutes after the dental injection to compose myself, then I would be OK." When asked what would make treatment worse, patients may answer, "They kept drilling even though I said it hurt. They told me it was only the vibration of the drill." Most fearful patients are primarily concerned with pain and embarrassment in front of the dentist.

Many patients find it helpful to know how long procedures will last. When drilling, the dentist can say, "I am going to work on your teeth for the count of five and then give you a break," or "I am going to work on your teeth for the count of two and then ask if you felt any pain." Then the dentist can count slowly while drilling. When patients know they have only a limited time to tolerate a procedure, they are less likely to become upset. It also allows the clinician to assess whether additional anesthetic might be needed (Box 3-3).

BOX 3-2

Patient Questions About Injections

How do you feel about injections (shots)?
What is the worst part of getting a shot? The pain? Just the idea?
What was the nature of the problem?
Did the anesthetic work? Did it wear off during treatment?
Was the tooth pulp involved?
Was an anesthetic even offered in periodontal treatment situations?
How did the dentist or dental hygienist handle the situation? Did the provider deny the pain?

BOX 3-3

Anesthesia and Periodontal Treatment

Periodontal care is a special situation. Many patients need to have scaling and root planing repeatedly over many years. This may be considered aversive treatment, and often a local anesthetic is not offered. Dental hygienists may be perceived as the source of fear. An alternative is to use a topical anesthetic with a periodontal probe for a full mouth examination. Also, a local anesthetic may be used before scaling and root planing for both maintenance patients and new patients.

The dentist needs to work closely with the dental hygienist in prescribing periodontal treatment. Preoperative medications for postoperative pain control or intraoperative sedation may be helpful. Postoperative telephone calls to assess patient comfort are also important. Often the dentist is unaware that a patient is encountering problems during periodontal treatment and dental hygiene visits.

One strategy, for example, is to drill for short periods while counting, interspersing the drilling with short breaks of 5 to 10 seconds. It is not necessary to interrupt the work. In fact, placing these breaks in the work reduces the amount of patient interruptions.

Patients with Special Problems

A smaller number of patients may have anxiety or mood disorders, which can make receiving dental treatment difficult. Working with these patients requires extra skills.[4] Many potential patients have untreated anxiety that manifests as panic attacks. These episodes can be quite frequent and mimic heart attacks. Patients may attribute them to a local anesthetic given by the dentist or to other external causes. Other patients who may be very difficult to treat have a gag reflex problem, which can occur both at the dental office and in other anxiety-provoking situations.

Patients with mood disorders may be depressed. The cardinal signs of depression are loss of affect, poor appetite, and difficulty sleeping. If working or functioning normally in society, the individual may not be difficult to treat if given special care. On the other hand, if the person is unemployed or receiving disability, care must be taken initially not to provide a complicated treatment plan. Goals should be modest and implemented in a step-by-step manner. Many of these patients lack the skills to master the dental care situation and may fail to cope well with decisions about treatment, or they may not tolerate the treatment itself. Last-minute cancellations are common.

Sexual and Physical Abuse

Research suggests that some of the distress seen in patients is attributable to abuse experienced during childhood or even to current abuse.[5] One patient treated could not tolerate the feelings of numbness from a mandibular block because it recreated feelings of once being choked. Other patients may suddenly behave like a child or appear as if they are hearing voices.

Although it is not necessary to ask every patient about abuse, it is important to recognize that it may explain behavior in the dental operatory that is otherwise a mystery. If the clinician sees such behavior, questioning should be done carefully. Most often, patients will appreciate the concern and empathy. Many of these patients will already have been in some form of therapy for the problem. If not, the dentist may be able to guide them to seek professional assistance. Posttraumatic stress syndrome is easier to treat when the trauma is recent and is more difficult when flashbacks and other symptoms are present.

Differing Ways Patients Express Fears

Just as patients may differ in *what* they fear, *how* they manifest fear and anxiety may also vary. Fear specialists suggest that anxiety is manifested in one or a combination of three channels. The first and most difficult to assess is *thought*. Patients may recall unpleasant experiences and become upset, even if the current dentist is doing everything right. The second channel is *behavior*. Children often show their distress by trying to escape. Adults are less likely to try to flee the chair but will curl their toes or grip the arms of the chair. Such people will also close their eyes and tighten the neck and facial musculature. They deny they are fearful. The third channel is *physiologic*. This is seen primarily in a rapid heart rate but can include a variety of autonomic responses, including sweating, dizziness, and nausea. Few patients show fear in all these ways at once. It can be distressing to the inexperienced clinician when a patient complains of chest pain (with normal vital signs) after an injection of local anesthetic but denies being fearful. This phenomenon of lack of concordance is common, and comprehensive assessment of the patient is important.

Exposure as a Goal

Anxious patients often recreate past dental treatment experiences in their minds when they enter a dental treatment environment. All the emotions of the previous experience surface. When questioned, many of these patients say, "It's not you." They seem to have no control over the emotion. Having control over the situation and mastering the problem are the goals of treatment. To do this, the patient must stay in the treatment situation and not flee. Fears are maintained when no new experiences replace unpleasant memories. Moreover, multiple positive experiences are required to undo even a single negative impact. The objective of all "fear treatments" is to have the patient experience dental treatment successfully. Such treatment will be stressful, and some patients in this category never become completely comfortable. Nevertheless, they can visit regularly and seek prevention-oriented care rather than emergency care. Developing this form of mastery is similar to learning to drive a car or ride a horse. Being a good dental patient requires this sense of mastery. Certain questions may help uncover the patient's concerns (Box 3-4).

> ### BOX 3-4
>
> ### Questions About Patient Concerns
>
> Do you find it difficult to relax in the dental chair?
> Do you sometimes find yourself "hanging on for dear life" or "white knuckling it" during certain procedures?
> Have you ever felt it was difficult to breathe or swallow while in the dental chair?
> Is there anything you can do to relax yourself in the dental chair?

Fortunately, many patients have learned stress management skills at work or in other areas of their personal lives. Asking about these skills may lead to a simple recommendation that the patient apply the same approach to dental treatment. The patient may have participated in a smoking cessation or similar program. Adapting existing strategies can be a shortcut to effective patient management.

When treating fearful patients, the dentist needs to construct a step-by-step treatment plan that places the shorter and less traumatic procedures first. Abscesses and endodontic problems should be treated symptomatically and definitive treatment postponed so that the patient can experience the easier procedures early in treatment. Willpower and tolerance for dental treatment are "built" on successful experiences.

Combining Nonpharmacologic and Pharmacologic Modalities

Pharmacologic agents always work better in an atmosphere where rapport and trust are well established, with expectations for successful treatment. Drugs are not a substitute for attentive care, and nonpharmacologic therapies may not be appropriate for many patients. The clinician needs to determine the patient's preferences. Some patients will avoid drugs at all costs. Others see pharmacologic aids as essential to coping with treatment. The clinician should try to match the patient's preferred approach to pharmacologic support whenever possible. The following analogy about headache remedies is useful: When people get a headache they have three basic choices. First, they can employ a drug-oriented solution—they take aspirin. Second, they can choose a nonpharmacologic solution—they can rest. Finally, some people do both—they take aspirin and rest. In most cases the patient's preferred management will work. So, too, with treatments for pain and anxiety associated with dental care.

Whether the dentist uses one strategy or a combination will depend primarily on the patient's preference. Some patients, perhaps out of fear, attempt to cope without adequate skills or agents, which will be successful only if the dental treatment is not complex or aversive. If the treatment requires cooperation and patience, a combined pharmacologic and cognitive or behavioral pain/stress reduction strategy is required. Whatever the decision, dental care should never be attempted if the patient is not adequately prepared to cope.

Sedative-hypnotic drugs administered orally in combination with nitrous oxide or given intravenously can be useful for patients who need extensive treatment. This approach can also be used if logistics are likely to cause difficulties for the patient (e.g., teenager who will miss too much school, worker whose boss complains about excessive sick leave). The approach used in the Dental Fears Research Clinic at the University of Washington, Seattle, differs from the common practice of using only pharmacology for sedation. Initially, the patient's fears are diagnosed, and a strategy is developed for desensitization or moderation of the fears. Then the dentist may perform simple procedures, often scaling and root planing with local anesthetic, to teach the patient to relax and breathe while receiving dental care. The patient establishes that he or she is an active participant in the process by showing up on time and practicing relaxation at home. When the patient appears well versed, a session of sedation is scheduled. At the same time, follow-up sessions with the dental hygienist or dentist are planned. The patient should see the sedation as a convenience to overcome the backlog of needed care rather than the solution to fears. There is little evidence that sedation alone effectively treats fear, and over the long term, the sedation-alone approach is relatively ineffective.

The ideal outcome of treatment is that the patient attributes success to personal coping rather than drug administration. Throughout psychiatry and medicine, patients who use drugs as a substitute for coping often find it difficult to continue treatment later if their anxieties reappear. Experience has shown that anxieties treated with drugs alone do recur.

Targeting the Treatment to the Symptoms

Pain and anxiety treatment is symptom oriented. If the problem is a function of how a patient acts (e.g., gripping the arms of the dental chair and waiting for the worst), a behavioral solution of relaxation may be very helpful and appropriate. If patients hold their breath when receiving a dental injection, a paced breathing exercise may be helpful. If their thoughts are dysfunctional, distraction may be helpful. If the noise of the drill triggers a response, earphones and a CD player may soothe the patient. Other patients are vigilant and distrustful. For them, good explanations and the opportunity to watch treatment in a mirror may be the most efficacious. The more that is discovered about the problem, the easier it is to make suggestions about what might work (Box 3-5).

Plan Multiple Strategies

Some strategies do not work every time. For example, the effects of nitrous oxide at a given concentration vary from visit to visit for the same person and between laboratory and clinic settings. Thus patients should be equipped with more than one coping strategy. Patients are asked to identify one strategy as primary and to practice that approach at home before their next visit. At the same time, they are asked to pick a backup strategy that they can use if they tire of the first one.

The Dental Team

Managing pain and anxiety is a team effort. The dentist is not alone in managing the fearful patient. Skilled clinicians use the dental assistant and dental hygienist to help prepare patients for treatment. An assistant can be trained to teach patients who use nitrous oxide how to breathe slowly and deeply and to employ a distraction strategy. This approach reduces side effects of nitrous oxide, avoids hyperventilation or breath holding, and is likely to result in more profound pain control at lower concentrations of gas. A skilled dental hygienist can teach patients to relax while receiving dental injections. The relaxed patient is less likely to become upset if a little topical anesthetic numbs the throat. Similarly, the wise dentist uses the assistant to cue an anxious patient to breathe during the dental injection and not to hold onto the arms of the chair during dental procedures.

Often the field of vision of the dentist is limited. It is helpful to have another person in the treatment area observe the rest of the patient's body and notify the dentist if a pain or distress reaction is evident. Dental assistants, dental hygienists, and office staff can debrief patients after treatment to learn what problems occurred during treatment and to seek solutions. Patients may reveal distress to the receptionist while denying it to the dentist. The dentist should always thank a patient if distress or unhappiness about treatment has been reported. Encouraging feedback allows the treatment team to adapt positively and be more successful.

Techniques that Work

Anxious patients need to be involved in active coping. It is often best to begin a session with a statement and then a question. "I know what I am going to be doing today with your tooth. What are you going to be doing to keep yourself comfortable?" If the patient does not have a strategy to practice actively during treatment, a failure is likely. The patient who says, "I'll just keep my mind blank," is a candidate to have negative thoughts about the dental care. It is much better to practice and use active coping techniques, as described next.

Enhancing Control and Information

In the dental treatment situation, patients must give up a certain amount of control over their body for treatment to be delivered. Many patients find this distressing and find that it increases their pain and discomfort during treatment. Information helps lessen this distress. The classic "Tell-show-do" approach advocated for children's dentistry works equally well with adults. Giving the patient a mirror to watch the treatment may be helpful, especially for the vigilant patient. For others it is like watching television and can be distracting. Asking permission before tipping the chair back or before giving an injection enhances patient control.

Patients also appreciate information about injections (Box 3-6), such as the following:

> Injections hurt for two reasons. First, there is the pain of the needle puncturing the oral tissue. We help control this pain by using topical ointments or drug patches. Second, there is the pain of injecting the fluid into the tissue. We help moderate this pain by injecting very slowly.

The following scenario often works well. The dentist takes out a syringe and needle set and demonstrates. Initially the plunger should be pushed hard, showing the patient how the fluid squirts across the room. Then the plunger can be pushed gently, with the solution dribbling out. The dentist can make an analogy of a garden hose. If the hose is turned on full volume and aimed into the dirt, it will make a hole. If a soft spray is used, it will do no damage. After such an explanation, most patients are more comfortable with injections. Then the dentist's only job is to use topical anesthetic effectively and inject extremely slowly. Spending nearly a minute injecting a full cartridge of anesthetic is not too slow. When finished, ask for feedback from the patient: "On a scale of 1 to 10, where 10 is very painful, how comfortable was the injection?"

Cues that signal the beginning and length of injections are helpful to the patient. The dentist can say

---

BOX 3-6

Syringes and the Anxious Patient

Explain why needles and syringes are so "big."
Explain why dentists inject so slowly.
"The needle is flexible and won't break. It does not go in all the way."
"The anesthetic makes you feel differently, but you can still swallow. Your muscles are still OK."

to the patient, "I am going to inject for the count of 10—one, two, three—and then be finished. If you experience any discomfort, I want you to tell me." Counting rarely interferes with the injection. Also, patients often thank the dentist for giving them this sense of control over time.

Information can be helpful to the patient during placement of an intravenous cannula. Extremely apprehensive patients anticipate pain, often because a previous experience with blood being drawn was painful and left them bruised. The dentist can explain the purpose of topical EMLA cream or subcutaneous lidocaine in reducing intravenous access pain. Explaining that the needle is actually withdrawn once the plastic catheter is in place also makes many nervous patients more comfortable.

Gagging is a common clinical problem, and control is an important factor. When faced with an impression tray, many normal children and adults become quite anxious. Gagging is the most common fear of children. It can be helpful to rehearse an impression with an empty tray before proceeding. Often the patient will gain some control from helping to hold the handle of the tray and may also benefit by knowing that the tray can be removed at any time if a signal is given, such as raising the hand. After practice with a tray, few patients request that it be removed prematurely, and the sense of safety and control over its removal is enough to accomplish the task. The patient should always be told how long the tray will be in the mouth and should be informed as the time passes.

The dental team should never leave a patient who is afraid of gagging unattended. The patient can sit up once the tray is in place and can be encouraged to hold the low-volume suction. Many patients like to hold the tray. When the patient is allowed this sense of safety, taking impressions is usually much less stressful.

Modifying Attention and Using Distraction

People have a remarkable ability to turn their attention away from objects and events. Every student knows how to daydream, and one can drive a car to a destination and not even remember the trip. The key to using distraction is to use it appropriately. Distraction works best when it is individualized, so the patient should be asked what is distracting. For one patient it may be listening to a CD of rock music; for another, the dentist telling stories about his or her

children may be best. Involved and complicated distractions are more effective. Soft background music does not work well. For children, stories and riddles are potential distractions. Distraction is not appropriate when a patient is upset.

Distraction is not a substitute for good local anesthesia; it is best used as a complement. Distraction also enhances the effectiveness of nitrous oxide.

Distraction works quite well with gaggers. It is a key element in almost every advocated technique. Simply engaging the interest of the patient in a story or one-way conversation is enough to divert attention away from concerns about choking.

Relaxation

Anxious patients, especially those anticipating the pain of injections, hold their breath. Tensing the musculature tends to increase pain. Such patients have their eyes tightly shut and are stiff, "holding on for dear life." A patient can be taught a simple exercise to identify when the muscles are tight and then to relax, easing the pain. The patient can be instructed to practice tensing and relaxing the facial and large body muscles several times a day between appointments. The patient should be cued to remember to relax in anticipation of the injection or other potentially distressing procedures. If the patient begins to tense when topical anesthetic is applied in anticipation of an injection, lightly touching the hand that is tensed can remind the patient to relax.

As with distraction, telling patients to relax when they are very upset may be perceived as denying pain or distress. If the situation is stressful, it is better to stop the procedure and reschedule. Before beginning again, the clinician should review the approach and problem solve with the patient.

Paced Breathing

Along with muscle relaxation, controlling the depth and rate of breathing is an important nonpharmacologic aid to reducing both pain and anxiety (Box 3-7). Because most patients who are afraid of injections hold their breath, encouraging breathing is important. On the other hand, shallow rapid breathing is counterproductive and can lead to dizziness and nausea. Instead, the patient should take a deep breath and then hold it for a slow count of five. The dentist or assistant can coach the patient to exhale very slowly, again counting to five. The assistant may

BOX 3-7

Patient Education: Paced Breathing

> Explain that improper breathing makes a person feel bad.
> Demonstrate slow, paced breathing.
> Practice paced breathing with the patient.
> Have the patient practice at home.

touch the patient's shoulder to cue breathing, pushing down on the out breath.

When a patient is becoming very upset, slow-paced breathing is the best method to calm the patient. The clinician can see this strategy working; when the breathing slows, so will the heart rate, and with it any palpitations that the patient feels. Breathing is very calming. Once the patient feels in control again, the problem can be solved and a decision made on whether the patient can proceed.

Paced breathing is important when using nitrous oxide or oral and intravenous medications that affect respiration. Patients who can effectively perform breathing exercises maintain oxygen saturation. Similarly, patients can use their breathing and relaxation skills during placement of an intravenous line.

Hypnosis

Hypnosis is a formalized method of applying the techniques of attention modification, paced breathing, and muscle relaxation. It has been employed in dentistry for more than 100 years. Highly regarded courses in hypnosis for clinicians are available on a regional basis from the American Society of Clinical Hypnosis. The courses are graded from beginner to advanced. A beginner's course will equip the clinician with skills that can be used the next day in practice. A hypnosis course is an easy way to practice talking to patients about a more comfortable way to experience dental treatment.

The process of helping a patient reach a hypnotic state is called *induction*, as described in the following example:

The patient should be relaxed and sitting up.
Dentist: Please make yourself comfortable. You must be comfortable to get relaxed. Do you feel comfortable now?
Patient: Yes.

Dentist: Now raise your arms over your head and then just let them drop into your lap. Good. You may have felt a moment of relaxation when you did that. Your whole body relaxed briefly. Please try it again. You may begin to sense that when you relax that your limbs get heavy. This heaviness is part of relaxation. Now try breathing slowly. Take a deep breath, hold your breath as you are comfortable, and let it out slowly. Each time you breathe in and out, you will get more and more relaxed. You may want to close your eyes.

The dentist can count while giving breathing and suggestions for relaxation as follows:

Dentist: I would like you to tighten your arm and hand muscles; make them stiff out in front of you. Now as I count, I want you to imagine first tightening and then loosening the muscles. One, feel the muscles of your hands tighten and your arms stiffen. Two, make them really tight. Three, now begin to loosen them a little. Take a deep breath and let it out slowly. Four, imagine your muscles getting heavy and much looser. Take another breath. Five, your arms may not feel so heavy that they begin to fall into your lap.

Once a patient becomes comfortable, the dental work can be started. The dentist should alert the patient about an upcoming noise, bump, or other action. Throughout the procedure the dentist can continue to encourage the patient to maintain the relaxed quiet state.

Often, hypnosis sessions end by the clinician giving the patient *posthypnotic suggestions*, which usually take the form of praising the patient for doing well and suggesting that the feeling of calm and painlessness of the session will continue in the period after treatment. The patient should be told that practice at home improves the effectiveness of hypnosis.

Biofeedback

A pulse meter can be extremely helpful to the clinician with an anxious patient. Heart rate is a simple indicator of physiologic upset. Many patients are dyssynchronous in their fear responses and may deny being upset even when they have rapid heart rates and perspiration on the upper lip. This may happen when patients are being pushed to proceed either by a clinician or a family member. If the heart rate is more than 10 beats/minute above a waiting room baseline, the patient is upset. When the rate is 110 or 120, patients experience pounding in the chest, and many will become much more visibly upset. Their responses can mimic cardiac problems. Thus the heart rate should be used as a cue to calm the patient with relaxation or breathing techniques. The clinician should never proceed when the heart rate is significantly elevated. Simply giving the patient a break for a few seconds or a drink of water may be sufficient.

Some patients find it helpful to monitor their own pulse using a pulse oximeter or a hand-held exercise pulse meter. Patients can be taught to monitor the heart rate and to institute breathing and relaxation exercises if the rate is increasing. They can also do this during breaks in treatment.

Controlling Thoughts

Patients with uncontrollable thoughts often "psyche" themselves with messages that they cannot tolerate treatment or that they are going to embarrass themselves or disrupt treatment, which in turn makes them more upset. Some patients find it helpful to adopt a mantra or a saying that they can repeat to themselves or aloud (e.g., I did OK last time, I'll do OK this time; I'm doing fine, my body is relaxed; I can do this). Some patients may have skills they can bring from another setting (e.g., yoga, martial arts). They may already have a "talk-to-myself" strategy and only need to be encouraged to use it during dental care.

Desensitization

Desensitization is the formal process from cognitive-behavioral psychology used earlier for patients who have long-standing fears and who need more practice to be successful dental patients. A hierarchy of stimuli is constructed related to the patient's fears. For example, an injection hierarchy might appear as follows:

1. Seeing the syringe across the room.
2. Seeing the syringe in the dentist's hand.
3. Touching the syringe in the dentist's hand.
4. Holding the syringe.
5. Looking at the syringe with the needle cap off.
6. Having the syringe in the mouth with the needle cap on.
7. Having the syringe in the mouth with the needle cap off.
8. Having a tiny amount of anesthetic administered.

When desensitization is employed, the patient is first taught relaxation and paced-breathing skills. Then each of the stimuli is presented in order. At each step of the hierarchy the patient must demonstrate that he or she can relax and not become too anxious before proceeding to the next step. Typically, a truly fearful patient will require one or two short visits to move through the hierarchy. In assessing whether to proceed, the clinician should remember to observe behavior, obtain self-reports of anxiety, and monitor physiologic parameters, especially heart rate. Unless all these channels are under control, the fear may persist.

Preventing Relapse

Most fearful patients can expect to have some of their nonadaptive thoughts and feelings return to some extent. The goal is not complete elimination of these, since this is often too time-consuming and may be unrealistic. Rather, the goal is for the patient to be able to return to the dentist's office. Because fears can return and prevent optimal dental visits, the dentist should schedule patients on shorter recall intervals at the beginning. The patient can receive oral hygiene recalls every couple of months during the immediate period after treatment. These return visits can help maintain rapport and can facilitate the patient returning when a problem occurs (e.g., broken cusp, toothache). Fearful patients appreciate home care instruction more than nonfearful patients because they often see it as a way to avoid the anxiety of extensive dental treatment.

Therapeutic Recommendations

It is important to recognize when a patient is too difficult to treat and should be referred. This is true for patients with mood and anxiety conditions, as well as for patients with physical disease. The difference is that patients with mental health problems may be embarrassed and may resist being stigmatized with the label of "it's in your head." Patients who have never been to a psychiatrist or psychologist are unlikely to take such a referral well.

With a difficult patient the dentist first should attempt to establish rapport and then should consider instituting simple prevention-oriented treatments. Analgesics and antibiotics can be used to alleviate pain and treat infections. Knowing more about the patient makes a successful referral more likely. Referrals for specific help in overcoming anxiety over injections or gagging that interferes with treatment will be better accepted than more general referrals.

Most problems with dental encounters can be overcome with a *cognitive-behavioral approach*. Although other techniques work, experience has demonstrated that these are the most efficient strategies. Often in only a few sessions, a skilled clinician can help a patient. The local psychological association or medical society can identify possible colleagues for referrals.

Referrals to mental health practitioners are preferred over prescribing sedating drugs or other medications. Medications used in this way are unlikely to cure the anxiety or pain and are often counterproductive.[6]

SUMMARY

Many potential dental patients are anxious. They often report pain during or after treatment. Management of pain and anxiety is generally successful when behavioral modification methods are used. These techniques are simple and can be readily incorporated into general and specialty practices. At the same time, anesthetics, analgesics, and sedative agents are useful complements to well-developed behavioral skills. Experience and skill in using a broad range of behavioral techniques and pharmacologic agents provide patients with more options and a safer and more comfortable treatment experience. Dentists with these skills are prepared to meet the needs of their patients.

References

1. Corah NL: Assessment of a dental anxiety scale, *J Dent Res* 43:496, 1969.
2. Murtomaa H, Milgrom P, Weinstein P, et al: Dentist perceptions and management of pain experienced by children during treatment: a survey of groups of dentists in the USA and Finland, *Int J Paediatr Dent* 6:25-30, 1996.
3. Nakai Y, Milgrom P, Mancl L, et al: Effectiveness of local anesthesis in pediatric dental practice, *J Am Dent Assoc* 131(12):1699-1705, 2000.
4. Milgrom P, Weinstein P, Getz T. *Treating fearful dental patients: a patient management handbook*, ed 2, Seattle, 1995, University of Washington Continuing Dental Education.
5. Walker EA, Milgrom P, Weinstein P, et al: Assessing abuse and neglect and dental fear in women, *J Am Dent Assoc* 127:485-490, 1996.
6. Kleinknecht RA: *Mastering anxiety: the nature and treatment of anxious conditions*, New York, 1991, Plenum Press.

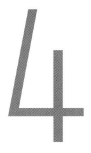

CHAPTER 4

Basic Physiologic Considerations

Daniel E. Becker
Bruce E. Bradley

CHAPTER OUTLINE

TABLE 4-1

Autonomic Control of Selected Effectors

Target	Sympathetic Effect (Adrenergic Receptor)	Parasympathetic Effect
Pupil (via iris)	Mydriasis (α)	Miosis
Gastrointestinal tone	Inhibitory (α, β_2)	Excitatory
Bronchioles	Dilation (β_2)	Constriction
Heart	Excitatory (β_1)	Inhibitory
Vessels	Dilation (β_2)	Insignificant
	Constriction (α)	
Airway secretions	Insignificant	Stimulation

Autonomic Nervous System

General Functions

The autonomic nervous system regulates all vital organs and is a target for many therapeutic, as well as adverse, drug effects. Unlike somatic (voluntary) efferent nerves, autonomic nerves exit the central nervous system and synapse with a second neuron that innervates the target organ. Only this second neuron, the postganglionic neuron, is germane to clinical practice.

Table 4-1 summarizes the most relevant parasympathetic and sympathetic innervations. Two general concepts are apparent from this table: (1) *sympathetic innervation* produces effects that are considered ideal during stress responses, and (2) *parasympathetic innervation* generates the opposite effects. Although most organs receive dual innervation, a significant exception is the absence of parasympathetic innervation to blood vessels and the ventricular myocardium. Both divisions are active simultaneously during stressful situations, with the dominant division establishing the net effect on each system. Whereas the sympathetic innervations dominate cardiovascular function, parasympathetic innervations dominate oropharyngeal secretions and gastrointestinal function. Several exceptions to these generalizations, including influences on metabolic processes, vasomotor tone, and secretion of sweat and tears, are intentionally omitted because they have little application to patient assessment, monitoring, and support during sedation and anesthesia (Box 4-1).

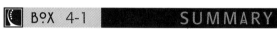

BOX 4-1 SUMMARY

Autonomic Considerations

Parasympathetic effects include pupil constriction (miosis), bronchoconstriction, stimulation of oral and airway secretions, and reduced heart rate and atrioventricular (AV) conduction.

Parasympathetic effects are mediated by acetylcholine. They are imitated by cholinergic agonists and cholinesterase inhibitors and inhibited by anticholinergic drugs.

Sympathetic effects are mediated via three adrenergic receptors: α-receptors mediate pupil dilation (mydriasis) and vasoconstriction; β_2-receptors mediate bronchodilation and vasodilation; and β_1-receptors mediate increase in heart rate, AV conduction, and contractility.

Sympathetic effects are mediated by norepinephrine and epinephrine. They are imitated by various adrenergic agonists and inhibited by adrenergic antagonists.

Synaptic Transmission and Pharmacologic Applications

Synaptic transmission consists of neuronal release of either acetylcholine or norepinephrine, each binding to specific membrane receptors on effector cells. It is the specific cholinergic or adrenergic receptor subtype that actually generates the biochemical events leading to the clinical effect; the neurotransmitter merely "activates the switch." These synapses are the

TABLE 4-2

Comparative Effects of Various Cholinergic Agonists and Antagonists on Selected Body Functions

	Gastrointestinal Tone	Gastric Secretion	Oral/Respiratory Secretions	Heart Rate
Cholinergic Agonists				
Methacholine	++	++	++	---
Bethanechol	+++	++	++	-
Pilocarpine	++	++++	++++	?
Cholinergic Antagonists				
Atropine	--	-	-	+++
Scopolamine	-	-	----	0
Glycopyrrolate	---	---	---	?, +

+, Relative stimulatory effect; −, relative inhibitory effect; ?, degree of influence not fully established.

TABLE 4-3

Commonly Prescribed Antihistamines and Psychotropic Agents Having Significant Anticholinergic Actions

Antihistamines	Tricyclic Antidepressants	Antipsychotics
Diphenhydramine (Benadryl)	Desipramine (Norpramin)	Chlorpromazine (Thorazine)
Hydroxyzine (Vistaril)	Amitriptyline (Elavil)	Thioridazine (Mellaril)
Promethazine (Phenergan)	Doxepin (Sinequan)	Fluphenazine (Prolixin)
	Nortriptyline (Pamelor)	Haloperidol (Haldol)
		Thiothixene (Navane)

target for pharmacologic interventions by appropriate receptor agonists and antagonists.

The synapses for parasympathetic and voluntary nerves are classified as cholinergic because these neurons release acetylcholine (ACh), which subsequently binds to either of two principal classes of cholinergic receptors: (1) nicotinic receptors found on skeletal muscle and (2) muscarinic receptors on autonomically innervated tissues. The activity of ACh within the synapse is brief because it is hydrolyzed instantaneously by acetylcholinesterase (AChE).

Cholinergic receptors are the sites of action for a variety of drugs used in clinical practice. Drugs acting as antagonists at nicotinic receptors on skeletal muscle are referred to as *neuromuscular blockers*. Drugs acting at muscarinic sites either as agonists or antagonists are referred to as cholinergic and an-

ticholinergic drugs, respectively (Table 4-2). Cholinergic drugs imitate parasympathetic effects, whereas anticholinergic drugs block this influence and thereby facilitate sympathetic dominance. Many sedative and psychotropic medications have significant anticholinergic actions that allow the dentist to anticipate their potential side effects. Within the central nervous system, cholinergic synapses are generally excitatory.[1] For this reason, anticholinergic agents produce sedative and antiemetic influences. Commonly prescribed antihistamines and psychotropic agents have significant anticholinergic actions (Table 4-3).

Two neurotransmitters function at adrenergic synapses: norepinephrine is released directly by sympathetic neurons, whereas epinephrine is distributed to the synapse after its release from the adrenal medulla. Sympathetic effects are mediated by three distinct receptors: alpha (α), beta-1 (β_1), and beta-2 (β_2) (Table 4-4).

Two processes account for the termination of the effects of adrenergic neurotransmitters. Norepinephrine, released by sympathetic nerves, is taken back into the neuronal endings (reuptake), where it is either stored in vesicles for reuse or oxidized by monoamine oxidase (MAO). In contrast, epineph-

rine from the adrenal medulla, or administered systemically, undergoes hepatic clearance by catecholamine O-methyltransferase (COMT) and MAO. For catecholamines, such as epinephrine and levonordefrin used with local anesthetics, COMT is most significant.[2,3]

Like cholinergic receptors, adrenergic receptors are the target for a variety of drugs that act as agonists and antagonists (Table 4-5). Their effects are predictable if one is familiar with the functions of the three principal adrenergic receptors (see Table 4-4). For example, a drug acting as an α-agonist constricts vessels, whereas an antagonist mediates vasodilation.

TABLE 4-4
Adrenergic Receptors and Functions

Receptor	Principal Location	Effect Mediated
α	Blood vessels	Vasoconstriction
β_1	Heart	Increased rate and contractility
β_2	Blood vessels	Vasodilation
	Bronchioles	Bronchodilation

TABLE 4-5
Selected Adrenergic Drugs

Drug	RECEPTOR AFFINITY		
	α	β_1	β_2
Agonists			
Epinephrine	+++	+++	++
Norepinephrine	+++	++	0,+
Levonordefrin	+++	++	0,+
Ephedrine	+	++	+
Phenylephrine	+++	0	0
Albuterol	0	0,+	+++
Antagonists			
Labetalol (Normodyne, Trandate)	–	– – –	– – –
Prazosin (Minipress)	– – –	0	0
Propranolol (Inderal)	0	– – –	– – –
Nadolol (Corgard)	0	– – –	– – –
Metoprolol (Lopressor)	0	– – –	0, –
Atenolol (Tenormin)	0	– – –	0, –
Esmolol (Brevibloc)	0	– – –	0, –

+ and – designates relative potencies as agonist or antagonist.

Cardiovascular System

Arterial Blood Pressure

Despite the complexity of cardiovascular physiology, its purpose is simple: it must perfuse vital organs and tissues with oxygenated blood. Arterial blood pressure fluctuates according to specific events in each cardiac cycle (Box 4-2). The pressure is greatest during ventricular systole (systolic blood pressure) and is attributed to ventricular ejection. At the completion of systole the ventricles enter a period of rest (diastole), and their pressure decreases to zero. However, arterial pressure does not decline this far because, on closure of the aortic valve, resistance within the arterial system maintains a diastolic pressure. This influence is described variably as aortic re-

◗ BOX 4-2   SUMMARY
Blood Pressure and Cardiac Cycle

Systolic blood pressure is a function of stroke volume. Heart rate compensates for cardiac output when stroke volume undergoes any significant change.

Stroke volume and therefore systolic blood pressure are directly related to myocardial contractility and preload (venous return).

Diastolic blood pressure is a function of arterial resistance.

An increase in arterial resistance elevates diastolic blood pressure. When resistance becomes excessive, it impedes cardiac ejection and creates afterload on the heart.

sistance, systemic vascular resistance, or peripheral resistance. Although blood volume and viscosity are contributory, vessel diameter and elasticity are the principal factors that determine the degree of arterial resistance and therefore diastolic pressure. Systolic and diastolic pressures can be visualized by examining ventricular and aortic pressure curves (Fig. 4-1).

Systolic blood pressure is sustained by cardiac output and therefore can be influenced by heart rate and stroke volume (Fig. 4-2, *A*). Of these two factors, *stroke volume* is most significant. Rate merely compensates for changes in stroke volume. Slow rates are common in well-trained athletes, but faster rates are required to sustain adequate cardiac output in patients with low stroke volumes (e.g., patients with heart failure).

Stroke volume is directly related to myocardial contractility, which is largely a function of intracellular calcium ions that increase after sympathetic activation of β_1-adrenergic receptors within the myocardium. However, the heart is centered within a closed system of veins and arteries, each having an influence on cardiac output. Venous return acts to *preload* each cardiac cycle and influences stroke volume according to the Frank-Starling principle. All striated muscles have an intrinsic ability to contract more forcefully when stretched, in this case by ve-

nous return. There is a limit to this direct relationship, however; a point is reached where, on further stretching, fibers are unable to respond and stroke volume diminishes. This critical limit is lower for patients with cardiac compromise (Fig. 4-2, *B*).

Normally, arterial resistance has little influence on stroke output of the heart. If resistance is severely elevated by hypertension or the heart is weak, however, the opposition imposed by arterial resistance can reduce stroke volume. Resistance to ventricular ejection is called *afterload* (see Fig. 4-2).

Many factors contribute to short-term and long-term regulation of cardiac function and arterial pressure. However, neural mechanisms that contribute to short-term regulation are most germane to this discussion. The sympathetic nervous system increases cardiac output, venous return, and arterial resistance. The vasomotor center, located in the pons and medulla, transmits excitatory and inhibitory impulses to sympathetic neurons that exit the spinal cord. Two neural reflexes are key in modulating activity of the vasomotor center.[4] The first consists of baroreceptors located in the carotid and aortic arches that respond to changes in mean arterial pressure. Increased pressure triggers afferent input to the vasomotor center that leads to a decrease in heart rate and arterial resistance. Conversely, low pressure

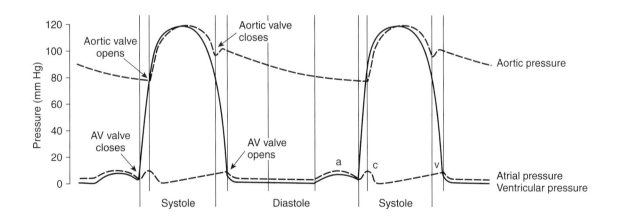

Fig. 4-1 Arterial blood pressure. As ventricular systole commences, ventricular pressure increases to 120 mm Hg, and the pressure is transmitted to the aorta. This is *systolic pressure* and is a function of ventricular systole. During ventricular diastole, ventricular pressure decreases to zero, but aortic pressure does not drop below 80 mm Hg. This is *diastolic pressure* and is essentially a function of arterial resistance. These pressures are transmitted throughout the arterial tree and are recorded indirectly using the familiar sphygmomanometer. *AV,* Atrioventricular. (Modified from Guyton AC, Hall JE: *Textbook of medical physiology,* ed 9, Philadelphia, 1996, WB Saunders.)

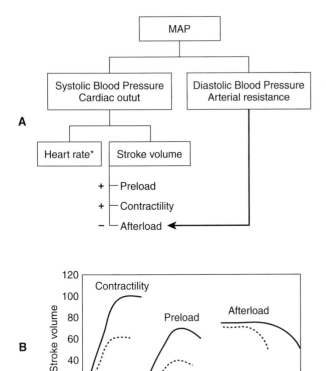

Fig. 4-2 A, Flow chart illustrates the central role of stroke volume in determining mean arterial pressure *(MAP).* Stroke volume is influenced by three principal variables. *Preload* (venous return) and *contractility* are positive influences, whereas *afterload* (arterial resistance) can have a negative influence. *Major MVo_2 determinants. **B,** In the normal heart *(solid lines),* contractility and preload are positive influences on stroke volume. Increasing either of these variables results in an increased stroke volume. Peripheral resistance has little influence on stroke volume unless it becomes excessive. In this case, stroke volume will diminish. In patients with heart failure, progressive weakening of the myocardium alters the heart's response to these variables *(dotted lines).* Contractility and preload have less ability to improve stroke volume, and arterial resistance has a more significant negative influence.

unleashes excitatory influences within the vasomotor center that increase overall cardiovascular tone.

Any increase in venous return to the right atrium triggers two reflexes, only one of which involves the vasomotor center. Locally, venous return stretches the right atrium and stimulates the sinoatrial (SA) node to accelerate the heart rate. More significant, however, is the activation of stretch receptors located within myocardium of the right atria. When activated, these receptors trigger the so-called Brainbridge reflex, which leads to stimulation of the vasomotor center and subsequent increase in heart rate and contractility.

Cardiac Cycle

The contractile events within a cardiac cycle must be carefully synchronized if function is to be normal. This responsibility is attributed to a specialized system of tissues that depolarizes spontaneously. These impulses spread directly onto myocardial cells, igniting them to depolarize and contract. Essential components of this specialized system, as well as the sequence of their conduction, commence with the SA node, spreading through the atrioventricular (AV) node, bundle of His, and Purkinje fibers. Because its spontaneous firing rate is greater than that of the others, the SA node normally functions as the heart's pacemaker. The intrinsic firing rates of all these tissues are influenced by autonomic innervations: sympathetic fibers increase the rates, and parasympathetic fibers decrease the rates.

Blood volumes associated with ventricular filling and ejection are illustrated in Fig. 4-3. Knowledge of these principles enables a better understanding of the status of patients who have chronic atrial fibrillation and heart failure. The amount of blood ejected by the atria ("atrial kick") contributes a relatively small portion of the total end-diastolic volume. For this reason, patients with chronic atrial fibrillation have little compromise in stroke volume unless their ventricular rate is too rapid to allow time for adequate passive filling. Generally, these patients are medicated with a digitalis preparation that slows ventricular rates. For patients with heart failure, consultation with the cardiologist regarding their ejection fraction can provide insight into their degree of decompensation.

Coronary Perfusion and Oxygen Demand

Arterial blood flow (perfusion) to most tissues is greatest during ventricular systole and results from the surge in pressure from ventricular ejection. However, terminal branches of the coronary system are embedded within the muscular wall of the heart

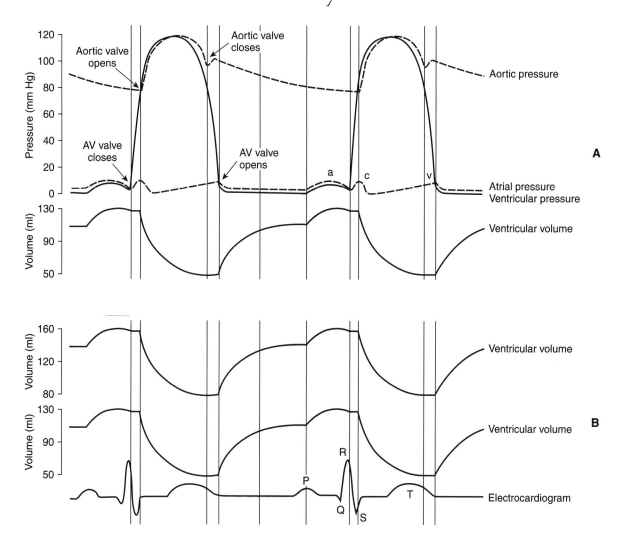

Fig. 4-3 A, Ventricular volumes. At the end of diastole, the left ventricle has filled with 130 ml of blood, called the end-diastolic volume (EDV). At the completion of systole, there is 50 ml of blood remaining as end-systolic volume (ESV). The stroke volume for this cycle is 80 ml and reflects the difference between EDV and ESV. Note how the ventricle accumulates an EDV for the subsequent cycle, starting with the ESV of 50 ml remaining from the previous cycle. Roughly two thirds of ventricular filling occurs passively, blood flowing from the atria before atrial systole. Only the final third of ventricular filling is actually attributed to atrial systole (i.e., "atrial kick"). **B,** Stroke volume versus ejection fraction. Ventricular volume curves shown have a stroke volume of 80 ml. In the upper tracing the stroke volume represents 50% of the 160 ml EDV; in the lower tracing it represents 62% of the 130 ml EDV. Hearts vary in size, and EDV varies with each cardiac cycle. The percentage of the EDV pumped during a cardiac cycle is referred to as the *ejection fraction* and more accurately reflects myocardial strength. Ejection fractions that fall below 0.54 indicate a progression in the severity of heart failure. (**A** modified from Guyton AC, Hall JE: *Textbook of medical physiology,* ed 9, Philadelphia, 1996, WB Saunders.)

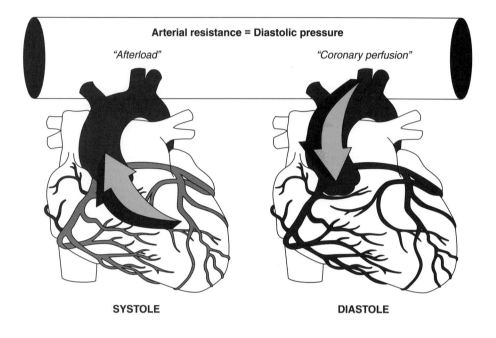

Fig. 4-4 Coronary perfusion. During systole, ventricles eject blood into the arterial system. During diastole, peripheral resistance provides backpressure, closing the aortic valve and perfusing the coronary system. Therefore peripheral resistance has negative and positive influences on cardiac function. It represents the afterload against which the ventricles must work to eject but also provides the backflow pressure required for coronary perfusion.

BOX 4-3   SUMMARY

Coronary Perfusion

Coronary blood flow is greatest during diastole and is driven by backpressure generated by aortic resistance (i.e., diastolic pressure).

Factors that increase myocardial demand for oxygen include heart rate, afterload, and preload, in order of their significance.

Normal cardiac function requires a balance between myocardial oxygen supply (perfusion) and myocardial oxygen demand. Tachycardias are detrimental in two ways: they diminish diastolic time during which coronary perfusion occurs, and they increase the demand for oxygen by myocardial cells.

Tachycardias can also result in hypotension because time for ventricular filling (preload) may be diminished to a point where stroke volume is compromised.

and are compressed during ventricular systole. For this reason, the greatest opportunity for perfusion of the coronary vessels occurs while the ventricles are at rest (diastole). During diastole, ventricular pressure drops to zero while resistance in the aorta and arterial tree (diastolic blood pressure) generates a backflow pressure that closes the aortic valve and drives blood into the coronary system[5] (Fig. 4-4). In summary, three principal factors influence coronary perfusion: patency of the coronary arteries, an adequate period of diastolic time for perfusion, and aortic resistance (Box 4-3). In addition to coronary artery disease, which reduces coronary patency, hypotension and rapid heart rates further compromise coronary perfusion. These variables must be considered when caring for patients who have coronary artery disease; virtually all coronary perfusion occurs during diastole, and there is little ability to increase perfusion during periods of emotional stress.

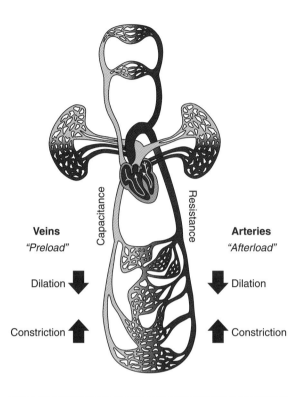

Veins
"Preload"

Arteries
"Afterload"

Capacitance

Resistance

Dilation

Dilation

Constriction

Constriction

Fig. 4-5 Vascular influences on cardiac function. Preload reflects myocardial tension during diastole and is influenced by venous return. Venous dilation lowers venous pressure, thereby decreasing return of blood to the heart; venous constriction increases return of blood. Afterload reflects myocardial tension during systole and is determined by the arterial resistance a heart must overcome to eject each stroke volume. Afterload is reduced by arterial dilation and increased by arterial constriction.

It is equally important to consider factors that create myocardial demand for oxygenated blood; the greater workload of a muscle, the greater the energy required. The two major factors that determine myocardial oxygen demand (MVO_2) are heart rate and wall tension (i.e., preload and afterload). The influence of venous and arterial tone on preload and afterload is illustrated in Fig. 4-5. In terms of wall tension, afterload has a greater influence than preload on MVO_2.[6] Therefore hypertension and accelerated heart rate introduce the greatest demand for adequate coronary perfusion. Conversely, the heart's required amount of oxygen is reduced by decreasing heart rate and blood pressure, both of which are primary objectives when managing patients who have coronary artery disease.

Respiratory System

Respiration is the vital function most susceptible to adverse outcome associated with conscious sedation and general anesthesia (Box 4-4). Drugs used for these procedures can depress cardiovascular function directly, but adverse cardiovascular events are more likely caused by respiratory depression. Essential aspects of respiration are organized into the following four categories of events: ventilation, gas exchange, vascular transport, and the control of ventilation.[7]

Ventilation

Ventilation pertains to the movement of gases between the atmosphere and the alveoli. Inspiration delivers oxygen found in room air to the alveoli, and expiration releases carbon dioxide (CO_2), the byproduct of cell metabolism, to the environment. An incredible volume of gas occupies the extensive labyrinth of tubes and passages in the respiratory tract. The total lung capacity in an average young man is approximately 5800 ml, which is subcategorized into so-called volumes and capacities and based on the proportion mobilized during various degrees of ventilatory effort (Fig. 4-6).

Functional residual capacity (FRC) reflects the volume of gas remaining in the lungs at the end of tidal respiration (see Fig 4-6). The oxygen content found in the FRC may be viewed as an oxygen reserve. If ventilation ceases, oxygen within this reserve continues to diffuse into the pulmonary capillaries. Therefore the duration of time from onset of apnea until hypoxemia is a function of the oxygen concentration found in the FRC. This is the basis for oxygenating a patient before neuromuscular blockade and tracheal intubation and for practicing oxygen supplementation during conscious sedation and anesthesia. If apnea occurs, more time will be available to initiate appropriate interventions. However, this potential benefit must be weighed against the false sense of security it conveys to the clinician relying on pulse oximetry to monitor respiratory status. Even if respiratory depression is significant, oxygenation will be adequate despite the presence of hypoventilation

BOX 4-4

Respiratory System

Ventilation is the movement of gases between the atmosphere and the alveoli. Ventilatory effort is controlled by the respiratory center in response to hypercapnia and hypoxemia, and can be depressed by sedatives, opioids, and general anesthetics.

The time from apnea until anoxia depends on oxygen concentration within the functional residual capacity. This volume is small in pediatric patients, and the concentration can be augmented by administration of supplemental oxygen.

Despite ventilatory effort, airway obstruction can impede oxygen delivery to tissues. Laryngeal edema, laryngospasm, and bronchospasm are examples of obstruction, each having a distinct pathogenesis and manner of treatment.

Oxygen and CO_2 are transported in blood primarily as oxyhemogloblin and bicarbonate ion, respectively. However, the pressures of unbound gas (ABGs) reflect respiratory status as follows:

1. Pa_{O_2} is normally 80 to 100 mm Hg and reflects oxygenation. Its value can be monitored noninvasively by extrapolating percent hemoglobin saturation as provided by pulse oximetry (Sp_{O_2}).
2. Pa_{CO_2} is normally 35 to 45 mm Hg and reflects ventilation. Its value can be monitored noninvasively by capnography, which samples P_{ETCO_2}.

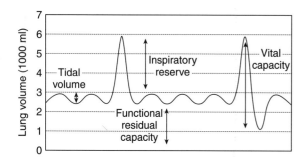

Volumes	Average (ml)	Capacities	Average (ml)
Tidal	500	Functional residual	2300
Inspiratory reserve	3000	Vital	4600

Fig. 4-6 Pulmonary ventilation is assessed by spirometry, which records volumes of gas moved into and out of the lungs during various ventilatory efforts. The average values illustrated are for young adult males; those for females are approximately 25% less.

and in arterial carbon dioxide tension (Pa_{CO_2}). During deep sedation and general anesthesia, the risk for significant respiratory depression and transient episodes of apnea justify oxygen supplementation and continuous assessment of ventilation. However, conscious sedation carries only minor risk, and the clinician may be wiser to expect patients to remain adequately oxygenated while breathing room air. Pe-

diatric conscious sedation is a notable exception, because children are at greater risk for airway obstruction and are more apt to experience transient episodes of apnea. Even more importantly, their FRC is much less than that in adults, and their oxygen demand is almost double that of an adult based on kilogram of weight. For these reasons, children should receive oxygen supplementation during all forms of sedation and general anesthesia.

Airway patency must be sustained to ensure adequate ventilation. This objective is the most essential caveat for the safe use of sedation and anesthesia. Along with standard measures for upper airway support, the clinician should be familiar with the pathophysiology and management of three conditions that have the potential to compromise airway patency: laryngeal edema, laryngospasm, and bronchospasm.

Laryngeal edema is a swelling of the mucosa lining the larynx. Like swelling in the sinuses and other mucous membranes, laryngeal edema results from inflammatory changes associated with infection or allergic responses. Treatment is predicated on administration of α-agonists that constrict blood vessels, thereby shrinking or decongesting the mucous membrane.

Laryngospasm occurs when skeletal muscle supporting the vocal cords contracts, often as a reflex to irritation by secretions or foreign bodies. Pharmacologic management requires the use of neuromuscular blockers, which relax skeletal muscle. Fortunately, positive-pressure oxygenation will generally force

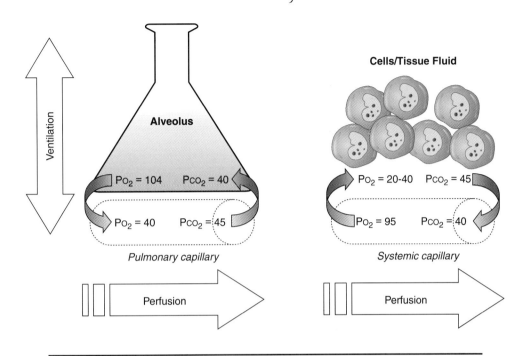

Fig. 4-7 Exchange of oxygen and CO_2 at the respiratory unit and at the tissue level obeys simple principles of diffusion. Diffusion gradients are established by differences in gas tensions at the respective locations illustrated. Adequate exchange within the lung depends on ventilation and perfusion. For this reason, abnormal arterial gas tensions may be attributed to either respiratory or cardiovascular dysfunction.

these muscles to relax, and drug administration is not required.

Bronchospasm is a contraction of smooth muscle that regulates the diameter of the lower airway. These episodes occur not only in patients with asthma but also during anaphylactoid reactions. Bronchial smooth muscle is innervated by autonomic nerves and requires the use of α_2-adrenergic agonists for relaxation.

Gas Exchange

Exchange of oxygen and CO_2 occurs at two locations, the alveoli and systemic tissues. In each case the exchange occurs with capillaries and follows principles of simple diffusion: gas moves from greater concentration or pressure to lesser concentration. Alveolar exchange occurs at so-called respiratory units, each composed of two single layers of squamous epthelium, the alveolus and the endothelium of the pulmonary capillaries. Normal

alveolar exchange is predicated on adequate ventilation and adequate perfusion of pulmonary capillaries. This is the key interface of cardiovascular and respiratory function for oxygenating arterial blood. For this reason, low arterial content of oxygen (hypoxemia) may be the result of either respiratory or cardiovascular compromise. At the tissue level, gases diffuse through capillary endothelium and the cell membranes within the particular tissue being perfused (Fig. 4-7).

Gas Transport

Approximately 98% of the total oxygen in arterial blood is bound to hemoglobin within the red blood cells. The remaining 2% is dissolved in plasma, where it produces a gas pressure referred to as *arterial oxygen* tension (Pao_2). Although most oxygen is transported within the bloodstream as oxyhemoglobin, it is unbound oxygen that actually enters the cells, driven by Pao_2. As oxygen enters cells, the Pao_2

declines but is replaced instantaneously by oxygen released from hemoglobin. The relationship between percent hemoglobin saturation and PaO_2 is illustrated in the oxygen-hemoglobin dissociation curve (Fig. 4-8). Under normal conditions, 98% of total hemoglobin in arterial blood is oxygenated, and PaO_2 is 95 mm Hg. At the tissue level, PaO_2 drops to 40 mm Hg, and hemoglobin saturation is reduced to approximately 70% to 75%, normal values for venous blood. Pulse oximetry measures the percent hemoglobin saturation in arterial blood, and the patient's PaO_2 is estimated according to the oxygen-hemoglobin dissociation curve.

CO_2 is transported in three manners: 70% as bicarbonate ion, 23% bound to hemoglobin (carbaminohemoglobin), and 7% dissolved in plasma.

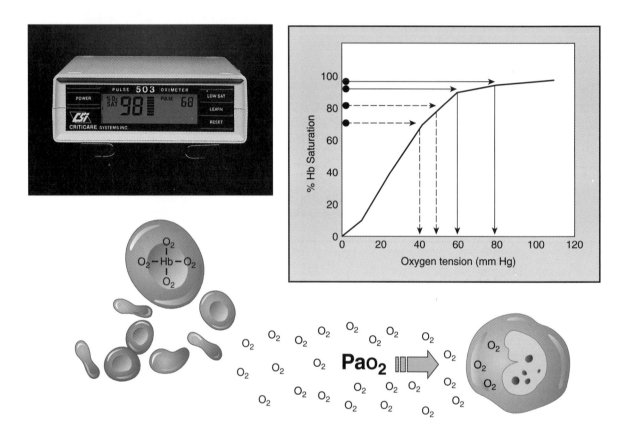

Fig. 4-8 Pulse oximetry and the oxygen-hemoglobin dissociation curve. Most of the oxygen transported in blood is bound to hemoglobin *(Hb)* found in red blood cells. The percent of total hemoglobin saturated with oxygen is plotted on the y axis of the oxygen-hemoglobin dissociation curve. This is the value that is measured by pulse oximeters (98% in this illustration). Any oxygen unbound to hemoglobin is dissolved in plasma, and it produces a tension that drives the oxygen into tissues. This tension is plotted on the x axis of the curve and is directly related to the percent hemoglobin saturation; the greater the hemoglobin saturation, the greater the oxygen tension. Because pulse oximetry provides the hemoglobin saturation percentage, the clinician must deduce the actual arterial oxygen tension (PaO_2) based on this curve. *Hypoxemia* is defined as a PaO_2 below 80 mm Hg. Note that this limit corresponds to a hemoglobin saturation of approximately 95%. At 90% saturation the sigmoid curve reaches its steepest portion and corresponds to a PaO_2 of 60 mm Hg. From this point on, hemoglobin desaturates more rapidly and the difference between the hemoglobin saturation percentage and PaO_2 is approximately 30. These values provide a useful clinical guideline while monitoring patients using pulse oximetry.

After leaving tissues as a byproduct of cell metabolism, most of the CO_2 enters red blood cells, where a portion of it combines with hemoglobin. However, most of it is instantaneously converted to carbonic acid by the enzyme carbonic anhydrase. The carbonic acid subsequently dissociates into hydrogen ions that bind to hemoglobin, whereas bicarbonate ions diffuse from the red cells into the plasma (Fig. 4-9). The portion of CO_2 that remains dissolved in venous blood creates a gas tension of 45 mm Hg. As it diffuses from pulmonary capillaries into the alveoli for expiration, the tension remaining in arterial blood ($Paco_2$) is approximately 40 mm Hg. This is approximately equal to the tension of CO_2 found in alveoli at the end of expiration, designated end-tidal CO_2 ($Petco_2$).

Respiratory status is evaluated medically by sampling arterial blood gases (ABGs). The normal range for Pao_2 is 80 to 100 mm Hg, which reflects oxygenation, and the range for $Paco_2$ is 35 to 45 mm Hg, which reflects ventilation. Hypoventilation is characterized as low Pao_2 (hypoxemia) and elevated $Paco_2$ (hypercarbia). If the patient breathes an enriched oxygen mixture, the Pao_2 will appear normal, but hypoventilation is detected by the elevated $Paco_2$. During sedation and anesthesia, these parameters of respiratory status can be monitored noninvasively using pulse oximetry and capnography. Oximetry assesses oxygenation by reporting percent hemoglobin saturation, and capnography samples $Petco_2$, thereby reflecting ventilation.

Control of Ventilation

The respiratory center consists of several groups of neurons located in the medulla and pons. The most

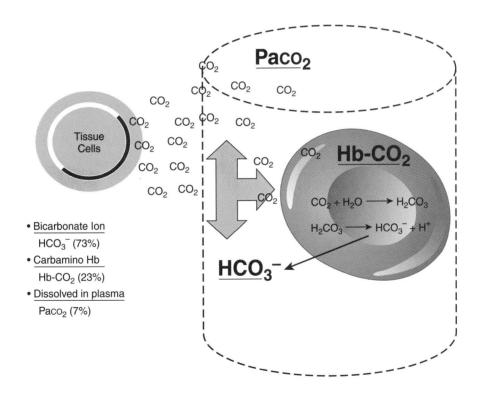

Fig. 4-9 CO_2 transport. CO_2 is a byproduct of cell metabolism. It leaves the tissues and enters capillaries, where it is transported in three manners. Within red blood cells it is combined with hemoglobin as carbaminohemoglobin *(Hb-CO$_2$)* or converted to bicarbonate ion (HCO$_3^-$) by reacting with water to form carbonic acid. The remainder is transported dissolved in plasma, which is reflected as CO_2 tension *(Paco$_2$)*.

important of these is the inspiratory group, which emits action potentials along descending tracts that ultimately excite contraction of the inspiratory muscles. This inspiratory region is activated by central and peripheral neural inputs (Fig. 4-10).

The most significant stimulus for ventilation is referred to as *central hypercapnic drive*. This mechanism is attributed to a chemosensitive area of neurons that stimulate the respiratory center when they become excited by hydrogen ions. Normally, hydrogen ions cannot penetrate the blood-brain barrier, but CO_2 can. On entering the tissue fluid of the medulla, CO_2 is converted to carbonic acid, which dissociates into hydrogen ions. Although hydrogen ions are the

actual stimulus for ventilation, their source is CO_2, and the mechanism is called hypercapnic drive by convention.

After 1 to 2 days of elevated PCO_2, the central chemosensitive area becomes tolerant to increases in hydrogen ion concentration (pH), and peripheral mechanisms assume a more prominent role. This is the basis for patients with chronic lung disease depending on peripheral hypoxemic drive. The carotid and aortic bodies not only contain baroreceptors, which regulate cardiovascular tone, but also contain chemoreceptors that sense significant decreases in PaO_2. When activated by hypoxemia, afferent impulses are conducted along glossopharyngeal and va-

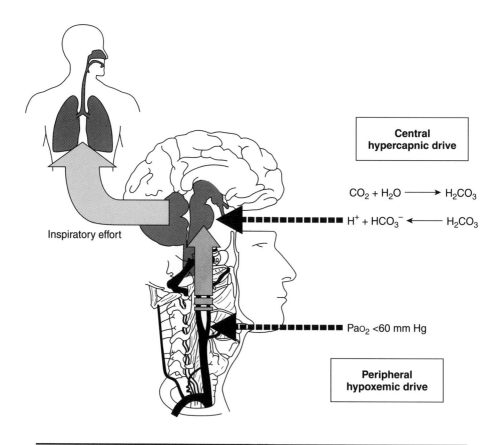

Central hypercapnic drive

$$CO_2 + H_2O \longrightarrow H_2CO_3$$

$$H^+ + HCO_3^- \longleftarrow H_2CO_3$$

Inspiratory effort

$PaO_2 < 60$ mm Hg

Peripheral hypoxemic drive

Fig. 4-10 Control of ventilation. The respiratory center is located in the medulla and initiates neural impulses to respiratory muscles that generate inspiratory effort. The respiratory center is stimulated by two principal mechanisms, so-called hypercapnic and hypoxemic drives. Receptors for hypercapnic drive are located within the respiratory center and are triggered by hydrogen ions produced by ionization of carbonic acid. Receptors for hypoxemic drive are located peripherally, within the carotid and aortic bodies, and sense arterial oxygen tensions below 60 mm Hg.

gal neurons to the inspiratory center, where excitatory output is generated. Although hypoxemic drive is normally a backup mechanism to central hypercapnic drive, it assumes primary significance in patients with chronic lung disease.

Sedatives, opioids, and general anesthetics all depress ventilation, but each has a predilection for depressing either hypercapnic or hypoxemic drive.[8] Opioids primarily depress the central chemosensitive area (hypercapnic drive), whereas inhalation anesthetics and benzodiazepines exert greater influence on chemoreceptors in the carotid and aortic bodies (hypoxemic drive).

Respiratory influences of central nervous system depressants are studied most often by measuring the response of patients to elevations in Pa_{CO_2}. Subjects are asked to breathe a controlled mixture of gas that contains a standard concentration of oxygen, but inspired CO_2 concentrations are gradually increased. During the control phase of a study, there is a compensatory increase in minute ventilation as Pa_{CO_2} rises progressively above 40 mm Hg (Fig. 4-11, *line A*). This is described as the standard CO_2 response curve. Some degree of respiratory depression is associated with normal sleep; minute ventilation does not increase until Pa_{CO_2} reaches 45 mm Hg (Fig.

4-11, *line B*). These data provide the basis for the conventional wisdom that normal physiologic sleep shifts the CO_2 response curve to the right 5 mm Hg. Opioids also have a dramatic influence on ventilation response (Fig. 4-11, *line C*). After subjects receive an opioid (e.g., morphine 10 mg, intravenously), the CO_2 response curve not only shifts further to the right, but its slope is also depressed. This implies not only that chemoreceptors are less sensitive to elevations in Pa_{CO_2}, but also that the additional neural traffic that ultimately triggers inspiratory effort is obtunded as well.

All classes of drugs used for conscious sedation and general anesthesia depress ventilation but differ in their intensity and mechanism.[9] It follows that combining drug classes not only enhances the effect at a single target tissue but also potentiates respiratory depression further by contributing influences at additional sites of respiratory control. These negative influences can be monitored continuously while titrating drugs intravenously, but they are entirely unpredictable after oral administration of predetermined doses. For this reason, regimens that combine sedatives and opioids should be avoided in oral or intramuscular sedation techniques and limited to those for intravenous conscious sedation.

SUMMARY

The physiologic principles addressed in this chapter are ideal and should be applied only to the normal, healthy patient. A patient's physiologic reserve is compromised by disease and also declines continuously with the normal aging process. The sum of these changes alters the responses the dentist can anticipate when sedating or anesthetizing the elderly patient. Diminished physiologic reserve not only alters time for onset and recovery but also increases the intensity of negative influences on cardiovascular and respiratory function. This information, and because renal and hepatic function declines 50% by age 65,[10] provides a scientific basis for the conventional recommendation that drug dosages be reduced by at least 50% in the elderly patient.

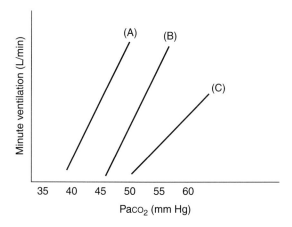

Fig. 4-11 CO_2 response curves. Central hypercapnic drive is the principal stimulus for ventilation. As arterial CO_2 tension increases, there is a compensatory increase in minute ventilation *(A)*. During normal sleep, chemoreceptors are less sensitive and do not respond until CO_2 tension reaches 45 mm Hg *(B)*. Opioids depress chemoreceptors further, with no noticeable response until CO_2 tension rises to 50 mm Hg *(C)*. (See text.)

References

1. Stoelting RK: *Pharmacology and physiology in anesthetic practice*, ed 2, Philadelphia, 1991, WB Saunders, p 624.
2. Lawson NW: Autonomic nervous system physiology and pharmacology. In Barash PG, Cullen BF, Stoelting RK, editors: *Clinical anesthesia*, ed 2, Philadelphia, 1992, JB Lippincott.

3. Hoffman BB, Lefkowitz RJ: Catecholamines, sympathomimetic drugs, and adrenergic receptor antagonists. In Hardman JG, Limbird LE, Molinoff PB, et al, editors: *Goodman and Gilman's the pharmacological basis of therapeutics,* ed 9, New York, 1996, McGraw-Hill.

4. Guyton AC, Hall JE: *Textbook of medical physiology,* ed 9, Philadelphia, 1996, WB Saunders, pp 209-220.

5. Berne RM, Levy MN: *Physiology,* ed 3, St Louis, 1993, Mosby, pp 510-517.

6. Stoelting RK: *Pharmacology and physiology in anesthetic practice,* ed 2, Philadelphia, 1991, WB Saunders, p 698.

7. Guyton AC, Hall JE: *Textbook of medical physiology,* ed 9, Philadelphia, 1996, WB Saunders, pp 477-536.

8. Keats AS: The effects of drugs on respiration in man, *Annu Rev Pharmacol Toxicol* 25:41-65, 1985.

9. Becker DE: The respiratory effects of drugs used for conscious sedation and general anesthesia, *J Am Dent Assoc* 119:153-156, 1989.

10. Montamat SC, Cusack BJ, Vestal RE: Management of drug therapy in the elderly, *N Engl J Med* 321:303-309, 1989.

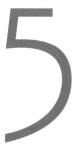

CHAPTER 5

Preoperative Assessment

DANIEL E. BECKER

CHAPTER OUTLINE

A thorough assessment of a patient's medical status is the standard of care when any medication is administered during dental care. Although this is true for procedures performed under local anesthesia alone, the information gathered may be viewed somewhat differently if the dentist is planning to use sedation or general anesthesia as adjuncts to dental treatment. The late Robert Dripps stated that satisfactory outcome of anesthesia is largely determined by the quality of preanesthetic and postanesthetic care.[1] If this tenet is accepted, preoperative assessment of the dental patient must assume paramount importance. Meticulous documentation of the patient's medical history and flawless baseline vital sign assessment are essential if the dentist is to reasonably estimate the patient's fitness for the anesthetic and treatment planned.

A system for classifying preoperative physical status was developed by the American Society of Anesthesiologists (ASA) in 1941 and was revised to its current form in 1974 (Box 5-1). Despite its universal acceptance as a standard in preoperative assessment, this system has been shown to lack scientific precision and might better be appreciated as a *guideline* rather than a standard.[2] In addition to the inherent inconsistency of any subjective rating, this particular system does not precisely define variables such as age, obesity, or the duration and nature of the surgery to be performed. For example, a 70-year-old ASA 3 patient undergoing a lengthy neurosurgical procedure would likely be a greater anesthetic risk than a 35-year-old ASA 3 patient about to have dental or plastic surgery.

Despite these shortcomings, the ASA classifications are a useful basis for decisions regarding the risks for sedation and anesthesia in the office. Classes 1 and 2 patients are generally acceptable candidates for in-office sedation and anesthetic care, whereas class 4 patients should be managed on an inpatient basis. Most class 3 patients who are well controlled by their medication can be safely managed in the office, but those with questionable stability are better managed in the hospital if a general anesthetic is required.

Recording the Medical History

Anesthetic History

The patient should be carefully questioned regarding past experiences with local and general anesthetics. Most patients vividly recall any unpleasant experiences, regardless of their true significance. For those having little or no experience with any form of anesthesia, questions regarding other family members may be helpful, since the patient may also be genetically or psychosocially predisposed to an adverse anesthetic outcome. This is especially true for general anesthetics. Finally, information regarding past hospitalizations is also helpful.

Current Medications

Information regarding a patient's medications not only provides insight regarding medical status but also may alert the dentist to possible drug interactions. Careful attention should be paid to any prescribed medications the patient is taking currently or has taken within the past month. The use of glucocorticosteroids for more than 2 weeks or similar duration, within the previous month or two, introduces a risk for adrenal atrophy that may indicate a need for steroid prophylaxis. This is true especially if extensive treatment is planned or a stormy postoperative course is anticipated. Finally, questioning should be directed to include any medications prescribed for which the patient may not be compliant.

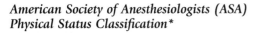

B⚬X 5-1

American Society of Anesthesiologists (ASA) Physical Status Classification*

Class	Description
1	Healthy patient
2	Mild systemic disease—no functional limitation
3	Severe systemic disease—definite functional limitation
4	Severe systemic disease that is a constant threat to life
5	A moribund patient who is not expected to survive for 24 hours with or without operation

Modified from Owens WD, Felts JA, Spitznagel EL: *Anesthesiology* 49:239-243, 1978.
*Addition of an "E" after each class indicates emergency surgery. Such a designation increases the surgical risk.

With only a few exceptions, there is little reason to discontinue any medication prescribed for cardiovascular disease. Diuretics should be withheld until after the appointment to minimize the immediate need for micturition. Their chronic use may be associated with hypokalemia and risk for cardiac arrhythmias, and any irregularity in the patient's baseline pulse should be viewed with suspicion. A serum potassium level should be measured if a general anesthetic is planned. Antihypertensive drugs can potentiate the hypotensive influences of sedatives and anesthetics, but the patient is at greater risk for acute hypertensive episodes if chronic medications other than diuretics are withheld. It is better to continue these medications and give particular attention to intraoperative monitoring and cautious ambulation after postural change. Unless significant bleeding is anticipated, the use of aspirin or other antiplatelet agents need not be withheld. This is also true for warfarin, provided the international normalization ratio (INR), formerly prothrombin time, is within standard therapeutic range. If extensive surgery is planned, the dentist should consult the prescribing physician regarding medication management.

Patients treated with β-blockers present a dilemma. Abrupt withdrawal may result in rebound hypertension, tachycardia, and chest pain. Unfortunately, β-blockade heightens sensitivity to vasopressors contained in local anesthetic solutions. Blockade of vascular β_2-receptors may potentiate vasoconstriction mediated by unopposed α-receptor activation. Dramatic episodes of hypertension and reflex bradycardia have been reported for patients medicated with nonselective β-blockers after receiving small doses of epinephrine or levonordefrin with local anesthetics.[3,4] Such responses are unlikely with cardioselective (β_1) blockers since, at conventional dosages, they do not block vascular β_2-receptors. For patients taking nonselective agents, either avoid the use of vasopressors entirely or limit the amount to that contained in one U.S. cartridge (i.e., 18 μg [epinephrine 1:100,000]). Provided the baseline blood pressure is not elevated, any increase will be tolerable. This dose can be repeated every 5 minutes provided blood pressure and pulse remain stable. Otherwise, additional anesthetic can be added to the area using a vasopressor-free preparation.

All chronically prescribed psychoactive agents should be continued. In most patients, therapeutic influence requires a steady-state serum concentration that has taken several weeks to establish. Furthermore, interrupting sedative-anxiolytics such as benzodiazepines may result in signs and symptoms of withdrawal. There are no major interactions with psychoactive drugs in anesthetic practice, other than monoamine oxidase inhibitors. The use of meperidine is contraindicated for patients taking this category of antidepressant because their interaction can precipitate seizure and a hypertensive crisis. Putative interactions regarding vasopressors and antidepressants have been overstated. Although indirect-acting sympathomimetics should be avoided, the judicious use of epinephrine or levonordefrin is not contraindicated for patients medicated with this or any of the remaining categories of antidepressants, including tricyclic antidepressants and selective serotonin reuptake inhibitors.

Often, patients are not questioned regarding use of nonprescription drugs, recreational drugs, and homeopathic supplements. Cough, cold, and allergy medications may have a direct impact on vital sign assessment, and they introduce risk for cardiac arrhythmias and drug interactions. The same is true for appetite suppressants, decongestants, and cocaine, since all are sympathomimetic amines. Recommendations for managing asymptomatic cocaine abusers are reasonable if there is evidence of excessive use of any sympathomimetic agent.[5] Avoid outpatient general anesthesia, opting instead for sedation and local anesthesia, and along with blood pressure and pulse, electrocardiography (ECG) monitoring of such patients is encouraged.

Patients who smoke are prone to episodes of coughing, in addition to well-established compromise on cardiovascular and respiratory function. Heavy smokers may have as much as 15% reduction in oxygen-binding sites on hemoglobin because carbon monoxide is present.[6] Heavy alcohol consumers may have a variety of organ dysfunctions, but diminished hepatic biotransformation of anesthetics should be anticipated.

The chronic use of opioids or other central nervous system (CNS) depressants, either prescribed or abused, should alert the clinician to possible dependence. In such cases, it is advisable to maintain the patient's current level of use. For those suspected of opioid dependence, it is wise to avoid the use of nalbuphine, pentazocine, or butorphanol because these particular opioids have mixed agonist-antagonist action that may precipitate a withdrawal syndrome.

History of Allergies

Even when a patient reports an allergic reaction, this does not necessarily preclude the use of the particular drug or drug class in question. Patients may label any adverse drug experience as an "allergic reaction." This is true not only for reactions to local anesthetics, which are more often attributable to syncope or symptoms related to use of vasopressors, but also for antibiotics, opioids, and nonsteroidal antiinflammatory drugs (NSAIDs), which frequently produce nausea and dyspepsia. Any report of allergy should be further questioned to clarify that signs and symptoms were consistent with hypersensitivity reactions (i.e., rash, pruritus, urticaria, airway compromise). Immediate allergic reactions are immunoglobulin E (IgE) mediated and must be confirmed serologically, but other mechanisms can produce signs and symptoms of equal consequence. For this reason, the patient's reaction should be presumed at least pseudoallergic in mechanism, pending confirmation by an allergist.

There are no convincing data confirming IgE-mediated reactions to local anesthetics. Nevertheless, patients have experienced at least "pseudoallergic" reactions to local anesthetics.[7] If an anesthetic is required before medical clearance can be obtained, the wisest choice would be either mepivacaine or prilocaine without vasopressors. If local anesthetics produce allergies, esters of benzoic acids may cross-react, but this would not be likely with amide local anesthetics.[8,9] Furthermore, by avoiding those solutions containing vasopressors, one avoids bisulfites that are included as antioxidants. Sensitivity to bisulfites is well established, especially among atopic patients.[10] An algorithm for managing patients with putative allergy to local anesthetics is provided in Fig. 5-1.

Nausea is the most common adverse reaction to codeine and its derivatives. However, IgE antibodies have been detected that react with several opioids, including codeine,[11] and nearly all opioids are capable of triggering degranulation of mast cells, leading to the direct release of histamine.[12,13] Until issues regarding cross-reactivity among opioids are resolved, a prudent approach would be to select alternatives that are molecularly dissimilar. For example, when clinical signs reported for a codeine reaction are al-

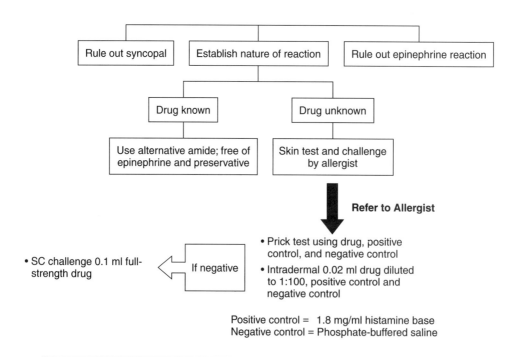

Fig. 5-1 Management of patients who claim allergy to local anesthetics. (Modified from de Shazo RD, Kemp SF: *JAMA* 278(22):1903, 1997.)

lergic in nature, one should select an agent that is dissimilar in structure (i.e., meperidine, fentanyl, nalbuphine, pentazocine).

Reputed allergic reactions to aspirin or other NSAIDs are most likely related to pseudoallergic mechanisms. Although their molecular structures may be strikingly dissimilar, all NSAIDs inhibit cyclooxygenases from converting arachidonic acid to prostaglandins. This shifts the arachidonic acid pathway toward another group of enzymes, lipoxygenases, which are not inhibited by the NSAIDs. These enzymes convert arachidonic acid into leukotrienes, and even subtle increases in these autacoids may lead to adverse reactions in atopic patients.[14,15] It is wise to substitute acetaminophen for patients who claim allergy to any of the NSAIDs.

Penicillins have been confirmed as producing both IgE-mediated and non-IgE-mediated reactions.[16] Patients rarely have serologic confirmation that their previous reaction was IgE mediated, leaving the clinician little recourse but to avoid all penicillins. Erythromycin and clindamycin are the most conventional alternatives. If necessary, cephalosporins can be prescribed, provided the reaction to penicillin was only pruritic or maculopapular. A history of urticaria (hives) or anaphylactoid symptoms are more convincing evidence that the patient's reaction to penicillin was truly IgE mediated, and in this case, one should refrain from prescribing any β-lactam derivative.[17,18]

Recent emphasis on infection control has contributed to an increased number of reports regarding latex allergy. Latex is a milky white sap obtained from rubber trees *(Hevea brasiliensis)* and is used in more than 40,000 medical products.[19] IgE-mediated reactions to latex have been confirmed, and a surprising number of allergic incidents have been reported, including anaphylaxis and death.[20-22] All standard medical history forms should be revised to include an inquiry regarding adverse reactions to rubber products.

Cardiovascular Disease

Ischemic Heart Disease

Ischemic heart disease is a condition whereby the myocardium is inadequately supplied with oxygenated blood. The pathogenesis reflects an imbalance between coronary artery supply and myocardial oxygen demand. Atherosclerosis is generally the primary coronary lesion, but plaque rupture, thrombosis, or vasospasm may all be superimposed. Myocardial oxygen demand is determined primarily by heart rate and systolic wall tension. The dentist cannot influence the severity of coronary lesions, but stress reduction and proper use of sedation can have a very beneficial effect on myocardial oxygen demand. Conversely, the indiscriminate use of vasopressors in local anesthetics increases myocardial oxygen demand.[23]

The nature and frequency of anginal episodes, prescribed medications, and the effectiveness of these medications are key items of information when assessing severity and stability of the patient's ischemic disease. Medications generally include antiplatelet agents, β-blockers, and vasodilators. A system for classification of angina has been proposed by the Canadian Cardiovascular Society (Box 5-2).[24] Classes 1 and 2 angina reflect a stable pattern and present little cardiovascular risk during dental procedures, provided standard stress reduction protocols are followed. Classes 3 and 4 angina reflect unstable patterns that present significant risk for either episodes of angina or plaque rupture leading to myocardial infarction. For these patients, consultation with the patient's physician should precede dental treatment. Standard care is to postpone elective procedures for any patient who had myocardial infarction during the previous 6 months. However, it is reasonable to expand this convention to include those having any invasive cardiac

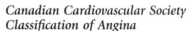

BOX   5-2

Canadian Cardiovascular Society Classification of Angina

Class	Description
1	Angina caused only by severe or prolonged exertion
2	Angina on moderate effort, such as walking uphill
3	Angina with mild exertion, resulting in marked limitation of ordinary activity; inability to walk two blocks or climb one flight of stairs
4	Angina with almost any activity or may occur at rest

Modified from Campeau L: *Circulation* 54:522, 1975.

procedure (e.g., angioplasty, coronary artery bypass grafting) even if infarction did not occur.

Congestive Heart Failure

Congestive heart failure is generally attributed to diminished myocardial contractility that manifests as a reduction in cardiac output and venous backup leading to peripheral edema and pulmonary congestion. Drugs used to manage these patients include digoxin, which provides a positive inotropic influence; diuretics, which counter edema; and vasodilators, which reduce preload and afterload on the compromised myocardium. Currently, angiotensin-converting enzyme (ACE) inhibitors (e.g., captopril [Capoten], lisinopril [Zestril], enalapril [Vasotec]) are regarded as vasodilators of choice, whereas the routine use of digoxin and diuretics is questionable.[25]

The patient with heart failure should be assessed for signs of peripheral edema and symptoms of pulmonary congestion, especially when reclined to a supine position. Careful attention should be given to blood pressure because sudden elevations can lead to venous backup and pulmonary congestion.

Hypertension

Hypertension is the most common cardiovascular disorder in developed countries. Myriad conditions confound an understanding of this disorder, and attempts at classification based on etiology are artificial (e.g., primary [essential] versus secondary hypertension). Primary hypertension accelerates the pathogenesis of atherosclerosis, but arterial stenosis produced by generalized atherosclerosis elevates the blood pressure of patients who would otherwise be normotensive. Regardless of its etiology or classification, consequences of hypertension manifest as end-organ damage, including heart failure, nephropathy, cerebrovascular disease, and retinopathy. Acute elevations in blood pressure are especially detrimental to patients with ischemic heart disease or heart failure.

Medical management of hypertensive patients includes the use of diuretics, β-blockers, and vasodilators. The most recent guidelines for diagnosis and management of hypertension are summarized in Table 5-1.[26] Formerly, the severity of hypertension was based on diastolic pressure, but current guidelines use whichever reading is highest, systolic or diastolic. The use of *stages* has replaced adjectives such as mild, moderate, and severe. There are no absolute guidelines regarding acceptable limits for elective dental treatment. However, guidelines for primary care physicians regarding further evaluation and referral are a reasonable reference. Keeping in mind that baseline readings in the dental office are most likely elevated, patients having pressures that do not exceed stage 2 in severity would appear acceptable for elective care, provided they are asymptomatic and free of significant cardiac or cerebrovascular disease. However, this guideline does not obviate the requirement for additional judgment. Whereas a general anesthetic

---

TABLE 5-1

Classification of Hypertension and Follow-up*

Systolic BP	Diastolic BP	Category	Follow-up
<130	<85	Normal	Recheck in 2 yr
130-139	85-89	High normal	Recheck in 1 yr
Hypertension			
140-159	90-99	Stage 1 (mild)	Confirm within 2 mo
160-179	100-109	Stage 2 (moderate)	Evaluate or refer within 1 mo
≥180	≥110	Stage 3 (severe)†	Evaluate or refer within 1 wk or immediately if indicated

From JNC VI: *Arch Intern Med* 157:2413-2446, 1997.
*If classification on the basis of systolic and diastolic blood pressure differ, use higher category for classification and follow-up recommendations.
†Previous guidelines (JNC V) included stage 4 (very severe, >209/119), which indicated immediate care.

may aggravate any degree of hypertension, especially during induction and emergence, sedation may actually prove beneficial. For patients with questionably high pressure, a sedative regimen can be administered and its influence on blood pressure assessed before continuing the proposed dental treatment.

Valvular Heart Disease

Valvular heart disease carries a significant risk for bacterial endocarditis but does not have a great impact on sedation and anesthesia except in the most severe cases. Prolapse and stenosis, with or without incompetence (regurgitation), are the principal lesions and most often involve the aortic and mitral valves. Stenosis compromises filling of the distal chamber, which may be further diminished with shortened filling time. For this reason, tachycardias should be avoided if patients have significant aortic stenosis because blood pressure could drop precipitously. Conversely, regurgitant flow is accentuated by slow heart rates and high pressure within the distal chamber. These fundamental pathophysiologic principles spawn two pragmatic caveats. Rapid heart rates should be avoided if patients have aortic or mitral stenosis, whereas slow rates and hypertension should be avoided if patients have valvular incompetence, such as that associated with mitral valve prolapse.[6]

Cardiac Pacemakers

Cardiac pacemakers are implanted in more than 1 million people in the United States, and each year more than 400 new pacemakers are implanted per million members of the population.[27] They are most often used in patients who have symptomatic supraventricular arrhythmias and heart blocks unresponsive to drug therapy. Pacemakers have two essential components: (1) a pulse generator powered by a lithium-iodine battery lasting 7 to 10 years and (2) pacing leads. These leads are stainless steel wires most often introduced via the subclavian or external jugular veins and guided to the cardiac chamber(s), where they are attached to an electrode anchored in the right atrium or ventricle. Asynchronous pacemakers generate impulses at a predetermined fixed rate. Synchronous or "on-demand" pacemakers are most common and activate when the patient's natural rate falls above or below a preset level. Pacemakers are classified using a three-letter code indicating the chamber paced, the chamber sensed, and the response delivered (Box 5-3). (Two additional letters may be included in the code but are not germane for our purposes.) The most versatile and widely used pacemaker uses a DDD code.[27] This particular device paces and senses both atria and ventricles and may trigger or inhibit activity depending on what is sensed.

Preanesthetic evaluation of patients with pacemakers should include the indication for pacing and a comment regarding its quality of performance. The type, date, and location of the pacemaker implanted also should be recorded. Any history of vertigo or syncope indicates dubious pacemaker function, and patients should be referred to their physician. Monitoring during sedation or anesthesia should reflect the function and integrity of the pacemaker. Ideally this is provided by continuous electrocardiography, but at the very least, a precordial stethoscope should be placed to continuously monitor rate and rhythm.

Pacemaker function can be altered by membrane threshold changes and by electrical potentials generated by skeletal muscle (myopotentials).[28,29] Hyperkalemia lowers membrane thresholds, making it easier for pacemakers to stimulate myocardial cells, whereas hypokalemia has the opposite influence on membranes, making it more difficult for pacemakers to activate a chamber. Likewise, action potentials radiating from skeletal muscle during episodes of shivering can inhibit normal sensing patterns.

Modern pacemakers have been improved to resist electromagnetic interference, but the dental office environment may still present some hazard. Ultrasonic prophylaxis units do not pose a danger, provided the

---

BOX 5-3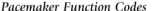

Pacemaker Function Codes

Chamber Paced	Chamber Sensed	Response
V (ventricle)	V (ventricle)	T (triggered or stimulated)
A (atrium)	A (atrium)	I (inhibited)
D (double or both)	D (double or both)	D (double or both)
	O (none)	R (reverse)
		O (none)

From Kusumoto FM, Goldschlager N: *N Engl J Med* 334:89-98, 1996.

instrument is not close to the implanted generator. However, electrocautery units have potential for pacemaker interference.[28] Influence from these units can be minimized by placing the grounding plate as far from the implanted generator as possible and making sure that the generator is never located between the grounding plate and the electrode tip of the cautery unit. Also, keep the current as low as possible, and limit pulse duration (1 second) and frequency (1 pulse/10 seconds).

Pharmacologic considerations and indications for sedation and anesthesia should not be changed only because of a pacemaker. Agents to counter brady-arrhythmias, such as atropine and isoproterenol, should be readily available for use should pacemaker failure occur. In the unlikely event that defibrillation or cardioversion would be necessary, the paddles should not be placed within 5 inches of the implanted generator.[28,29]

TABLE 5-2

Index of Cardiac Risk*

Condition	Identifying Factors	Points
Ischemic heart disease	Myocardial infarction within 6 mo	10
	Myocardial infarction >6 mo earlier	5
	Class III angina	10
	Class IV angina	20
Congestive heart failure	S₃ gallop, jugular distention, or pulmonary edema	11
Arrhythmias	PVCs >5/min	7
	Rhythm other than NSR	7
Valvular disease	Significant aortic stenosis	3
Miscellaneous	Other systemic disease	3
	Age >70	5

Modified from Goldman L, Caldera DL, et al: *N Engl J Med* 297:845-850, 1977; and Detsky AS, Abrams HB, et al: *J Gen Intern Med* 1:211, 1986.
PVC, Premature ventricular contraction; *NSR,* normal sinus rhythm.
*Index of cardiac risk is based on four classes according to the following point values: class I, 0-5 points; class II, 6-12 points; class III, 13-25 points; class IV, >25 points. This method was shown to be a more sensitive predictor of cardiac events than the overall ASA physical status classification method. Class IV patients are at a statistically greater risk for minor and major cardiac events during noncardiac surgery under general anesthesia.

Cardiac Risk

Cardiac risk as presented by Goldman et al is a method for specific estimation of risk for patients having cardiovascular disease (Table 5-2).[30] Using this method, class IV patients (scoring >25 points) exhibited a significant incidence of both minor and life-threatening cardiac complications. This Goldman index was modified by Detsky et al to include unstable angina, providing a useful adjunct for assessing the cardiac risk of patients about to receive outpatient dental treatment.[31] A history of myocardial infarction within the previous 6 months cannot be used for point tabulation because elective dental treatment is contraindicated for these patients. A reasonable policy would be to contraindicate treatment for a class IV patient and secure a medical consultation for those in class III. If any uncertainty exists, consultation may also be desirable for questionable class II patients (Box 5-4).

Respiratory Disease

Asthma

Asthma is an increased responsiveness of the tracheobronchial tree to a variety of intrinsic and extrinsic stimuli. It is now appreciated that chronic inflammation sustains irritability of smooth muscle directly and indirectly via mucous secretion.[32] Patients should be questioned regarding factors that precipitate wheezing

BOX 5-4   SUMMARY

Patient Management of Cardiovascular Disease

Continue all medications. (Diuretics can be withheld to obviate immediate need for micturition.)

Be alert for vasopressor interactions with nonselective β-blockers.

Although ECG monitoring is standard care during general anesthesia, it should be considered during sedation for any patient whose stability is questionable or if procedure is extensive (e.g., multiple implants with sinus grafting, complete odontectomy, and alveoloplasty).

Maintain pulse and blood pressure within normal limits throughout procedure.

Local anesthesia must be profound. If not attainable, reschedule under general anesthetic.

and their medications, which generally include glucocorticoid drugs and sympathomimetic agents. In general, drugs that release histamine should be avoided. Although opioids are notorious in this regard, their effects are not deleterious to asthma patients. In fact, they may actually be desirable because they depress airway reflexes. Formerly, antihistamines (H_1 blockers) and anticholinergics were believed to increase mucous viscosity and were therefore contraindicated in patients with asthma or chronic obstructive pulmonary disease (COPD). This concern has been dispelled, however, and the anticholinergics are currently enjoying a reprise for chronic therapy.[33-35]

Chronic Obstructive Pulmonary Disease

COPD is a generic term used to describe patients who have airflow obstruction resulting from chronic bronchitis or emphysema. The condition may be accompanied by airway hyperactivity (i.e., an asthmatic component), but this condition alone is not regarded as COPD.[32,36] Depending on the relative proportion of each disease component, patients may be hypercapnic or hypoxemic or may have some degree of right-sided or left-sided heart failure (Box 5-5 and Table 5-3).

CNS depressants must be used cautiously in these patients, most notably the opioids, which depress central carbon dioxide drive, and the inhalation anesthetics, which have a profound effect on peripheral hypoxemic drive.[37] Often these patients, chronic "lungers," tolerate chronically elevated carbon dioxide levels, which shift their principal respiratory control to peripheral hypoxemic drive. This raises a concern regarding oxygen supplementation for such patients since elevated fractional inspired oxygen content (FIO_2) may depress ventilatory response (Box 5-6). However, concentrations that do not exceed 40% are generally well tolerated and can be maintained using a nasal cannula at flow rates of 1 to 4 L/min based on the following formula[32]:

$$FIo_2 = 20 + 4 \times L/min$$

Thus a nasal cannula delivering an oxygen flow of 3 L/min would provide 32% FIo_2 (20 + [4 × 3]).

TABLE 5-3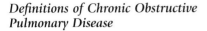

Distinguishing Features of Chronic Obstructive Pulmonary Disease

	Predominant Emphysema	Predominant Bronchitis
Dyspnea	Severe	Mild
Sputum	Scanty, mucoid	Copious, purulent
$Paco_2$	35-40	50-60
Pao_2	65-75	45-60
Cor pulmonale	Rare	Common

From Honig EG, Ingram RH Jr: Chronic bronchitis, emphysema, and airway obstruction. In Fauci AS, Braunwald E, Isselbacher KJ, et al, editors: *Harrison's principles of internal medicine,* ed 14, New York, 1998, McGraw-Hill.

BOX 5-6 **SUMMARY**

Patient Management of Respiratory Disease

Continue all medications and bring to the appointment any inhalers used as needed. This does not include long-acting bronchodilators and steroid inhalers that are administered once or twice daily. These provide no immediate relief.

Consider possible adrenal atrophy if using prednisone more than 10 mg/day. (Inhaled glucocorticoid drugs are not a concern.)

Schedule late-morning appointments, which allow patient to clear mucous secretions that accumulate during the night.

Avoid oxygen supplementation at FIo_2 greater than 40%. This could depress hypoxemic respiratory drive, which is significant for patients with COPD.

BOX 5-5

Definitions of Chronic Obstructive Pulmonary Disease

Either or both of the following conditions may be present:
Chronic bronchitis: Chronic productive cough for 3 months in each of 2 successive years
Emphysema: Abnormal permanent enlargement of the air spaces distal to the terminal bronchioles, accompanied by destruction of their walls and without obvious fibrosis

From the American Thoracic Society: *Am J Respir Crit Care Med* 152:77s-120s, 1995.

Liver and Kidney Disease

Liver and kidney disease must be relatively severe to adversely influence the biotransformation and elimination of drugs used briefly for sedation or general anesthesia. Interest is more appropriately directed toward postoperative bleeding and infection control. If concern arises regarding electrolyte status, appropriate laboratory or physician consultation is encouraged.

Neurologic Disorders

In general, a history of neurologic dysfunction is not a major concern, provided the condition is medically controlled. The epileptic patient should be maintained on the prescribed anticonvulsant regimen and consideration given to the fact that most of these medications are sedative in nature. Phenobarbital is well documented as an inducer of hepatic microsomal activity, which may shorten the duration of drugs used for sedation and anesthesia.

Parkinson's Disease

Patients with Parkinson's disease have a defect in central dopaminergic activity. Their medications should be maintained and use of antidopaminergic agents avoided. This would include phenothiazine and butyrophenone derivatives such as promethazine and droperidol, respectively. Since cholinergic input inhibits central dopaminergic transmission, anticholinergic agents may be useful adjuncts. In this regard, diphenhydramine, a histamine (H_1) receptor blocker with anticholinergic activity, is an attractive addition to sedative and anesthetic regimens for patients with Parkinson's disease. It has proven efficacy for countering extrapyramidal symptoms mediated by antidopaminergic agents.[38]

Alzheimer's Disease

Although poorly understood, Alzheimer's disease is a dementia related to a defect in central cholinergic transmission. For this reason, it is prudent to avoid the use of centrally acting anticholinergic agents. If such an agent is required, glycopyrrolate is most appropriate because its quaternary structure confers water solubility and does not cross the blood-brain barrier, limiting its CNS distribution.

Multiple Sclerosis

Multiple sclerosis is characterized as a demyelination process, most likely related to an autoimmune mechanism. Patients experience localized or generalized neurologic deficits that undergo periods of remission and exacerbation. Of special concern is autonomic involvement, which may predispose the patient to bradycardia and hypotension. Elective dental care should be scheduled during periods of remission and additional consideration given to any history of glucocorticosteroid use by the patient to control the disorder.

Obesity

The obese patient requires a variety of considerations when contemplating sedation and general anesthesia. Obese patients may self-medicate with sympathomimetic agents for appetite suppression, which introduces concerns regarding drug interactions addressed at the beginning of this chapter. Intravenous access is one of the most perplexing aspects of providing sedation and anesthesia for obese patients. Relaxing the patient using orally administered benzodiazepines or nitrous oxide inhalation is useful when difficulty is anticipated.

Obesity is most accurately measured using the body mass index (BMI):

$$BMI = weight\ (kg)/Height\ (m^2)$$

Using this index, grades of obesity have been defined and offer an arbitrary basis for assigning such patients to ASA risk categories (Fig. 5-2). Obesity is associated with myriad cardiovascular, pulmonary, and metabolic derangements.[39,40] These must be suspected, even if the medical history is negative.

Assessment of airway and pulmonary status should be the initial consideration during preoperative evaluation. Obese patients often have short, thick necks and remarkably small mouths, which contribute to airway obstruction and difficulties in intubation. Diaphragmatic breathing can be severely compromised by the large quantity of abdominal fat, making chair position an important consideration. Obesity is associated with a reduction in functional residual capacity, which may lower baseline arterial oxygen tensions. Severely and morbidly obese patients should not be candidates for office intravenous sedation or general anesthesia because of the significant risk for catastrophic airway problems. Serious

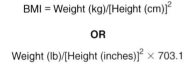

BMI = Weight (kg)/[Height (cm)]^2

OR

Weight (lb)/[Height (inches)]^2 × 703.1

Grade of Obesity	BMI
0	<25
I	25-29.9
II	30-40
III	>40

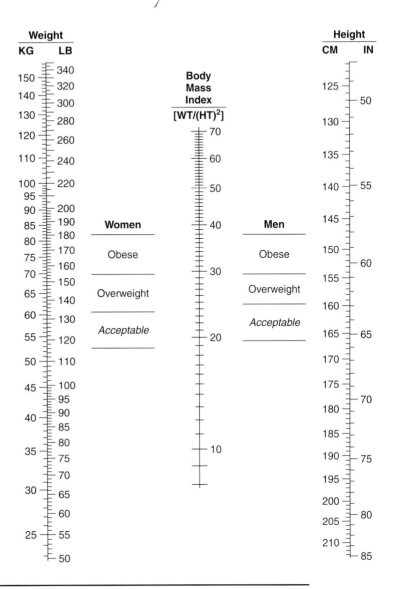

Fig. 5-2 Grading obesity based on body mass index *(BMI)*. Grade II patients should be regarded as at least ASA 2 or 3 risk, depending on severity of concomitant conditions. Grade III patients are morbidly obese and should be considered as ASA 4. (From Bray GA: Obesity. In Fauci AS, Braunwald E, Isselbacher KJ, et al, editors: *Harrison's principles of internal medicine,* ed 14, New York, 1998, McGraw-Hill; and Buckley FP: Anesthesia and obesity and gastrointestinal disorders. In Barash PG, Cullen BF, Stoelting RK, editors: *Clinical anesthesia,* ed 3, Philadelphia, 1997, Lippincott-Raven.)

consideration should be given to general anesthesia with awake tracheal intubation in a hospital where inpatient postoperative management is available.

Cardiovascular compromise is common in obese patients, especially hypertension. Varying degrees of cardiomegaly may be evident, attributed to left ventricular hypertrophy, and diminished cardiac reserve can result in poor exercise tolerance. Increased myocardial oxygen consumption and several systemic metabolic derangements increase the risk of ischemic heart disease. Abnormal glucose tolerance and unpredictable responses to insulin are also frequent complications with obesity, and fatty infiltration may alter liver function.

Pulmonary aspiration is an ever-present danger when administering a general anesthetic to obese patients. This is explained in part by the high incidence of hiatal hernia and gastroesophageal reflux associated with obesity. Furthermore, the obese patient has increased gastric acidity, volume, and intragastric pressure.[40] Preoperative use of anticholinergic drugs, histamine (H_2) receptor antagonists, and metoclopramide should be considered to reduce gastric acidity and volume.

Endocrine Derangements

Diabetes Mellitus

Diabetes mellitus is a disorder of carbohydrate metabolism that results from defects in insulin secretion, insulin action, or both (Box 5-7).[41] In type 1 diabetes an individual has absolute insulin deficiency and requires insulin replacement. In type 2 diabetes an individual produces inadequate amounts of insulin and exhibits varying degrees of tissue resistance.

BOX 5-7   **SUMMARY**

Patient Management of Diabetes Mellitus

Schedule early-morning appointments if possible.

Type 2 patients: Withhold oral hypoglycemic agents or insulin until they can drink or consume food.

Type 1 patients: Have patients administer half their normal AM dose of insulin and then the remaining half after food is consumed.

Use D5W IV infusion to avoid hypoglycemia. A brief period of mild hyperglycemia is of no consequence.

Although unconventional, if light sedation is planned, it may be preferable that the patient consume a normal light breakfast and take his or her medications as normal. If deep sedation or general anesthesia is planned, normal nothing-by-mouth (NPO) guidelines must be followed. In this case, clear liquids are permitted up to 3 hours before the procedure, and hypoglycemic medications are used as suggested.

Type 2 diabetics are generally managed with diet or oral hypoglycemic agents, but some may require insulin replacement. A person with well-controlled type 2 diabetes poses little concern for the dentist administering anesthesia other than ensuring the patient does not become hypoglycemic. The same can be said for type 1 patients who have reasonable glycemic control, provided they have no evidence of end-organ compromise. Diabetes contributes to myriad angiopathies and neuropathies that compromise cardiovascular and renal status. In addition to coronary artery disease and hypertension, the patient with diabetes may have increased risk for bradycardia and hypotension associated with vasovagal responses or sudden postural change. Patients with diabetes who have a poor history of glycemic control and evidence of significant end-organ damage should be considered only for light sedation and local anesthesia in the ambulatory setting.

Thyroid Disorders

Most patients with a history of thyroid disorder are controlled and present in a euthyroid state. In this case, there is little concern regarding conscious sedation and anesthesia. However, patients who have questionable control, whether hypoactive or hyperactive, are a concern. The hypothyroid patient is very sensitive to CNS depressants, with risks for hypoventilation, hypothermia, and hypoglycemia. Patients medicated with thyroid replacement (e.g., Synthroid) may be functionally hyperthyroid if they are ingesting an excessive amount. Careful attention to preoperative vital signs is essential because hypertension and tachycardia are indicative of hyperthyroid status. These patients should not receive local anesthetics that contain vasopressors because they are at risk for *thyroid storm*, a hypermetabolic state that includes hyperthermia, hypertension, and cardiac arrhythmias. Treatment of such patients should be delayed until a euthyroid state can be confirmed.

Adrenocortical Derangements

Adrenocortical derangements are complex and require that a stable condition be confirmed with the patient's endocrinologist. Concern is directed most often to secondary hypocorticism caused by prolonged glucocorticoid therapy. If any doubt exists regarding hypothalamic-pituitary-adrenal (HPA) axis function, a prophylactic dose of cortisol 100 to

200 mg or its equivalent should be added to the normal regimen preoperatively. Single doses of glucocorticoid drugs are virtually free of adverse effects.

Neuromuscular Disease

Muscular Dystrophies

Muscular dystrophies are degenerative disorders of striated muscle that present a constant threat to ventilatory function. The Duchenne type is the most severe and typically compromises cardiac and skeletal muscles. Such patients must be hospitalized if sedation or general anesthesia is required.

Myasthenia Gravis

Myasthenia gravis is an autoimmune disorder consisting of circulating antibodies against cholinergic receptors on skeletal muscle (i.e., nicotinic receptors). As might be predicted, patients with myasthenia gravis are exquisitely sensitive to competitive neuromuscular blockers, and their response to depolarizing agents is unpredictable. Cholinesterase inhibitors (e.g., pyridostigmine) are used to manage this disorder, with possible parasympathomimetic side effects such as bradycardia and bronchoconstriction. In addition, these patients are highly susceptible to ventilatory depression. Consequently, deep sedation and general anesthesia are best avoided in the office. Light sedation techniques may be used, provided the patient's respiratory status is well monitored.

Physical Assessment and Laboratory Testing

Baseline information regarding vital signs is an essential component of the medical record. It not only aids in assessing the patient's medical status but also provides essential reference data during intraoperative monitoring. Ideally the information is gathered during an interview appointment, when the patient is less likely to be apprehensive about treatment.

Along with the patient's age, weight, and height, essential vital signs should include blood pressure, pulse, and respiratory pattern. A manual blood pressure device should be used rather than automated units. The latter devices are convenient adjuncts for intraoperative monitoring, but all have a potential for occasional malfunction, especially during periods of medical urgency. The clinician should not discontinue using standard manual equipment because it is "obsolete."

The patient should be questioned regarding physical stamina, including exertional or postural dyspnea, and any history of lightheadedness or syncopal events. The dentist should also note any visual impressions of cardiovascular, respiratory, or neurologic compromise, including evidence of distended jugular veins, edema of extremities, or elevated nail beds. Noting equilateral pupil responses to the dental light is also useful baseline information for patients with significant evidence of mental impairment. A system for assessing functional capacity can be a useful adjunct when assessing patients with questionable ASA or cardiac index.[42,43] The Duke Activity Status Index is provided in Table 5-4.

The routine use of laboratory batteries should be discouraged since, in the absence of specific indications, they seldom contribute additional safety to patient care.[44-48] The usefulness of routine 12-lead electrocardiograms has also been clarified.[49] In the absence of cardiac disease, an ECG provides little useful

TABLE 5-4

Duke Activity Status Index (DASI) *

Activity	Weight†
Personal care (dress, eat, bath, toilet)	2.75
Walk around in house	1.75
Walk 1-2 blocks (level ground)	2.75
Climb a flight of stairs	5.5
Run short distance	8
Light work: dusting, wash dishes	2.7
Moderate work: vacuuming, sweeping	3.5
Yard work: raking, weeding, mowing	4.5
Sexual relations	5.25
Golf, bowling, dancing, doubles tennis	6
Swim, singles tennis, basketball, ski	7.5

From Hlatky MA, Boineau RE, et al: *Am J Cardiol* 64:651-654, 1989; and Hollenberg SM: *Chest* 115:51s-57s, 1999.
*Using this system, Hollenberg has suggested the following values for assessing functional capacity: >7, excellent; 4-7, moderate; <4, poor.
†Based on metabolic equivalents: 1 MET = 3.5 ml/kg/min oxygen utilization.

Condition suspected	Hgb/Hct (male)	Hgb/Hct (female)	WBC	Platelets	PT/PTT	BT	Electrolytes	BUN/creat	Serum glucose	LFTs	Hep screen	Albumin/total pro	Dipstick UA	UA with micro	ABG	Pulse oximetry	Bedside PFTs	TFTs	Chest x-ray	ECG	Serum HCG	HIV screen	T & C	Med. consult
Procedure																								
Minor (anticipate low blood loss)																								
Major (anticipate high blood loss)	■	■																					○	
Age (years)																								
<45		■											■											
45-60		■											■							▲				▲
>60	■	■											■						■	■				▲
Associated condition																								
Cardiovascular disease	■	■						■								■			■	■				
Pulmonary disease															■		■		■	■				▲
Malignancy			●	●	■	●				■									■					▲
Hepatobiliary disease					■					■														▲
Renal disease	■	■					■	■						■										▲
Bleeding disorder	■	■		■	■	■																		▲
Diabetes							■	■	■					■										
Thyroid disease							■					●						■						▲
H/O hepatitis					■					■	■													▲
Smoking history	■	■													▲	■	■		■					
H/O exposure to TB or high risk group																			■					
H/O exposure to HIV or high risk group																						◆		
Radiation therapy			■																■	▲	◆			
Infectious process			■																					
Poor nutrition status												■												
Suspected pregnancy																					■			
Medications																								
Diuretics							■	■																
Digitalis							■	■												■				
Corticosteroids							■		■															
Anticoagulants	■	■			■																			
NSAIDs/ASA						■																		
ACE inhibitor							■																	

■ Suggested by the literature
● Obtain in leukemias
▲ Obtain, depending on clinical examination and practitioners expertise
○ In elective surgery, practitioner may elect to obtain autologous blood
◆ Controversial, may need consent from patient

Hgb/Hct	Hemoglobin/Hematocrit
WBC	White blood count
PT	Prothrombin time
PTT	Partial thromboplastin time
BT	Bleeding time
Electrolytes	Na, K, Cl, CO_2
BUN	Blood urea nitrogen
Creat	Creatinine
LFTs	Liver function tests
Hep screen	Viral hepatitis screen
Albumin/total pro	Albumin/serum total protein
ABG	Arterial blood gas
PFTs	Pulmonary function tests
TFTs	Thyroid function tests
T & C	Type & cross-match
Med. consult	Medicine consult
H/O	History of
NSAIDs	Nonsteroidal antiinflammatory drugs
ASA	Aspirin

Fig. 5-3 Protocol for ordering laboratory tests for patients undergoing oral and maxillofacial surgery. (From Wagner JD, Moore DL: *J Oral Maxillofac Surg* 49:177-182, 1991.)

TABLE 5-5

Suggestions for Laboratory Testing in Oral and Maxillofacial Surgery Patients*

Age	Test
6 mo-50 yr	None
50-64 yr	Hematocrit within 6 mo
65-74 yr	Hematocrit within 6 mo
	ECG within 1 yr
>74 yr	Hematocrit within 6 mo
	ECG within 1 yr
	BUN and glucose within 6 mo

Modified from Roizen MF, Fischer SP: Preoperative evaluation: adults and children. In White PF, editor: *Ambulatory anesthesia and surgery,* Philadelphia, 1997, WB Saunders.
*Protocol for ordering laboratory tests for patients undergoing conscious sedation in the ambulatory setting. These suggestions presume the patient is healthy or has only mild, well-controlled disease (ASA 1 or 2). When appropriate, additional tests should be considered based on medical status.

information in patients under 40 to 45 years of age. However, if deep sedation or general anesthesia is planned, a 12-lead tracing is generally encouraged for men over 40 years of age and women over 55. Wagner and Moore[50] have provided an excellent review of preoperative testing for the patient undergoing oral and maxillofacial surgery (Fig. 5-3). It is much more common, however, for patients undergoing ambulatory dental procedures to receive conscious sedation and local anesthesia. Requirements for laboratory testing in this population remain unclear, but reasonable suggestions are summarized in Table 5-5.

References

1. Dripps RD, Eckenhoff JE, Vandam LD: *Introduction to anesthesia: the principles of safe practice,* Philadelphia, 1988, WB Saunders, p 13.
2. Owens WD, Felts JA, Spitznagel EL: ASA physical status classifications: a study of consistency of ratings, *Anesthesiology* 49:239-243, 1978.
3. Foster CA, Aston SJ: Propranolol-epinephrine interaction: a potential disaster, *Plast Reconstr Surg* 72:74-78, 1983.
4. Mito RS, Yagiela JA: Hypertensive response to levonordefrin in a patient receiving propranolol: report of a case, *J Am Dent Assoc* 116:55-57, 1988.
5. Passasch TJ, McCarthy FM, Jastak JT: Cocaine and sudden cardiac death, *J Oral Maxillofac Surg* 47:1188-1191, 1989.
6. Vandam LD, Desai SP: Evaluation of the patient and preoperative preparation. In Barash PG, Cullen BF, Stoelting RK, editors: *Clinical anesthesia,* Philadelphia, 1989, JB Lippincott.
7. Jackson D, Chen AH, Bennett CR: Identifying true lidocaine allergy, *J Am Dent Assoc* 125:1362-1366, 1994.
8. Anderson JA, Adkinson NF Jr: Allergic reactions to drugs and biologic agents, *JAMA* 258:2891-2899, 1987.
9. Schatz M: Adverse reactions to local anesthetics, *Immunol Allergy Clin North Am* 12:585-609, 1992.
10. Schwartz HJ, Gilbert IA, et al: Metabisulfite sensitivity and local dental anesthesia, *Ann Allergy* 62:83-86, 1989.
11. Harle DG, Baldo BA, et al: Anaphylaxis following administration of papaveretum. Case report: implication of IgE antibodies that react with morphine and codeine, and identification of an allergenic determinant, *Anesthesiology* 71:489-494, 1989.
12. Flacke JW, Flacke WE, et al: Histamine release by four narcotics: a double-blind study in humans, *Anesth Analg* 66:723-730, 1987.
13. Weiss ME, Adkinson NF, Hirshman CA: Evaluation of allergic drug reactions in the perioperative period, *Anesthesiology* 71:483-486, 1989.
14. Babu KS, Salvi SS: Aspirin and asthma, *Chest* 118(5):1470-1476, 2000.
15. Weiss ME: Drug allergy, *Med Clin North Am* 76:857-882, 1992.
16. Erffmeyer JE: Reactions to antibiotics, *Immunol Allergy Clin North Am* 12:633-648, 1992.
17. Donowitz GR, Mandell GL: Beta-lactam antibiotics (2 parts), *N Engl J Med* 318:419-426, 490-500, 1988.
18. Shepherd GM: Allergy to beta-lactam antibiotics, *Immunol Allergy Clin North Am* 11:611-633, 1991.
19. Warpinski JR, Folgert J, et al: Allergic reaction to latex: a risk factor for unsuspected anaphylaxis, *Allergy Proc* 12:95-102, 1991.
20. Holzman RS: Latex allergy: an emerging operating room problem, *Anesth Analg* 76:635-641, 1993.
21. Kelly KJ, Kurup VP, et al: The diagnosis of natural rubber latex allergy, *J Allergy Clin Immunol* 93:813-816, 1994.
22. Misselbeck WJA, Gray KR, Uphold RE: Latex induced anaphylaxis: a case report, *Am J Emerg Med* 12:445-447, 1994.
23. Troullos ES, Dionne RA, et al: Plasma epinephrine levels and cardiovascular response to high administered doses of epinephrine contained in local anesthesia, *Anesth Prog* 34:10-13, 1987.
24. Campeau L: Grading of angina pectoris, *Circulation* 54:522, 1975 (letter).
25. Cohn JN: The management of chronic heart failure, *N Engl J Med* 335:490-498, 1996.
26. The Sixth Report of the Joint National Committee on Detection, Evaluation, and Treatment of High Blood Pressure (JNC VI), *Arch Intern Med* 157:2413-2446, 1997.
27. Kusumoto FM, Goldschlager N: Cardiac pacing, *N Engl J Med* 334:89-98, 1996.

28. Bloomfield P, Bowler GMR: Anaesthesia management of the patient with a permanent pacemaker, *Anaesthesia* 44:42-46, 1989.

29. Zaidan JR: Pacemakers, *Anesthesiology* 60:319-334, 1984.

30. Goldman L, Caldera DL, et al: Multifactorial index of cardiac risk in noncardiac surgical procedures, *N Engl J Med* 297:845-850, 1977.

31. Detsky AS, Abrams HB, et al: Predicting cardiac complications in patients undergoing noncardiac surgery, *J Gen Intern Med* 1:211, 1986.

32. American Thoracic Society: Standards for the diagnosis and care of patients with chronic obstructive pulmonary disease (COPD), *Am J Respir Crit Care Med* 152:77s-120s, 1995.

33. Gross NJ: Anticholinergic agents in COPD, *Chest* 91:52s-57s, 1987.

34. Gross NJ: Ipratropium bromide, *N Engl J Med* 319:486-494, 1988.

35. Popa V: Pharmacodynamic aspects of chlorpheniramine-induced bronchodilation, *Chest* 93:952-959, 1988.

36. Honig EG, Ingram RH Jr: Chronic bronchitis, emphysema, and airway obstruction. In Fauci AS, Braunwald E, Isselbacher KJ, et al, editors: *Harrison's principles of internal medicine*, ed 14, New York, 1998, McGraw-Hill.

37. Keats AS: The effects of drugs on respiration in man, *Ann Rev Pharmacol Toxicol* 25:41-65, 1985.

38. Stone DJ, DiFazio CA: Sedation for patients with Parkinson's disease undergoing ophthalmologic surgery, *Anesthesiology* 68:821, 1988.

39. Bray GA: Obesity. In Fauci AS, Braunwald E, Isselbacher KJ, et al, editors: *Harrison's principles of internal medicine*, ed 14, New York, 1998, McGraw-Hill.

40. Buckley FP: Anesthesia and obesity and gastrointestinal disorders. In Barash PG, Cullen BF, Stoelting RK, editors: *Clinical anesthesia*, ed 3, Philadelphia, 1997, Lippincott-Raven.

41. American Diabetes Association: Report of the Expert Committee on the Diagnosis and Classification of Diabetes Mellitus, *Diabetes Care* 20:1183-1197, 1997.

42. Hlatky MA, Boineau RE, et al: A brief self-administered questionnaire to determine functional capacity (The Duke Activity Status Index), *Am J Cardiol* 64:651-654, 1989.

43. Hollenberg SM: Preoperative cardiac risk assessment, *Chest* 115:51s-57s, 1999.

44. Schein OD, Katz J, et al: The value of routine preoperative medical testing before cataract surgery, *N Engl J Med* 342:168-175, 2000.

45. Narr BJ, Hansen TR, Warner MA: Preoperative laboratory screening in healthy Mayo patients: cost-effective elimination of tests and unchanged outcomes, *Mayo Clin Proc* 66:155-159, 1991.

46. Fleisher LA: Preoperative evaluation. In Barash PG, Cullen BF, Stoelting RK, editors: *Clinical anesthesia*, ed 3, Philadelphia, 1997, Lippincott-Raven.

47. Gold BS, Fleisher LA: Management of outpatients with pre-existing diseases. In White PF, editor: *Ambulatory anesthesia and surgery*, Philadelphia, 1997, WB Saunders.

48. Roizen MF, Fischer SP: Preoperative evaluation: adults and children. In White PF, editor: *Ambulatory anesthesia and surgery*, Philadelphia, 1997, WB Saunders.

49. Goldberger AL, O'Konski M: Utility of the routine electrocardiogram before surgery and on general hospital admission, *Ann Intern Med* 105:552-557, 1986.

50. Wagner JD, Moore DL: Preoperative laboratory testing for the oral and maxillofacial surgery patient, *J Oral Maxillofac Surg* 49:177-182, 1991.

PART

II

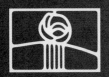

PHARMACOLOGIC CONSIDERATIONS

CHAPTER 6

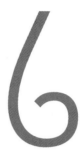

Local Anesthetics

JOHN A. YAGIELA

CHAPTER OUTLINE

Local anesthetics applied in appropriate concentrations reversibly depress conduction in peripheral nervous tissue. Because of their enviable record of efficacy and safety in producing insensibility to pain in discrete regions of the body, local anesthetics are administered in more ways than perhaps any other group of therapeutic agents. Since all excitable tissues are susceptible to local anesthetic block, these drugs also are used systemically as antiarrhythmic agents and as adjuncts for general anesthesia.

Cocaine, the original local anesthetic, was first injected for mandibular anesthesia by William Halsted several months after Carl Koller's demonstration of its anesthetic property was made public on September 15, 1884.[1] Pioneers such as Halsted, James Corning, and August Bier soon developed many of the basic techniques for administration still used today.[2] The liabilities of cocaine anesthesia also were soon recognized. Heinrich Braun employed formulations containing epinephrine to retard absorption of the local anesthetic from the injection site, and Alfred Einhorn developed procaine and other nonaddictive alternatives to cocaine.[3] Table 6-1 catalogs important landmarks in the development of local anesthesia.

Mechanism Of Local Anesthesia

All local anesthetics in clinical practice inhibit nerve conduction by interfering with the entry of sodium (Na^+) ions through Na^+ channels in the nerve cell membrane. The typical sodium channel in nervous tissue is composed of three polypeptides, a large α subunit (260 kDa) and two much smaller β subunits (β1, 36 kDa; β2, 33 kDa). The α subunit constitutes the channel itself and contains the necessary components for channel functioning. The β subunits modulate channel opening and mediate cell-cell interactions. The β subunits are structurally similar to cell adhesion molecules and may account for the aggregation of Na^+ channels at the nodes of Ranvier.[4]

The structure of the Na^+ channel's α subunit is that of a large polypeptide that comprises four homologous domains (I through IV), each of which includes six α-helical segments (S1-S6) spanning the plasma membrane (Fig. 6-1). The S4 segments are unusual in that they contain multiple positively charged amino acid residues (arginine, lysine) that are normally attracted to the electronegative cytoplasmic side of the membrane. The peptide linkages between the S5 and S6 segments incorporate the so-called *P loops* that form the outer vestibule of the pore. The P loops are

TABLE 6-1

Pioneers and Landmarks in the Development of Local Anesthesia

Year	Person	Contribution
1859	Niemann	Isolation of cocaine in pure form; recognition of its topical anesthetic property
1884	Koller	Clinical introduction of cocaine topical anesthesia
1884	Halsted	Clinical introduction of cocaine regional anesthesia
1885	Corning	Application of tourniquet to retard cocaine absorption; first use of spinal anesthesia
1898	Bier	Spinal anesthesia via lumbar puncture
1901	Braun	Use of epinephrine as "chemical tourniquet"
1904	Einhorn	Synthesis of procaine
1908	Bier	Intravenous regional anesthesia with procaine
1920	Cook Laboratory	Marketing of anesthetic cartridge and syringe
1943	Löfgren	Synthesis of lidocaine
1947	Novocol Company	Marketing of dental aspirating syringe
1957	Ekenstam	Synthesis of bupivacaine
1959	Cook-Waite, Roehr Company	Marketing of disposable sterile needle

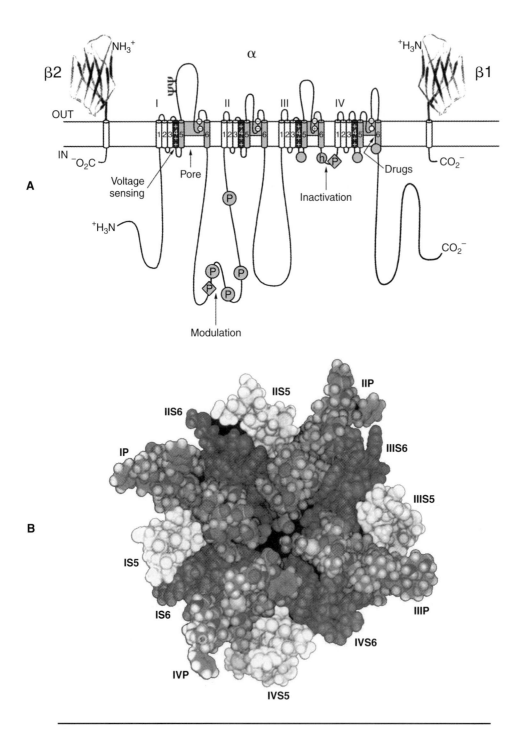

Fig. 6-1 The sodium channel. **A,** Primary structure (unfolded view). The numbered cylinders in the membrane represent the transmembrane segments. The bold lines indicate the relative lengths of polypeptide connectors. Each *P* indicates a phosphorylation site for protein kinase A *(circles)* and protein kinase C *(diamonds)*. Unlettered circles are sites implicated in forming the receptor for the inactivation gate *(h)*. (From Catterall WA: *Neuron* 26:13-25, 2000.) **B,** Molecular model of the sodium channel pore (external view). The P loops (P) and transmembrane segments *(S)* forming the outer vestibule of the pore are shown. (From Lipkind GM, Fozzard HA: *Biochemistry* 39:8161-8170, 2000.)

supported by the S5 and S6 segments, as predicted by detailed structural analysis of a bacterial K[+] channel (see Figure 6-1).[5] The S6 segments also line the inner portion of the channel. A phenylalanine residue on the IV/S6 segment is critical for local anesthetic binding.[6-7] It has also been suggested that a phenylalanine moiety exists in the cytoplasmic loop that links the III/S6 and IV/S1 segments and forms the inactivation gate of the Na[+] channel interact with the aromatic ring of local anesthetics.[8]

The Na[+] channel typically cycles through three primary configurations during an action potential. In the quiescent nerve, most Na[+] channels are in a resting, closed state. Partial depolarization of the membrane caused by electrotonic currents traveling in front of an advancing action potential induces the voltage-sensing S4 segments independently to spiral outward, carrying with them approximately 12 positive charges across the membrane.[4] Once all the S4 segments have moved, the channel becomes open to Na[+] entry, leading to an explosive depolarization and propagation of the action potential. Almost immediately, however, these same channels become inactivated, preventing continued Na[+] influx regardless of any further stimulation. The molecular basis for inactivation is the rapid attachment of the III/S6-IV/S1 linker peptide to a hydrophobic site on the inner surface of the pore exposed by the outward rotation of the IV/S4 segment.[4] Reversion from the refractory inactivated state to the responsive resting state occurs only after the membrane is repolarized and the IV/S4 segment has returned to its resting position.

Local anesthetics binding to the Na[+] channel disrupt the normal cycling process. If sufficient channels are blocked over a sufficient length of nerve, the action potential is prevented from proceeding down the neuron. Fig. 6-2 illustrates a developing anesthetic block in a single neuron.

It is not yet established how local anesthetic binding to the channel prevents Na[+] entry. Physical occlusion of the channel pore may occur, but analysis of gating currents (which are created by movements of the S4 segments) suggests that a predominant mechanism is prevention of the conformational transitions that underlie Na[+] channel function. Local anesthetics diminish gating currents in concert with their potential to inhibit the action potential.[9-10] The resultant inability of the channel to open precludes regeneration of the action potential whether or not the local anesthetic physically blocks the pore.

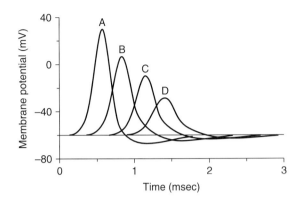

Fig. 6-2 Developing local anesthetic block in a single neuron. *A,* Normal action potential. *B,* Incipient local anesthetic block. The height of the action potential falls as sodium channels are prevented from opening. The rate of conduction is likewise inhibited. *C,* Progressive decline in the action potential in response to the developing local anesthetic block. *D,* Cessation of axonal conduction. Enough channels are blocked that electrotonic depolarization of the adjacent, unaffected membrane is insufficient to generate a self-replicating action potential.

Because clinically useful local anesthetics are fairly heterogeneous in structure, it is safe to conclude that the channel binding site lacks the stereospecificity normally ascribed to a drug receptor. (The term "local anesthetic receptor" is in fact rarely used.) Nevertheless, the location of the binding site within the pore itself places some structural limitations on drugs intended for use as local anesthetics. As illustrated by lidocaine (Fig. 6-3), the typical local anesthetic is amphiphilic, with a lipophilic aromatic ring structure at one end of the molecule and a hydrophilic amino group at the other end, which confers water solubility to the drug when charged by the reversible binding of a hydrogen ion. An intermediate linkage consisting of an amide, ester, or ether moiety bonded to a short alkyl chain provides the appropriate separation between the lipophilic and hydrophilic ends. Consistent with the need to have both sufficient water solubility to avoid precipitation on injection into interstitial fluid and satisfactory lipid solubility to penetrate the hydrophobic nerve sheath and axolemma, local anesthetics have *dissociation constants* (pK$_a$) in the 7.5 to 9.0 range, which permits the neutral and charged forms to coexist at tissue pH. Size constraints cluster the molecular weights of these drugs to between 200 and 300 Da.

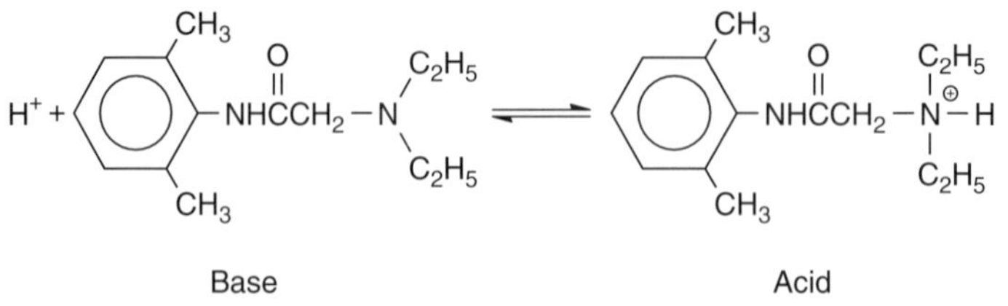

Fig. 6-3 Structural formulas of lidocaine in the uncharged, base form and in the charged, acidic form. Assuming a tissue pH of 7.4 and a dissociation constant (pK_a) of 7.8, the acid:base ratio is 2.5:1 (72% of the drug is charged, and 28% is uncharged), as calculated by the Henderson-Hasselbalch equation ($pH = pK_a + \log[\text{base/acid}]$).

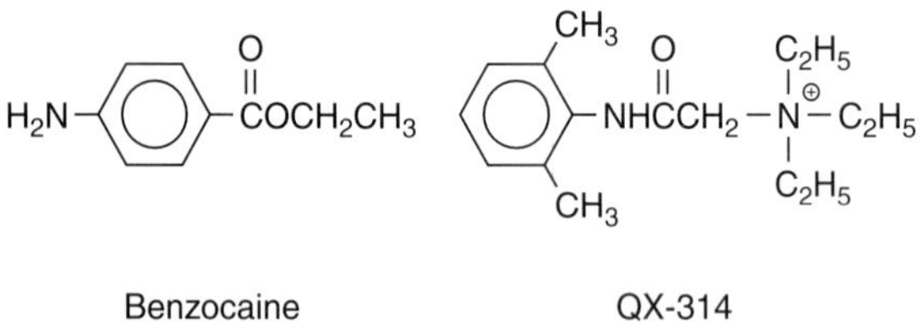

Fig. 6-4 Structural formulas of the nonamphiphilic local anesthetics benzocaine and QX-314.

Two drugs differ in structure from the typical local anesthetic (Fig. 6-4). *Benzocaine* is a topical local anesthetic lacking the amino terminus of its parent drug, procaine; *QX-314*, a drug used solely for research purposes, is the permanently charged, quaternary amine derivative of lidocaine. Largely insoluble in aqueous media, benzocaine is unsuitable for parenteral injection. Unable to penetrate the nerve sheath, QX-314 is only active when injected into the axoplasm. An important corollary of these findings is that both the free base and charged acidic forms of the conventional local anesthetic can block Na^+ channels.

Factors that Influence Local Anesthetic Blockade

Although local anesthetics act similarly to inhibit nerve conduction in vitro, a number of variables exist that strongly influence the degree and even the type of blockade observed clinically. Variables such as con-centration and dose are easily controlled; others, such as potency, are inherent features of the anesthetic selected; and still others (e.g., tissue pH, barriers to anesthetic spread) are intrinsic to the patient. Several determinants of local anesthetic activity have been extensively studied and deserve special comment.

Anesthetic Potency and "Minimum Inhibitory Concentration"

Local anesthetics vary in their innate ability to block nerve conduction. Experimental studies and clinical observations agree that anesthetic potencies differ by more than tenfold.[11] As revealed in Table 6-2, anes-thetic potency is most closely associated with the lipid:buffer distribution coefficient (Q), which esti-mates the relative tendency for an anesthetic to asso-ciate with the nerve membrane at a given tempera-ture and pH.[12]

In a manner analogous to the minimum alveolar concentration (MAC) for general anesthetics, at-tempts have been made to define local anesthetic po-tency in terms of the "minimum blocking concen-tration" (C_m), the lowest concentration necessary for blocking a given nerve in vitro within a selected time-frame. Unfortunately, this approach has proved un-satisfactory. As discussed later, the concentration re-quired for anesthesia is highly dependent on the length of nerve exposed to the anesthetic, the amount of impulse traffic flowing through the nerve, and the physiologic state of the nerve. Variables in drug distribution and differences in anesthetic sus-ceptibility independent of fiber type further weaken the concept of C_m as a useful predictor of local anes-thetic effect.

TABLE 6-2

Physicochemical and Clinical Properties of Local Anesthetics

Drug	PK$_a$*	Rate of Onset	Q*	Relative Potency†	Duration of Anesthesia	MW	Phasic Block‡
Amides							
Prilocaine	7.8	Fast	55	2	Moderate	220	Low
Lidocaine	7.8	Fast	110	2	Moderate	234	Medium
Bupivacaine	8.1	Medium	560	8	Long	288	High
Esters							
Procaine	8.9	Medium	3	1	Short	236	Medium
Tetracaine	8.4	Medium	541	8	Long	264	Medium

*pK$_a$ (dissociation constant) and Q (octanol:buffer distribution coefficient) measured at 36° C in buffered (pH 7.4) isotonic saline solution (except for prilocaine, which are extrapolated from values taken at 25° C. (Data from Strichartz GR, Sanchez V, Arthur GR, et al: *Anesth Analg* 71:158-170, 1990.)

†Tonic block; peripheral nerve in vitro. (Data from Covino BG: Toxicity and systemic effects of local anesthetic agents. In Strichartz GR, editor: *Local anesthetics: handbook of experimental pharmacology,* vol 81, Berlin, 1987, Springer-Verlag.)

‡ Potency determined in peripheral nerve in vitro. (Data from Courtney KR, Strichartz GR: Structural elements that determine local anesthetic activity. In Strichartz GR, editor: *Local anesthetics: handbook of experimental pharmacology,* vol 81, Berlin, 1987, Springer-Verlag.)

Differential Nerve Block and Critical Length

The notion that anesthetic susceptibility varies with fiber size arose from the discovery that the rate of onset of cocaine anesthesia in the peripheral nerve was diameter dependent.[13] It gained strong support from observations of patients receiving spinal and epidural anesthesia who lost autonomic control and the sensations of nociception and temperature (small fiber functions) but maintained motor control and the sensations of touch and pressure (large fiber functions).

In a seminal paper, Franz and Perry[14] found that an absolute differential nerve block could be obtained, but only when the length of axon exposed to the local anesthetic was restricted (e.g., to 2 mm). Given that a minimum of three nodes had to be fully blocked before conduction would fail, and that the internodal distance varies with fiber diameter, they concluded that there is a size-dependent "critical length" of anesthetic exposure necessary to block a given nerve. Small fibers would be blocked before large fibers because small areas of effective concentrations of anesthetic would be achieved in peripheral nerves before large areas, and small fibers would be affected longer because small areas of effective concentrations would persist longer into the recovery phase. An absolute differential block, however, would

be expected only when anatomic barriers to diffusion limited anesthetic exposure, as in the case of epidural anesthesia.[15] With the demonstration[16] that C_m varies inversely with the length of axon exposed up to 3 cm, the critical length hypothesis has been modified by Fink[15] to apply to situations, such as subarachnoid anesthesia, in which decremental conduction occurring over more than three nodes may still result in differential blockade because smaller fibers would have more nodes affected, leading to a progressive decline in the action potential to below threshold.

Intensity and Frequency of Stimulation

In the early stages of anesthetic block, patients sometimes lose sensitivity to small painful stimuli, such as pin pricks, but remain responsive to more intense stimuli, such as surgical incisions. A number of explanations may account for this finding, including that the stronger stimulus undoubtedly activates more fibers, some of which are not yet blocked by the anesthetic. In the case of topical or infiltration anesthesia, in which the anesthetic is locally active, a more intense stimulus may lead to greater initial depolarization of the free nerve endings, overcoming the inhibitory effect of the local anesthetic.

Frequency-dependent block, otherwise referred to as *use-dependent block* or *phasic block*, denotes an *increase* in anesthetic effect as a nerve is repeatedly stimulated. Depending on the local anesthetic agent and the rate of nerve stimulation, frequency-dependent block can vary enormously, from contributing little to the anesthetic effect to providing virtually all of it. Frequency-dependent block is presumably contingent on the relative ability of the anesthetic agent to reach and leave the site of action within the Na+ channel, as influenced by the various conformational states of the channel. Drugs such as QX-314, which are permanently charged, can only reach the site of action when the channel is open (or at least partially activated) and are highly dependent on the frequency of stimulation for blocking the nerve.* Benzocaine, which lacks a positive charge, is largely devoid of frequency-dependent blocking activity. For typical anesthetics, which can exist in both charged and uncharged forms, pK_a and, in particular, molecular weight are positively correlated with the tendency to cause frequency-dependent block.[19] Bupivacaine, which is high in both attributes (see Table 6-2), elicits this effect.

The importance of frequency-dependent block is easily illustrated. For example, because nervous transmissions encoded in repeated bursts of depolarization are more susceptible to anesthetic action than are transmissions that occur at low frequency, local anesthetics may block noxious stimuli and sympathetic nervous system outputs preferentially over somatomotor activity simply because of differences in transmission frequency.[20] Additionally, the antiarrhythmic action of lidocaine may be ascribed to a selective development of Na^+ channel inhibition during ventricular tachycardia, and the cardiotoxic effect of bupivacaine may be correlated in part with its tendency to cause frequency-dependent block at even resting heart rates.[21]

Blockade of Other Channels

In addition to reducing Na^+ permeability, local anesthetics can impede ion movement through other channels similar in structure to the Na^+ channel. Differential nerve blockade may occur when these other channels modulate nerve conduction. For example, selective inhibition of an outward potassium (K^+) current by a local anesthetic could prevent full repolarization and result in residual Na^+ channel inactivation. Bupivacaine is especially potent in blocking K^+ channels, which may explain the special sensitivity of small axons to conduction block with this drug.[22]

Inflammation and Tissue pH

Clinical observations and experimental reports agree that the presence of inflammation can greatly impair local anesthetic efficacy. Inflammation is associated with a number of physiologic and pathologic disturbances. For example, increased local blood flow in the inflamed tissue may enhance systemic uptake of local anesthetic and prevent anesthetic concentrations from developing within axons. The most publicized disturbance influencing local anesthetic action is tissue acidity. A low pH in the extracellular space impairs the ability of local anesthetics to cross the nerve sheath and membrane because it reduces the proportion of anesthetic in the lipophilic, free base form. A fall in pH from 7.4 to 6.4, for example, reduces the proportion of the base form of lidocaine in the extracellular fluid from 28% to 4%, a sevenfold reduction. Not only would this effect retard the onset of anesthesia, it could preclude anesthesia altogether. Should the intraneuronal pH be unaffected by the inflammation, the concentration of local anesthetic will be depressed even after full equilibration by "ion trapping" within the interstitial space. Some evidence exists, however, that the pH and buffering capacity of inflamed tissues are not necessarily reduced[23] and that other reasons for local anesthetic failure must exist.

Hyperalgesia is commonly associated with inflammatory states. Prostaglandins, kinins, and other substances produced during inflammation activate nociceptors directly and/or make them more responsive to additional stimuli. In clinical situations where local anesthetic blockade is incomplete, the enhanced recruitment of fibers for a given operative stimulus may lead to the perception of pain. Several studies have suggested that certain chemicals produced during inflammation may directly interfere with conduction blockade.[24] These substances may include peptides, prostaglandins, and derivatives of adenosine. The finding that Na+ channels are sub-

---

*Cardiac Na^+ channels are unique in that positively charged local anesthetics can reach their site of action after external application.[17,18] Single amino-acid substitutions in the IV/S6 segment can open up hydrophilic pathways in neuronal Na^+ channels or close them in cardiac channels.

ject to phosphorylation raises the possibility of direct hormonal regulation of neuronal depolarization (see Figure 6-1, *A*).[4]

Uptake, Distribution, and Elimination

The processes of absorption, distribution, metabolism, and excretion should be considered because they dictate whether systemic effects will follow local anesthetic administration. The rate of absorption from the injected tissue also plays a role in the duration of anesthesia.

A number of variables influence the uptake of local anesthetics. These include the affinity of the anesthetic for the local tissues, the tissue blood flow, the effect of the anesthetic agent on the local circulation, and the coadministration of a vasoconstrictor. In general, drugs injected for dental anesthesia are absorbed fairly rapidly, with peak plasma concentrations occurring within 15 to 30 minutes.

As a local anesthetic is absorbed into the systemic circulation, a portion of it is reversibly bound to plasma proteins, principally α_1-acid glycoprotein and, to a lesser extent, albumin. The local anesthetic also is taken up by red blood cells. Plasma protein binding appears to be related to the lipid:buffer distribution coefficient. About 95% of the highly lipophilic etidocaine and bupivacaine is bound at nontoxic concentrations; comparable figures for the moderately lipophilic lidocaine and the modestly lipophilic prilocaine are 70% and 55%, respectively.[25] The blood: plasma ratio follows a reverse relationship, with prilocaine exhibiting a value of 1.0, lidocaine 0.84, and the two lipophilic drugs below 0.75.

Once the anesthetic is absorbed, it is distributed to virtually all tissues of the body. Normally, the rate of distribution is sufficiently fast with respect to absorption that transient toxic concentrations do not occur in any specific tissue. If the drug is injected intravascularly, however, a pattern of sequential distribution emerges in which the anesthetic is first taken up by the lungs, quickly distributed to other organs with relatively large blood supplies (rapidly equilibrating tissues: brain, heart, liver, kidneys, spleen), and then redistributed to muscle and fat (Fig. 6-5).[26] Although the lungs serve a potentially useful role in buffering an injected bolus of anesthetic within the first minute,[27] the rapid uptake of drug into the brain and heart can lead to exaggerated yet short-lived systemic effects.

The metabolic fate of local anesthetics depends on their chemical classification. Procaine, benzocaine, tetracaine, and related ester derivatives of *p*-aminobenzoic acid are predominantly hydrolyzed by plasma pseudocholinesterase. Hepatic esterase activity is more important with certain other ester anesthetics. In all instances, however, hydrolysis results in the loss of local anesthetic activity.

The normally rapid hydrolysis of procaine-like drugs in plasma (elimination half-time of procaine can be as low as 43 seconds) has inhibited pharmacokinetic studies of ester local anesthetics. Drugs known to retard ester metabolism include the anticholinesterase agents (e.g., neostigmine, echothiophate), several insecticides (e.g., parathion), and, surprisingly, amide local anesthetics (especially bupivacaine).[25] Of course, the greatest deficit in ester metabolism occurs in individuals with deficient pseudocholinesterase activity.

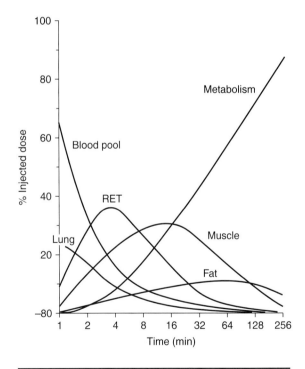

Fig. 6-5 Distribution and metabolism of lidocaine after an intravenous infusion lasting 1 minute. *RET,* Rapidly equilibrating tissues (including the brain, heart, liver, and kidneys). Metabolism indicates the percentage of the injected dose that has been metabolized. (From Benowitz N, Forsyth RP, Melmon KL, et al: *Clin Pharmacol Ther* 16:87-98, 1974.)

Amide anesthetics typically undergo a complex pattern of biotransformation. Other than prilocaine, which is metabolized in part by the lung and/or kidney, and articaine, which is largely hydrolyzed in the plasma, amides are broken down exclusively in the liver. The initial reaction usually involves microsomal N-dealkylation, converting the tertiary amine of drugs such as lidocaine and bupivacaine to secondary amines. Often these initial metabolites retain significant activity and contribute to systemic reactions. A second N-dealkylation may occur, or the molecule may be hydrolyzed (and inactivated) by hepatic amidase activity. Prilocaine, a secondary amine, largely undergoes hydrolysis without prior N-dealkylation. Hydroxylation of the aromatic ring may take place any time during this sequence, and a high proportion of the derivatives is conjugated with glucuronic acid. Articaine is unique among the local anesthetics in that it is an amide with an ester side chain on the aromatic moiety. Hydrolysis of the ester linkage by plasma enzymes yields articainic acid. Articainic acid is largely devoid of efficacy and toxicity.

Terminal anesthetic metabolites, which are much less lipid soluble than the parent drugs, are excreted principally in the urine. Very little local anesthetic is excreted unchanged.

The pharmacokinetic profile of amide local anesthetics (Table 6-3) bears no obvious relationship to any single physicochemical property (see Table 6-2).[28-30] Whereas etidocaine and bupivacaine share similar half-times of elimination, etidocaine enjoys a significantly greater hepatic clearance than does bupivacaine but is also sequestered much more by peripheral tissues. The unusually large clearance of prilocaine reflects the extrahepatic elimination of the drug. Because the hepatic clearances of lidocaine and etidocaine approach 75% of the total liver blood flow, anything that alters liver blood flow may affect local anesthetic metabolism. On the positive side, a high-protein meal can increase lidocaine metabolism 20% on average by stimulating portal circulation.[31] More important, however, are situations in which metabolism is impaired. Disorders known to decrease liver blood flow include cirrhosis, congestive heart failure, and hypotension. Hypotensive patients in the sitting position may be especially prone to local anesthetic toxicity because an acute fall in the apparent volume of distribution has been linked to an 80% increase in the peak lidocaine concentration after intravenous (IV) injection.[32] Drugs that have the potential to lower hepatic blood flow include the

TABLE 6-3

Pharmacokinetic Parameters of Amide Local Anesthetics in Humans *

Drug	$t_{1/2}$ (min)	V_{Dss} (L)	Cl (L/min)
Lidocaine	96	91	0.95
Mepivacaine	114	84	0.78
Prilocaine	93	261	2.84
Bupivacaine	162	73	0.58
Etidocaine	162	133	1.11

*$t_{1/2}$, Elimination half-time; V_{Dss}, volume of distribution at steady state; *Cl*, clearance.
Data from Punnia-Moorthy A: *Br J Anaesth* 61:154-159, 1988; Brown RD: *Br Dent J* 151:47-51, 1981; and Arthur GR: Pharmacokinetics of local anesthetics. In Strichartz GR, editor: *Local anesthetics: handbook of experimental pharmacology,* vol. 81, Berlin, 1987, Springer-Verlag.

β-adrenergic blocking drug propranolol. However, a direct effect on local anesthetic metabolism probably accounts for most of the 50% reduction in lidocaine clearance caused by propranolol[33] and most if not all of the similar reduction caused by the H_2-antihistamine cimetidine.[34] Old age also has been shown to retard lidocaine metabolism; the deficit may be caused by an impairment in hepatic clearance[35] or an increase in the apparent volume of distribution.[36]

Systemic Effects

Once absorbed into the systemic circulation, a local anesthetic may interact with Na^+ channels in all excitable tissues. Neurons in the central nervous system (CNS) are probably the most responsive, but prominent actions also include the heart and vasculature. Not all systemic reactions involve Na^+ conductance changes, however, which raises the possibility for nonexcitable tissues to interact with local anesthetics.

Central Nervous System

Dose-dependent effects of local anesthetics on the CNS are listed in Table 6-4, using lidocaine as a representative drug. Blood concentrations routinely associated with clinical doses in dentistry cause only minimal alterations in mental activity. Even the IV

TABLE 6-4

Effects of Lidocaine on the Central Nervous System and Cardiovascular System

Concentration (μg/ml)	CNS Effect*	CVS Effect*
<5	Anticonvulsant activity mild sedation, analgesia	Antiarrhythmic activity, mild increases in mean BP with similar increases in cardiac output or peripheral vascular resistance
5-10	Lightheadedness, slurred speech, drowsiness, euphoria nausea, dysphoria, sensory disturbances, diplopia, muscle twitching	
10-15	Disorientation, uncontrollable tremors, respiratory depression, tonic-clonic seizures	Cardiovascular instability
15-20	Coma, respiratory arrest	
>20		Profound myocardial depression, vasodilation, cardiovascular collapse

CNS, Central nervous system; CVS, cardiovascular system; BP, blood pressure.
*CNS and CVS effects are listed in approximate order of occurrence with increasing blood concentration.

injection of 1 mg/kg lidocaine to control ventricular tachyarrhythmias, which typically results in a peak blood concentration of up to 4.5 μg/ml,[37] normally elicits only potentially beneficial effects in the CNS, such as analgesia, anticonvulsant activity, and perhaps mild sedation. Increasingly excessive dosages and blood concentrations, however, start to depress vital areas of the brain. Thus confusion, somnolence, and respiratory depression may develop. Excitatory phenomena—dysphoria, auditory and visual disturbances, and signs of motor hyperactivity—also occur, arising from the selective depression of inhibitory centers within the cerebral cortex. These excitatory responses tend to predominate and evolve into generalized seizures when the amygdaloid complex is sufficiently released from tonic inhibition to begin depolarizing spontaneously. Direct inhibition of the γ-aminobutyric acid A (GABA$_A$) receptor complex by local anesthetics may produce this effect.[38] Postictally, complete respiratory arrest may ensue in response to cerebral hypoxia, hypercarbia, and the continued uptake of the local anesthetic into the brain.

Cardiovascular System

Cardiovascular reactions to local anesthetics stem from direct actions on the heart and vascular smooth muscle, from direct actions on sympathetic neurons, and from changes in autonomic function mediated via the CNS. The coadministration of a vasoconstrictor such as epinephrine has an additional influence on the ultimate clinical response.

Local Anesthetics. As in the CNS, blood concentrations typically observed after regional anesthesia produce only benign alterations in cardiovascular function (see Table 6-4). A centrally mediated increase in sympathetic nervous activity is presumed to be responsible for the mild increase in heart rate, cardiac output, and mean arterial blood pressure reported in some studies.[39] Alternatively, a modest increase in peripheral vascular resistance brought on by a direct stimulation of vascular smooth muscle may predominate, leading to a small decrease in cardiac output.[37] The antiarrhythmic efficacy of lidocaine depends on several cardiac actions.[40] Ectopic pacemaker activity is reduced or eliminated because the drug inhibits spontaneous depolarization during phase 4 of the cardiac action potential. Ventricular tachyarrhythmias are aborted because lidocaine reduces membrane responsiveness to depolarizing stimuli in a frequency-dependent manner. An increase in the effective refractory period:action potential duration ratio also helps regularize ventricular conduction.

Adverse cardiovascular responses to local anesthetics are generally not manifested unless the blood concentration reaches the convulsant range (10 to 15 µg/ml for lidocaine). Both hypertensive and hypotensive reactions occur, representing different interplays of the direct depressant actions of the drug on the myocardium, centrally mediated disturbances in autonomic function, and the effects of hypoxia and hypercarbia. With lidocaine and most other local anesthetics, the dose required to induce cardiac arrest experimentally is several times greater than the dose that produces respiratory arrest. Therefore profound myocardial depression, vascular dilatation, and cardiovascular collapse are unlikely to occur clinically if the patient's ventilation is adequately supported.

This generalization, however, may not hold true for long-acting anesthetics such as bupivacaine and etidocaine. Some animal investigations and clinical case reports indicate that these drugs may cause fatal cardiac arrhythmias at dosages similar to those that trigger seizures and respiratory arrest, especially if hypercarbia, acidosis, and hypoxia are also present.[41-42] As previously mentioned, the penchant for these drugs to induce frequency-dependent block may underlie this enhanced cardiotoxicity. The exact mechanism, however, remains to be determined, and investigators are finding evidence to support several disparate theories, from inhibition of myocardial energy production[43] to proposals of a CNS origin for cardiac arrhythmias.[44-45]

Most amide local anesthetics are racemic drugs. With the discovery that the pronounced cardiotoxicity of bupivacaine is largely associated with its R (+) enantiomer, efforts were made to develop S (−) congeners.[46] Levobupivacaine and ropivacaine (an analogue of levobupivacaine in which the butyl side chain is replaced with a propyl moiety) are now available as alternatives to bupivacaine. Interestingly, although these drugs are less disruptive of cardiac function when given intravenously, direct infusion into the left main coronary arteries of sheep shows no significant differences in toxicity.[47]

Vasoconstrictors. Studies over the last two decades have overturned a once widely held tenet in clinical dentistry that the amount of epinephrine injected during local anesthesia is low compared to the endogenous release of the hormone and therefore has little or no effect systemically. Fig. 6-6 collates findings from six studies on the effect of intraoral injection of lidocaine with epinephrine on the resting venous plasma concentration of epinephrine.[48-53] With an overall mean epinephrine baseline of 39 pg/ml,

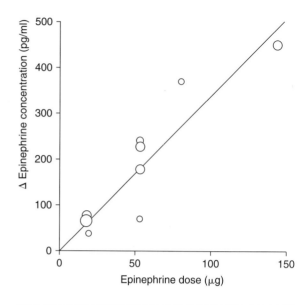

Fig. 6-6 Changes in venous plasma epinephrine after intraoral injection of 2% lidocaine with 1:100,000 epinephrine (1:25,000 for the 80-µg dose). Each circle indicates the mean value of a group of subjects; the relative size of the circle is proportional to the number of subjects in the group ($N = 6$ to 14). (Data from various sources.[48-53])

regression analysis reveals a linear increase with injected epinephrine such that a single dental cartridge of 2% lidocaine with 1:100,000 epinephrine doubles the baseline titer. Venous plasma concentrations associated with the injection of 100 to 150 µg of epinephrine, which often occurs in oral and periodontal surgery, produce concentrations equivalent to that present during heavy exercise.[54]

The absorption of even the small amounts of epinephrine contained in one or two dental cartridges evokes modest but reproducible increases in stroke volume and cardiac output and comparable decreases in peripheral vascular resistance.[55-56] Blood pressure and heart rate are most often minimally affected by these low doses. However, with toxic doses, as may occur when a large volume of anesthetic is accidentally injected into the blood stream, dramatic increases in blood pressure and changes in heart rate (tachycardia, reactive bradycardia, arrhythmias) can develop. Such changes are more likely to occur in patients with preexisting cardiovascular disease and in individuals taking medications likely to augment adrenergic action (e.g., tricyclic antidepressants, non-specific β-adrenergic blockers).[57]

Comparative information is not readily available for levonordefrin, the primary vasoconstrictor alternative to epinephrine. Levonordefrin may be absorbed in sufficient concentrations after intraoral injection to elicit systemic reactions. Because levonordefrin does not strongly stimulate vasodilative β$_2$-adrenergic receptors, it is more likely to increase peripheral vascular resistance and mean blood pressure and reflexively reduce cardiac output and heart rate in dental patients. At toxic doses, epinephrine and levonordefrin exhibit similar pharmacologic profiles.

Miscellaneous Effects

An interesting array of miscellaneous actions has been ascribed to local anesthetics.[11] For example, local anesthetics have been shown to augment neuro-muscular blockade in combination with either depolarizing or nondepolarizing agents. Both pre- and postjunctional effects probably contribute to this action; in the case of succinylcholine, the aforementioned ability of local anesthetics to inhibit pseudo-cholinesterase may add another dimension to the potentiation.

The ability of amide local anesthetics to perturb calcium metabolism allows these drugs to cause vascular smooth muscle contraction in clinical concentrations and once raised the possibility that malignant hyperthermia might be triggered in susceptible patients. Numerous lines of evidence now indicate this concern is unjustified.[58] Local anesthetics are myotoxic, however, if injected into or adjacent to skeletal muscle.[59] A dose-dependent action on bronchial smooth muscle is similar to that observed in vascular smooth muscle, with low concentrations causing constriction and high concentrations causing dilation.

Methemoglobinemia is a special problem with prilocaine but may be also caused by benzocaine and possibly lidocaine.[60-61] Metabolites of these drugs (*o*-toluidine in prilocaine) upset the balance between oxidation of the iron in hemoglobin to the ferric (Fe^{+3}) state and its enzymatic reduction back to the ferrous (Fe^{+2}) form. Cyanosis occurs when the methemoglobin concentration exceeds 1.5 g/dl. Although no association between congenital forms of methemoglobinemia and local anesthetic-induced cyanosis has been drawn, prilocaine should be avoided in such individuals, and benzocaine should be used sparingly. Potentially positive inter-actions between local anesthetics and blood include an antithrombotic effect after surgery,[62] an inhibition of neutrophil function,[63] and a reduction of albumin extravasation in burn injuries.[64]

No discussion of the physiologic consequences of local anesthesia would be complete without mentioning the most common cause of systemic disturbances: psychogenic reactions. Intraoral injection is widely perceived by patients as the single most stressful procedure encountered in routine dentistry. Common responses to this stress include pallor, sweating, nausea, headache, palpitation, hyperventilation, and syncope. Although these reactions as a group are easily managed, life-threatening responses, including cardiac arrest, may occur.[65] The more pronounced a reaction is, the more likely it will be misdiagnosed as a drug allergy.

True allergic reactions to local anesthetics are now quite rare in dentistry. The almost complete abandonment of ester anesthetics for regional anesthesia and the removal of paraben preservatives from local anesthetic cartridges are responsible for this improvement in patient safety. The possibility remains, however, for patients to exhibit hypersensitivity to sulfites contained in some anesthetic solutions. Sodium metabisulfite and acetone sodium bisulfite prevent the oxidation of adrenergic vasoconstrictors. Although isolated case reports may describe true allergic reactions,[66] most patients affected by sulfites have asthma and airways hyperreactive to sulfur dioxide, a breakdown product of inhaled or ingested sulfites.[67] In the most sensitive of these individuals, the response threshold for bronchial constriction is in the 0.5 to 1 mg range, roughly comparable to what is present in a single dental cartridge. Initial use of sulfite-containing anesthetics in the threshold range to gauge patient sensitivity coupled with stepped increases in future appointments is a useful strategy for hyperreactors; total restriction is necessary in the rare but truly allergic patient.

Therapeutic Suggestions For Drug Selection

The selection of drugs for local anesthesia is ideally based on considerations of safety, efficacy, and duration of effect. Amides are the only local anesthetics currently marketed for use in single-dose cartridges. Although the amides differ somewhat in relative toxicity, safety issues assume prominence only with respect to certain patients, such as allergic individuals, young children, patients on certain drugs, and

TABLE 6-5

Average Durations of Local Anesthesia

Preparation	MAXILLARY INFILTRATION		INFERIOR ALVEOLAR BLOCK	
	Pulpal Tissue	Soft Tissue	Pulpal Tissue	Soft Tissue
2% Lidocaine HCl; 1:100,000-1:50,000 epinephrine	60	170	85	190
2% Mepivacaine HCl; 1:20,000 levonordefrin	50	130	75	185
3% Mepivacaine	25	90	40	165
4% Prilocaine	20	105	55	190
4% Prilocaine; 1:200,000 epinephrine	40	140	60	220
0.5% Bupivacaine; 1:200,000 epinephrine	40	340	240	440
1.5% Etidocaine; 1:200,000 epinephrine	30	280	240	470
4% Articaine; 1:100,000 epinephrine	60	190	90	230

patients with significant cardiovascular disease. None of these formulations have been proved to differ from the rest in nerve block efficacy, and variances in the rate of onset are more dependent on the technique of administration than on the drug injected (with the possible exception of bupivacaine, whose onset may be delayed by 1 to 2 minutes). Thus drug selection for intraoral anesthesia often devolves into a decision based on the duration of effect.

Duration

Table 6-5 summarizes the durations of pulpal and soft tissue anesthesia after maxillary supraperiosteal injection ("infiltration") and inferior alveolar nerve block. Three crucial factors govern the duration of anesthesia. The first is the presence of a vasoconstrictor. Epinephrine and levonordefrin are powerful α-adrenergic receptor agonists and strongly reduce blood flow in the area of injection. This action helps to retain the local anesthetic locally, giving it time to accumulate in neuronal tissues, from which it slowly diffuses. Prolongation of anesthesia occurs uniformly with maxillary supraperiosteal injections, but the failure of epinephrine to alter prilocaine anesthesia in

the mandible underscores the second governing factor, the site of injection.

Site-specific influences on local anesthesia are often overlooked, as in the mistaken use of formulations without a vasoconstrictor to "shorten" the duration of mandibular soft-tissue anesthesia after inferior alveolar nerve block and drugs such as bupivacaine for "long-duration" pulpal anesthesia after maxillary supraperiosteal injection. With intraligamentary or intraosseous anesthesia, formulations with vasoconstrictors are significantly more effective in providing anesthesia for a clinically useful duration.[68-70]

The third important variable affecting duration is the anesthetic agent itself. The effect of lidocaine without epinephrine is so evanescent in the maxilla that it is not considered a useful agent for pulpal anesthesia. Its moderately high lipid:buffer distribution coefficient cannot overcome the local vasodilation it produces at the injection site. Bupivacaine and etidocaine (both with epinephrine, Fig. 6-7), on the other hand, are so lipid soluble that that they can provide up to 8 hours of postsurgical pain relief after inferior alveolar nerve block and can reduce the number of oral analgesic doses taken by the patient.[71] This same lipophilicity, however, reduces their use-

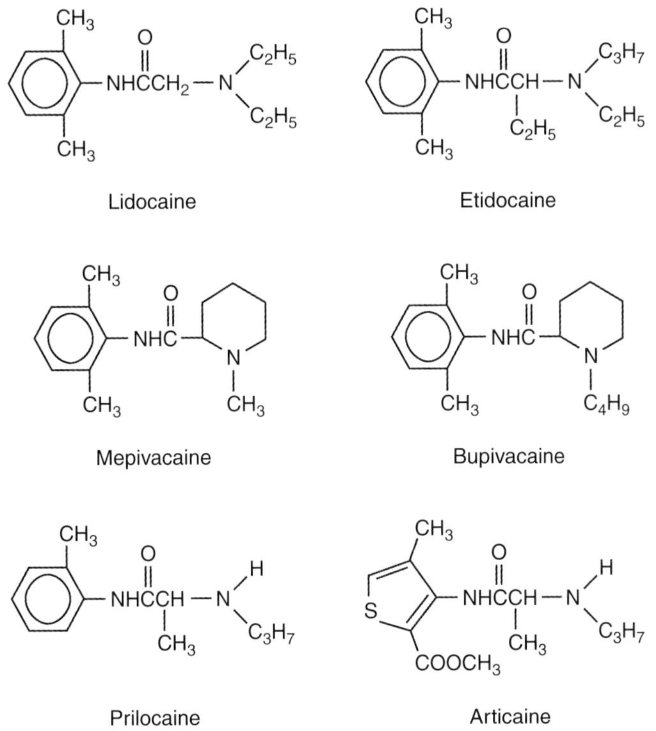

Fig. 6-7 Structures of the tertiary amino-amide anesthetics lidocaine and mepivacaine with their respective long-acting congeners etidocaine and bupivacaine and the secondary amino-amide anesthetic prilocaine with its thiophene analogue, articaine.

fulness for maxillary pulpal anesthesia, since avid uptake by supraperiosteal tissues hampers diffusion to the superior dental plexus.[72]

Dosage

Most often with young children, but occasionally with adults receiving extensive treatments, dosage limitations for the various clinically available formulations must be considered in drug selection. Table 6-6 lists maximum dosage recommendations in product information approved by the Food and Drug Administration and, in parentheses, generally lower limits found in the United States Pharmacopeia Drug Information (USPDI).[73] Although the dosage limits reported by the manufacturer are presumably based on comparative animal experiments and limited human studies, the more restrictive suggestions arise from concerns that the generous blood supply to the orofacial region may result in more rapid drug absorption and higher peak blood concentrations than would occur with identical doses administered elsewhere.

In particular, dosage considerations constrain use of the 3% mepivacaine and 4% prilocaine and articaine formulations in small children. With 50% more local anesthetic per cartridge in 3% mepivacaine than in 2% mepivacaine with 1:20,000 levonordefrin, maximum recommended doses can easily be reached in the young child requiring multiple restorations. Selection of the 3% formulation in an attempt, largely futile, to shorten the duration of mandibular anesthesia and prevent lip and tongue biting, coupled with failure to heed dosage limitations, has proved to be a prescription for disaster.[74] Death and permanent brain injury have also resulted because of a failure to appreciate the additive nature

TABLE 6-6

Maximum Recommended Doses of Local Anesthetics*

Drug	Trade Name	Maximum Dose (mg/kg)	Maximum Adult Dose (mg)
Lidocaine	Alphacaine	4.5†	300†
	Lignospan Standard	7 (4-5 in children)‡	500 (100-150 in children)‡
	Lignospan Forte		
	Octocaine		
	Xylocaine		
Mepivacaine	Arestocaine	6.6 (5-6 in children†)	400 (180‡ and 270† in children)
	Carbocaine		
	Isocaine		
	Polocaine		
	Scandonest		
Prilocaine	Citanest Plain	8	600
	Citanest Forte		
Bupivacaine	Marcaine	—	90‡§
Etidocaine	Duranest	8 (5.5)‡	400‡
Articaine	Septocaine	7 (5 for ages 4-12)‡	—

*From product information approved by the Food and Drug Administration. Children dosages have not been established for bupivacaine or etidocaine. Values in parentheses are the generally more conservative guidelines listed in the United States Pharmacopeia Drug Information (USPDI).
†Without vasoconstrictor.
‡With vasoconstrictor.
§The maximum recommended dose for nondental use is 225 mg.

of local anesthetics and other CNS depressants.[75] Small children again are at special risk because they are often unable to cooperate with extensive dental treatment and therefore are administered sedative drugs to facilitate their care.

Vasoconstrictor

Except in situations where there is a desire to limit the duration of maxillary anesthesia, the decision to use a local anesthetic formulation without a vaso-constrictor (e.g., 3% mepivacaine, 4% prilocaine) is usually made to enhance patient safety. Four groups of patients are at increased risk of adverse reactions to vasoconstrictors: (1) patients hypersensitive to sulfites (discussed previously); (2) patients hyperreactive to adrenergic amines; (3) patients taking drugs that can potentially interact with adrenergic amines; and (4) patients with significant cardiovascular disease.

Some individuals appear to be unusually responsive to vasoconstrictors, especially epinephrine. These patients tend to be highly anxious before injection, however, and it is not clear whether the vasoconstrictor causes the reaction or merely augments the effect of endogenously released hormone. Anxiety, tremulousness, palpitation, and a feeling of chest compression are variably reported. Selecting a formulation without a vasoconstrictor, with lower concentrations of epinephrine, or with levonordefrin in place of epinephrine (which may be less likely to cause symptoms of cardiac stimulation in some patients) may help to minimize this problem, but reducing stress (by limiting the number of procedures planned and therefore the dosage required) and providing sedation as indicated should also be considered.

Several potentially adverse drug interactions involve the adrenergic vasoconstrictors used in dental local anesthetics (Table 6-7).[76-77] Although com-

TABLE 6-7

Drug Interactions Involving Local Anesthetics and Vasoconstrictors

Drug	Interacting Drug	Effect and Recommendation
Local anesthetics	Alcohol, CNS depressants, centrally acting antihypertensives and muscle relaxants, opioids, antidepressants, antipsychotics, antihistamines, $MgSO_4$ (parenteral)	Increased CNS and respiratory depression may occur. Use cautiously.
	Antiarrhythmic drugs (e.g., quinidine)	Increased cardiac depression may occur. Use cautiously.
	Antimyasthenics (e.g., neostigmine)	Local anesthetics may antagonize the effects of antimyasthenic drugs on muscle contractility. Treat patients in consultation with physician.
	Amiodarone, β-blockers (e.g., propranolol), cimetidine	Metabolism of amides in liver is reduced. Use cautiously.
Vasoconstrictors (epinephrine, levonordefrin)	General anesthetics (e.g., halothane, thiopental)	Increased possibility of cardiac arrhythmias exists with some agents. Consult with anesthesiologist.
	Tricyclic antidepressants (e.g., imipramine, amitriptyline), maprotiline	Sympathomimetic effects may be enhanced. Use epinephrine cautiously. Avoid levonordefrin.
	Nonselective β-blockers (e.g., propranolol), adrenergic neuron blockers (e.g., guanethidine), COMT inhibitors (e.g., entacapone)	Hypertensive and/or cardiac reactions are more likely. Use cautiously.
	Phenothiazines (e.g., promethazine), butyrophenones (e.g., haloperidol), α-blockers (e.g., prazosin)	Vasoconstrictor action is inhibited, which may lead to hypotensive responses. Use cautiously.
	Cocaine	Arrhythmias and hypertensive responses possible. Avoid concurrent use.

CNS, Central nervous system; *MgSO₄,* magnesium sulfide; *COMT,* catechol-*o*-methyltransferase.
Local anesthetics and vasoconstrictors include all formulations available in cartridge form for dental use in the United States. The term "use cautiously" indicates that the interaction is rare or not usually dangerous and that careful administration within recommended dosage limits and increased surveillance of drug effects should suffice to avoid serious toxicity.

monly cited in the dental literature, monoamine oxidase inhibitors are excluded because of strong evidence that no interactions occur with either exogenously administered epinephrine or levonordefrin.[57]

The use of epinephrine and related drugs in patients with cardiovascular disease has been debated in dentistry for decades. The marketing of effective anesthetic formulations without vasoconstrictors in the 1960s altered the character of this debate, and research since then has helped to clarify the pharmacology of adrenergic amines in medically compromised patients. Nevertheless, there is still no simple answer to drug selection. Patients with hypertension that is well controlled by medication should be able to tolerate regular doses of epinephrine (assuming no interfering drug interactions); patients with unstable angina pectoris or cardiac arrhythmias may be at risk from receiving even small amounts of vasoconstrictor. One recent study[78] has demonstrated that supraperiosteal injection of two cartridges of 2% lidocaine with 1:100,000 epinephrine produces the same metabolic workload as light exercise (e.g., raking leaves, walking at 2 miles/hour) and therefore should be tolerated by patients with that level of exercise capacity. Nevertheless, a statement made jointly by the American Heart Association and the American Dental Association concerning patients with ischemic heart disease still provides a good summary for this issue:[79]

> Vasoconstrictor agents should be used in local anesthesia solutions during dental practice only when it is clear that the procedure will be shortened or the analgesia rendered more profound. When a vasoconstrictor is indicated, extreme care should be taken to avoid intravascular injection. The minimum possible amount of vasoconstrictor should be used.

Articaine

As the most recent addition to the local anesthetic armamentarium in the United States, articaine deserves special comment. Currently the drug is available only as a 4% solution with 1:100,000 epinephrine and has a profile of action most similar to that of 2% lidocaine with 1:100,000 epinephrine. Claims have been made that this formulation of articaine enjoys a higher success rate than other available local anesthetic preparations for dentistry and that buccal supraperiosteal injection of articaine can provide palatal anesthesia in the maxilla and pulpal and lingual anesthesia in the mandible. None of these claims has been proved in properly controlled clinical trials.[80-81] Nevertheless, articaine has taken over 90% of the dental anesthesia market in Germany, where it was introduced in 1976, and is now the leading local anesthetic in Canada (marketed in 1983). The possibility cannot be ruled out that a small percentage of patients (e.g., those with acute pulpitis) may be anesthetized more successfully using 4% articaine with epinephrine because of the formulation's high concentration of local anesthetic. This high concentration may also explain why articaine (and 4% prilocaine) is also more likely than other formulations to cause nerve damage after inferior alveolar-lingual nerve block injection.[82]

References

1. Liljestrand G: The historical development of local anesthesia. In Lechat P, editor: *International encyclopedia of pharmacology and therapeutics*, vol 1, New York, 1971, Pergamon.
2. Fink BR: Leaves and needles: the introduction of surgical local anesthesia, *Anesthesiology* 63:77-83, 1985.
3. Clark JH: History of regional anesthesia. In Jastak JT, Yagiela JA, editors: *Regional anesthesia of the oral cavity*, St Louis, 1981, Mosby.
4. Catterall WA: From ionic currents to molecular mechanisms: the structure and function of voltage-gated sodium channels, *Neuron* 26:13-25, 2000.
5. Lipkind GM, Fozzard HA: KcsA crystal structure as framework for a molecular model of the Na+ channel pore, *Biochemistry* 39:8161-8170, 2000.
6. Ragsdale DS, McPhee JC, Scheuer T, et al: Common molecular determinants of local anesthetic, antiarrhythmic, and anticonvulsant block of voltage-gated Na^+ channels, *Proc Natl Acad Sci U S A* 93:9270-9275, 1996.
7. Li HL, Galue A, Meadows L, et al: A molecular basis for the different local anesthetic affinities of resting versus open and inactivated states of the sodium channel, *Mol Pharmacol* 55:134-141, 1999.
8. Kuroda Y, Miyamoto K, Tanaka K, et al: Interactions between local anesthetics and Na^+ channel inactivation gate peptides in phosphatidylserine suspensions as studied by 1H-NMR spectroscopy, *Chem Pharm Bull (Tokyo)* 48:1293-1298, 2000.
9. Neumcke B, Schwarz W, Stämpfli R: Block of Na channels in the membrane of myelinated nerve by benzocaine, *Pflügers Arch* 390:230-236, 1981.
10. Cahalan MD, Almers W: Interactions between quaternary lidocaine, the sodium channel gates, and tetrodotoxin, *Biophys J* 27:39-56, 1979.
11. Covino BG: Toxicity and systemic effects of local anesthetic agents. In Strichartz GR, editor: *Local anesthetics: handbook of experimental pharmacology*, vol 81, Berlin, 1987, Springer-Verlag.
12. Strichartz GR, Sanchez V, Arthur GR, et al: Fundamental properties of local anesthetics. II. Measured octanol:buffer partition coefficients and pK_a values of clinically used drugs, *Anesth Analg* 71:158-170, 1990.
13. Gasser HS, Erlanger J: The role of fiber size in the establishment of a nerve block by pressure or cocaine, *Am J Physiol* 88:581-591, 1929.
14. Franz DN, Perry RS: Mechanisms for differential block among single myelinated and nonmyelinated axons by procaine, *J Physiol (Lond)* 236:193-210, 1974.
15. Fink BR: Mechanisms of differential axial blockade in epidural and subarachnoid anesthesia, *Anesthesiology* 70:851-858, 1989.
16. Raymond SA, Steffensen SC, et al: The role of length of nerve exposed to local anesthetics in impulse blocking action, *Anesth Analg* 68:563-570, 1989.
17. Balser JR: Structure and function of the cardiac sodium channels, *Cardiovasc Res* 42:327-338, 1999.
18. Sunami A, Glaaser IW, Fozzard HA: Structural and gating changes of the sodium channel induced by mutation of a residue in the upper third of IVS6, creating an external access path for local anesthetics, *Mol Pharmacol* 59:684-691, 2001.

19. Courtney KR, Strichartz GR: Structural elements that determine local anesthetic activity. In Strichartz GR, editor: *Local anesthetics: handbook of experimental pharmacology,* vol 81, Berlin, 1987, Springer-Verlag.

20. Scurlock JE, Meymaris E, Gregus J: The clinical character of local anesthetics: a function of frequency-dependent conduction block, *Acta Anaesthesiol Scand* 22:601-608, 1978.

21. Clarkson CW, Hondeghem LM: Evidence for a specific receptor site for lidocaine, quinidine, and bupivacaine associated with cardiac sodium channels in guinea pig ventricular myocardium, *Circ Res* 56:496-506, 1985.

22. Brau ME, Nau C, Hempelmann G, et al: Local anesthetics potently block a potential insensitive potassium channel in myelinated nerve, *J Gen Physiol* 105:485-505, 1995.

23. Punnia-Moorthy A: Buffering capacity of normal and inflamed tissues following the injection of local anaesthetic solutions, *Br J Anaesth* 61:154-159, 1988.

24. Brown RD: The failure of local anaesthesia in acute inflammation: some recent concepts, *Br Dent J* 151:47-51, 1981.

25. Arthur GR: Pharmacokinetics of local anesthetics. In Strichartz GR, editor: *Local anesthetics: handbook of experimental pharmacology,* vol 81, Berlin, 1987, Springer-Verlag.

26. Benowitz N, Forsyth RP, Melmon KL, et al: Lidocaine disposition kinetics in monkey and man. I. Prediction by a perfusion model, *Clin Pharmacol Ther* 16:87-98, 1974.

27. Jorfeldt L, Lewis DH, Löfström JB, et al: Lung uptake of lidocaine in healthy volunteers, *Acta Anaesthesiol Scand* 23:567-574, 1979.

28. Tucker GT, Mather LE: Pharmacokinetics of local anaesthetic agents, *Br J Anaesth* 47:213-224, 1975.

29. Tucker GT, Mather LE: Clinical pharmacokinetics of local anaesthetics, *Clin Pharmacokinet* 4:241-278, 1979.

30. Arthur GR, Scott DHT, Boyes RN, et al: Pharmacokinetic and clinical pharmacological studies with mepivacaine and prilocaine, *Br J Anaesth* 51:481-485, 1979.

31. Elvin AT, Cole AFD, Pieper JA, et al: Effect of food on lidocaine kinetics: mechanism of food-related alteration in high intrinsic clearance drug elimination, *Clin Pharmacol Ther* 30:455-460, 1981.

32. Feely J, Wade D, McAllister CB, et al: Effect of hypotension on liver blood flow and lidocaine disposition, *N Engl J Med* 307:866-869, 1982.

33. Bax NDS, Tucker GT, Lennard MS, et al: The impairment of lignocaine clearance by propranolol: major contribution from enzyme inhibition, *Br J Clin Pharmacol* 19:597-603, 1985.

34. Jackson JE, Bentley JB, Glass SJ, et al: Effects of histamine-2 receptor blockade on lidocaine kinetics, *Clin Pharmacol Ther* 37:544-548, 1985.

35. Abernethy DR, Greenblatt DJ: Impairment of lidocaine clearance in elderly male subjects, *J Cardiovasc Pharmacol* 5:1093-1096, 1983.

36. Nation RL, Triggs EJ: Lignocaine kinetics in cardiac patients and aged subjects, *Br J Clin Pharmacol* 4:439-448, 1977.

37. Klein SW, Sutherland RIL, Morch JE: Hemodynamic effects of intravenous lidocaine in man, *Can Med Assoc J* 99:472-475, 1968.

38. Sugimoto M, Uchida I, Fukami S, et al: The alpha and gamma subunit-dependent effects of local anesthetics on recombinant GABA$_{(A)}$ receptors, *Eur J Pharmacol* 401:329-337, 2000.

39. Löfström JB: Physiological effects of local anaesthetics on circulation and respiration. In Löfström JB, Sjöstrand U, editors: *Local anaesthesia and regional blockade: monographs in anaesthesiology,* vol 15, Amsterdam, 1988, Elsevier.

40. Dowd FJ, Matheny JL: Introduction to cardiovascular pharmacology: antiarrhythmic drugs. In Yagiela JA, Neidle EA, Dowd FJ, editors: *Pharmacology and therapeutics for dentistry,* ed 4, St Louis, 1998, Mosby.

41. Albright GA: Cardiac arrest following regional anesthesia with etidocaine or bupivacaine, *Anesthesiology* 51:285-287, 1979.

42. Rosen MA, Thigpen JW, Shnider SM, et al: Bupivacaine-induced cardiotoxicity in hypoxic and acidotic sheep, *Anesth Analg* 64:1089-1096, 1985.

43. Stark F, Malgat M, Dabadie P, et al: Comparison of the effects of bupivacaine and ropivacaine on heart cell mitochondrial bioenergetics, *Anesthesiology* 88:1340-1349, 1998.

44. Thomas RD, Behbehani MM, Coyle DE, et al: Cardiovascular toxicity of local anesthetics: an alternative hypothesis, *Anesth Analg* 65:444-450, 1986.

45. Heavner JE: Cardiac dysrhythmias induced by infusion of local anesthetics into the lateral cerebral ventricle of cats, *Anesth Analg* 65:133-138, 1986.

46. Foster RH, Markham A: Levobupivacaine: a review of its pharmacology and use as a local anaesthetic, *Drugs* 59:551-579, 2000.

47. Chang DH, Ladd LA, Copeland S, et al: Direct cardiac effects of intracoronary bupivacaine, levobupivacaine, and ropivacaine in sheep, *Br J Pharmacol* 132:649-658, 2001.

48. Goldstein DS, Dionne R, Sweet J, et al: Circulatory, plasma catecholamine, cortisol, lipid, and psychological responses to a real-life stress (third molar extractions): effects of diazepam sedation and inclusion of epinephrine with the local anesthetic, *Psychosomat Med* 44:259-272, 1982.

49. Chernow B, Balestrieri F, Ferguson CD, et al: Local dental anesthesia with epinephrine, *Arch Intern Med* 143:2141-2143, 1983.

50. Dionne RA, Goldstein DS, Wirdzek PR: Effects of diazepam premedication and epinephrine-containing local anesthetic on cardiovascular and plasma catecholamine responses to oral surgery, *Anesth Analg* 63:640-646, 1984.

51. Cioffi GA, Chernow B, Glahn RP, et al: The hemodynamic and plasma catecholamine responses to routine restorative dental care, *J Am Dent Assoc* 111:67-70, 1985.

52. Troullos ES, Goldstein DS, Hargreaves KM, et al: Plasma epinephrine levels and cardiovascular response to high administered doses of epinephrine in local anesthesia, *Anesth Prog* 34:10-13, 1987.

53. Knoll-Köhler E, Frie A, Becker J, et al: Changes in plasma epinephrine concentrations after dental infiltration anesthesia with different doses of epinephrine, *J Dent Res* 68:1098-1101, 1989.

54. Cryer PE: Physiology and pathophysiology of the human sympathoadrenal neuroendocrine system, *N Engl J Med* 303:436-444, 1980.

55. Kennedy WF Jr, Bonica JJ, Ward RJ, et al: Cardiorespiratory effects of epinephrine when used in regional anesthesia, *Acta Anaesthesiol Scand Suppl* 23:320-333, 1966.

56. Kaneko Y, Ichinohe T, Sakurai M, et al: Relationship between changes in circulation due to epinephrine oral injection and its plasma concentration, *Anesth Prog* 36:188-190, 1989.

57. Jastak JT, Yagiela JA: Vasoconstrictors and local anesthesia: a review and rationale for use, *J Am Dent Assoc* 107:623-630, 1983.

58. Minasian A, Yagiela JA: The use of amide local anesthetics in patients susceptible to malignant hyperthermia, *Oral Surg Oral Med Oral Pathol* 66:405-415, 1988.

59. Yagiela JA, Benoit PW, Buoncristiani RD, et al: Comparison of the myotoxic effects of lidocaine with epinephrine in rats and humans, *Anesth Analg* 60:471-480, 1981.

60. Ludwig SC: Acute toxic methemoglobinemia following dental analgesia, *Ann Emerg Med* 10:265-266, 1981.

61. Spielman FJ, Anderson JA, Terry WC: Benzocaine-induced methemoglobinemia during general anesthesia, *J Oral Maxillofac Surg* 42:740-743, 1984.

62. Borg T, Modig J: Potential anti-thrombotic effects of local anaesthetics due to their inhibition of platelet aggregation, *Acta Anaesthesiol Scand* 29:739-742, 1985.

63. Azuma Y, Shinohara M, Wang PL, et al: Comparison of inhibitory effects of local anesthetics on immune functions of neutrophils, *Int J Immunopharmacol* 22:789-796, 2000.

64. Cassuto J, Nellgård P, Stage L, et al: Amide local anesthetics reduce albumin extravasation in burn injuries, *Anesthesiology* 72:302-307, 1990.

65. Abraham ZA, Lees DE: Two cardiac arrests after needle punctures in a patient with mitral valve prolapse: psychogenic? *Anesth Analg* 69:126-128, 1989.

66. Schwartz HJ, Sher TH: Bisulfite sensitivity manifesting as allergy to local dental anesthesia, *J Allergy Clin Immunol* 75:525-527, 1985.

67. Simon RA: Sulfite sensitivity, *Ann Allergy* 56:281-288, 1986.

68. Kaufman E, LeResche L, Sommers E, et al: Intraligamentary anesthesia: a double-blind comparative study, *J Am Dent Assoc* 108:175-178, 1984.

69. Edwards RW, Head TW: A clinical trial of intraligamentary anesthesia, *J Dent Res* 68:1210-1214, 1989.

70. Replogle K, Reader A, Nist R, et al: Anesthetic efficacy of the intraosseous injection of 2% lidocaine (1:100,000 epinephrine) and 3% mepivacaine in mandibular first molars, *Oral Surg Oral Med Oral Pathol Oral Radiol Endod* 83:30-37, 1997.

71. Danielsson K, Evers H, Holmlund A, et al: Long-acting local anaesthetics in oral surgery: clinical evaluation of bupivacaine and etidocaine for mandibular nerve block, *Int J Oral Maxillofac Surg* 15:119-126, 1986.

72. Danielsson K, Evers H, Nordenram Å: Long-acting local anesthetics in oral surgery: an experimental evaluation of bupivacaine and etidocaine for oral infiltration anesthesia, *Anesth Prog* 32:65-68, 1985.

73. USP Dispensing Information: *Drug information for the health care professional*, vol 1, ed 20, Englewood, Colo, 2000, Micromedex.

74. Berquist HC: The danger of mepivacaine 3% toxicity in children, *J Calif Dent Assoc* 3(9):13, 1975.

75. Goodson JM, Moore PA: Life-threatening reactions after pedodontic sedation: an assessment of narcotic, local anesthetic, and antiemetic drug interaction, *J Am Dent Assoc* 107:239-245, 1983.

76. Yagiela JA: Adverse drug interactions in dental practice: interactions associated with vasoconstrictors, *J Am Dent Assoc* 130:701-709, 1999.

77. Yagiela JA: COMT inhibitors and epinephrine: a new drug interaction? *Pulse* 33:1,4, 2001.

78. Niwa H, Satoh Y, Matsuura H: Cardiovascular responses to epinephrine-containing local anesthetics for dental use: a comparison of hemodynamic responses to infiltration anesthesia and ergometer-stress testing, *Oral Surg Oral Med Oral Pathol Oral Radiol Endod* 90:171-181, 2000.

79. Kaplan EL, editor: *Cardiovascular disease in dental practice*, Dallas, 1986, American Heart Association.

80. Haas DA, Harper DG, Saso MA, et al: Lack of differential effect by Ultracaine (articaine) and Citanest (prilocaine) in infiltration anaesthesia, *J Can Dent Assoc* 57:217-223, 1991.

81. Malamed SF, Gagnon S, Leblanc D: Efficacy of articaine: a new amide local anesthetic, *J Am Dent Assoc* 131:635-642, 2000.

82. Haas DA, Lennon D: A 21-year retrospective study of reports of paresthesia following local anesthetic administration, *J Can Dent Assoc* 61:319-320, 323-326, 329-330, 1995.

CHAPTER 7

Therapeutic Uses of Non-Opioid Analgesics

RAYMOND A. DIONNE
CHARLES BERTHOLD
STEPHEN A. COOPER

CHAPTER OUTLINE

The management of pain and inflammation in dentistry has several unique features. Pain not only signals tissue injury but also impedes most dental procedures, delays the resumption of normal activities after dental surgical procedures, and lessens the likelihood of patients seeking dental procedures in the future. Although pain during therapy is usually adequately controlled by local anesthesia, postoperative pain control is often inadequate either because of insufficient pain relief or unacceptable side effects. Inadequate pain control can lead to overuse of medication or too-frequent readministration of prescribed drugs. Side effects from opioids, such as drowsiness, nausea, and vomiting, occur with greater frequency in ambulatory dental patients than in nonambulatory hospitalized patients. In addition, inadequate pain control during the immediate postoperative period may contribute to the development of hyperalgesia,[1] leading to greater pain at later time points during recovery. Pain associated with dentistry also contributes to apprehension about future dental care to the extent that patients frequently report being very nervous or terrified at the prospect of dental care.[2] These considerations indicate that optimal analgesic therapy for ambulatory dental patients should be efficacious with a minimum incidence of side effects, and, ideally, should lessen the prospect of pain associated with future dental therapy.

Nonsteroidal antiinflammatory drugs (NSAIDs) are the mainstay of therapy for the management of acute dental pain. They have also been evaluated for chronic orofacial pain, for minimizing edema after surgical procedures, and for endodontic pain. When used as directed, over-the-counter (OTC) dosing regimens for ibuprofen, ketoprofen, or naproxen sodium are safe and effective for most patients with a wide variety of dental pain conditions.[3] The toxicity associated with chronic high dose NSAID administration is well documented, suggesting the need to carefully weigh the benefit-to-risk relationship for each therapeutic indication. The new generation of selective cyclooxygenase-2 (COX-2) inhibitors holds promise for achieving the therapeutic effects of traditional NSAIDs without the toxic renal and gastrointestinal (GI) effects but have not been adequately studied for dental indications or for large numbers of subjects. The use of NSAIDs for dentistry are presented with their documented toxic effects to suggest rational uses and therapeutic applications that should be reevaluated in future studies.

Salicylates

Salicylates, in the form of willow bark, were introduced to medicine as analgesics in 1763. Salicyclic acid was derived from salicin, the active agent in willow bark, in 1838. The synthesis of acetylsalicylic acid (aspirin) eventually resulted in the displacement of salicylate derived from naturally occurring sources (Box 7-1). Since its introduction in 1899, aspirin has been widely used for its analgesic, antipyretic, antiinflammatory, and antirheumatic effects. Only recently has the probable mechanism of action of salicylates been identified as the inhibition of prostaglandin synthesis, which blocks the initial oxygenation of arachidonic acid by cyclooxygenase.

Aspirin

Aspirin is a weak acid that is well absorbed from the GI tract when taken orally. Its ability to dissociate favors absorption from the stomach, but it is principally absorbed from the small intestine because of its greater surface area. Acetylsalicylic acid is rapidly metabolized to salicylic acid by plasma and gastric esterases. Salicylate, an active form of aspirin, is widely distributed in the body, metabolized mainly in the liver by conjugation, and excreted in the urine mostly as salicyluric acid.

Although the efficacy of aspirin has been accepted for several generations based on more than 100 years of clinical use, controlled studies have documented its efficacy for dental pain only during the past 20 years. A double-blind controlled study demonstrated that aspirin 650 mg was more effective than codeine 30 mg and placebo in relieving postoperative pain from third molar extractions.[4] The ceiling analgesic

---

■ BOX 7-1   SUMMARY

Salicylates

Aspirin produces gastric irritation and increases bleeding time at therapeutic doses.

NSAIDs should not be administered to patients with a history of allergy to aspirin.

Diflunisal is an alternative to aspirin and other NSAIDs when prolonged duration of action represents a therapeutic benefit.

dose was originally thought to be 650 mg. A dose of aspirin 1200 mg, however, had a significantly greater analgesic effect than aspirin 600 mg when evaluated in the oral surgery model.[5] Numerous studies have shown the efficacy of aspirin in the relief of dental pain, and it is a standard of comparison for other oral analgesics. Aspirin is generally accepted to be as potent as acetaminophen in terms of its analgesic and antipyretic effects, but the antiinflammatory property of acetaminophen is considered to be weak. Aspirin is more effective than codeine 60 mg [4] but is less efficacious than ibuprofen 400 mg.[6]

Aspirin has several side effects that frequently cause people to substitute other nonopioids. The most commonly reported side effects are epigastric distress, nausea, ulceration, and, less frequently, vomiting. Aspirin-induced GI injury results from two known mechanisms. Local irritation of the mucosal lining allows diffusion of acid into the mucosa with subsequent tissue damage. In addition, gastric prostaglandins that inhibit secretion of acid and promote secretion of cytoprotective mucus are inhibited by aspirin. For this reason, aspirin is contraindicated for patients with GI ulcers. Through its inhibition of prostaglandin synthesis, aspirin has also been shown to affect platelet function, which may result in prolonged bleeding time when aspirin is used after surgery. Aspirin should not be given to patients with liver disease, hypothrombinemia, hemophilia, or vitamin K deficiency, and it should also be avoided in patients who are taking anticoagulant drugs.

Allergic reactions to aspirin are uncommon but are more frequently seen in persons with asthma, nasal polyps, or a history of an allergic reaction to other aspirin-like drugs (including NSAIDs). Aspirin interactions with insulin or oral hypoglycemic agents may result in a greater hypoglycemic effect; an alternative nonopioid analgesic should be considered for patients taking one of these agents.

Aspirin is commonly available in effervescent, plain tablet, sustained-release, and enteric-coated forms. The effervescent form of aspirin (Alka-Seltzer) gives a higher peak plasma concentration than the plain tablet or sustained-release preparations.[7] Absorption from enteric-coated tablets is slower and occasionally incomplete and could lead to a slower onset of pain relief. Thus rapid onset, which is often critical for acute pain, is best achieved with the effervescent form of aspirin. The relationship between plasma levels and therapeutic effect is indirect, and no fixed dose, schedule, or dosage form will provide the desired result in all patients. The maximum recommended dosage is 650 mg every 4 hours (3900 mg/day) or 500 to 1000 mg every 4 hours, up to a maximum dosage of 4000 mg/day.

Diflunisal

Diflunisal, a salicylic acid derivative (5-[2,4-difluropheny]salicylic acid), is more effective than aspirin and has fewer GI and hematologic adverse effects. Evaluation in the oral surgery model demonstrates that diflunisal has greater peak analgesia than aspirin 650 mg and a duration of effect up to 12 hours, making a twice-daily dosing regimen possible.[8] In another oral surgery study, mean bleeding time for the group increased by 53%, but the increase did not exceed the upper limit of normal bleeding time for any patient.[9] The tendency for intraoperative or postoperative bleeding did not increase. These studies indicate that diflunisal is an alternative to aspirin and other NSAIDs in situations where prolonged duration of action presents a therapeutic benefit.

Acetaminophen and Phenacetin

Acetaminophen and phenacetin are derivatives of acetanilide, which was introduced to medical practice in the 1800s as an analgesic and antipyretic but was soon abandoned because of toxicity (cynanosis from methemoglobinemia). Phenacetin was subsequently developed as a less toxic alternative to acetanilide. Acetaminophen is the active metabolite of phenacetin and has been widely used as an alternative to aspirin for the treatment of mild-to-moderate pain (Box 7-2). Phenacetin was primarily used in combination with aspirin and caffeine (APC tablets), but it was removed from the U.S. market because of its possible relationship to renal papillary necrosis.

BOX 7-2   SUMMARY

Acetaminophen

Acetaminophen is as potent as aspirin but has fewer side effects.

Acetaminophen is the preferred analgesic when salicylates or NSAIDs are contraindicated.

Acetaminophen

Acetaminophen is generally thought to be as potent as aspirin, but it has fewer side effects. The mechanism of action of acetaminophen remains unclear because it is only a weak inhibitor of peripheral prostaglandin synthesis and appears to be active in the central nervous system (CNS). It does not inhibit platelet aggregation. Its antiinflammatory properties have not been well demonstrated, although it significantly reduced swelling compared with placebo in a postextraction study.[10] Acetaminophen has been shown to be as potent as aspirin after third molar extraction.[11] Increasing the dose of acetaminophen to 1000 mg increases analgesia, and this dose is superior to codeine 60 mg.[12]

Acetaminophen is indicated for the relief of mild-to-moderate pain of dental origin. It is the preferred analgesic for patients in whom salicylates and NSAIDs are contraindicated because of GI disease, aspirin hypersensitivity, or prolonged bleeding time.

Preexisting liver disease increases the likelihood of a serious hepatotoxic reaction to an overdose of acetaminophen. Acetaminophen is well tolerated at therapeutic doses and has no common adverse effects. An overdose greater than 10 g may cause serious, irreversible hepatic toxicity, which can be fatal in some patients. If overdose is suspected, acetylcysteine (Mucomyst) should be administered within 24 hours under a physician's direction.

The usual dosage is 650 mg every 4 to 6 hours, not to exceed 4000 mg/day. Acetaminophen is also available in 500-mg tablets and caplets for administration 3 to 4 times daily, not to exceed 4000 mg/day.

Nonsteroidal Antiinflammatory Drugs

Knowledge of the clinical pharmacology of NSAIDs is based largely on studies performed in the oral surgery model.[4] Ibuprofen, the prototype of the NSAID class, has demonstrated analgesic activity over a dose range from 200 to 800 mg with a duration of activity from 4 to 6 hours.[6,13] When given before the onset of pain, ibuprofen suppresses the onset of pain and lessens the severity.[14,15] Ibuprofen suppresses swelling over the initial 2- to 3-day postoperative course when edema formation associated with the inflammatory process is most prominent. Interactions with the release of β-endorphin have been demonstrated both intraoperatively during surgical stress and during postoperative pain, suggesting that NSAIDs can modify the neurohumoral responses to

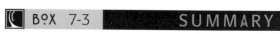

pain.[16,17] The wealth of data from clinical trials using NSAIDs makes it one of the most well-studied drug classes for acute inflammatory pain in ambulatory patients (Box 7-3).

Ibuprofen

Ibuprofen is the prototype of the NSAID class of analgesics that was first introduced to clinical practice in the United States in 1974. It is particularly useful for conditions in which aspirin or acetaminophen does not result in adequate pain relief or where the use of opioid-containing combinations would likely result in CNS or GI side effects. It is widely prescribed for acute and chronic orofacial pain in doses of 600 to 800 mg and as a nonprescription analgesic in 200- to 400-mg dosages up to 1200 mg/day.

A 400-mg dose of ibuprofen has been found superior to aspirin 650 mg, acetaminophen 600 to 1000 mg, and combinations of aspirin and acetaminophen plus codeine 60 mg.[6,18,19] A single dose of ibuprofen 400 mg or administration of multiple doses up to 5 days postoperatively was superior to dihydrocodeine 30 mg in the oral surgery model.[20,21] Administration of doses greater than 400 mg is not likely to result in greater peak relief, but increased drug blood levels may modestly prolong the duration of effect.[13]

Ibuprofen is comparable to other NSAIDs when evaluated in the oral surgery model. Ibuprofen 400 mg produces analgesia similar to meclofenamate sodium 100 mg but with a lower incidence of stomach pain and diarrhea.[22] Ibuprofen 200 mg results in similar onset and peak analgesia but has a shorter duration than naproxen sodium 220 mg when evaluated up to 12 hours after a single dose.[23] The shorter duration demonstrated has little clinical significance, since the normal dosing interval for low-dose ibuprofen is every 4 to 6 hours. The 400-mg dose of ibuprofen was also similar to a suspension formulation of diclofenac in a study with large sample sizes ($n = 80$ to 83) sufficient to detect differences.[24] No advantage could be demonstrated between tablets and soluble formulations of ibuprofen 200 mg, 400 mg, and 600 mg evaluated up to 6 hours postoperatively.[25] No dose-related difference could be demonstrated in this study between the 400-mg and 600-mg dose of either formulation, supporting the generalization that there is little advantage in increasing the dose of ibuprofen to 600 mg. Recent evidence suggests that solubilized ibuprofen has a faster onset of effect when compared with acetaminophen.[26]

Ibuprofen has also been evaluated for dental pain of other causes. Periodontal surgery involves elevation of a surgical flap often extending over a quarter of the mouth or more, osseous reshaping, and implantation of materials to replace bone lost to the disease process and can last 2 to 3 hours. Ibuprofen in doses of 200 and 400 mg was demonstrated to be superior to placebo in a single dose, 6-hour observation after periodontal surgery.[27] Comparison of ibuprofen 600 mg given either immediately before periodontal surgery or after the procedure demonstrated a suppression of pain intensity compared with placebo over the first 8 hours after surgery.[28] No clinical studies have reported a noticeable increase in postsurgical bleeding.

Patients undergoing orthodontic tooth movement can experience varying degrees of discomfort, especially over the first few days after placement or adjustment of orthodontic devices. Administration of a single dose of ibuprofen 400 mg compared with aspirin 650 mg and placebo demonstrated that both active drugs suppressed pain compared with placebo up to 7 days after placement of orthodontic devices.[29] Ibuprofen was superior to aspirin at most intervals during the first 2 days, which suggests that it is more effective for suppressing the inflammatory response normally seen after orthodontic adjustments.

A less well-characterized indication for the use of NSAIDs is the management of endodontic pain. Acute pain from pulpal or periapical tissues is a major reason why patients seek urgent dental care. Although the management of pain with endodontic treatment is primarily aimed at removing the necrotic or inflamed tissue, a variety of proinflammatory mediators are released and may contribute to postoperative discomfort. Mechanical debridement and the use of canal medicaments also contribute to periapical inflammation that persists beyond the duration of local anesthesia. Although the results of analgesic studies using the oral surgery model should generalize to endodontic pain, a few studies have directly addressed the use of NSAIDs for endodontic procedures.

Ibuprofen was compared with a wide variety of treatments after an endodontic procedure (root canal obturation), but none of the nine active treatments could be differentiated from placebo.[30] This result may reflect a lack of assay sensitivity for this model, since only 4% of the patient sample ($N = 411$) developed moderate or severe pain, and the remainder reported having either no pain or mild pain. Endodontic pain has previously been demonstrated as being sensitive to the effects of NSAIDs,[31] but only when subjects who are symptomatic before the procedure are included in the analyses. Most patients who have no pain before an endodontic procedure report little pain postoperatively.[32]

Naproxen and Naproxen Sodium

Naproxen is also a propionic acid derivative but is longer-acting than ibuprofen. It is the only NSAID administered as a pure enantiomer, the S (+) isomer. It is available in two formulations, with the sodium salt being more rapidly absorbed than naproxen. The different formulations should not be used concomitantly because they both circulate in the plasma as the naproxen anion, and the resultant additive plasma concentration increases the possibility of dose-related adverse effects. An initial loading dose of 500 to 550 mg is used to reach therapeutic levels more rapidly, and subsequent doses of 250 to 275 mg are given at 6- to 8-hour levels. A single 550-mg dose of naproxen sodium has greater analgesic activity than aspirin 650 mg and has a lower incidence of side effects.[33] A repeat-dose comparison of naproxen 500 mg twice/day with aspirin 650 mg for 3 days after oral surgery also demonstrated greater efficacy and fewer side effects for naproxen.[34] For dental pain, naproxen 550 mg was found more efficacious than aspirin 325 mg plus codeine 60 mg.[35] This combination, however, is half the normal therapeutic dose of aspirin and codeine when used in combination (i.e., acetaminophen 650 mg plus codeine 60 mg). Both preoperative naproxen and naproxen administered 30 minutes after oral surgery suppress pain over the first 8 hours after surgery.[36] The lack of a parallel placebo group, however, makes it difficult to determine if this result represents an equal suppression of postoperative pain by treatment regimens or a lack of assay sensitivity.

OTC naproxen sodium is available in a formulation containing 220 mg with a recommended dosage of 1 to 2 tablets twice/day. Naproxen's long half-life is an advantage if effective pain relief is achieved, but in patients with inadequate relief, the long half-life prevents administration of a second dose for 8 to 12 hours. A review of 48 randomized, double-blind, clinical studies (25 in the dental pain model) indicates no overall difference in the rate of adverse events seen for naproxen sodium compared with placebo, ibuprofen, or acetaminophen.[37] These data suggest that OTC naproxen is well tolerated even when administered without professional supervision.

Ketoprofen

Ketoprofen is chemically related to other proprionic acid derivatives with analgesic and antipyretic properties. It acts peripherally via inhibition of prostaglandin and leukotriene synthesis (similar to other NSAIDs) but is also thought to act centrally.[38] Ketoprofen is as effective as an analgesic for the relief of mild-to-moderate pain in doses ranging from 25 to 150 mg with greater efficacy than aspirin 650 mg[39] or codeine 90 mg.[40] Ketoprofen 25 mg is therapeutically equivalent to ibuprofen tablets 400 mg (Fig. 7-1) in the oral surgery model.[39]

Ketoprofen has been administered locally to the site of injury, although it is not an indicated route of administration, to decrease systemic exposure to NSAIDs. A 10-mg formulation placed directly into an extraction site 1 hour after oral surgery resulted in significantly less analgesia compared with placebo. Peripheral administration of the 10-mg dose also resulted in greater analgesia than oral administration of the same dose formulation.[41] These data indicate that administration of an NSAID to a peripheral site of tissue injury results in greater analgesia than oral administration and suggest the potential for less drug toxicity through lower circulating drug levels.

Etodolac

Etodolac is indicated as an analgesic based on activity in the oral surgery model and has a more favorable profile of GI safety. In a dose-range study (50, 100, and 200 mg), the analgesic effect of the 200-mg dose of etodolac was significantly greater than placebo for vir-

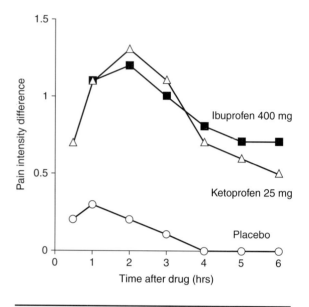

Fig. 7-1 Analgesic equivalency of ibuprofen and ketoprofen at usual analgesic doses.

tually all measures of analgesia. Although the 200-mg dose of etodolac was similar in efficacy to aspirin, it resulted in a duration that was approximately twice as long. All study medications were equally well tolerated.[42] A study comparing etodolac 300 mg to the combination of acetaminophen with hydrocodone for postoperative pain after periodontal surgery found the drugs to be equivalent over the first 8 hours.[43] Etodolac administered preoperatively, however, suppressed the time to the first postoperative dose of medication, supporting the value of preventive analgesic treatment in this model. These data suggest therapeutic equivalence for etodolac to other commonly used analgesics.

Etodolac is reported to be tenfold more selective for COX-2 compared with its effect on COX-1. This sparing of COX-1 activity gives rise to greater gastric tolerance, which has been demonstrated in many studies.[44] These limited data in the oral surgery model suggest that etodolac is useful as an analgesic for dental indications with a prolonged duration of action and favorable GI safety with repeated administration.

Ketorolac

Ketorolac is the only NSAID approved for parenteral administration for the short-term management of moderate-to-severe pain, and it has been used successfully even in selected pediatric cases. It is comparable to intramuscular (IM) meperidine 100 mg and IM morphine 10 mg in a number of analgesic models with similar onset and analgesic efficacy, and it is longer-acting.[45,46] Ketorolac causes less drowsiness, nausea, and vomiting than morphine 12 mg.[47] The ability of injectable ketorolac to overcome the slower onset of orally administered drugs combined with analgesic efficacy comparable to parenteral opioids and reduced side effects (Fig. 7-2) suggests that it is preferred for the management of pain not adequately controlled by other NSAIDs or opioid combinations. This parenteral route of administration, however, limits its use for ambulatory patients to the initial dose before discharge.

Local administration of injectable ketorolac 30 mg in endodontic emergency patients after pulpotomy produced significant analgesic effects.[48] An interesting observation was demonstration of analgesic effects for the mandibular infiltration, contrary to the poor efficacy usually reported for local anesthetic infiltration in the mandible. Also, the presence of inflammation did not hinder the analgesic effect of ketorolac infiltration, nor did the injection result in any tissue irritation. These data, although gathered from only one study, suggest that the intraoral injection of ketorolac may be a useful adjunct for the management of endodontic pain, especially in cases where local anesthetic administration is ineffective because of inflammation or injections located at a mandibular site.

Ketorolac is also available for oral administration at a dosage of 10 mg every 4 to 6 hours; the total daily dose should not exceed 40 mg. Labeling now recommends that oral ketorolac be used only when the injectable form has first been administered. For oral surgery pain, a single dose of oral ketorolac 10 mg is superior to acetaminophen 600 mg and acetaminophen 600 mg plus codeine 60 mg but is therapeutically equivalent to ibuprofen 400 mg.[49] Oral administration of ketorolac results in faster absorption than after IM administration.[50] The lower recommended oral dose (10 mg) compared with the parenteral dose (30 to 60 mg), however, results in much lower peak blood levels with less analgesia than parenteral ketorolac.

Meclofenamate Sodium

Meclofenamate sodium is an NSAID with analgesic, antiinflammatory, and antipyretic activity. It acts simultaneously to inhibit both the cyclooxygenase and

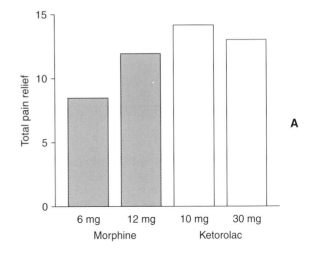

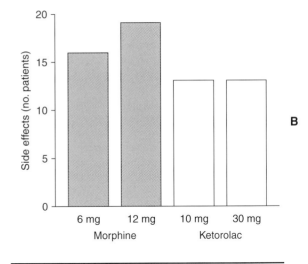

Fig. 7-2 Demonstration of analgesic efficacy for the NSAID ketorolac approximately equivalent to therapeutic doses of morphine **(A)** but with a lower incidence of side effects **(B).**

lipoxygenase pathways, resulting in reduced formation of prostaglandins and leukotrienes.[51] In the oral surgery model, meclofenamic acid results in analgesia superior to aspirin,[52] acetaminophen,[53] and acetaminophen plus codeine.[53] Unlike other NSAIDs, it does not significantly interfere with platelet aggregation or prolonged bleeding. This drug is not commonly used for acute pain in clinical practice because of the incidence of diarrhea with repeated dosing.

Piroxicam

Piroxicam is an oxicam NSAID. Its plasma half-life has been estimated at 45 hours, allowing once-daily dosing, with peak plasma concentration occurring 2 to 4 hours after oral administration.[54] Piroxicam in single doses of 20 to 40 mg has been shown to produce analgesia approximately equivalent to aspirin 648 mg with a longer duration.[55] Piroxicam (40 mg) preoperatively before third molar surgery (under general anesthesia) significantly reduced the number of those patients requiring opioid analgesia and also reduced the doses of paracetemol over the first 24 hours postoperatively.[56] These limited data suggest that piroxicam has less efficacy than other NSAIDs but has a longer duration of action. Longer duration does not necessarily represent a therapeutic advantage because patients will often take pain-relief medications before the recommended dosing interval if analgesia is inadequate, introducing the possibility of cumulative GI damage.[57] Piroxicam is not commonly used in clinical practice because of these limitations.

Preventive Analgesia

Most studies in which an NSAID is administered orally after onset of pain demonstrate an onset of activity within 30 minutes and peak analgesic activity at 2 to 3 hours after drug administration (Box 7-4). An early attempt to optimize ibuprofen analgesia in the immediate postoperative period after local anesthesia offset involved administration of the drug before oral surgery. This allows sufficient time for drug absorption during the surgical procedure and the 1- to 2-hour duration of standard local anesthetics postoperatively. Preoperative administration of ibuprofen 400 mg increased the time to the first postoperative dose of analgesic by approximately 2 hours compared with placebo pretreatment.[14] A subsequent study demonstrated that preoperative administration of ibuprofen 800 mg significantly lowered pain intensity over the first 3 hours after surgery as the residual effects of the local anesthetic dissipated.[15] Administration of a second dose of ibuprofen 4 hours after the initial dose extended this preventive analgesic effect to result in less pain than placebo, acetaminophen (given both preoperatively and postoperatively), or acetaminophen plus codeine 60 mg (administered postoperatively). The ability to suppress the onset and lower the intensity of postoperative pain up to 8 hours is repli-

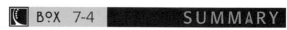

BOX 7-4 SUMMARY

Preventive Analgesia

Administration of NSAIDs in the perioperative period before local anesthetic offset delays the onset of postoperative pain and lowers its intensity.

Blockade of prostanoids formed by constitutive COX-1 during and immediately after surgery is less important than suppression of the products of inducible COX-2 during the first few hours after surgery.

cable[58,59] and extends to the use of other NSAIDs, such as flurbiprofen.[60]

Comparison of ibuprofen administration before periodontal surgery versus administration immediately after surgery demonstrated that both groups experienced a significant delay in pain onset compared with placebo.[28] A similar study in the oral surgery model using naproxen also could not differentiate between preoperative or postoperative administration,[36] suggesting that preoperative administration is not critical for suppressing pain onset. Recognition of the induction of COX-2 in the postoperative period[61] suggests that blockade of the formation of prostanoids released during surgery by constitutive COX-1 is less important than suppression of COX-2 and prostanoid release during the postoperative period. Consistent with this observation is the demonstration that both preoperative and postoperative administration of ibuprofen 800 mg are equally effective at suppressing pain and prostaglandin E_2 (PGE_2) levels at the extraction site (Fig. 7-3).[62] Ibuprofen and other NSAIDs given before the induction of COX-2 and subsequent release of prostanoids as a preventive analgesic strategy suppress pain in the immediate postoperative period and inhibit peripheral and central hyperalgesia that cause pain at later intervals.

Analgesic Activity of Ibuprofen Isomers

The biologic actions of NSAIDs often reside partly or exclusively in one of the enantiomers. When 2-arylpropionic acids, such as ibuprofen, are tested for cyclooxygenase inhibition in vitro, the activity resides almost exclusively in the S (+) isomer. Ibuprofen is synthesized and administered clinically as a racemic mixture of the S (+) and R (−) isomers. A unidirectional conversion of the inactive R (−) isomer to the

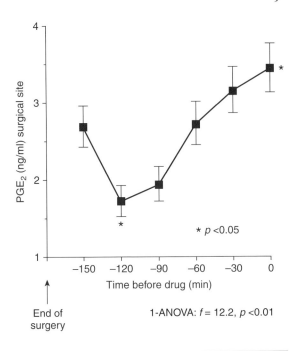

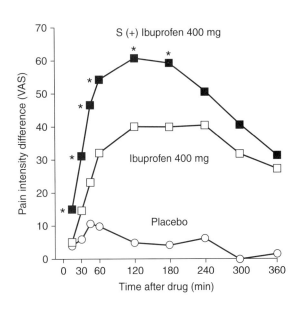

Fig. 7-3 Mean levels of prostaglandin E_2 (PGE_2) after oral surgery as collected by a microdialysis probe placed under the mucoperiosteal flap.

Fig. 7-4 Greater analgesia after administration of the S (+) isomer of ibuprofen compared with racemic ibuprofen at the same dose.

pharmacologically active S (+) isomer results in metabolic activation of the racemic drug. When given in equal amounts of the S (+) isomer (i.e., racemic ibuprofen 400 mg versus S [+] isomer 200 mg), both drugs should be essentially the same. The racemic mixture may even have a slightly longer duration of action because conversion of the R (−) isomer is converted to the S (+) isomer over time. Conversely, conversion of racemic ibuprofen to the active S (+) isomer may contribute to variability in analgesia among individuals and may explain the poor relationship observed between plasma concentrations of ibuprofen and clinical response for acute pain[13] and rheumatoid arthritis.[63] Administration of 400 mg of S (+) ibuprofen results in greater analgesia than an equivalent milligram dose of racemic ibuprofen (Fig. 7-4), presumably a result of the twofold greater amount of the active S (+) isomer.

Recognition of the differential effects of the two enantiomers of ibuprofen suggests that any delay in onset associated with administration of racemic ibuprofen is because less of the S (+) enantiomer is given. The resulting delay in hepatic conversion of the inactive form results in therapeutic levels of the active isomer. Similarly, the peak analgesic effect of racemic ibuprofen may be limited by the concentration of the S (+) isomer achieved by the balance among the amount administered in the racemic mixture, incomplete conversion of the R (−) isomer to the S (+) isomer, and faster renal elimination of the R (−) isomer than the S (+) isomer. Differences among individuals in the therapeutic response to racemic ibuprofen may be related to variability in the pharmacokinetic activation of the active isomer of ibuprofen.

NSAID-Opioid Combinations

Although ibuprofen and related NSAIDs have proved effective for dental pain, their lack of a central effect and their inability to enhance analgesia with increasing doses has led to combining ibuprofen with orally effective opioids, a reinvention of the classic analgesic combination (Box 7-5). Results, however, generally have been disappointing.

▉ B⚬X 7-5 — SUMMARY

Nonsteroidal Antiinflammatory–Containing Combinations

> Combining an NSAID with an opioid results in additive analgesia but has increased side effects, especially in ambulatory patients.
>
> A full therapeutic dose of each ingredient in the combination is needed to achieve a genuine therapeutic advantage.
>
> One tablet of the fixed-dose combination of ibuprofen 200 mg and hydrocodone 7.5 mg should be administered with ibuprofen 200 to 400 mg to result in the normal analgesic dose of ibuprofen and an additive effect of the opioid with acceptable side effects.

Ibuprofen Plus Codeine

Cooper[64] evaluated the combination of a single dose of ibuprofen 400 mg plus codeine 60 mg compared with each drug alone, placebo, and the combination of aspirin 650 mg plus codeine 60 mg. Although the ibuprofen plus codeine combination resulted in slightly higher mean hourly analgesic scores and produced substantially greater analgesia than codeine 60 mg, the combination did not produce significantly greater analgesia than ibuprofen 400 mg alone. Comparison of ibuprofen 400 mg plus codeine 60 mg with ibuprofen 400 mg in another study demonstrated significant differences on several, but not all, derived measures of analgesic activity.[65] Side effects were more frequent after the opioid-containing combination but consisted of minor adverse events such as drowsiness and "faintness." McQuay[66] demonstrated a 30% increase in analgesic effect with the addition of codeine 20 mg to ibuprofen 400 mg in a crossover study with two doses of the drugs being evaluated. With this lower dose of codeine, no tendency for greater incidence of adverse effects was detected, and more than 70% of subjects expressed a preference for the combination.

These and other similar studies provide a basis for adding codeine to a 400-mg dose of ibuprofen as needed to produce additive analgesia but will result in a dose-related increase in side effects. A minimum dose of codeine 20 to 30 mg is needed in combination with ibuprofen 400 mg to produce detectable additive analgesia with minimum side effects.

Administration of a traditional dose of codeine 60 mg in combination with ibuprofen 400 mg may produce additive analgesia but for a relatively short duration of 1 to 2 hours, which also produces a significant increase in the incidence of side effects (Fig. 7-5). In the absence of a marketed fixed dose combination, it may be more practical to initiate analgesic treatment with ibuprofen 400 to 600 mg on a fixed schedule and dispense 30-mg tablets of codeine to be taken as needed for pain not adequately controlled by the NSAID. This strategy will result in exposing the opioid to only those patients in need of additional pain relief, thus resulting in a more favorable therapeutic ratio than exposing all patients to opioid side effects. Prescribing codeine as a single entity (i.e., not in a fixed combination with another drug) requires careful adherence to regulations associated with Schedule II opioids.

Ibuprofen Plus Hydrocodone

Ibuprofen plus hydrocodone reportedly produced an additive effect at the marketed doses according to studies conducted for the manufacturer. However, no information is available, comparing the combination of ibuprofen 200 mg plus hydrocodone 7.5 mg with ibuprofen 400 to 600 mg alone. Demonstration of superiority for the combination to either hydrocodone 7.5 mg alone or ibuprofen 200 mg alone is insufficient evidence that the marketed combination is superior to OTC NSAIDs (ibuprofen, naproxen, ketoprofen), aspirin, acetaminophen, or prescription doses of ibuprofen or other NSAIDs. Even if analgesic equivalency was established for the combination compared with ibuprofen 400 to 600 mg or its equivalent, it is likely that a greater incidence of CNS and GI side effects would occur in the opioid-containing combination.

The therapeutic advantage for the use of an ibuprofen-hydrocodone combination rests in adding a normal therapeutic dose of ibuprofen (400 to 600 mg) with a dose of the opioid that produces additive analgesia with a tolerable incidence of side effects. Combining one tablet of the marketed fixed dose combination with one to two tablets of nonprescription ibuprofen would result in a combination containing ibuprofen 400 to 600 mg and hydrocodone 7.5 mg. Extrapolating from a dose-response comparison of ibuprofen and oxycodone,[67] it is likely that hydrocodone 7.5 mg would result in a marginal additive analgesic effect in com-

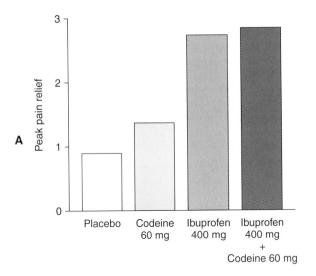

A

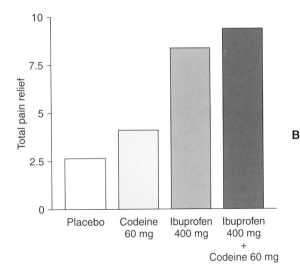

B

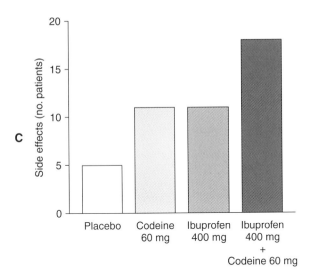

C

Fig. 7-5 Lack of additive peak analgesic efficacy for codeine 60 mg in combination with ibuprofen 400 mg **(A)** or total pain relief **(B)** but with an increased incidence of side effects attributable to the codeine **(C).**

bination with ibuprofen 400 mg but with a greater incidence of side effects than use of the ibuprofen alone (Fig. 7-6). The use of two tablets of the marketed, fixed-dose formulation in an ambulatory patient population would likely result in additive analgesia that would be greater than either drug alone but would also likely produce an excessive amount of adverse effects. The currently marketed, fixed-dose combination of ibuprofen and hydro-

codone should be reserved for clinical situations where ibuprofen 400 to 600 mg provides inadequate pain relief. Patients should be instructed to take one tablet of the combination with one 200-mg OTC tablet of ibuprofen every 4 to 6 hours, not to exceed the recommended maximum dosage of the combination or the recommended daily maximum dosage for ibuprofen (2400 mg/24-hour period) (Box 7-5).

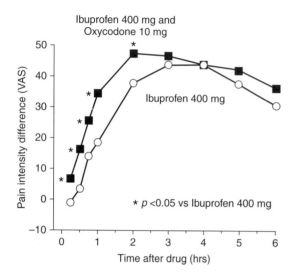

Fig. 7-6 Additive effect of oxycodone 10 mg in combination with ibuprofen 400 mg at early time points only.

Cyclooxygenase-2 Inhibitors

Research into the pathophysiology of inflammatory pain led to recognition that at least two forms of the COX enzyme are responsible for the formation of products of the arachidonic acid cascade. One form, characterized as *COX-1*, is responsible for the normal homeostatic functions of prostaglandins in the GI tract that maintain mucosa integrity, initiate platelet aggregation, and regulate renal blood flow. The other form, *COX-2*, was initially thought to be induced only during inflammation and to contribute to the pain, edema, and tissue destruction associated with acute inflammation, rheumatoid arthritis, and osteoarthritis. Researchers now recognize that the COX-2 enzyme is also expressed in the brain and kidneys and plays a still as-yet-undefined physiologic role in these tissues.

The NSAIDs spectrum of activity reflects their generally accepted mechanism to suppress the activity of both the COX-1 and COX-2 isoforms of cyclooxygenase with resultant decreased formation of products of the arachidonic acid cascade. Observations that COX-1 is constitutively distributed throughout the body, whereas COX-2 expression is limited to a few specialized tissues and is induced during inflammation lead to the hypothesis that COX-1 is primarily responsible for the adverse GI effects of existing dual COX-1/COX-2 inhibitors. On the other hand, COX-2 mediates the synthesis of prostanoids during patho-

BOX 7-6   SUMMARY

COX-2 Inhibitors

Celebrex has less analgesic efficacy than ibuprofen and should not be used until further studies demonstrate a therapeutic advantage for dental applications.

Rofecoxib is approximately equivalent to ibuprofen for analgesia but has less potential for GI toxicity and bleeding with repeated administration.

logic processes. This hypothesis suggests that dual COX-1/COX-2 inhibitors, such as ibuprofen, produce both therapeutic and toxic effects at therapeutic doses, whereas selective COX-2 inhibitors should have therapeutic effects largely devoid of NSAID toxicity.

Two drugs now on the market are highly selective for COX-2 suppression at the doses administered clinically with minimum effects on COX-1 activity. The specificity of rofecoxib for COX-2 versus COX-1 inhibition was demonstrated in males administered dosages up to 375 mg daily for 14 days.[68] Significant dose-related inhibition of PGE_2 was produced without inhibition of thromboxane formation, providing evidence that rofecoxib is a selective inhibitor of COX-2 in humans without evidence of COX-1 inhibition in doses eightfold higher than doses associated with clinical efficacy. The expectation is that they will provide therapeutic efficacy comparable to current NSAIDs but without the GI and renal toxicity that contributes directly to the morbidity and mortality associated with chronic NSAID administration.

Single doses of celecoxib were demonstrated in the oral surgery model of acute pain to be superior to placebo (at all doses reported in published abstracts) and comparable to aspirin 650 mg but were generally less effective than standard doses of naproxen and ibuprofen (for the first 4 to 6 hours). In multiple dose studies conducted in patients after orthopedic and general surgery, celecoxib's analgesic efficacy was inconclusive. As a consequence of these data, celecoxib did not receive FDA approval for the management of acute pain because it fails to satisfy the criteria of demonstrating analgesic efficacy in at least two different pain models. Celecoxib was more effective than placebo for the treatment of osteoarthritis and was approved and marketed for this indication.

Rofecoxib appears to have greater analgesic efficacy than celecoxib based on the results of studies in the oral surgery model (Box 7-6). Rofecoxib was

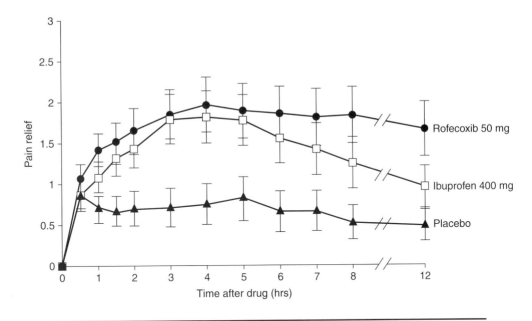

Fig. 7-7 Comparison of the analgesic effects of the COX-2 inhibitor rofecoxib with analgesic effects of ibuprofen 400 mg and placebo.

compared with ibuprofen 400 mg and placebo in a single-dose study in the oral surgery model of acute pain using traditional analgesic endpoints and the two-stopwatch method for estimating analgesic onset (Fig. 7-7). The total pain relief and sum of the pain intensity difference score during 8 hours after a single 50-mg dose of rofecoxib was superior to placebo but not distinguishable in this study from ibuprofen 400 mg.[69] The median time to onset of pain relief was indistinguishable for rofecoxib (0.7 hour) and ibuprofen (0.8 hour), but significantly fewer subjects in the rofecoxib group required additional analgesic within 24 hours than in either the placebo or ibuprofen groups. In a second study comparing rofecoxib in doses of 12.5, 25, and 50 mg to naproxen 550 mg and placebo, a clear dose response was demonstrated for analgesia.[70] The 25- and 50-mg doses of rofecoxib were numerically superior but statistically indistinguishable from naproxen for both pain relief and pain intensity difference. In both studies, the incidence of clinical and laboratory adverse experience were similar.

Both celecoxib and rofecoxib when used clinically appear to have reduced risk for producing GI perforations, ulcers, and bleeding compared with traditional NSAIDs, such as ibuprofen, diclofenac, and indomethacin. It should be noted that the standard

NSAID warnings regarding GI and renal toxicity also extend to the COX-2 selective inhibitors until greater experience has been gained with these new molecular entities.

In view of the modest analgesic activity demonstrated for celecoxib (Celebrex) and its failure to be approved for an acute pain indication, dentists should avoid using this drug until more clinical experience has been gained and new studies are conducted that demonstrate clear evidence of analgesic activity in the oral surgery model.

The data published in abstract form for rofecoxib provide clear evidence of an acute analgesic effect in replicate studies in two models of acute pain and selectivity for COX-2 inhibition. The drug is well tolerated after single doses and does not appear to inhibit COX-1–mediated platelet aggregation. These data provided a basis for approval of rofecoxib as the first selective COX-2 inhibitor indicated in the United States for the management of acute pain (up to a maximum of 5 days) and for the treatment of osteoarthritis. The analgesic activity for a 50-mg dose of rofecoxib should be comparable to that of ibuprofen 400 mg. Although the expected GI safety of rofecoxib is predicted to be less than that of dual COX-1/ COX-2 inhibitors such as ibuprofen, its effect on the kidneys is yet to be determined. The analgesic dose of rofecoxib (a single 50-mg dose over 24 hours) is greater than the recommended dose for rheumatoid arthritis and osteoarthritis (12.5 to 25 mg) because of a greater incidence of side effects with repeated doses (e.g., extremity edema). This dosage could present a problem if pain occurs before the 24-hour remedication time.

For most dental procedures, patients are adequately managed on nonprescription doses of NSAIDs at a nominal cost to the patient. In addition, patients have usually been previously exposed to aspirin, acetaminophen, or OTC formulations of ibuprofen, making it unlikely that they will experience an idiosyncratic or allergic response when given one of these drugs after a dental procedure. These considerations suggest that although the new selective COX-2 inhibitor rofecoxib holds promise for analgesic efficacy with greater safety than traditional NSAIDs, it would be prudent to wait until additional clinical experience in patients with osteoarthritis substantiates their putative safety advantage.

Effects on Edema

The acute postoperative sequelae of dental procedures includes other signs of inflammation resulting from tissue injury, most prominently edema. Although synthetic analogs of endogenous corticosteroid drugs are used extensively to control the sequelae of both acute and chronic inflammation, their use postoperatively is tempered by their ability to suppress the immune system, thereby increasing the risk of infection. NSAIDs have a more selective mechanism of action than glucocorticoids and a more favorable side effect profile, suggesting that drugs of this class may inhibit inflammation without the risks of corticosteroid administration. Ibuprofen produced a trend for reduced swelling in comparison to placebo when given for 3 days at a dosage of 400 mg 3 times/day.[71] Administration of ibuprofen 600 mg 4 times/day for 2 days also showed a trend toward suppressed edema formation at 48 hours after oral surgery.[59] A retrospective analysis of the data from two studies done in series evaluating the effects of two NSAIDs (ibuprofen and flurbiprofen) permitted the conclusion that NSAIDs significantly suppress edema formation after oral surgery compared with placebo.[59] A more recent study concluded that the combination of ibuprofen 400 mg 3 times/day and methylprednisolone 32 mg reduced swelling by

greater than 50% compared with placebo.[72] The lack of separate groups receiving either ibuprofen alone or methylprednisolone does not permit any conclusion about the contribution of ibuprofen to the total reported effect on swelling.

Although they are somewhat inconclusive, the observations from the two studies in which ibuprofen was administered alone demonstrated a reduction in swelling compared with placebo with minimal side effects and no evidence of interference with healing or perioperative bleeding.

Recommendations for Use of NSAIDs in Dentistry

NSAIDs are one of the most widely used drug classes for dental pain along with aspirin, acetaminophen, and codeine. They are generally more efficacious than these standard drugs in most studies, presumably resulting from the inflammatory cause of most dental pain and NSAIDs' prominent antiinflammatory effects. A single dose of ibuprofen 400 mg is usually more effective than combinations of aspirin or acetaminophen plus an opioid (usually codeine or oxycodone) and has fewer side effects. When possible, NSAID therapy is preferable for ambulatory patients who generally experience a higher incidence of side effects after receiving an opioid. NSAIDs also modestly suppress swelling after surgical procedures, providing additional therapeutic benefit without the potential liabilities of administering steroids (Fig. 7-8). These considerations and the vast experience gained through 25 years of clinical use make ibuprofen the drug of choice for dental pain for patients who do not have any contraindications to its use.

Limitations to orally administered NSAIDs for dental pain include delayed onset when compared with an injectable opioid, the inability to consistently relieve severe pain, and an apparent lack of effectiveness when given repeatedly for chronic orofacial pain. The best strategy for minimizing pain onset is administration of an NSAID before the postoperative induction of COX-2. For patients who do not receive satisfactory relief from an NSAID alone, combining it with an opioid may provide additive analgesia, but it will also be accompanied by more frequent side effects. The optimum balance for individual patients can be best achieved by supplying them with an NSAID to be taken at specified intervals and a separate prescription for codeine 30 mg to

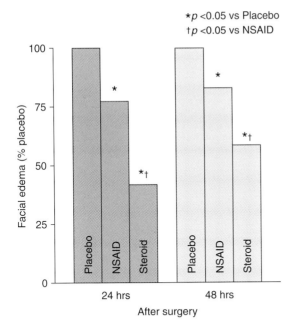

Fig. 7-8 Effects of NSAIDs on postoperative edema.

be taken if needed and titrated between one and two tablets to achieve pain relief with minimum side effects. A fixed-dose combination of ibuprofen 200 mg and hydrocodone 7.5 mg is problematic unless coadministered with additional ibuprofen.

Repeated doses of an NSAID for chronic orofacial pain should be reevaluated because of its apparent lack of efficacy, the potential for serious GI and renal toxicity with repeated dosing, and its potential for tolerance with repeated dosing. The lack of suitable alternatives predicts the continued use of ibuprofen and other NSAIDs for this patient population; however, their use should be limited to a short trial and should be discontinued if signs of GI or renal toxicity are noted.

References

1. Gordon SM, Dionne RA, Brahim J, et al: Blockade of peripheral neuronal barrage reduces postoperative pain, *Pain* 70:209-215, 1997.
2. Dionne RA, Gordon SM, McCullagh LM, et al: Assessment of clinical needs for anesthesia and sedation in the general population, *J Am Dent Assoc* 129:167-173, 1998.
3. Doyle G, Furey S, Berlin R, et al: Gastrointestinal safety and tolerance of ibuprofen at maximum over-the-counter use, *Aliment Pharmacol Therap* 13:897-906, 1999.
4. Cooper SA, Beaver WT: A model to evaluate mild analgesics in oral surgery outpatients, *Clin Pharmacol Ther* 20:241-250, 1976.
5. Seymour RA, Rawlins MD: Efficacy and pharmacokinetics of aspirin in postoperative pain, *Br J Clin Pharmacol* 13:807, 1982.
6. Cooper SA, Needle SE, Kruger GO: Comparative analgesic potency of aspirin and ibuprofen, *J Oral Surg* 35:898-903, 1977.
7. Petersen JK, Husted SE, Pedersen AK, et al: Systemic availability of acetylsalicylic acid in human subjects after oral ingestion of three different formulations, *Acta Pharmacol Toxicol* 51:285, 1982.
8. Forbes JA, Calderazzo JP, Bowser MW, et al: A 12-hour evaluation of the analgesic efficacy of diflunisal, aspirin, and placebo in postoperative dental pain, *J Clin Pharmacol* 22:89-96, 1982.
9. Chapmen PJ, Macleod AWG: The effects of diflunisal on bleeding time and platelet aggregation in a multidose study, *Int J Oral Maxillofac Surg* 16: 448-453, 1987.
10. Lokken P, Skjelbred P: Analgesic and antiinflammatory effects of paracetamol evaluated by bilateral oral surgery, *Br J Clin Pharmacol* 10:253S, 1980.
11. Skjelbred P, Album B, Lokken P: Acetylsalicylic acid versus paracetamol: effect on postoperative course, *Eur J Clin Pharmacol* 12:257, 1977.
12. Quiding H, Oikarinen V, Sane J, et al: Analgesic efficacy after single and repeated doses of codeine and acetaminophen, *J Clin Pharmacol* 24:27, 1984.
13. Laska EM, Sunshine A, Marrero I, et al: The correlation between blood levels of ibuprofen and clinical analgesic response, *Clin Pharmacol Ther* 40:1-7, 1986.
14. Cooper SA: Five studies on ibuprofen for postsurgical dental pain, *Am J Med* 77A:70-77, 1984.
15. Dionne R, Cooper SA: Evaluation of preoperative ibuprofen on postoperative pain after impaction surgery, *Oral Surg Oral Med Oral Pathol* 45:851-856, 1978.
16. Dionne RA, Campbell RL, Cooper SA, et al: Suppression of postoperative pain by preoperative administration of ibuprofen in comparison to placebo, acetaminophen, and acetaminophen plus codeine, *J Clin Pharmacol* 23:37-43, 1983.
17. Troullos E, Hargreaves KM, Dionne RA: Ibuprofen elevates immunoreactive beta-endorphin levels in humans during surgical stress, *Clin Pharmacol Ther* 62:74-81, 1997.
18. Dionne RA, McCullagh L: The S (+) isomer of ibuprofen suppresses plasma β-endorphin coincident with analgesia in humans, *Clin Pharmacol Ther* 63:694 -701, 1998.
19. Jain AK, Ryan JR, McMahon G, et al: Analgesic efficacy of low-dose ibuprofen in dental extraction, *Pharmacotherapy* 6:318-322, 1986.
20. Forbes JA, Barkaszi BA, Ragland RN, et al: Analgesic effect of fendosal, ibuprofen, and aspirin in postoperative oral surgery pain, *Pharmacotherapy* 4:385-391, 1984.

21. Frame JW, Evans CRH, Flaum GR, et al: A comparison of ibuprofen and dihydrocodeine in relieving pain following wisdom teeth removal, *Br Dent J* 166:121-124, 1989.

22. McQuay HJ, Carroll D, Guest PG, et al: A multiple dose comparison of ibuprofen and dihydrocodeine after third molar surgery, *Br J Oral Maxillofac Surg* 31:95-100, 1993.

23. Hersh EV, Cooper SA, Beets N, et al: Single dose and multidose analgesic study of ibuprofen and meclofenamate sodium after third molar surgery, *Oral Surg Oral Med Oral Pathol* 76:680-687, 1993.

24. Kiersch TA, Halladay SC, Koschik M: A double-blind, randomized study of naproxen sodium, ibuprofen, and placebo in postoperative dental pain, *Clin Ther* 15:845-854, 1993.

25. Seymour RA, Ward-Booth P, Kelly PJ: Evaluation of different doses of soluble ibuprofen and ibuprofen tablets in postoperative dental pain, *Br J Oral Maxillofac Surg* 34:110-114, 1996.

26. Bakshi R, Frenkel G, Dietlein G, et al: A placebo-controlled comparative evaluation of diclofenac dispersible versus ibuprofen in postoperative pain after third molar surgery, *J Clin Pharmacol* 34:225-230, 1994.

27. Packman E et al: Onset of ibuprofen liquigel (400 mg) compared to acetaminophen caplets (1000 mg) in the treatment of tension headache, *J Clin Pharmacol* 38:876, 1998.

28. Vogel RI, Gross JI: The effects of nonsteroidal antiinflammatory analgesics on pain after periodontal surgery, *J Am Dent Assoc* 109:731-734, 1984.

29. Vogel RI, Desjardins PJ, Major KVO: Comparison of presurgical and immediate postsurgical ibuprofen on postoperative periodontal pain, *J Periodontol* 63:914-918, 1992.

30. Ngan P, Wilson S, Shanfeld J, et al: The effect of ibuprofen on the level of discomfort in patients undergoing orthodontic treatment, *Am J Orthod Dentofacial Orthop* 106:88-95, 1994.

31. Torabinejad M, Cymerman JJ, Frankson M, et al: Effectiveness of various medications on postoperative pain following complete instrumentation, *J Endod* 20:345-354, 1994a.

32. Flath RK, Hicks ML, Dionne RA, et al: Pain suppression after pulpectomy with preoperative flurbiprofen, *J Endod* 13:339-347, 1987.

33. Torabinejad M, Dorn SO, Eleazer PD, et al: Effectiveness of various medications on postoperative pain following root canal obturation, *J Endod* 20:427-431, 1994b.

34. Sevelius H, Segre E, Bursick K: Comparative analgesic effects of naproxen sodium, aspirin, and placebo, *J Clin Pharmacol* 20:480-485, 1980.

35. Sindet-Pedersen S, Petersen JK, Gotzsche PC, et al: A double-blind, randomized study of naproxen and acetylsalicylic acid after surgical removal of impacted third molars, *Int J Oral Maxillofac Surg* 15: 389-394, 1986.

36. Reudy JA: A comparison of the analgesic efficacy of naproxen and acetylsalicylic acid-codeine in patients with pain after dental surgery, *Scand J Rheumatol* 2(suppl):60-63, 1973.

37. Sisk AL, Grover BJ: A comparison of preoperative and postoperative naproxen sodium for suppression of postoperative pain, *J Oral Maxillofac Surg* 48:674-678, 1990.

38. DeArmond B, Francisco CA, Lin JS, et al: Safety profile of over-the-counter naproxen sodium, *Clin Ther* 17:587-601, 1995.

39. Willer J, De Broucker T, Bussel B, et al: Central analgesic effect of ketoprofen in humans: electrophysiological evidence for a supraspinal mechanism in a double-blind and cross-over study, *Pain* 38:1-7, 1989.

40. Cooper SA, Berrie R, Cohn P: Comparison of ketoprofen, ibuprofen, and placebo in a dental surgery pain model, *Adv Ther* 5:43-53, 1988a.

41. Mehlisch D, Frakes L, Cavaliere ME, et al: Double-blind comparison of single oral doses of ketoprofen, codeine, and placebo in patients with moderate to severe dental pain, *J Clin Pharmacol* 24:486-492, 1984.

42. Dionne RA, Gordon S, Tahara M, et al: Analgesic efficacy and pharmacokinetics of ketoprofen administered into a surgical site, *J Clin Pharmacol* 139:131-138, 1999.

43. Nelson SL, Bergman SA: Relief of dental surgery pain: a controlled 12-hour comparison of etodolac, aspirin, and placebo, *Anesth Prog* 32:151-156, 1985.

44. Tucker PW, Smith JR, Adams DF: A comparison of 2 analgesic regimens for the control of postoperative periodontal discomfort, *J Periodontol* 67:125-129, 1996.

45. Dvornik DM: Tissue selective inhibition of prostaglandin biosynthesis by etodolac, *J Rheumatol* 24(suppl 47):40-47, 1997.

46. Stanski DR, Cherry C, Bradley R, et al: Efficacy and safety of single doses of intramuscular ketorolac tromethamine compared with meperidine for postoperative pain, *Pharmacotherapy* 10(suppl):40S-44S, 1990.

47. Spindler JS, Mehlisch D, Brown CT: Intramuscular ketorolac and morphine in the treatment of moderate to severe pain after major surgery, *Pharmacotherapy* 10(suppl):51S-58S, 1990.

48. O'Hara DA, Fragen FJ, Kinzer M, et al: Ketorolac tromethamine as compared with morphine sulfate for treatment of postoperative pain, *Clin Pharmacol Ther* 41:556-561, 1987.

49. Penniston SG, Hargreaves KM: Evaluation of periapical injection of ketorolac for management of endodontic pain, *J Endod* 22:55-59, 1996.

50. Forbes JA, Kehm CJ, Grodin CD, et al: Evaluation of ketorolac, ibuprofen, acetaminophen, and an acetaminophen-codeine combination in postoperative oral surgery pain, *Pharmacotherapy* 10(suppl 6 pt 2):94s-105s, 1989.

51. Jung D, Mroszczak EJ, Wu EJ: Pharmacokinetics of ketorolac and *p*-hydroxyketorolac following oral and intramuscular administration of ketorolac tromethamine, *Pharmaceut Res* 6:62-65, 1989.

52. Boctor AM, Eickhoct M, Pugsley TA: Meclofenamate sodium is an inhibitor of both the 5-lipoxygenase and cyclooxygenase pathways of the arachidonic acid and cascade in vitro, *Prosta Leuko Med* 23:229-238, 1985.

53. Markowitz NR, Young SK, Rohere MD, et al: Comparison of meclofenamate sodium with buffered aspirin and placebo in the treatment of postsurgical dental pain, *J Oral Maxillofac Surg* 43:517-522, 1988c.

54. Cooper SA, Firestein A, Cohn P: Double blind comparison of meclofenamate sodium with buffered aspirin and placebo in the treatment of postsurgical dental pain, *J Clin Dent* 1:31-34, 1988c.

55. Desjardins PJ: Analgesic efficacy of piroxicam in postoperative dental pain, *Am J Med* 84(suppl 5A):35-41, 1988.

56. Hutchinson GL, Crofts SL, Gray IG: Preoperative piroxicam for postoperative analgesia in dental surgery, *Br J Anaesth* 65:500-503, 1990.

57. Henry D, Drew A, Beuzeville S: Adverse drug reactions in the GI system attributed to ibuprofen. In Rainsford KD, Powanda MC, editors: *Safety and efficacy of nonprescription (OTC) analgesic and NSAIDs*, London, 1998, Kluwer Academic Publishers, pp 19-45.

58. Berthold CW, Dionne RA: Clinical evaluation of H1 receptor and H2 receptor antagonists for acute postoperative pain, *J Clin Pharmacol* 33:944-948, 1993.

59. Troullos ES, Hargreaves KM, Butler DP, et al: Comparison of nonsteroidal antiinflammatory drugs, ibuprofen and flurbiprofen, to methylprednisolone and placebo for acute pain, swelling, and trismus, *J Oral Maxillofac Surg* 48:945-952, 1990.

60. Dionne RA: Suppression of dental pain by the preoperative administration of flurbiprofen, *Am J Med* 80:41-49, 1986.

61. Seibert K, Zhang Y, Leahy K, et al: Pharmacological and biochemical demonstration of the role of cyclooxygenase-2 in inflammation and pain, *Proc Natl Acad Sci U S A* 91:12013-12017, 1994.

62. Roszkowski MT, Swift JQ, Hargreaves KM: Effect of NSAID administration on tissue levels of immunoreactive prostaglandin E_2, leukotriene B_4, and (S)-flurbiprofen following extraction of impacted third molars, *Pain* 73: 339-345, 1997.

63. Grennan DM, Aarons L, Siddiqui M, et al: Dose-response study with ibuprofen in rheumatoid arthritis: clinical and pharmacokinetic findings, *Br J Clin Pharmacol* 15:11-316, 1983.

64. Cooper SA, Engle J, Ladov M, et al: Analgesic efficacy of an ibuprofen-codeine combination, *Pharmacotherapy* 2:162-167, 1982.

65. Petersen JK, Hansson F, Strid S: The effect of an ibuprofen-codeine combination for the treatment of patients with pain after removal of lower third molars, *J Oral Maxillofac Surg* 51:637-640, 1993.

66. McQuay HJ, Carroll D, Watts PG, et al: Codeine 20 mg increases pain relief from ibuprofen 400 mg after third molar surgery: a repeat dosing comparison of ibuprofen and an ibuprofen-codeine combination, *Pain* 37:7-13, 1989.

67. Dionne RA: Additive analgesic effects of oxycodone and ibuprofen in the oral surgery model, *J Oral Maxillofac Surg* 57:673-678, 1999.

68. Van Hecken A, Depre M, Ehrich E, et al: Demonstration of specific COX-2 inhibition by MK-966 in humans with supratherapeutic doses, *Clin Pharmacol Ther* 65:164, 1999 (abstract).

69. Brown J, Morrison BW, Christensen S, et al: MK-0966 50 mg versus ibuprofen 400 mg in postsurgical dental pain, *Clin Pharmacol Ther* 65:118, 1999a (abstract).

70. Fricke JF, Morrisson BW, Fite S, et al: MK-966 versus naproxen sodium 550 mg in postsurgical dental pain, *Clin Pharmacol Ther* 645:119, 1999 (abstract).

71. Lokken P, Olsen I, Bruaset I, et al: Bilateral surgical removal of impacted third molar teeth as a model for drug evaluation: a test with ibuprofen, *Eur J Clin Pharmacol* 8:209-216, 1975.

72. Schultze-Mosgau S, Schmelzeisen R, Frolich JC, et al: Use of ibuprofen and methylprednisolone for the prevention of pain and swelling after removal of impacted third molars, *J Oral Maxillofac Surg* 53:2-7, 1995.

CHAPTER 8

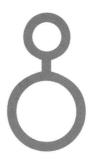

Opioid Analgesics and Antagonists

DANIEL A. HAAS

CHAPTER OUTLINE

The opioid class of drugs has played a major role in providing pain control for dental patients. Knowledge of these agents expanded in 1973 with the discovery of specific receptors for morphine. Given that morphine is an extract of a plant, the presence of these receptors led to the question: Why would humans have specific receptors for an exogenous chemical? It was more logical that these receptors must be present for endogenous substances. Therefore the search for these compounds followed and led to the discovery of the endogenous opioid peptides in 1975. It is now known that many of these naturally occurring compounds exist. The effects of opioid analgesics are mediated through these receptors and mimic many of the actions of these endogenous peptides. This chapter will review the pharmacology of the opioid class of drugs and their role in dentistry.

Terminology and Classification

These drugs have been referred to interchangeably as narcotics, opiates, or opioids. Although *narcotic* describes a primary action of these agents, it is no longer the preferred term. *Opiate* is correctly used to describe derivatives of opium, such as morphine. The term *opioid*, originally defined as "opiate-like," is now used to include both true opiates and opiate-like agents. It is a more correct pharmacologic term, since these drugs act through the opioid receptors. Thus the term *narcotic* is being superseded by the term *opioid*, and these drugs are now more correctly referred to as *opioids* or *opioid analgesics*.[1-4]

Opioids may be classified by either their chemical structure or their action on opioid receptors (Box 8-1). Classification by structure, such as semisynthetic and synthetic, is illustrated in Box 8-2 and may

be helpful in determining whether a patient has a cross-allergy to another opioid. It may be assumed that a documented allergy to one opioid within one classification group would rule out the use of another opioid within that same group. For example, a true allergy to codeine would contraindicate the use of oxycodone; however, meperidine could be used.

The second classification is based on opioids' action on opioid receptors. As described in Chapter 2, a drug may be an agonist, a partial agonist, an agonist/antagonist, or an antagonist. This classification is illustrated in Box 8-3 and will be used in this chapter.

The opioid receptors are present for the endogenous opioids, which are subdivided into three families: enkephalins, endorphins, and dynorphins. These are peptides with wide distribution throughout the central nervous system (CNS) and are derived from a precursor peptide. Enkephalins are found throughout the CNS but particularly in sites important in the transmission of pain. The prototype for the endorphins is β-endorphin, which is primarily concentrated in the anterior pituitary and is formed by the cleavage of proopiomelanocortin. Dynorphins also have a wide distribution and are found in the primary afferents in the dorsal horn of the spinal cord and throughout the brain.

BOX 8-1   SUMMARY

Opioid Classification

> Opioid drugs mimic the action of naturally occurring compounds.
> Endogenous opioids are classified as endorphins, enkephalins, and dynorphins.
> Opioids may be categorized by their chemical structure or by action on receptors.

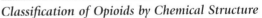

BOX 8-2

Classification of Opioids by Chemical Structure

Phenanthrenes	Alfentanil
Morphine	Sufentanil
Codeine	Remifentanil
Oxycodone	
Hydrocodone	**Phenylheptylamines**
Hydromorphone	Propoxyphene
Dihydrocodeine	Methadone
Oxymorphone	
Nalbuphine	**Morphinans**
Buprenorphine	Butorphanol
Heroin	Levorphanol
Phenylpiperidines	**Benzomorphans**
Meperidine	Pentazocine
Fentanyl	

BOX 8-3

Classification of Opioids by Action on Receptors*

Agonists	Heroin
Morphine	Propoxyphene
Codeine	(Darvon)
Oxycodone (Percodan,	Methadone
Percocet)	
Hydrocodone (Lortab)	**Agonist/Antagonists**
Hydromorphone	Pentazocine (Talwin)
(Dilaudid)	Nalbuphine (Nubain)
Oxymorphone	Butorphanol (Stadol)
(Numorphan)	Buprenorphine
Dihydrocodeine	(Buprenex)
(Synalgos)	Dezocine (Dalgan)
Meperidine (Demerol)	
Fentanyl (Sublimaze)	**Antagonists**
Alfentanil (Alfenta)	Naloxone (Narcan)
Sufentanil (Sufenta)	Naltrexone (Trexan)
Remifentanil (Ultiva)	Nalmefene (Incystene)
Levorphanol	Nalorphine
(Levo-Dromoran)	

*Generic names are listed with trade names in parentheses.

Pharmacokinetic Considerations

Opioids are well absorbed by most routes of administration. However, their bioavailability when given orally can be low because of significant first-pass metabolism in the liver. Therefore the oral dose needs to be much higher than the parenteral dose for that agent (Box 8-4). Equivalent oral and intramuscular doses for analgesia for a number of commonly used opioids are shown later in this chapter (see Table 8-1). Codeine and oxycodone have a relatively low first-pass effect, which is the reason for their common use as oral analgesics.

Opioids are primarily biotransformed in the liver by glucuronidation. The metabolites are generally inactive, with the exception of those from meperidine and morphine. One of meperidine's metabolites is normeperidine, which can lead to seizures in susceptible patients. Morphine-6-glucuronide is believed to have analgesic action on its own. The minority of opioids that are esters, such as heroin and remifentanil, are hydrolyzed by tissue esterases. Opioid metabolites are primarily excreted by the kidneys.

Pharmacokinetic Considerations

High first-pass effect results in large differences between oral and parenteral doses.

Appropriate adjustments must be made when prescribing for patients who have reduced hepatic function.

Effects Of Opioid Receptor Stimulation*

Mu-1	**Kappa**
Supraspinal analgesia	Supraspinal analgesia
Euphoria	Spinal analgesia
Nausea/vomiting	Sedation
Miosis	Constipation
Tolerance	Miosis
Pruritus	Psychotomimetic
Mu-2	**Delta**
Spinal analgesia	Supraspinal analgesia
Sedation	Spinal analgesia
Constipation	Nausea/vomiting
Respiratory depression	Respiratory depression
	Tolerance
	Pruritus

Adapted from Reisine T, Pasternak G: Opioid analgesics and antagonists. In Hardman JG, Limbird LE, Molinoff PB, et al, editors: *Goodman and Gilman's the pharmacological basis of therapeutics,* ed 9, New York, 1996, McGraw-Hill; Coda BB: Opioids. In Barash PG et al, editors: *Clinical anesthesia,* ed 3, Philadelphia, 1996, Lippincott-Raven; Pasternak GW: *Clin Neuropharmacol* 16:1-18, 1993.
*This box summarizes *reported* effects, the knowledge of which continues to evolve. Therefore this box represents only the current understanding of receptor actions.

Pharmacodynamics: Actions and Effects of Opioids

The mechanism of action of the opioids is stimulation of the opioid receptors. Opioid receptors are divided into the subtypes mu, kappa, and delta. Each of these is further subdivided into a number of subtypes, such as mu-1, mu-2, kappa-1, kappa-2, kappa-3, and so on.

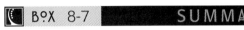

BOX 8-6 SUMMARY

Opioid Effects

Analgesia	Antitussive
Sedation	Nausea and vomiting
Mood alteration	Constipation
(euphoria or	Miosis
dysphoria)	Biliary tract spasm
Respiratory depression	Histamine release
Tolerance	Chest wall rigidity
Physical dependence	Neuroendocrine

TABLE 8-1

*Opioid Receptor Selectivity**

	Mu	Kappa	Delta
Morphine	+	+	+
Fentanyl	+	•	+
Pentazocine	−/+	+	•
Nalbuphine	−/+	+	•
Butorphanol	−/+	+	•
Naloxone	−	−	−

Adapted from Kalant H: Opioid analgesics and antagonists. In Kalant H, Roschlau WHE, editors: *Principles of medical pharmacology,* ed 6, Oxford, UK, 1998, Oxford University Press; and Reisine T, Pasternak G: Opioid analgesics and antagonists. In Hardman JG, Limbird LE, Molinoff PB, et al, editors: *Goodman and Gilman's the pharmacological basis of therapeutics,* ed 9, New York, 1996, McGraw-Hill.
+, Agonist; −, antagonist; −/+, agonist/antagonist or partial agonist; •, no effect or no known effect.
*This table summarizes what is currently known about receptors, which continues to evolve. Therefore the above table only represents the current understanding of receptor selectivity.

BOX 8-7 SUMMARY

Effects of Opioids

Opioid drugs produce myriad effects, primarily by activating mu opioid receptors.

Ambulation potentiates nausea and vomiting. Advise patients to limit activity or remain recumbent for the first hour or two after consumption of postoperative analgesics, especially when using higher doses.

Opioids produce tolerance and physical dependence with chronic use. They do not produce addiction, although such behavior may be fostered in susceptible patients.

Respiratory depression can be a significant, dose-limiting consideration in elderly patients or in those with significant respiratory disease.

The sigma receptor is not classified as an opioid receptor, although it can be stimulated by many opioids. This latter receptor is believed to elicit psychotomimetic responses such as dysphoria and hallucination.

The opioid receptors have a wide distribution throughout the CNS and, to a lesser extent, in peripheral tissues. They appear to be coupled to G-proteins and elicit changes in the second messenger cAMP system and calcium and potassium ion channels.[1] Recent research has shown that opioid receptors act-

ing at peripheral sites have analgesic and other anti-inflammatory effects. These actions are noted primarily in inflamed tissue. All three receptor types are present peripherally.

Opioid receptors are involved in a wide range of physiologic action. They appear to subserve an endogenous analgesia system and influence cardiovascular, respiratory, gastrointestinal, genitourinary, endocrine, and immunologic systems. The actions of receptor stimulation vary and are summarized in Box 8-5. Receptor selectivity among a number of agents is summarized in Table 8-1.

In general terms, opioids inhibit neuronal activity. All opioids share the following specific properties, as summarized in Box 8-6, with varying degrees of expression among the different agents. Specific differences will be addressed in the discussion of the individual drugs (Box 8-7).

Analgesia

Analgesia is the primary effect of all opioids. The analgesia that is obtained can be profound and results from a combination of both an increase in pain threshold, which inhibits pain perception, and an increase in pain tolerance. This latter feature is important and is characterized by the finding that even if the patient still can feel pain, it is not as distressing.

Mu-1, kappa-3, and delta receptor agonists induce analgesia by action in the brain, whereas stimulation of mu-2, kappa-1, and delta-2 opioid receptors can induce analgesia by action in the spinal cord.[2] This latter mechanism is used when opioids are administered epidurally or spinally into the subarachnoid space.

Opioids inhibit the release of substance P from the synapses of the dorsal root ganglia and decrease afferent transmission of pain sensation. Of the neurons that mediate pain, opioids inhibit the response of C fiber stimulation to a greater degree than that of A delta fibers, which is a result of opioid inhibition of the excitatory postsynaptic potential that should result from C fiber stimulation. Opioids can also cause analgesia by stimulating receptors in the periaqueductal gray of the midbrain and the raphe nucleus of the medulla oblongata, whose neurons project down to the spinal cord. Therefore both the ascending and descending pathways of analgesia are affected.

For use as analgesics for postoperative dental pain, opioids should always be prescribed with a non-opioid. As mentioned in Chapter 7, a therapeutic dose of an NSAID can provide better analgesia than codeine 60 mg and very often is the only analgesic required. Nevertheless, if it is determined that the pain will not be relieved by a non-opioid alone, then it is reasonable to add an opioid to the regimen. Codeine or oxycodone are the first considerations as oral agents because they have favorable first-pass characteristics. If they are ineffective, other agents, such as hydromorphone, hydrocodone, or dihydrocodeine, may be considered. In circumstances of a documented allergy to one of the phenanthrene group, such as codeine, it is reasonable to consider an opioid from another group, such as meperidine or pentazocine.

Sedation

Opioids can induce drowsiness and mental clouding. It is believed that sedation is mediated by mu-2 and kappa receptor stimulation. Profound sedation may result when other CNS depressants, such as the benzodiazepines, are given with opioids. Physicians often take advantage of this effect when inducing conscious or deep sedation, so that addition of an opioid will likely reduce the amount of benzodiazepine required. Conversely, however, this characteristic can be a disadvantage because it may be easier to overly sedate a patient.

Mood Alteration

The mood alteration may manifest as either a euphoria or a dysphoria. The euphoria experienced is a detached, foggy, euphoric sensation. The euphoria found with opioids differs from that found with other drugs, such as amphetamines, which provide a stimulation effect. It is believed that the euphoria is mediated by the mu receptors, whereas the potential for dysphoria is mediated by kappa and possibly sigma receptor stimulation.

Respiratory Depression

All opioids depress respiration. This important action is caused by a dose-dependent decrease in the response of the respiratory center to carbon dioxide. The slopes of the alveolar ventilatory response to carbon dioxide are reduced and shifted to the right, which means that there is less ventilation per amount of carbon dioxide. (A more thorough explanation can be found in Chapter 4.) Respiratory depression is commonly the cause of death from acute opioid overdose. High doses can totally block spontaneous respirations without necessarily inducing unconsciousness. This effect may be seen in low-to-medium doses when given to susceptible patients, such as the elderly, and it is potentiated by other CNS depressants.

Clinically, this is seen as a decrease in rate of breathing with a compensatory increase in tidal volume. In high enough doses the patient becomes apneic, although capable of responding to a command to initiate breathing. $Paco_2$ is elevated. Because of these respiratory effects, administration of opioids to patients with respiratory disorders, such as chronic obstructive pulmonary disease, must be done with caution. Severe forms of respiratory disease may be considered a contraindication to their use.

Tolerance

Administration of any of the opioids can lead to tolerance, which is characterized by a decreased response to the same dose of a particular drug after repeated administrations. Therefore dose increases are required to yield a consistent effect. Tolerance usually does not manifest until after several weeks of repeatedly taking therapeutic doses, with frequent large doses being most likely to induce tolerance. The range can be as marked as thirty-five-fold the normal dose.[5] Tolerance develops simultaneously for most opioid effects (e.g., analgesia, sedation, respiratory depression), but there is little tolerance of the constipating influences. For this reason, chronically medicated patients may receive staggering doses of opioids on a daily basis and are spared from respiratory depression, but they must contend with troublesome aspects of constipation.

Physical Dependence

Physical dependence may result from opioid use. It is attributed to an adaptation of homeostatic mechanisms in response to repeated use of a drug. An opioid-dependent patient will require continued administration of the drug to maintain normal homeostatic balance. If administration of the drug is stopped abruptly, a withdrawal syndrome follows spontaneously. The syndrome can be suppressed by drug replacement. Withdrawal can be severe and may present with pilo-erection or goose-flesh (hence the term *cold turkey*), rhinorrhea, lacrimation, yawning, myalgia, hyperventilation, hyperthermia, mydriasis, vomiting, diarrhea, anxiety, and hostility. Administration of opioids for conscious sedation or general anesthesia will not induce a physically dependent state.

Addiction

Drug addiction is a behavior syndrome that includes a compulsion to continue using a substance despite a lack of medical necessity and significant substance-related problems. Although tolerance and physical dependence are inevitable consequences of chronic use of opioids, they should not, by themselves, imply that the patient is "addicted." This distinction is important, because patients with severe and/or chronic pain sometimes are deprived of adequate opioid medication simply because they show evidence of tolerance or dependence.[6] Once their medical condition improves, the majority of patients who are tolerant and dependent on opioids are successfully withdrawn from their medication by reducing the dosage every 2 to 3 days. Terminology has confused this issue further because *chemical or substance dependency* has largely replaced the more pejorative term *addiction*. Nevertheless, addiction is a neuropsychiatric condition that exists independently of the drug used. Addiction may be fostered by opioid consumption but is not induced by a specific pharmacodynamic mechanism.

Antitussive Effect

Opioids are very effective at depressing the cough reflex, often in subanalgesic doses. When used for anes-

thesia, this effect may be of value in the immediate postoperative period or for procedures such as bronchoscopy. Dextroisomers, such as dextromethorphan, are often used as antitussives because they are less likely to induce other unwanted opioid actions.

Nausea and Vomiting

Nausea and vomiting is a common adverse side effect of any opioid, with no documented differences among the different agents. Nausea is due to direct stimulation of the chemoreceptor trigger zone, which is in the area postrema in the floor of the fourth ventricle of the medulla. In addition to opioid receptors, this site also has serotonergic, dopaminergic, histaminergic, and muscarinic receptors. Furthermore, there is also input from the vestibular apparatus, and therefore the nausea and vomiting is characteristically exacerbated if the patient is ambulatory. High-dose opioids appear to inhibit the vomiting center. In addition, the opioid antagonist naloxone will not reverse nausea and vomiting but instead can trigger it.

Constipation

Opioids depress peristaltic contractions, thereby suppressing diarrhea and leading to constipation. Clinically, this effect is dose-dependent and is noted more with repeated administration as given for postoperative analgesia.

Biliary Spasm

Opioid administration may induce spasm of the biliary smooth muscle. Bile duct pressure increases and can lead to epigastric distress that may mimic angina-like pain. This effect is noted particularly with morphine and may be secondary to the release of histamine.

Histamine Release

Many opioids, particularly morphine, are capable of releasing histamine from circulating basophils and tissue mast cells. Conversely, fentanyl does not have this action. Histamine release may not be mediated by opioid receptors because it is not reversed by opioid antagonists. It is a clinically relevant action, since morphine administration leads to vasodilation and a decrease in systemic vascular resistance, which may lead to hypotension.

Miosis

All opioids except for meperidine induce miosis, which is caused by the drug's effect on the nucleus of the oculomotor nerve. Pinpoint pupils are often a sign of opioid overdose.

Chest Wall Rigidity

The administration of intravenous opioids has been associated with chest wall rigidity. This is characterized by an increase in muscle tone, which can lead to severe truncal stiffness. It appears to be more prevalent with rapid administration and higher doses, in the elderly, and when nitrous oxide is coadministered. The mechanism for this effect is believed to be mediated by mu-receptor stimulation of neurons in the basal ganglia. Treatment can consist of either administration of naloxone or neuromuscular blockers.

Neuroendocrine Effects

Opioids induce endocrine effects through actions in the thalamus and hypothalamus. They inhibit the release of luteinizing hormone releasing hormone (LHRH) so that LH and follicle-stimulating hormone (FSH) release from the pituitary is reduced. Consequently, testosterone secretion is reduced. Decreased libido, ejaculate volume, and sperm motility result in males. Anovulatory cycles or amenorrhea may occur in females. Prolactin secretion is also stimulated.

Analysis of Specific Agents

A brief summary of the specific opioids follows. A comparison of opioids used in analgesia is shown in Table 8-2. Table 8-3 compares opioids used for sedation or general anesthesia.

Agonists

The actions of agonists can be predicted based on the effects listed in Box 8-6. A summary of agents commonly used follows, with only differentiating characteristics being emphasized. When used orally for analgesia, the opioids described have a duration of action approximating 4 hours.

Morphine. The prototypical opioid is morphine. Its onset of peak action following intravenous administration is prolonged because of a delay in crossing

TABLE 8-2

*Comparison of Opioids Used Orally for Postoperative Analgesia**

Drug	Recommended Oral Dose (mg, every 4 to 6 hrs)	EQUIVALENT ANALGESIC DOSE (MG)	
		PO	IM
Morphine	Not commonly used in this context	20-60	10
Codeine	60	200	120
Oxycodone	5-10	30	10
Hydromorphone	2-4	7.5	1.5
Meperidine	100	300	75
Pentazocine	50	180	60
Hydrocodone	5-10		
Dihydrocodeine	32		

Adapted from US Pharmacopeia Drug Information Index, 2001, Rockville, Md, USP; and Dionne RA: New approaches to preventing and treating postoperative pain, *J Am Dent Assoc* 123:27-34, 1992. *PO*, orally; *IM*, intramuscularly.
*The equivalent analgesic doses for severe pain are listed only to allow for comparison of potencies. Although administration of these doses results in equal analgesic effect, they will be more likely to induce the adverse effects as described earlier. Therefore they are *not* meant to be used as recommended doses for postoperative dental pain.

the blood-brain barrier, which is a result of its poor lipid solubility and high degree of ionization at plasma pH. Cardiovascular effects are notable in that morphine administration results in relative stability. Even high doses, such as 1 mg/kg given to supine and normovolemic patients, are unlikely to significantly alter myocardial contractility or blood pressure. These doses will, however, predispose a patient to orthostatic hypotension or syncope. Bradycardia can result and may be secondary to brainstem stimulation of the vagus or caused by a direct depressant effect at the sinoatrial (SA) node of the heart.[7]

Peak onset of respiratory depression from morphine is approximately 30 minutes. Caution is therefore warranted for patients with a history of chronic obstructive lung disease or other causes of decreased

TABLE 8-3

Comparison of Opioids Used for Sedation/Anesthesia

Drug	Equivalent Potent Dose (mg)	Time to Peak Analgesic Effect by IV (min)	Duration of Analgesic Action*	Protein Binding	Clearance
Morphine	10	20	4-5 hr	26%-36%	Renal
Meperidine	100	5-7	2-4 hr	70%	Hepatic/renal
Fentanyl	0.125	3-5	30-60 min	79%-87%	Hepatic
Alfentanil	0.5	1-2	5-10 min	89%-92%	Hepatic
Sufentanil	0.02	2	5 min	93%	Hepatic
Remifentanil	0.02	<1	<5 min	70%	Hydrolysis
Pentazocine	30	15-30	2-3 hr	Moderate	Renal
Nalbuphine	10	30	3-4 hr	?	Renal
Butorphanol	2	30	2-4 hr	High	Renal

Adapted from Coda BB: Opioids. In Barash PG et al, editors: *Clinical anesthesia,* ed 3, Philadelphia, 1996, Lippincott-Raven; US Pharmacopeia Drug Information Index, 2001, Rockville, Md, USP; Stoelting RK: Opioid agonists and antagonists. In *Pharmacology and physiology in anesthetic practice,* Philadelphia, 1991, JB Lippincott.
IV, Intravenous.
*The duration of action is dose-dependent and may vary.

BOX 8-8 — SUMMARY

Opioid Agonists and Agonist/Antagonists

Codeine and its derivatives are prodrugs. Only 10% of an administered dose is converted to the active morphine derivative. They are less effective for patients who are taking cimetidine or the antidepressants fluoxetine and paroxetine.

Opioid agonists are equivalent in their analgesic efficacy and propensities to produce side effects. They have staggering differences in their potencies, and reputed differences are largely attributable to failure to compare equally potent doses.

Agonist/antagonists activate kappa, rather than mu, opioid receptors. There is a ceiling to these effects, which makes them less effective analgesics but less likely to produce severe respiratory depression or dependence.

Agonist/antagonists block mu opioid receptors, which can produce abrupt withdrawal in patients who depend on conventional agonists.

Meperidine should not be prescribed for more than 2 to 3 days because it is converted to normeperidine, a CNS stimulant with an extremely long elimination half-life. This statement is also true for propoxyphene, which is converted to norpropoxyphene.

respiratory reserve. Morphine administration may also lead to increased intracranial pressure and an increase in the tone of smooth muscle, which can affect the sphincter of Oddi. Histamine release is common, and therefore one should use morphine cautiously or not at all in patients with a history of asthma.

Morphine has been widely used as an adjunct to general anesthesia, but because of the delay in onset and long duration of action, it is not particularly suited for outpatient sedation or anesthesia. It is also used for severe chronic pain as is found in cancer. It is normally not used for routine postoperative pain in dentistry. In general anesthesia it has a recommended dose of 0.1 mg/kg when used as an adjunct.

Codeine. Codeine is the most commonly used opioid in dentistry (Box 8-8). It is used as a postoperative analgesic but is not usually used for sedation or anesthesia. It has the lowest first-pass effect of the opioids, and therefore absorption by the oral route is relatively good, with a bioavailability of approximately 60%. Its onset of action orally is approximately 30 to 45 minutes and is slightly more rapid when given intramuscularly.

Codeine has exceptionally low affinity for opioid receptors, and its analgesic effect is caused by its demethylation to morphine (Fig. 8-1). Only 10% of the administered dose is converted to this active form, but the remaining prodrug has antitussive properties and can trigger nausea and vomiting within the chemoreceptor trigger zone.[2] For this reason, codeine 120 mg is regarded as equivalent to morphine 10 mg, and doses large enough to provide relief from more severe pain produce an unacceptably high incidence of nausea. Also, the hepatic cytochrome enzymes responsible for demethylation of codeine and its derivatives (CYP-2D6) are inhibited by cimetidine (Tagamet), fluoxetine (Prozac), and paroxetine (Paxil). Patients medicated with these drugs are unlikely to benefit from codeine derivatives.[8]

Appropriate substitutions on the morphine molecule result in the formation of derivatives with greater potency, such as hydromorphone (Dilaudid) and oxymorphone (Numorphan). Like codeine, hydrocodone and oxycodone are prodrugs, and approximately 10% of an administered dose is converted to the respective morphine derivative. Equally potent intramuscular doses have been established, but the equivalent oral doses for hydrocodone and oxycodone are empiric estimations.

The recommended adult dose for analgesia is 30 to 60 mg, although in the dental pain model there has been little effect noted in doses less than 60 mg. Although it is possible to gain additional analgesia above 60 mg, this is often considered to be a practical ceiling because there is a greater increase in the unwanted side effects described previously. Occasionally, doses of 90 mg may be required. Orally it is available as 15-, 30-, or 60-mg tablets as either codeine phosphate or sulfate.

Oxycodone. Oxycodone is chemically related to morphine and codeine. The oral absorption is relatively good. It has similar applications as codeine, with the noted difference being an increased potency. It is commonly prescribed as 5-mg doses in combination with acetaminophen (Percocet) or as approximately 2.5- or 5-mg doses with aspirin (Percodan). It is also available alone in 5-mg tablets (Roxicodone). The recommended dose for analgesia is

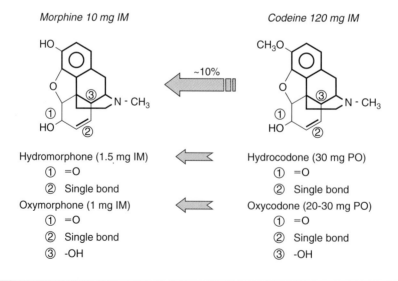

Morphine 10 mg IM   Codeine 120 mg IM

Hydromorphone (1.5 mg IM)
  ① =O
  ② Single bond
Oxymorphone (1 mg IM)
  ① =O
  ② Single bond
  ③ -OH

Hydrocodone (30 mg PO)
  ① =O
  ② Single bond
Oxycodone (20-30 mg PO)
  ① =O
  ② Single bond
  ③ -OH

Fig. 8-1 A simple methyl group at the phenolic hydroxyl position distinguishes codeine and its derivatives from their morphine counterparts. This substitution drastically reduces their binding to mu receptors but does not diminish their antitussive effect or their ability to produce nausea and vomiting.

5 to 10 mg. It is usually considered only if it is determined that codeine is not sufficiently potent for postoperative analgesia, and an opioid is indicated.

Hydrocodone. This opioid is used as an analgesic. Its characteristics are similar to those of codeine. It is formulated in combination as a 5-mg dose with aspirin (Lortab ASA) or a 2.5-, 5-, 7.5-, or 10-mg dose with acetaminophen. The adult dose is 5 to 10 mg.

Dihydrocodeine. This opioid is available in a 16-mg dose as an analgesic in combination with acetaminophen or aspirin (Synalgos). Its characteristics are similar to those of codeine. The adult therapeutic dose is 32 mg.

Hydromorphone. Hydromorphone (Dilaudid) is very potent but can play a role for short-term use as an analgesic for postoperative dental pain. It is more commonly used for severe pain as found in cancer. In dentistry, hydromorphone may be considered when opioids such as codeine or oxycodone have not been effective. Significant abuse potential exists, so hydromorphone should be prescribed in limited quantities only. This drug is not a primary choice for analgesia but should represent an alternative when all other options have proven to be ineffective. The recommended dose for relief of severe pain is 2 to 4 mg. It is available in a 1-, 2-, 4-, or 8-mg tablet.

Meperidine. Meperidine (Demerol) is a purely synthetic drug, derived from the phenylpiperidine family. Traditionally, it has been the most widely used opioid for outpatient sedation and anesthesia in dentistry. It is characterized by having atropine-like properties in addition to its opioid agonist effects. The vagolytic actions may result in a decrease in upper respiratory tract secretions and an increase in heart rate, although these effects are minimal in the usual doses administered for sedation.

At equivalent analgesic doses, meperidine has the same effects as morphine. It differs from morphine in having a shorter duration of action, more complex biotransformation, and greater lipid solubility. Meperidine has a high hepatic extraction ratio, leading to increased doses being required if this drug is administered orally. Cardiovascular effects of meperidine administration include hypotension secondary to negative inotropism, decreased systemic vascular resistance, and decreased venous return.[7] Meperidine has been shown to have a direct depressant effect on myocardial contractility. The hemodynamic responses are variable. Orthostatic hypotension is commonly seen because of interference with compensatory sympathetic reflexes. Both bradycardia and tachycardia have been reported to occur secondary to meperidine administration.

One of the metabolites is normeperidine, which has been associated with toxicity, particularly in patients with hepatic and renal disease where elimination is impaired. This toxicity is seen as CNS excitation, such as agitation, seizures, or hallucinations. It may also be seen in patients concurrently on monoamine oxidase inhibitors (MAOIs) or amphetamines. Potential interactions between meperidine and amphetamines include increased risk of hypotension, possibly leading to cardiovascular collapse, severe respiratory depression, and convulsions. Potential interactions between meperidine and MAOIs can be similar but are particularly characterized by unpredictable excitatory effects such as seizures, hypertension followed by cardiovascular collapse, or rigidity. Meperidine is contraindicated in patients having taken an MAOI within the past 2 weeks.

The typical dose administered for sedation approximates 1 mg/kg, often not exceeding 100 mg. At doses of 50 to 100 mg it can be expected to have a duration of action of 30 to 45 minutes. High doses are not used in general anesthesia because they have prominent negative inotropic effects.

Although meperidine has excellent analgesic properties when given parenterally, its high first-pass effect makes it a poor choice when used orally. As can be seen in Table 8-2, it is less potent than codeine when used in this manner. The high first-pass effect leads to an excess of the potentially toxic metabolite normeperidine when used orally. This problem is exacerbated by normeperidine's half-life of 15 to 20 hours, which leads to accumulation and therefore predisposes the patient to toxicity. Meperidine is, however, indicated when an opioid is required for patients with a true allergy to codeine or oxycodone. The recommended adult dose for analgesia is approximately 100 mg.

Propoxyphene. Propoxyphene (Darvon) is a weak opioid agonist that binds primarily to the mu receptor. One of its metabolites is norpropoxyphene, which has a half-life of 30 hours and therefore can lead to accumulation. This metabolite can lead to toxicity manifesting in CNS signs and symptoms. As an oral analgesic, doses of 90 to 120 mg are considered equivalent to codeine 60 mg.[2] It is available either alone or in combination with acetaminophen or aspirin.

Fentanyl. Fentanyl (Sublimaze) is a synthetic opioid agonist that is an analog of meperidine. It is 75 to 125 times more potent than morphine in analgesic effect. It is characterized by a rapid onset and short duration of action after a single dose when compared with morphine or meperidine. Fentanyl's high lipid solubility contributes to its rapid onset as it readily crosses the blood-brain barrier, particularly when compared with morphine. It also has a high hepatic extraction ratio and is not used orally. High lipid solubility leads to significant concentration of this drug in fatty tissues. Subsequently, slow release from muscle and fat leads to a longer plasma half-life, in spite of its short duration of action. Fentanyl's short duration of action is analogous to that of thiopental because it is caused by redistribution into lipid, and repeated doses will lead to accumulation and increased duration of action and effect.

In doses under 10 μg/kg, no significant change in hemodynamic variables is found, with relatively little effect on myocardial contractility.[7] Histamine is not released. Fentanyl is a potent respiratory depressant, but this usually lasts only 5 to 15 minutes if doses under 100 μg are given. Chest wall rigidity has been reported but is unlikely to occur if fentanyl is administered slowly. Reports have stated that when the rate is 30 to 80 μg per minute, no rigidity should result. The lack of histamine release makes it preferable in patients predisposed to bronchospasm. Precautions include contraindication for use in patients having taken an MAOI within the past 2 weeks, for reasons similar to those for meperidine.

Fentanyl is indicated for either anesthesia or sedation and is particularly suited for short procedures. The dose range for sedation is in the order of 1 μg/kg. At this dose, it can be expected to have a duration of action of 30 to 60 minutes. Advantages of fentanyl over other opioids include cardiovascular stability, relatively short duration of action, and lack of histamine release.

Doses of 1 to 2 μg/kg intravenously provide analgesia. Doses of 2 to 10 μg/kg can be given as an adjunct to volatile agents to minimize cardiovascular responses to specific stimuli. Doses in the range of 50 to 150 μg/kg have been used alone to produce general anesthesia.

Alfentanil. Alfentanil (Alfenta) is an analog of fentanyl that is 5 to 10 times less potent and is characterized by a rapid elimination half-life, which results in a duration of action that is about one-third that of fentanyl. It has a rapid onset of action because of a low pKa that leads to a high proportion of un-ionized drug at physiologic pH. For bolus administration, the recovery from alfentanil will be more rapid than that found with fentanyl or sufentanil. No difference can be expected on short infusions. The termination of effect is due to hepatic biotransformation and redistribution, similar to fentanyl or thiopental, but alfentanil is not prone to significant accumulation after continuous infusion.

Alfentanil has been used primarily in general anesthesia with little documentation for use in sedation. It can be used for both induction of anesthesia after bolus administration and maintenance by infusion. Doses of 150 to 250 μg/kg administered rapidly intravenously will induce general anesthesia in approximately 45 seconds. This should be followed by infusion at a rate of 0.5 to 1 μg/kg/min.

Sufentanil. Sufentanil (Sufenta) is an analog of fentanyl that is 5 to 10 times as potent and has a rapid recovery after infusion. It is more lipid-soluble compared with fentanyl but shares its properties of hepatic biotransformation with a high hepatic extraction ratio. Cardiovascular effects are similar to those found with fentanyl. Histamine is not released. Sufentanil is primarily used in general anesthesia. As with fentanyl and alfentanil, it can be used for both induction of anesthesia following bolus administration and maintenance by infusion. Induction may be accomplished by doses of 8 to 30 μg/kg. For maintenance a loading dose of 0.5 to 8 μg/kg may be considered followed by increments of 10 to 50 μg as needed.

Remifentanil. Remifentanil (Ultiva) is a new selective mu-receptor agonist used as an adjunct in general anesthesia. It is characterized by a rapid onset and a very short duration of action. This ultrashort duration of action is not from redistribution of the drug but is caused by its metabolism, which is unique in that it is hydrolyzed by plasma and tissue esterases. Administration is similar to sufentanil and alfentanil in that it is given by intravenous infusion.

Remifentanil is 22 to 47 times more potent than alfentanil.[3]

Opioid Agonist/Antagonists

Drugs in this group have antagonist properties at mu opioid receptors and produce their effects by activating kappa receptors. They lack the efficacy of pure agonists. These agents have been reported to have ceiling effects on respiratory depression in that continued increases in dose will not correlate with a continued depression in respiration. These drugs will inhibit the action of other opioid agonists that may be administered subsequently and can induce withdrawal in patients dependent on conventional agonists.

Pentazocine. Pentazocine (Talwin) was the first of this category of opioid to have widespread use. This synthetic derivative of benzomorphan has weak antagonist activity in addition to agonist effects. Pentazocine depresses myocardial contractility, but myocardial oxygen demand is greater because of increases in peripheral resistance, blood pressure, and the concentration of plasma catecholamines. Although the antagonist action is weak, it is sufficient to precipitate opioid withdrawal reactions. It would be expected to have a ceiling effect on respiratory depression and visceral pain. Adverse reactions include potential for psychotomimetic effects, such as disorientation, confusion, depression, hallucinations, and dysphoria. Doses that produce sedation have also been associated with diaphoresis and dizziness.

Pentazocine has been used for outpatient sedation procedures in doses approximating 0.5 mg/kg, usually to a maximum of 30 mg. In these doses it can be expected to have a duration of action of 1 hour. Intraoperative use in general anesthesia appears limited.

Pentazocine has clinical use for analgesia as an alternative to codeine or oxycodone. It is indicated when an opioid is required for patients with a true allergy to codeine or oxycodone. The recommended adult dose for analgesia is approximately 50 mg.

Nalbuphine. Nalbuphine (Nubain) is a synthetic compound related to oxymorphone and naloxone. Its analgesia and duration of action are similar to that of morphine. Respiratory depression is reported to have a ceiling effect after a dose of 30 mg. Unlike the effects of pentazocine and butorphanol, nalbuphine does not increase blood pressure or heart rate. For sedation or anesthesia, nalbuphine may be used in doses of 0.1 mg/kg, up to a usual maximum of 10 mg.

Butorphanol. Butorphanol (Stadol) is 5 to 8 times as potent as morphine. It is reported that the increases in respiratory depression are not dose-related, because of the ceiling effect. Cardiovascular effects have been reported as increased myocardial oxygen consumption secondary to increased cardiac work. Major side effects include the usual opioid adverse actions and psychotomimetic effects. Butorphanol has been used for outpatient sedation in doses approximating 0.02 mg/kg, usually to a maximum of 2 mg. Intraoperative use in general anesthesia appears limited.

Opioid Antagonists

Naloxone. Naloxone (Narcan) is an antagonist at all opioid receptors blocking the action of any of the agonists or agonist/antagonists mentioned previously. It is a valuable drug to be used for emergency reversal of opioid-induced effects. After intravenous administration, its onset of action is 1 to 2 minutes; after intramuscular administration, its onset is 2 to 5 minutes. It is not used orally. Its duration of action is dose- and route-dependent. It is also dependent on the extent of the overdose of the opioid in question. Intravenous administration may provide 45 minutes of effect, and intramuscular administration may provide a more prolonged effect.

Naloxone should be used with caution. All opioid receptors are antagonized, and therefore all opioid actions are reversed. Particular concern should be given to patients with cardiac irritability whose condition may worsen, as well as the opioid-dependent patient. Convulsions have been reported to occur, as well as ventricular tachycardia, ventricular fibrillation, and alterations in blood pressure.

The primary indication for using naloxone is in the treatment of opioid-induced respiratory depression, chest wall rigidity, or sedation that is prolonged or too deep. Therapeutic doses range from 0.1 mg up to 2.0 mg, and final doses of 0.4 to 0.8 mg are common. It is best administered intravenously by titrating slowly in 0.1 mg increments to effect. Duration of action is short, so that repeat doses may need to be administered every 5 minutes. Unfortunately, the short duration may allow for resumption of the opioid-agonist actions if its duration of action exceeds that of naloxone. Therefore these patients must continue to be monitored closely.

Naltrexone. This antagonist is similar to naloxone, except it can be used orally and is longer-acting. It has therapeutic use in the management of opioid dependence and alcoholism.

Clinical Considerations

Rational Use

Opioids are used for postoperative analgesia or as adjuncts in sedation and anesthesia. For postoperative analgesia they should be considered only if the use of one of the non-opioid analgesics is maximized, as described in Chapter 7. This rationale is based on knowing that the adverse effects of non-opioids are usually more easily tolerated compared with the adverse effects of opioids (Box 8-9). Although effective parenterally, their high first-pass effect leaves opioids less effective when administered orally. This effect is illustrated in Table 8-1, which compares equally potent doses when administered orally and parenterally.

If it is determined that an opioid is necessary, codeine should be the first to consider. Concurrent with a non-opioid, doses of 30 mg to as much as 90 mg for an adult are recommended.[9-11] If this addition of codeine is insufficient, the next opioid to consider is oxycodone. This drug is most commonly available with either aspirin (in Percodan) or acetaminophen (in Percocet). It is more potent than codeine and is indicated when an opioid is required but codeine has been proven to be ineffective. Doses of 5 to 10 mg are suggested. Hydrocodone in doses of 5 to 10 mg or dihydrocodeine in a dose of 32 mg can also be considered.

Formulations combining acetaminophen or aspirin with codeine, oxycodone, hydrocodone, dihydrocodeine, or pentazocine are available and popular because of ease of administration. However, this may be their only advantage because the relative doses of non-opioid to opioid are often inappropriate. When using these combination analgesics, one should continue to use the principle of maximizing the non-opioid before the opioid. As an example, the use of three tablets of acetaminophen (APAP) with codeine (Tylenol no. 2) will provide acetaminophen 900 mg with codeine 45 mg, which is preferable to one APAP with codeine

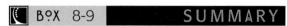

(Tylenol no. 4), which will provide acetaminophen 300 mg with codeine 60 mg. A reasonable alternative is to prescribe codeine separately with clear instructions that it be taken with the non-opioid.

Other opioids should be used less often to manage postoperative pain. Meperidine or pentazocine should be reserved for those situations where an allergy to codeine or oxycodone is confirmed, and it is felt that an opioid is necessary. Hydromorphone should be reserved for those rare situations where all other analgesics have proven ineffective, and a very short course of opioid is felt to be necessary.

For general anesthesia or parenteral sedation, agents such as fentanyl or meperidine are commonly used. The actions of sedation, mood alteration, and analgesia can complement the use of other agents, such as the benzodiazepines. Specific regimens will be discussed in Chapters 16 and 17. Generally healthy patients, such as those who are ASA class 1 or 2, with normal or high cardiac outputs require larger doses of opioids than do ASA class 3 patients, those with cardiovascular disease, or the elderly. Therefore doses should be reduced in these latter patients.

Additional considerations in the use of opioids include reports of allergy and use in geriatric and chemically dependent patients.

Allergy

As with reports of allergy to any medication, it is imperative that the practitioner follow through to confirm that it is a true allergy as opposed to either a patient self-diagnosis or a misdiagnosis by the patient's physician or dentist. The commonly found adverse effect of nausea and vomiting after taking any of the opioids, such as codeine taken for analgesia, has led many patients to assume an allergic reaction to the drug. Also, morphine's ability to release histamine often contributes to a misdiagnosis of allergy. This histamine release can induce pruritus that resembles part of an allergic response. One may assume an accurate diagnosis if the patient's history is consistent with the signs and symptoms of a true immune-mediated response or if the patient has had proper allergy testing and has been positively diagnosed.

It must be assumed that patients who are allergic to codeine will be allergic to all other drugs in that structural class (see Box 8-2). Therefore a history of allergy to codeine, morphine, oxycodone, hydromorphone, or hydrocodone may be considered to contraindicate use of any other in this class. In this case, the patient could consider switching to any of the pure synthetics, such as fentanyl, meperidine, or pentazocine.

Geriatric Patients

Elderly patients may be more sensitive to the effects of opioids, which include exaggerated CNS effects and respiratory depression. Furthermore, they may have age-related impairment of renal and hepatic function. These factors lead to the conclusion that initial doses of opioids must be reduced in the geriatric patient. In general, it has been recommended that if opioids are to be used, the physician or dentist should consider an initial dose of one-half of the drug usually administered. In cases where concomitant disease is present, minimizing the dose or avoiding use of opioids for outpatient procedures may be prudent.

Opioid-Dependent Patients

Patients who are currently dependent on opioids may require an increased dose because of tolerance. Agonist/antagonists should be avoided because they can precipitate withdrawal. Patients recovering from chemical dependency (addiction) may also require higher doses, depending on how long they have been drug-free. Any mood-altering drug must be administered with caution because it may rekindle the abusive behavior. When managing postoperative pain for such a patient, it is wise to consult with his or her medical practitioner. However, opioids are not con-

traindicated when they are part of a regimen for general anesthesia or sedation. Whenever possible, the use of the shorter-acting opioids, such as fentanyl, is preferable.

SUMMARY

Opioids play a role in postoperative analgesia in dentistry. They should be considered if the use of non-opioids by themselves is ineffective or likely to be ineffective. In this case, opioids should not be used alone but in combination with those analgesics.

Opioids also have a role in sedation or general anesthesia when, without their use, excessive doses of another CNS depressant would be required. Opioids offer the advantages of profound analgesia and sedation with minimum cardiovascular effects. Their durations of action are relatively short, and therefore they may deepen the level of sedation without prolonging the duration. Ideally, administration of the opioid should be timed so that the peak effect coincides with the most painful part of the procedure.

Concurrently opioids should be used judiciously. They are all strong respiratory depressants and can lead to nausea, vomiting, and possible chest wall rigidity. In the severely medically compromised or elderly patient, the physician or dentist may need to either reduce the dose or completely eliminate opioid administration.

After careful patient selection, opioids can be a valuable adjunct in the management of pain and the delivery of sedation and anesthesia.

References

1. Kalant H: Opioid analgesics and antagonists. In Kalant H, Roschlau WHE, editors: *Principles of medical pharmacology,* ed 6, Oxford, UK, 1998, Oxford University Press.
2. Reisine T, Pasternak G: Opioid analgesics and antagonists. In Hardman JG, Limbird LE, Molinoff PB, et al, editors: *Goodman and Gilman's the pharmacological basis of therapeutics,* ed 9, New York, 1996, McGraw-Hill.
3. Coda BB: Opioids. In Barash PG et al, editors: *Clinical anesthesia,* ed 3, Philadelphia, 1996, Lippincott-Raven.
4. Pasternak GW: Pharmacological mechanisms of opioid analgesics, *Clin Neuropharmacol* 16:1-18, 1993.
5. Way WL, Way EL, Fields HL: Opioid analgesics and antagonists. In Katzung BG, editor: *Basic and clinical pharmacology,* ed 6, New York, 1995, Appleton-Lange.
6. O'Brien CP: Drug addiction and drug abuse. In Hardman JG, Limbird LE, Molinoff PB, et al, editors: *Goodman and Gilman's the pharmacological basis of therapeutics,* ed 9, New York, 1996, McGraw-Hill.

7. Bailey PL, Stanley TH: Pharmacology of intravenous narcotic anesthetics. In Miller RD, editor: *Anesthesia,* New York, 1990, Churchill Livingstone.

8. Abramowicz M, Rizack MA, et al: *Med Lett* 41(1056):61-62, 1999.

9. US Pharmacopeia Drug Information Index, 2001, Rockville, Md, USP.

10. Dionne RA: New approaches to preventing and treating postoperative pain, *J Am Dent Assoc* 123:27-34, 1992.

11. Stoelting RK: Opioid agonists and antagonists. In *Pharmacology and physiology in anesthetic practice,* Philadelphia, 1991, JB Lippincott.

CHAPTER 9

Anxiolytics and Sedative-Hypnotics

Daniel E. Becker
Paul A. Moore

CHAPTER OUTLINE

Depending on the dose administered, drugs classified as anxiolytics and sedative-hypnotics have the ability to calm a patient and relieve anxiety (anxiolysis), promote drowsiness (sedation), and induce sleep (hypnosis). Confusion in terminology and classification can be attributed more to marketing strategies based on pharmacokinetic profiles than to unique effects produced by these agents. For example, the benzodiazepine triazolam (Halcion) is marketed for treatment of insomnia yet useful for the relief of anxiety. In contrast, diazepam (Valium) was initially marketed as an anxiolytic and formulated in doses appropriate for this purpose. Although 2 to 10 mg of diazepam are appropriate anxiolytic doses, higher doses are usually required for conscious or deep sedation. Marketing strategies aside, the pharmacodynamics of all sedatives follow a classic dose-response pattern so that low

doses impart a calming (anxiolytic or ataraxic) effect, greater doses produce sedation, and high doses can induce loss of consciousness (Fig. 9-1).

The benzodiazepine diazepam has been reputed to have skeletal muscle relaxant properties, but at therapeutic doses this effect is likely an extension of its anxiolytic properties. Distinct central mechanisms for anxiolysis, sedation, and skeletal muscle relaxation have been postulated, but these claims remain equivocal. In addition, some benzodiazepines and barbiturates have well-established anticonvulsant properties.

The anxiolytic and sedative-hypnotic agents also have several dose-related side effects in common. As might be expected, high doses of any central nervous system (CNS) depressant can produce loss of consciousness and depress respiration and cardiovascular tone. These detrimental effects are more likely after doses designed to induce deep sedation than anxiolysis. Chronic use of CNS depressants may result in drug dependence, and after abrupt discontinuation, a withdrawal syndrome may occur. Certain patients may paradoxically experience excitation rather than sedation, but an explanation for this peculiar response has not been confirmed. However, it occurs with greater frequency among pediatric and geriatric patients.

A large number of sedatives and anxiolytics are available. Benzodiazepines are prescribed most frequently; antiemetics, antihistamines, and occasionally barbiturates are also used in dental practice. Principal characteristics by which the three groups can be compared are summarized in Table 9-1. This chapter addresses major pharmacologic features of

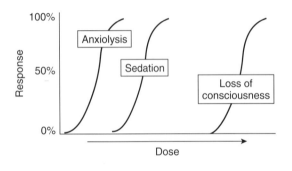

Fig. 9-1 Dose response curves demonstrating potential for producing anxiety relief before other signs of CNS depression (sedation, loss of consciousness) by titrating dose.

TABLE 9-1 📋

Comparisons of Three Classes of Sedative Drugs

	Benzodiazepines	Barbiturates	Antihistamines
Sedative-anxiolytic efficacy	+++	+++	++
Side effects*	++	+++	+
Anticonvulsant	+++	+++	0
Anterograde amnesia	+++	0	0
Anticholinergic	0	0	++
Antiemetic	0	0	++

+, Relative activity; *O*, no activity.
*Side effects are similar qualitatively but differ in frequency and intensity.

these drug classes (Box 9-1). Detailed information regarding drug selection and dosages for various indications are provided in subsequent chapters of this text.

Benzodiazepines

Benzodiazepines are the most commonly prescribed anxiolytic and sedative drugs because their efficacy as anxiolytics and sedatives is unsurpassed, and they produce a relatively low incidence of side effects. The therapeutic effect of benzodiazepines is attributed to their ability to potentiate the inhibitory influences of an endogenous neurotransmitter, gamma-aminobutyric acid (GABA).

Pharmacodynamics: Actions and Effects

GABA is the principal inhibitory neurotransmitter in the mammalian brain.[1] The GABA receptor is located within a large protein complex that surrounds chloride ion channels (chloride ionophores) found in neuronal cell membranes. When GABA binds to this receptor, the channel opens, allowing greater numbers of chloride ions to enter the cell. This influx of negative ions hyperpolarizes the neuron, rendering it less responsive to excitatory signals.

Specific binding sites for benzodiazepine (BZ) receptors are located within this same chloride ion channel complex. When activated by benzodiazepines, BZ receptors alter the configuration of GABA

receptors so that their affinity for GABA is enhanced, and there is a greater influx of chloride ions. It is significant that when used alone, benzodiazepines are incapable of opening chloride ion channels; they merely enhance the ionophore (channel) response to GABA (Fig. 9-2). Some researchers have suggested that this effect is an explanation for the relative safety of benzodiazepines.[2] The intensity of their effect is ultimately determined by a finite quantity of GABA, the brain's normal endogenous neurotransmitter.

At least two subtypes of BZ receptors have been isolated: BZ_1 and BZ_2. Researchers have proposed that BZ_1 receptors mediate sedation and possibly anxiolysis and have little influence on cognitive functions (e.g., amnesia).[3] This effect introduces the possibility that future benzodiazepine derivatives may produce more specific clinical effects. Already this concept has been promoted for quazepam

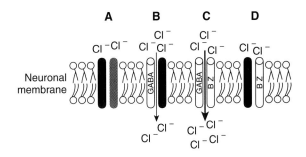

Fig. 9-2 Benzodiazepine action. **A,** Neuronal cell membranes contain channels (ionophores) through which various ions enter and exit neurons. One such channel is the so-called *chloride ionophore,* surrounded by dense complexes of protein. **B,** These protein complexes include receptors by which endogenous ligands can regulate the size of the ionophore. One such receptor is the so-called *GABA receptor.* When activated by GABA, the receptor opens chloride ionophore, allowing an influx of chloride ions. The neuron's membrane potential becomes more negative, and this hyperpolarization renders it less responsive to excitatory neurotransmitters. For this reason, GABA is regarded as an inhibitory neurotransmitter. **C,** Binding sites (receptors) for benzodiazepines are located within this GABA-chloride ionophore complex. Provided GABA is attached to its receptors, benzodiazepine *(BZ)* binding results in an even greater opening of the chloride ionophore. Benzodiazepines are said to potentiate the influence of GABA-mediated opening of chloride channels. **D,** Notice that benzodiazepines cannot influence the chloride channel if GABA is not present on its receptor.

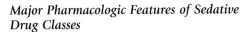

Major Pharmacologic Features of Sedative Drug Classes

Sedatives are generalized CNS depressants; they do not depress selected functions.

Sedatives produce their effects in a dose-response manner; as the dose is increased, patients experience anxiolysis, sedation, and ultimately hypnosis.

Benzodiazepines and barbiturates are effective as both anxiolytics and sedatives. Antihistamines are less effective but have antiemetic effects.

Barbiturates are more effective as hypnotics but are less safe.

(Doral), a relatively selective agonist for BZ_1 receptors. It is heralded as an excellent sedative for insomnia, having little risk for anterograde amnesia. As researchers continue to uncover additional receptor subtypes, there will be further clarification regarding distinct mechanisms that contribute in varying degrees to the sedative-hypnotic, muscle relaxant, anxiolytic, and anticonvulsant effects of benzodiazepines.

All benzodiazepines exhibit comparable efficacy as sedatives and anxiolytics. In addition to their sedative-anxiolytic effects, benzodiazepines also produce anterograde amnesia. Once recovered, patients have difficulty recalling events that occurred while they were sedated. It is significant that the patient, although sedated, was conscious when these events occurred. For example, a patient rendered unconscious by methohexital will not recall a palatal injection of lidocaine. The patient is not experiencing anterograde amnesia; he or she was unconscious. A patient sedated with a benzodiazepine might cry out while receiving a palatal injection but will usually not recall the event when questioned postoperatively.

Compared with other CNS depressants, such as barbiturates and opioids, benzodiazepines have minimal influence on respiration and cardiovascular function. The rapid intravenous administration of hypnotic doses may result in transient episodes of apnea or hypotension, but these events have little consequence unless patients are compromised medically. In fact, the most striking advantage of the benzodiazepines is their remarkable margin of safety.

Even huge doses are rarely fatal. Although suicide attempts with the benzodiazepines are relatively frequent, serious sequelae are rare unless other drugs are taken concomitantly.[4,5] A few deaths have been reported at doses greater than diazepam or chlordiazepoxide 700 mg.[6] Despite their margin of safety, caution must be exercised when using benzodiazepines in patients with chronic respiratory disorders, such as chronic obstructive pulmonary disease (COPD) or obstructive sleep apnea.

Pharmacokinetic Considerations

Differences among benzodiazepines are largely pharmacokinetic and include the degree of lipid solubility, elimination half-life, and pattern of clearance. These characteristics are the principal basis for selection because they influence the time of onset and the duration of effect (Table 9-2).

The most striking difference among benzodiazepines is their pattern of clearance. Some are biotransformed to active metabolites that have extended elimination half-lives, often longer than the parent drug. Metabolism of benzodiazepines is the result of a variety of hepatic phase 1 reactions: demethylation, hydroxylation, and oxidation. With the exceptions of lorazepam and oxazepam, benzodiazepines are metabolized by hepatic oxidative enzymes. The resulting metabolites, some of which retain anxiolytic activity, are then conjugated and eliminated primarily through renal excretion. Final disposition of the active and inactive metabolites occurs through conju-

TABLE 9-2

Characteristics of Selected Benzodiazepine and Miscellaneous Sedative-Anxiolytics[3]

Drug	Active Molecule(s)	T½ (hr)	Peak Onset Oral (hr)*
Diazepam (Valium)	Diazepam, Nordazepam	20-80	0.5-2
Lorazepam (Ativan)	Lorazepam	10-20	2-4
Triazolam (Halcion)	Triazolam	1.5-5.5	1-2
Alprazolam (Xanax)	Alprazolam	6-27	1-2
Chloral hydrate (Noctec)	Trichloroethanol	7-10	0.5-1
Hydroxyzine (Vistaril)	Hydroxyzine	3	0.5-3
Zolpidem (Ambien)	Zolpidem	1.4-4.5	1.6
Zaleplon (Sonata)	Zaleplon	1	1

*Peak onset is based on time until peak serum concentrations are achieved. Sedative effects are noticeable before peak onset. Rapid onset reflects high lipid solubility, which also shortens duration caused by redistribution to peripheral adipose tissue.

gation reactions, principally with glucuronic acid. Oxazepam and lorazepam are noteworthy in that their elimination pathway is via a one-step conjugation reaction, yielding water-soluble, pharmacologically inactive metabolites that are excreted in the urine and are not significantly affected by altered liver function.[7]

Although these metabolites may accumulate following repeated administration, this accumulation does not necessarily prolong the actual duration of their therapeutic effect. After single doses, such as those administered for preoperative sedation, the onset and duration are related most to the drug's lipid solubility. Drugs with greater lipid solubility have fast onset caused by rapid absorption and diffusion through the blood-brain barrier. Also, the duration of effect will be shorter because they distribute to adipose tissue, lowering the serum concentration and promoting redistribution from the brain. After repeated administration, elimination half-life may assume a more significant influence on the duration of clinical effect.[8]

The parent drugs and metabolites of benzodiazepines vary remarkably in their elimination half-lives. Unfortunately, some authors have created a misconception by categorizing them as short-, intermediate-, and long-acting based solely on this pharmacokinetic parameter. One has only to compare lorazepam (Ativan) and diazepam (Valium) to confirm the inaccuracy of this contention (see Table 9-2). Lorazepam is not converted to active metabolites, and its $T_{1/2}$ is shorter than that of diazepam and its metabolite, nordazepam. Still, the onset for lorazepam is slower, and its duration of clinical effect is longer because it is less lipid-soluble than diazepam. $T_{1/2}$ is not without any influence on duration, but it is less significant than lipid solubility.

Issues regarding active metabolites and half-lives provide a therapeutic enigma for physicians when prescribing benzodiazepines for insomnia. Agents that are highly lipid-soluble and have short elimination half-lives would appear to be more desirable than long-acting agents, presumably because there is less potential for daytime impairment. However, studies have not yet confirmed this assumption. Although certain patients may prefer short-acting agents, others experience rebound insomnia and anxiety the following day. Researchers have suggested that, for these latter individuals, agents having longer half-lives may be preferred. The decline in their serum concentration is more gradual, which may

provide a residual anxiolytic effect throughout the ensuing day.[8] These considerations also might be applicable to the use of these agents for preoperative sedation.

Selected Agents

The popularity of benzodiazepines for conscious sedation is a consequence of their large margin of safety and the ability to provide relief of anxiety without producing gross sedation. Numerous agents that differ primarily by their rates of onset and elimination are available (Box 9-2). Commonly used oral benzodiazepines in dentistry include diazepam (Valium), triazolam (Halcion), and lorazepam (Ativan). Midazolam (Versed) is frequently administered intravenously for conscious sedation. Recently an oral formulation has been approved for marketing in the United States.

Diazepam. Of the currently available benzodiazepines, diazepam is probably the most well known. For two decades after its introduction in the 1970s, it

---

> ▣ **B◦X 9-2**   **SUMMARY**
>
> ### *Benzodiazepines*
>
> Benzodiazepines produce their effects by acting as agonists at BZ receptors, which potentiate the body's natural inhibitory neurotransmitter, GABA. They are not GABA agonists.
>
> Little qualitative difference is found among benzodiazepines in terms of their efficacy as anxiolytics or sedatives.
>
> Great variation occurs among benzodiazepines in terms of their active metabolites and the elimination half-lives for parent drugs and metabolites.
>
> The half-life of a given agent does not predict the duration of its sedative effect after a single, preoperative dose. However, agents that have prolonged elimination time might produce residual lethargy in elderly patients.
>
> After a single dose, agents that have the greatest lipid solubility provide the fastest onset and the shortest duration, regardless of their elimination half-life.
>
> Flumazenil is a benzodiazepine antagonist that can be used to reverse excessive somnolence or respiratory depression attributed to any benzodiazepine.

was one of the top 10 drugs prescribed in the United States. It is formulated for oral and parenteral administration and is an effective and safe anxiolytic agent for use in dental practice.

The pharmacokinetic profile of diazepam is less than ideal. It has a relatively slow onset when administered either intramuscularly or orally. Intravenous use of diazepam is associated with thrombophlebitis at the injection site. Diazepam's elimination half-life is prolonged, and its primary metabolite, nordazepam (formerly desmethyldiazepam), retains significant CNS depressant activity. These properties limit its use in anesthesia and anxiety control where rapid onset and recovery is preferred.

Lorazepam. Lorazepam (Ativan) is a 1,4 benzodiazepine derivative that has been used extensively as an anxiolytic and sedative before anesthesia. Both oral and injectable formulations are available. Because this benzodiazepine metabolizes directly to an inactive conjugate, adverse drug reactions from drug interactions and liver impairment are rarely reported. After a single oral dose, peak plasma concentrations are established in 1 to 2½ hours, and the elimination half-life ranges from 8 to 25 hours. Bioavailability after oral administration has been calculated to be 93%.[7]

Lorazepam is most useful when rapid onset of activity is not essential and when prolonged sedation is indicated. In a double-blind comparison trial, oral triazolam was found to have a sedation onset of 60 minutes compared with 120 minutes for lorazepam. Six hours after drug administration, sleepiness persisted only for subjects in the lorazepam group.[9] Its use for sedation in critical care centers has been advocated because it has minimal cardiovascular and respiratory depressant effects, inactive metabolites, and few side effects.[10] Impairment of psychomotor skills has been found to continue for 12 hours after lorazepam administration as compared with 7 hours for diazepam.[11] The use of lorazepam for relief of fear and anxiety before outpatient dental procedures is limited because rapid onset of sedation is usually required, and prolonged psychomotor impairment that outlasts most dental procedures may extend recovery times.

Triazolam. Triazolam (Halcion) is chemically related to diazepam and is indicated for the treatment of insomnia. Its rapid onset, short duration of action, and lack of active metabolites also make it a nearly ideal

antianxiety medication for dental outpatients. When administered sublingually, triazolam produces even greater anxiolytic effects than oral administration of an equivalent dose without any detectable increase in side effects or psychomotor impairment.[12] Some clinicians are reluctant to use it for sedation, however, because they are unfamiliar with this application and are influenced by controversial claims as reported in the media concerning the drug.

Triazolam in a dose of 0.25 mg has proven effective as a preanesthetic medication before general anesthesia, plastic surgery, and oral surgery. A comparison of 0.125, 0.25, or 0.5 mg administered an hour before oral surgery demonstrated significant anxiety reduction for the two higher doses but prolonged psychomotor impairment after the 0.5 mg dose.[13] Administration of triazolam 0.25 mg in combination with 40% nitrous oxide resulted in anxiety relief comparable to a mean dose of diazepam 19 mg but with faster postoperative recovery for the triazolam-nitrous oxide combination.[13] Oral triazolam has also been demonstrated to be more effective than oral diazepam when administered to anxious patients before an endodontic procedure.[14] These studies indicate that oral triazolam is an anxiolytic agent comparable in efficacy to intravenous diazepam but without the potential toxicity of parenteral drug administration.

Orally or sublingually administered triazolam in doses of 0.25 to 0.5 mg does not produce any adverse changes in respiration, heart rate, or blood pressure.[12-14] In safety studies with healthy volunteers, even unusually high doses of triazolam (2 to 4 mg) did not depress the respiratory response to carbon dioxide or affect cardiovascular dynamics.[15,16] The absence of any reports of respiratory depression, despite the millions of doses administered, indicates that a single dose of triazolam is unlikely to produce respiratory distress in dental patients. The most common side effects reported after triazolam administration include drowsiness, light-headedness, and incoordination. Most adverse effects attributed to triazolam occur when doses are higher (0.5 to 1.5 mg) than the suggested dose for dental outpatients (0.25 mg), when given to the elderly, or when administered chronically with inadequate medical supervision.

Flumazenil. Flumazenil (Romazicon) is a benzodiazepine antagonist that effectively reverses somnolence and respiratory depression mediated at BZ

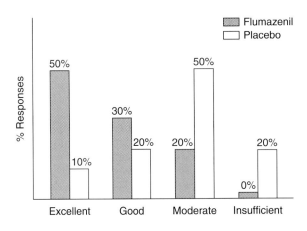

Fig. 9-3 Observer assessment of the reversal of IV sedation 5 minutes after administration of flumazenil (0.1 mg/ml) or placebo.

receptors. Clinical trials using flumazenil to reverse the CNS depression associated with intravenous diazepam sedation for third molar extractions have demonstrated its efficacy (Fig. 9-3).[17,18] It is available as a 0.1-mg/ml concentration in 5-ml and 10-ml vials. Although intended for intravenous administration in 0.2-mg increments up to 1 mg, it may be injected submucosally as well. To manage excessive somnolence or respiratory depression, attention should be given first to standard airway support, including supplemental oxygenation. This can be followed by submucosal injection of flumazenil 0.3 mg and can be repeated in 5 to 10 minutes if necessary. Flumazenil is contraindicated in patients who are dependent on benzodiazepines or those who have a history of seizure disorders.

Barbiturates

Like benzodiazepines, barbiturates potentiate the action of GABA. However, barbiturates also alter ion fluxes directly and also potentiate several additional neurotransmitters. These additional actions may explain their poor selectivity and low therapeutic index compared with those for benzodiazepines.[2] Using doses intended to produce anxiolysis or sedation, barbiturates are no more effective than benzodiazepines. However, when inducing general anesthesia, barbiturates are more predictable. Although this effect may be an advantage when inducing un-

consciousness, it provides little advantage for conscious sedation. For the most part, barbiturates are used only as anticonvulsants (phenobarbital) and for deep sedation or general anesthesia (thiopental, methohexital). Their use as sedatives for insomnia or preoperative sedation has been supplanted almost entirely by benzodiazepines. Among their many drawbacks for chronic use is a tendency to stimulate the activity of hepatic microsomal enzymes. This is particularly true for phenobarbital, which significantly shortens the activity of other drugs that may be administered concurrently. Another drawback is that painful stimuli may incite delirium and agitation, especially when used for preoperative sedation.[2]

The use of barbiturates for pediatric sedation is limited for three reasons: (1) their reputed ability to induce paradoxical excitement, (2) the limited therapeutic dosage range, and (3) the lack of available reversing agents. Inadequate doses are not effective and may cause disinhibition (i.e., cause an uncooperative child to be more unmanageable). Even at higher doses in the therapeutic range, a few children, particularly when stimulated, will demonstrate paradoxical excitation. These apparent stimulatory effects after administration of sedative-hypnotics are seen in less than 5% of pediatric patients and may be caused by either the barbiturate's hyperalgesic properties or respiratory depression and subsequent agitation. In addition, the CNS depressant effects seen with barbiturate overdose are not easily managed. Benzodiazepines and opioids have specific pharmacologic antagonists (flumazenil and naloxone) that can be administered to reverse the level of CNS depression. Barbiturates are nonspecific membrane depressants, and at the present time, specific reversal agents have not been developed. These disadvantages and the availability of benzodiazepines have resulted in a significant decrease in the use of barbiturates for pediatric sedation.

Antihistamines

When antihistamines are prescribed as antipruritics for various allergic disorders, sedation is often a troublesome side effect. However, this effect can be exploited when treating insomnia or preoperative anxiety. Antihistamines are less effective than benzodiazepines or barbiturates as anxiolytics or sedatives, so they cannot be recommended as primary agents for conscious

☾ BOX 9-3   SUMMARY
Barbiturates, Antihistamines,
and Nonbenzodiazepines

> Barbiturates have no advantage over benzodiazepines as sedatives or anxiolytics and do not produce anterograde amnesia.
>
> Barbiturates are more effective and predictable hypnotics but carry a greater risk for respiratory depression.
>
> Antihistamines are less effective sedatives than benzodiazepines but produce antiemetic effects.
>
> Antihistamines produce anticholinergic effects and should be avoided in elderly patients who have dementia.
>
> The newer so-called *nonbenzodiazepines* have no real advantage over traditional benzodiazepines and are identical in most respects.

sedation (Box 9-3). The sedative effect of antihistamines is attributed to their action as antagonists at histaminergic and cholinergic receptor sites, countering the normal excitatory influences of these respective neurotransmitters within the CNS.

Histamine and acetylcholine are among several neurotransmitters associated with neural pathways involved in nausea and vomiting. For this reason, antihistamines are useful antiemetic agents. Hydroxyzine (Vistaril) and promethazine (Phenergan) are prescribed most often, but other antihistamines are equally effective. Promethazine may be more effective in some cases of nausea and vomiting because it also blocks dopamine, a neurotransmitter associated with the chemoreceptor trigger zone adjacent to the vomiting center within the medulla. Emetic influences of opioids are attributed in part by activating these dopaminergic pathways. Unfortunately, dopamine antagonists also block dopamine receptors within the basal ganglia, which may initiate so-called *extrapyramidal symptoms* that mimic the skeletal muscle tremors and rigidity seen in Parkinson's disease. Obviously, drugs such as promethazine must be avoided in patients with overt parkinsonism. Furthermore, all agents with anticholinergic actions should be avoided if possible in elderly patients who have significant symptoms of dementia. This caution is predicated on information that Alzheimer's disease is attributed in part to inadequate levels of acetylcholine.

Miscellaneous Agents

Chloral Hydrate

Chloral hydrate is most often prescribed for oral sedation in children. It was first introduced by Liebig in 1832 and is the oldest and best-studied pediatric sedative. Considering present concerns and restrictions regarding parenteral sedation techniques, the usage of oral sedative agents, such as chloral hydrate, is likely to continue. As a halogenated derivative of acetaldehyde, chloral hydrate is highly lipid-soluble and carries greater CNS depressant properties than acetaldehyde. Because of tissue irritability, formulations of chloral hydrate are administered orally and rectally only.

The sedative-hypnotic activity of chloral derivatives probably results from the common metabolite trichloroethanol (TCE). Chloral hydrate is rapidly metabolized to TCE and to a lesser extent to trichloroacetic acid (TCA). Plasma levels of chloral hydrate are nearly undetectable immediately after administration. Peak plasma concentrations of TCE are reached in 20 to 60 minutes. The plasma half-life of TCE is estimated to be 8 hours. Both TCA and TCE are eliminated as glucuronide conjugates.[19,20]

Although definitive studies in children are sparse, it is generally assumed that therapeutic doses of chloral hydrate have minimum effects on respiratory and cardiovascular function. In adults, a 20 mg/kg-dose causes no significant change in arterial blood pressure or heart rate and changes in respiratory function (e.g., PCO_2, respiratory rate, tidal volume) are comparable to natural sleep. Patients who have asthma may be somewhat more sensitive to chloral hydrate's minimal respiratory depressive properties. The CO_2 chemoreceptor response appears to be unchanged in infants administered chloral hydrate 50 mg/kg.

The primary pharmacologic effect of chloral hydrate is CNS depression. Signs and symptoms after ingestion of increasing doses of chloral hydrate progress from relaxation, lethargy, drowsiness, and hypnosis to loss of consciousness and coma. Adverse effects to chloral hydrate administration are rare. When used as a hypnotic, untoward reactions occur in about 2% of the cases. Overt CNS depression, characterized by disorientation and prolonged drowsiness, account for half of these reactions. Hypersensitivity reactions, gastrointestinal (GI) disturbances, CNS excitation, headache, hepatic decompensation, and coagulation disturbances have also been reported. Reactions to chloral hydrate in dental patients are generally similar, although dose-related reactions, such as prolonged CNS depression and vomiting, appear more frequently in younger ambulating populations. With excessively high doses of chloral hydrate (i.e., 75 mg/kg or more), a significant incidence of vomiting has been reported. Therapeutic doses of chloral hydrate are generally limited to 50 to 60 mg/kg. The maximum recommended dose in children, irrespective of body weight, is 1000 to 1500 mg.

Dosages required to produce effective sedation are generally irritating to the GI mucosa, and patients may become delirious and combative when provoked by pain.[2] Unfortunately, this has been the case when this agent is used to manage highly recalcitrant pediatric dental patients. Although alternative sedative therapies are now available, chloral hydrate continues to be popular among pediatric dentists, a practice that originated before the introduction of barbiturates and benzodiazepines.

Zolpidem and Zaleplon

Zolpidem (Ambien) and zaleplon (Sonata) are the most recent agents introduced for the short-term management of insomnia. Their molecular structures are modified from benzodiazepines but are distinguished as nonbenzodiazepines by pharmaceutical industry marketing as a strategy to capitalize on negative views regarding benzodiazepines. They bind to benzodiazepine receptors, exhibiting some preference for the BZ_1 subtype, which implies that they produce less anterograde amnesia. Their effects are reversed by the benzodiazepine antagonist, flumazenil. Clinical considerations regarding these agents are identical to those discussed for benzodiazepines, and their pharmacokinetics closely resemble those for triazolam (Halcion). They have considerable lipid solubility that provides a rapid onset and short duration, short elimination half-lives (<4 hours), and no active metabolites.[3]

Therapeutic Recommendations

The proper use of sedatives for the management of situational anxiety and for conscious sedation is thoroughly addressed in subsequent chapters. The following section addresses special considerations regarding the use of sedatives for selected patients.

Use in Pregnancy

The adverse drug reactions during pregnancy may affect either the mother or the fetus. Hypersensitivity, allergy, or toxicity reactions to the mother may compromise her health and limit her ability to support a pregnancy. Adverse drug effects specific to the health of the fetus may include congenital defects, low birth weight, complications during delivery, and postnatal drug dependency. These effects are usually specific to the timing of drug administration during pregnancy (first, second, or third trimester), the dose given, and the duration of therapy. Fortunately, dental drug therapies are usually administered for a limited time and are generally less likely to cause complications during pregnancy. Product information sheets provided with prescription and nonprescription drugs, as well as drug information in the *Physician's Desk Reference* (PDR), generally include use-in-pregnancy information and ratings.

Administration of any of the CNS depressants commonly used for sedation therapy during pregnancy is problematic because they generally cross placental barriers to inhibit neuronal function in the developing fetus. Of the antianxiety drugs commonly prescribed, the benzodiazepine diazepam (Valium) has been most frequently assessed. Human investigations have noted an association between diazepam exposure during pregnancy and oral clefts,[21] and these associations have been carried over to the other, less frequently used benzodiazepines. Confirmation of these reports has not always been possible,[22] and recent articles have challenged any concern in the matter.[23,24] Although a single dose exposure compared with chronic therapy throughout a pregnancy would suggest only minimum risk for teratogenicity after benzodiazepine anxiolytic use and sedation/anesthesia, overall the evidence strongly cautions against their use during pregnancy.[25]

Drug and chemical exposure during pregnancy is believed to account for only about 1% of congenital malformations. Delivery complications and birth defects associated with pregnancy are more commonly caused by poor nutrition, smoking and alcohol consumption, diseases, genetic predisposition, and age. Maintaining a healthy life style, including optimum oral health, is essential for women who are currently pregnant or who are planning a pregnancy. When dental treatment is necessary to maintain oral health, selecting the safest agents, limiting the duration of the drug regimens, and minimizing dosages are the fundamental principles for safe therapy.

Pediatric Patients

Because of modifications in drug pharmacodynamics and pharmacokinetics, pediatric and geriatric patients may respond differently to anxiolytic and sedative-hypnotic drugs. The most obvious anatomic difference between the adult and pediatric patient is body size. An increased awareness for dosage adjustment in pediatric patients has developed in the last few years within dentistry. In pediatric sedation and anesthesia for children under 2 years of age who are infrequently treated, Clark's weight-based rule (child's dose = adult dose × child's weight/150 lb) usually proves to be satisfactory. Fixed pediatric dosage recommendations for a given age range are no longer endorsed for anesthetic and sedative agents. Available data reinforces the belief that serious adverse reactions in pediatric sedation are commonly caused by inadequate dosage reduction.[26]

Children's responsiveness to anesthetics and sedatives may differ from that of adults because of differences in pharmacokinetics or pharmacodynamics. These differences vary among drugs and are generally impossible to predict. For example, infants appear relatively more sensitive to morphine, possibly because of an immature barrier between the blood and the brain. Alternatively, relatively high doses of atropine are usually well tolerated by children. Fortunately, differences in drug absorption, distribution, and excretion occur primarily in the perinatal period and are usually not relevant to office practice, where treatment is usually limited to children over 2 years of age. It has been reported that young children may be unexpectedly sensitive to the CNS depressants used for dental anesthesia.

Geriatric Patients

The use of benzodiazepines in elderly patients is associated with an increase risk of falls and hip fractures.[27] Both an increased sensitivity to the agents and delay in the elimination of benzodiazepines is known to be prolonged and magnify the effects of benzodiazepines. Sedation in elderly patients is best administered in reduced doses or with titratable techniques.

References

1. Bloom FE: Neurotransmission and the central nervous system. In Hardman JG, Limbird LE, Molinoff PB, et al, editors: *Goodman and Gilman's the pharmacological basis of therapeutics*, ed 9, New York, 1996, McGraw-Hill.

2. Hobbs WR, Rall TW, Verdoorn TA: Hypnotics and sedatives: ethanol. In Hardman JG, Limbird LE, Molinoff PB, et al, editors: *Goodman and Gilman's the pharmacological basis of therapeutics*, ed 9, New York, 1996, McGraw-Hill.

3. Olin BR, Hebel SK, Dombek CE, editors: *Drug facts and comparisons*, 2001, St Louis, JB Lippincott (Facts and Comparisons).

4. Jatlow P, Dobular K, Bailey D: Serum diazepam concentrations in overdose, *Am J Clin Pathol* 72:571-577, 1979.

5. Greenblatt DJ, Allen MD, et al: Acute overdosage with benzodiazepine derivatives, *Clin Pharmacol Ther* 4:497-514, 1977.

6. Baldessarini RJ: Drugs and the treatment of psychiatric disorders: psychosis and anxiety. In Hardman JG, Limbird LE, Molinoff PB, et al, editors: *Goodman and Gilman's the pharmacological basis of therapeutics*, ed 9, New York, 1996, McGraw-Hill.

7. Greenblatt DJ: Clinical pharmacokinetics of oxazepam and lorazepam, *Clin Pharmacokinet* 6:89-105, 1981.

8. Greenblatt DJ, Miller LG, Shader RI: Neurochemical and pharmacokinetic correlates of the clinical action of benzodiazepine hypnotic drugs, *Am J Med* 88:18s-24s, 1990.

9. Thomas D, Tipping T, Halifax R, et al: Triazolam premedication: a comparison with lorazepam and placebo in gynaecological patients, *Anaesthesia* 41:692-697, 1986.

10. Young C, Knudsen H, Hilton A, et al: Sedation in the intensive care unit, *Crit Care Med* 28(3):854-866, 2000.

11. Seppala T, Kortilla K, Hakkinen S, et al: Residual effects and skills related to driving after a single oral administration of diazepam, medezepam, and lorazepam, *Br J Clin Pharm* 3:831-841, 1976.

12. Kaufman E, Hargreaves KM, Dionne RA: Comparison of oral triazolam and nitrous oxide to placebo and intravenous diazepam for outpatient premedication, *Oral Surg Oral Med Oral Pathol* 75:156-164, 1993.

13. Berthold CB, Dionne RA, Corey SE: Comparison of sublingually and orally administered triazolam for premedication prior to oral surgery, *Oral Surg Oral Med Oral Pathol Oral Radiol Endod* 84:119-124, 1997.

14. Ehrich DG, Lundgren JP, Dionne RA, et al: Comparison of oral triazolam, diazepam, and placebo as outpatient premedication for endodontic patients, *J Endodontics* 23:181-184, 1997.

15. Elliott HW, Navarro G, Nikka N, et al: Early phase I evaluation of sedative, hypnotics, or minor tranquilizers. In Kagan F, Harwood T, Rickels K, et al, editors: *Hypnotics: methods of development and evaluation*, New York, 1975, Spectrum, p 87.

16. Gottschalk LA, Elliott HW: Effects of triazolam and flurazepam on emotions and intellectual function, *Res Commun Psychol Psychiatry Behav* 1:575, 1976.

17. Finder RL, Moore PA, Close JM: Flumazenil reversal of conscious sedation with intravenous fentanyl and diazepam, *Anesth Prog* 42:11-16, 1995.

18. Bloom JW, Chernik DA, Davidson AB, et al: Reversal of central benzodiazepine effects by flumazenil after conscious sedation produced by intravenous diazepam, *Clin Therapeutics* 14:895-909, 1992.

19. Moore PA: Therapeutic assessments of chloral hydrate premedication in pediatric dentistry, *Anesth Prog* 31:191-195, 1984.

20. Moore PA, Mickey EA, et al: Sedation in pediatric dentistry: a practical assessment procedure, *J Am Dent Assoc* 109:564-569, 1984.

21. Safra JM, Oakley GP: Association between cleft lip with or without cleft palate and neonatal exposure to diazepam, *Lancet* 2:478-480, 1975.

22. Rosenberg L, Mitchell AA, et al: Lack of relation of oral clefts to diazepam use during pregnancy, *N Engl J Med* 309:1282-1285, 1983.

23. Koren G, Pastuszak A, Ito S: Drugs in pregnancy, *N Engl J Med* 338:1128-1137, 1998.

24. Rosen MA: Management of anesthesia for the pregnant surgical patient, *Anesthesiology* 91:1159-1163, 1999.

25. Moore PA: Selecting drugs for the pregnant dental patient, *J Am Dent Assoc* 129:1281-1286, 1998.

26. Goodson JM, Moore PA: Life-threatening reactions following pedodontic sedation: an assessment of narcotic, local anesthetic, and antiemetic drug interaction, *J Am Dent Assoc* 107:239-245, 1983.

27. Herings RM, Stricker BH, et al: Benzodiazepines and the risk of falling leading to femur fractures: dosage more important than elimination half-life, *Arch Intern Med* 155 (16):1801-1807, 1995.

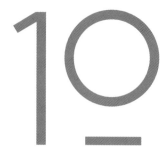

General Anesthetics

Daniel E. Becker

In 1920 Guedel described ether anesthesia according to four stages, each reflecting greater depression of brain function: *stage I*, analgesia; *stage II*, delirium; *stage III*, surgical anesthesia; and *stage IV*, medullary paralysis and death. These stages are merely of historical interest; they are not observed reliably with modern agents and techniques. Stage II, or delirium, is often used to describe excitatory events that frequently occur during slow induction or emergence from unconsciousness, but they are too unpredictable and inconsistent to attribute directly to modern general anesthesia.

General anesthesia is a drug-induced state characterized by an absence of perception to all sensations. The mechanism of general anesthesia remains controversial. Anesthetics may influence synaptic transmission by potentiating neurotransmitter release at inhibitory synapses or by inhibiting excitatory synapses. Despite the poor understanding of general anesthesia at the molecular level, much is known about the effects produced by the variety of drugs used alone or, more often, in combination.

Most anesthesiologists agree that general anesthesia requires three principal components, sometimes described as the anesthetic triad: (1) *unconsciousness* (hypnosis), (2) *analgesia* (areflexia), and (3) *skeletal muscle relaxation*.[1,2] Many of the agents classified by convention as general anesthetics do not accomplish all three of these objectives. The volatile inhalation agents come closest but only at doses that depress the brain to such a degree that vital functions are placed in jeopardy. The term *anesthetic* is used spuriously when describing potent sedative-hypnotics or opioids that produce only one component of complete general anesthesia. For example, thiopental provides hypnosis, but a surgical stimulus evokes autonomic and somatic reflexes that confirm absence of analgesia and muscle relaxation. Likewise, potent opioids provide analgesia and areflexia, but hypnosis is unreliable; controlled ventilation is required because of respiratory depression. For these reasons the most common approach is to (1) induce unconsciousness with a potent sedative-hypnotic or inhalation agent, (2) provide analgesia with an opioid, and (3) produce muscle relaxation using a neuromuscular blocking agent.

Regardless of the agent or regimen employed, the following approach is a practical guide for evaluating depth of anesthesia.[1] Surgical anesthesia is not present if (1) eyelids respond when eyelashes are stroked, (2) respirations are irregular, or (3) the patient is swallowing. Loss of eyelash reflex and presence of rhythmic respiration indicate onset of anesthesia, whereas tightness of the jaw and gagging indicate that depth is inadequate. Analgesia is inadequate if a surgical stimulus evokes an increase in respiratory rate, heart rate, or blood pressure. As anesthesia deepens, these responses are reduced or abolished, and a reduction in tidal volume and blood pressure will generally follow with increasing depth of anesthesia.

Inhalation Anesthetics

The inhalation agents are most deserving of the title "general anesthetics." They are excellent hypnotics and at higher concentrations produce varying degrees of analgesia and skeletal muscle relaxation. Although the mechanism for their anesthetic effect is unresolved, effects are directly related to their tension (partial pressure) in brain tissue. This follows an equilibration between tensions in the inspired gas, the alveoli, and the arterial blood.

Pharmacokinetics

When a constant tension of anesthetic gas is inhaled, its uptake and distribution are inversely related to the solubility of the agent in blood and tissues, expressed as the *blood:gas partition coefficient*. Gases with low solubility achieve tension rapidly in the blood phase of distribution, driving the concentration of the agent into the brain. This same principle applies to elimination of anesthetic gases, only in reverse. When administration of anesthetic gas is discontinued, the alveolar gas tension is washed out because no gas is coming from the anesthetic machine, and equilibration proceeds from the tissue to venous blood to alveoli for elimination by expiration (see Chapter 14, Fig. 14-1). Any elimination attributed to biotransformation is negligible for all anesthetic gases except halothane, 10% to 30% of which undergoes hepatic biotransformation to inactive metabolites.[3] Therefore inhalation anesthetics having the lowest blood:gas coefficients exhibit the most rapid onset and termination of effects.[4] These gases are most suited for patients who require intermittent alterations in anesthetic depth (Table 10-1).

TABLE 10-1

Comparison of Inhalation Anesthetics*

Anesthetic Agent	Blood:Gas Coefficient	Minimum Alveolar Concentration (MAC) (%)
Nitrous oxide	0.47	104
Sevoflurane	0.69	1.71
Desflurane	0.42	6
Isoflurane	1.46	1.15
Enflurane	1.91	1.7
Halothane	2.54	0.77

Data from Barash PG, Cullen BF, Stoelting RK, editors: *Clinical anesthesia*, ed 3, Philadelphia, 1997, Lippincott-Raven.
*Patients 21 to 65 years of age.

Minimum Alveolar Concentration

The dose of an anesthetic gas is expressed as its percentage in the inspired mixture. To compare the relative potencies of anesthetic gases, anesthesiologists have accepted a measure known as *minimum alveolar concentration* (MAC), which represents the percentage or concentration of the gas at 1 atmosphere that renders 50% of patients unresponsive to a surgical stimulus. It is analogous to the effective dose for 50% of patients (ED_{50}), expressed in milligrams for other drugs. Nitrous oxide (N_2O) is the least potent of the anesthetic gases, with a MAC of 104. It was extrapolated from studies conducted in a hyperbaric chamber because its MAC cannot be achieved at normal atmospheric pressure (see Table 10-1). Many variables can alter the MAC in a given patient (Box 10-1).

MAC reflects an adequate dose for only 50% of patients; successful clinical anesthesia may require 0.5 to 2.0 MAC for individual patients. More than 90% of all patients become anesthetized after administration of 1.3 MAC,[1,2] and presumably, 1.5 to 2.0 MAC is required to ensure anesthesia in all patients. Furthermore, the doses of anesthetic gases are generally additive; 0.5 MAC of one agent added to 0.5 MAC of another provides 1 MAC. Based on this principle, as well as the effects of other central nervous system (CNS) depressants on MAC, anesthesiologists often provide anesthesia using single inhaled anesthetics or mixtures equaling 0.8 to 1.2

BOX 10-1

Factors that Alter Minimum Alveolar Concentration (MAC)

Factors Increasing MAC
Fever
CNS stimulants
Decreasing age
Chronic alcoholism

Factors Decreasing MAC
Hypothermia
CNS depressants, including acute alcohol ingestion
Increasing age
Severe hypercapnia ($Paco_2$ >90 mm Hg)
Severe hypoxemia (Pao_2 <40 mm Hg)
Severe anemia (Hct <10%)

Data from Barash PG, Cullen BF, Stoelting RK, editors: *Clinical anesthesia*, ed 3, Philadelphia, 1997, Lippincott-Raven.
CNS, Central nervous system; *Paco₂*, carbon dioxide tension in arterial blood; *Pao₂*, oxygen tension in arterial blood; *Hct*, hematocrit.

BOX 10-2 SUMMARY

Pharmacokinetics of Inhalation Anesthetics

The onset and termination of anesthesia using inhalation agents is inversely related to solubility in blood. Low blood:gas coefficient correlates with rapid onset and rapid recovery.

Inhalation agents have comparable efficacy, provided they are administered in equivalent doses.

Doses of inhalation agents are expressed as units called MAC, which represent the minimum alveolar concentration required to produce unresponsiveness to surgical stimulation in 50% of patients.

MAC, in combination with intravenous sedatives and opioids.

Finally, it must be emphasized that MAC is a measure of the *dose-response* for an inhalation agent in producing anesthesia. Incremental increases in MAC do not predict with any precision the influence on respiratory or cardiovascular function. For example, 0.5 MAC does not necessarily produce half the influences on blood pressure as 1.0 MAC (Box 10-2).

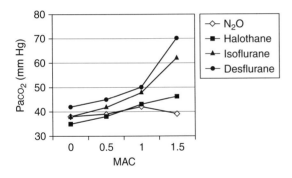

Fig. 10-1 Relative respiratory depression of inhalation anesthetics. A general comparison of respiratory depression is reflected in elevation of carbon dioxide tension in arterial blood *(Paco$_2$)*. Although not depicted, sevoflurane closely resembles isoflurane in respiratory influence. *MAC,* Minimum alveolar concentration; *N$_2$O,* nitrous oxide.

Systemic Effects

At equipotent concentrations (MAC), anesthetic efficacy is identical regardless of the agent or mixture selected. Their effects on the lungs, heart, and circulation, as well as less apparent actions on other organs, are similar qualitatively but differ in their intensity and the specific parameter they target. Side effects always accompany general anesthesia, and accurate knowledge of these properties is required for safe management of the patient. Data comparing the effects of inhalation anesthetics are obtained from healthy volunteers and will vary in patients who are ventilated, who have respiratory or cardiac disease, or who are medicated with drugs having cardiovascular effects.

Respiratory Effects. All inhalation agents depress ventilation, and their influence on ventilatory response to *hypoxemia* is greater than that for hypercapnia. Concentrations less than 0.5 MAC have minimal influence on hypercapnic drive, but the dose-response becomes more significant at higher concentrations, leading to apnea at concentrations of 1.5 to 2.0 MAC. In contrast, as little as 0.1 MAC produces a 50% to 70% reduction in ventilatory response to hypoxemia.[5,6] Inhalation agents tend to increase respiratory rate but depress tidal volume.[4-8] Their net influence on minute ventilation is reflected in the degree of hypercapnia that occurs during ad-

BOX 10-3 SUMMARY

Respiratory Effects of Inhalation Anesthetics

All inhalation agents increase respiratory rate and decrease tidal volume.

Most agents decrease net ventilation (minute ventilation); N$_2$O is the exception.

All inhalation agents have a more profound effect on hypoxemic drive (carotid bodies) than central hypercapnic drive.

Halothane, isoflurane, and sevoflurane have bronchodilating properties.

BOX 10-4 SUMMARY

Cardiovascular Effects of Inhalation Anesthetics

Inhalation anesthetics reduce MAP; N$_2$O is the exception.

Isoflurane, desflurane, and sevoflurane increase heart rate and decrease SVR but have little effect on cardiac output.

Halothane does not increase heart rate or decrease SVR. It lowers MAP by decreasing stroke volume.

Halothane is most active in sensitizing the heart to excitatory influences of sympathomimetic amines such as epinephrine.

SVR, Systemic vascular resistance.

ministration. N$_2$O is distinguished because its effects are least significant (Fig. 10-1 and Box 10-3).

In addition to their effects on central respiratory centers and carotid bodies, inhalation anesthetics have varied effects on the respiratory tract, especially the ability to relax bronchial smooth muscle. Halothane, isoflurane, and sevoflurane are most effective in this regard.[4,7] They are not so effective as to replace β$_2$-agonists as emergency bronchodilators, but they are useful agents for providing general anesthesia to patients having histories of asthma or reactive chronic obstructive pulmonary disease (COPD).

Cardiovascular Effects. Inhalation anesthetics produce a dose-dependent reduction in *mean arterial pressure* (MAP) (Boxes 10-4 and 10-5). Again, nitrous oxide is the exception.[8,9] Agents differ in the specific

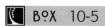

Comparison of Inhalation Anesthetics

Halothane induction is smooth but somewhat slower than other agents. It does not irritate the larynx, and it relaxes bronchial smooth muscles. Its principal drawbacks are cardiac sensitization to epinephrine, risk for halothane hepatitis, and its frequent mention in cases of malignant hyperthermia.

Isoflurane has a more pungent odor than halothane, but supplemental intravenous agents can overcome this shortcoming. The depth of anesthesia can be adjusted rapidly with isoflurane due to its low solubility. Cardiac output is well sustained, and systemic (including coronary) vessels dilate. Arrhythmias are uncommon, and epinephrine can be used in greater amounts for hemostasis than with halothane. Isoflurane is metabolized to only a minimal extent, with no reports of hepatic or renal toxicity.

Desflurane and *sevoflurane* have the most rapid onset and recovery of all inhalation anesthetics, a major advantage for outpatient use. Otherwise, they have little advantage over isoflurane and are more expensive.

Nitrous oxide (N_2O) is a weak agent with no muscle relaxant activity. Due to its low potency, high concentrations are required even to approach MAC. However, N_2O is nonirritating and has modest analgesic efficacy, and the onset of and recovery from its effects are very rapid. It causes little or no toxicity during ordinary clinical use. For procedures less than 1 hour, it is extremely useful in adjunct with potent intravenous agents. N_2O has minimal effects on respiratory and cardiovascular function; adding it to other inhalation agents reduces their dose and negative influences.

---

physiologic parameter they target; heart rate, myocardial contractility, and systemic vascular resistance (SVR). For example, halothane has little effect on SVR but reduces arterial pressure by decreasing stroke volume. The influence of sevoflurane is intermediate, between halothane and isoflurane (Fig. 10-2).[4,7-9]

Halothane does not increase plasma catecholamine concentrations, but it sensitizes the heart to the influences of these and other sympathomimetic amines. It is not dose dependent and occurs regardless of the concentration of halothane administered. Other inhalation agents are not a concern, but halothane can predispose a patient to cardiac dysrhythmias, and it is potentiated if hypercarbia is present and by thiopental.[4,7] The influence of methohexital has not been studied. The precise mechanism for this sensitization is unclear, but it is diminished when patients are premedicated with α-blocking and β-blocking agents,[10] suggesting that effects on the heart's conduction system and α/β-receptor responsiveness play a role.

During dental treatment, attention must be given to elevated catecholamine levels attributed to stress and pain and those associated with the use of vasopressors included in local anesthetic solutions and the gingival retraction cord. Although children tolerate greater doses of epinephrine than adults, the con-

ventional guideline when using halothane is to limit epinephrine doses to 2 μg/kg and 1 μg/kg if thiopental is also administered.[3]

Miscellaneous Effects. When considering therapeutic and adverse effects of drugs, both parent drug and metabolites must be considered; inhalation anesthetics are no exception. The respiratory and cardiovascular influences of inhalation anesthetics are attributed primarily to the parent drug administered. In some cases, however, a portion of an inhalation anesthetic is hepatically converted to metabolites, which may produce other toxic effects.

Most inhalation anesthetics in current use are relatively inert, but some are more prone than others to be metabolized. Certain of these metabolic products have been implicated in renal and hepatic toxicity. Other than a reduction in glomerular filtration that follows a decline in MAP and cardiac output, renal considerations are of little concern. Methoxyflurane (Penthrane) was an exception, but it is no longer in use. Despite modern agents having fluorinated structures, levels of fluoride that follow their limited biotransformations are insignificant and have not been implicated in nephrotoxicity.[7]

Mild *hepatotoxicity* can follow the use of any inhalation anesthetic because these drugs depress res-

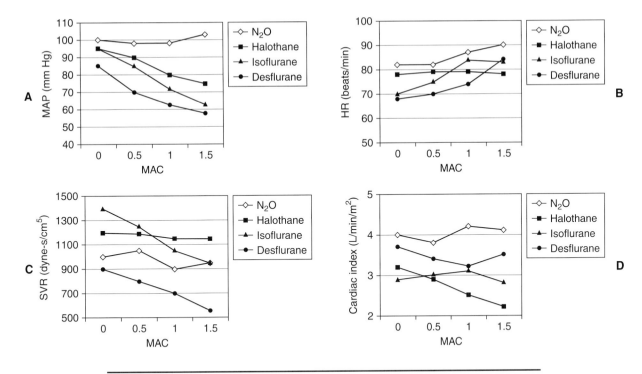

Fig. 10-2 Relative hemodynamic effects of inhalation anesthetics. **A,** Mean arterial pressure *(MAP)*. **B,** Heart rate *(HR)*. **C,** Systemic vascular resistance *(SVR)*. **D,** Cardiac index, or cardiac output adjusted for weight (body size). *MAC,* Minimum alveolar concentration; *N_2O,* nitrous oxide.

piration and arterial blood pressure. This toxicity is attributed to reduced oxygenation of hepatocytes and manifests clinically as nausea, lethargy, fever, and minor elevations in liver transaminases.[4,7] Although the incidence of this effect is estimated to be as high as 20% after the use of halothane, it is self-limiting.

Of greater concern is *halothane hepatitis,* a rare form of toxicity that may lead to massive hepatic necrosis and death. Its incidence has been estimated as 1 in 30,000 halothane exposures. Halothane hepatitis is believed to have an immune-mediated mechanism because 70% of patients who experience the condition are found to have antibodies that react against proteins found in their hepatocytes. Presumably these patients are genetically predisposed by having proteins that can be transformed to an immunogenic state by reactive metabolites of halothane.[4,7]

Other anesthetics are biotransformed to similar metabolites, but in most cases this accounts for less than 1% of their clearance, in contrast to 10% to 30%

for halothane. Nevertheless, patients who have developed this reaction to halothane have experienced hepatitis after exposure to other halogenated anesthetics. The unpredictable occurrence of this syndrome is a principal reason that the use of halothane has declined. The newest inhalation anesthetic, *sevoflurane,* does not produce these reactive metabolites and is an acceptable agent for patients who have experienced this reaction.[7] A regimen of N_2O and intravenous agents is also an alternative.

Inhalation anesthetics have varying influences on relaxation of skeletal muscle tone, one of the three requirements of clinically successful anesthesia. Isoflurane, desflurane, and sevoflurane provide twice the degree of skeletal muscle relaxation observed with halothane. N_2O has no effect.

Influences on skeletal muscle can be detrimental. *Malignant hyperthermia* is a hypermetabolic disorder of skeletal muscle that can be triggered by succinylcholine and most inhalation anesthetics. Nitrous oxide, local anesthetics, ketamine, and propofol are not associated with this disorder. Although largely a genetic condition, variants of classic malignant hyperthermia have been reported in individuals without genetic predisposition. Nevertheless, a personal or family history of anesthetic experience is the most effective means of avoiding this potential complication.

Intravenous Anesthetics

Intravenous (IV) "anesthetics" have a misleading title; no one agent has all the requirements for a complete general anesthetic (Box 10-6). Barbiturates and propofol produce hypnosis but have no analgesic properties. Doses great enough to obviate visceral reflexes that follow a surgical stimulus also depress respiratory and cardiovascular function to a dangerous level. Although opioids have excellent analgesic properties, doses required to produce reliable hypnosis inevitably cause apnea. Nevertheless, these agents are valuable components of multidrug anesthetic regimens, thus they are commonly viewed as anesthetics.

Sedative-Hypnotics

Numerous sedative-hypnotics can be used to induce unconsciousness, but ultrashort-acting barbiturates and propofol are used most often. They can be used alone for relatively painless procedures requiring unconsciousness or combined with local anesthetics and/or opioids to ensure analgesia. They are an excellent choice for ambulatory surgery.

Sedative-hypnotics have high lipid solubility, which ensures a rapid onset of action. After single-dose or intermittent-bolus injections, the duration of effect is brief because it is not governed by metabolism. As the drug distributes to adipose tissue and other less perfused tissues, plasma concentration is reduced, and the concentration in the brain declines due to redistribution. Therefore *distribution* rather than elimination half-life more accurately reflects the duration of their hypnotic effect. After repeated doses or continuous infusions, the duration increases because peripheral sites become saturated and the decline in plasma concentration becomes more dependent on the drug's metabolism (Table 10-2).

Pharmacologically, these drugs are sedatives, not general anesthetics, and they are useful for conscious sedation (see Chapter 16). Table 10-3 lists doses for conscious sedation and general anesthesia.[4,11,12]

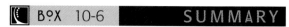

BOX 10-6   SUMMARY
Intravenous Anesthetics

Ultrashort-acting barbiturates, benzodiazepines, and propofol are sedative-hypnotics that can induce unconsciousness but cannot be used alone to provide general anesthesia. Analgesia must be provided by local anesthetics or opioids.

All sedative-hypnotics produce a dose-dependent depression of respiration and blood pressure. When using lower doses for conscious sedation, side effects are less significant.

The duration of effect for intravenous anesthetics depends more on drug distribution than elimination, but slow elimination may contribute to delays in full recovery.

Ketamine is unique among these agents because it produces a dissociative state and is an excellent analgesic. It does not produce respiratory depression, and airway reflexes remain intact. Delayed recovery and postoperative nausea and vomiting are drawbacks.

High doses of opioids can produce complete analgesia, but hypnosis is unreliable and respiratory depression is severe.

Barbiturates. *Thiopental* and *methohexital* are ultrashort-acting barbiturates that produce their hypnotic effect by interacting with gamma-aminobutyric acid (GABA). The GABA receptor complex regulates chloride ion influx, leading to polarization of neuronal membranes. Barbiturates not only potentiate the action of GABA on the chloride channels but also have a direct effect on chloride ion conductance. Although they are known to bind with specific receptors on this complex, no agent-specific antagonist is available for clinical use.

Thiopental and methohexital are almost entirely metabolized in the liver to inactive, water-soluble metabolites that are excreted in urine. Metabolism is more rapid for methohexital, and recovery after prolonged administration is faster than that after thiopental. Higher doses based on body weight are required in children due to more rapid hepatic clearance. Conversely, lower doses must be used in elderly persons.

Barbiturates are noted for their paradoxical excitation, especially in elderly patients and those in pain. Small doses appear to lower the pain thresh-

TABLE 10-2

Properties of Intravenous Agents after Induction Doses

	Thiopental	Methohexital	Propofol	Ketamine
Induction dose (mg/kg)	3-6	1-3	1.5-2.5	1-2
Distribution half-life (min)	2-4	5-6	2-4	11-16
Elimination half-life (hr)	11	4	1-3 (4-23)*	2-4
Onset (sec)	<30	<30	15-45	45-60
Duration (min)	5-10	5-10	5-10	10-20
Heart rate	↑	↑↑	↔↓	↑↑
Blood pressure	↓	↓	↓↓	↑↑
Ventilation	↓	↓	↓↓	↔

*Data using three-compartment model, in which redistribution from poorly perfused tissue sites delays elimination but poses little clinical influence.

old, giving a hyperalgesic impression, but this has not been confirmed in controlled studies. These properties make them less desirable than benzodiazepines for sedation.

The barbiturates have similar influences on respiration and cardiovascular function. They produce dose-dependent depression of the respiratory center and reduce the primary response to hypercapnia. After induction doses, MAP is reduced by 10 to 20 mm Hg, with a compensatory increase in heart rate of 15 to 20 beats/minute. The drop in pressure is attributed to venodilation after depression of the central vasomotor center. Any depression of arterial resistance or myocardial contractility is minimal and offset by baroreceptor reflexes.[4] Thiopental, but not methohexital, stimulates histamine release, which may contribute to hypotension.

Two forms of *porphyria*, variegate and acute intermittent, constitute an absolute contraindication to the use of barbiturates. In these conditions, barbiturates may precipitate a widespread demyelination of nerves and disseminated lesions throughout the CNS, resulting in pain, weakness, and paralysis that may be life threatening.[1]

Propofol. The action of propofol is similar to that of barbiturates; it potentiates GABA effects within the GABA receptor complex. The most distinguishing property of propofol relates to its pattern of clearance. It is rapidly biotransformed to inactive metabolites not only in liver but also in multiple tissue sites yet to be clearly defined. After prolonged administration, redistribution from storage sites does not de-

TABLE 10-3

Serum Concentrations and Doses for Conscious Sedation and Anesthesia

	Sedation	Anesthesia
Methohexital		
Serum concentration (μg/ml)	1-3	6-15
Loading dose (mg/kg)	0.2-1	1-2.5
Infusion (μg/kg/min)	25-75	75-200
Propofol		
Serum concentration (μg/ml)	1-2	4-6
Loading dose (mg/kg)	0.2-1	1-2.5
Infusion (μg/kg/min)	25-75	75-200
Ketamine		
Serum concentration (μg/ml)	0.1-1	1-4
Loading dose (mg/kg)	0.2-1	1-2
Infusion (μg/kg/min)	10-30	30-90

lay drug clearance, and recovery is rapid, which is a striking advantage over barbiturates.

Propofol's respiratory and cardiovascular influences are more pronounced than those of barbiturates. After induction doses, transient apnea occurs in 25% of patients and is further potentiated by opioids.

It depresses the respiratory response to hypercapnia and hypoxemia; the latter is observed even at low doses used for conscious sedation.[13] Reduction in blood pressure is attributed to depressed sympathetic outflow and includes a reduction in arterial resistance and myocardial contractility.

Propofol formulations support growth of bacteria and have been implicated in the transmission of nosocomial infections after careless practices. There should be little concern, provided standard aseptic practices are followed and opened vials or ampules are discarded at the end of the day.

Propofol is well suited for conscious sedation.[4,11-13] At these lower doses, adverse respiratory and cardiovascular influences are minimal. Due to its brief duration, however, it is used most efficiently when administered by continuous infusion. Shafer[14] compared continuous infusion rates for propofol when used for sedation versus anesthesia (Table 10-4).

A mechanism has not been established, but propofol has notable antiemetic efficacy, and postoperative nausea and vomiting are less frequent when propofol is a component of the anesthetic regimen. At low doses, such as a 10-mg dose followed by a 10-μg/kg/min infusion, propofol has been effective in managing chemotherapy-induced nausea.[7]

Benzodiazepines. Diazepam, lorazepam, and midazolam have been used to induce unconsciousness for anesthesia. However, large doses are required. The slow clearance of *diazepam* and its metabolites result in delayed recovery. *Lorazepam* has less lipid solubility, which results in a relatively slow onset, but its metabolites are not active as sedatives. *Midazolam* is most suitable due to its high lipid solubility, rapid clearance, and lack of active sedative metabolites. Compared with other classes of sedative-hypnotics, benzodiazepines have the least influence on respiratory and cardiovascular function, which makes them a consideration for severely compromised patients. They are the only class of sedatives that can be reversed by a specific antagonist, *flumazenil*. Generally, the benzodiazepines are used more often for conscious sedation (see Chapter 9).

Ketamine

Of the IV agents, ketamine comes closest to fulfilling the requirements of a complete anesthetic. It produces a unique form of unconsciousness described as *dissociation* that resembles catalepsy. In many pa-

TABLE 10-4

Infusion Rates for Propofol in Conscious Sedation and Total Intravenous Anesthesia (TIVA)

Duration and Dose	Sedation	TIVA
First 10 min (μg/kg/min)	25-75	150-300
10 min-2 hr (μg/kg/min)	25-60	125-260
Over 2 hr (μg/kg/min)	25-50	75-150
Serum concentration (μg/ml)	0.5-1.5	6-9

Data from Shafer SL: *J Clin Anesth* 5(6 suppl 1):145-215, 1993.

tients, the eyes remain open, with slow nystagmus and intact ocular reflexes. Ketamine's mechanism is attributed to an antagonist action at *N*-methyl-D-aspartate (NMDA) receptors, a class of glutamate receptor that regulates communication between limbic and thalamocortical systems. Ketamine produces analgesia, presumably at mu opioid receptors, which is apparent at doses well below those required for dissociation. However, it fails to produce skeletal muscle relaxation. Patients present varying degrees of skeletal muscle hypertonia along with nonpurposeful movement unrelated to any stimulus.

Ketamine is metabolized extensively in liver to several inactive metabolites excreted in urine. One metabolite, norketamine, is active and its accumulation during prolonged administration contributes to delayed recovery.

Ketamine does not depress minute ventilation, and responses to hypercapnia and hypoxemia remain unaltered. It is an excellent bronchodilator, and all airway reflexes remain virtually intact. Ketamine stimulates salivation, and patients should be premedicated with an anticholinergic such as glycopyrrolate to prevent airway irritation and laryngospasm.

Despite a direct negative influence on the heart, ketamine stimulates sympathetic outflow from the CNS and inhibits neuronal uptake of norepinephrine. Plasma epinephrine and norepinephrine concentration is elevated within 2 minutes after administration of ketamine.[7] Therefore the cardiovascular influences of ketamine are excitatory and include elevations in arterial pressure and heart rate. For this reason, ketamine should not be used in patients with hypertension, tachyarrhythmias, or ischemic heart disease.

Emergence from ketamine anesthesia is associated with delirium, which can be prevented by premedication with benzodiazepines. The incidence of emergence delirium is enhanced by atropine, droperidol, and other agents with central anticholinergic action.

Opioids

Opioids are generally included in anesthetic regimens to provide analgesia and offset sympathetic responses to surgical stimuli (see Chapter 8). For cardiac surgery, very large doses of opioids may be infused to obtain anesthesia. For example, morphine in doses of 1 to 3 mg/kg induces analgesia and unconsciousness; respiratory depression is severe, however, and ventilation must be mechanically controlled. The addition of N_2O or other inhalation agents ensures unconsciousness, and neuromuscular blocking agents are added to provide skeletal muscle relaxation.

References

1. Hardman JG, Limbird LE, Molinoff PB, et al, editors: *Goodman and Gilman's the pharmacological bases of therapeutics*, ed 9, New York, 1996, McGraw-Hill.

2. Chung DC, Lam AM: *Essentials of anesthesiology*, ed 3, Philadelphia, 1997, WB Saunders.

3. Yagiela JA, Neidle EA, Dowd FJ, editors: *Pharmacology and therapeutics for dentistry*, ed 4, St Louis, 1998, Mosby.

4. Barash PG, Cullen BF, Stoelting RK, editors: *Clinical anesthesia*, ed 3, Philadelphia, 1997, Lippincott-Raven.

5. Dahan A, van den Elsen MJ, Berkenbosch A, et al: Effects of subanesthetic halothane on the ventilatory responses to hypercapnia and acute hypoxia in healthy volunteers, *Anesthesiology* 80(4):727-738, 1994.

6. Yacoub O, Doell D, Kryger MH, et al: Depression of hypoxic ventilatory response by nitrous oxide, *Anesthesiology* 45(4):385-389, 1976.

7. Stoelting RK: *Pharmacology and physiology in anesthetic practice*, ed 3, Philadelphia, 1999, Lippincott-Raven.

8. Eger EI: *Nitrous oxide*, New York, 1985, Elsevier.

9. Weiskopf RB, Cahalan MK, Eger EI Jr, et al: Cardiovascular actions of desflurane in normocarbic volunteers, *Anesth Analg* 73(2):143-156, 1991.

10. Maze M, Smith CM: Identification of receptor mechanism mediating epinephrine-induced arrhythmias during halothane anesthesia in the dog, *Anesthesiology* 59:322-326, 1983.

11. Miller RD, editor: *Anesthesia*, ed 5, Philadelphia, 2000, Churchill Livingstone.

12. White PF, editor: *Ambulatory anesthesia and surgery*, Philadelphia, 1997, WB Saunders.

13. Smith I, White PF, Nathanson M, et al: Propofol: an update on its clinical use, *Anesthesiology* 81(4):1005-1043, 1994.

14. Shafer SL: Advances in propofol pharmacokinetics and pharmacodynamics, *J Clin Anesth* 5(6 suppl 1):14S-21S, 1993.

PART

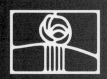

Intraoperative Management of Pain and Anxiety

CHAPTER 11

Monitoring

John P. Lawrence
Hideo Matsuura

This chapter explores important issues of patient monitoring and some of the basic principles of monitoring technology. Before discussing monitoring and equipment, the standards that ensure the safest conditions for patients in any type of environment need to be considered. Several professional organizations have developed monitoring guidelines to ensure safety for patients who receive anesthetic drugs and to minimize the potential for adverse litigation. Failure to follow established published standards of care leaves the clinician vulnerable to adverse anesthetic outcomes, unsatisfied patients, and unfavorable litigation outcomes.

Terminology and Principles

In this chapter an *anesthetic* is defined as a mood-altering medication administered for a surgical or dental procedure. The health professional administering these medications has the general title of *anesthetist* to avoid confusion among different training backgrounds, as might occur with "physician," "dentist," or "nurse anesthetist."

The level of anesthetic depth will be classified in traditional terms as either conscious sedation or general anesthesia. The patient who receives *conscious sedation* is alert (conscious), breathes spontaneously, and easily follows verbal commands. The moment a patient begins to lapse into unconsciousness, either temporarily or for prolonged periods, that level of anesthesia is classified as *general anesthesia.*

The terms "unconscious" sedation and deep sedation have been widely used, and considerable misconception surrounds this level of anesthesia. Use of the term "deep sedation" leads to the misleading impression that deep sedation bears little resemblance to general anesthesia. This misconception leads to a lack of appreciation for the vulnerable state of a patient who is unconscious due to anesthetic medications. In this chapter the dichotomous terms *conscious sedation* and *general anesthesia* are used to ensure clarity of presentation, simplify understanding of guidelines, eliminate misleading impressions of the anesthetic state, and ensure optimal care for all patients.

The most important principle of monitoring is that one individual must be charged with the task of watching the patient at all times. No piece of electronic equipment can replace a trained, vigilant professional capable of intervening to care for a patient. A comprehensive record should be kept to identify subtle changes in a patient's vital signs. The record also can be referred to in the future to support further anesthesia care, assist billing, and provide evidence in the event of litigation.

Monitoring instruments available for use today have minimal utility unless used consistently, operated and applied properly, and interpreted correctly. The individual charged with the responsibility of being the anesthetist must be capable of using monitors appropriately and must have sufficient training to administer anesthetics safely. If the monitors are not used properly, they not only have little value but may even endanger the patient because their use can lead to a false sense of security. The electronic circuitry of monitoring technology is not capable of ensuring adequate oxygenation, ventilation, and circulation. Only the anesthetist is capable of assimilating all the information and ensuring the safety of the anesthetized patient.

All patients who are anesthetized need to have a brief history and physical examination performed and baseline vital signs measured. These vital signs include the pulse, blood pressure, respiratory rate, oxygen saturation, and temperature. After conclusion of the surgical or dental procedure, vital signs should be measured for as long as necessary to ensure complete resolution of the anesthetic state.

Monitors

The monitors available for use can be categorized according to what they monitor, specifically oxygenation, ventilation, circulation, temperature, and level of neurologic alertness. These items are listed in the order of relative importance in which they should be evaluated. When deprived of *oxygenation*, brain damage will occur in 4 to 5 minutes, with death shortly thereafter. *Ventilation* is the next priority because it is intimately coupled with oxygenation and acid-base balance. *Circulation* is generally not the first system to be altered by anesthetics but is a vital concern. *Temperature* is generally not significantly altered unless the surrounding environment has an extremely different temperature or the patient's normal thermoregulatory mechanisms are impaired, such as during general anesthesia.

Oxygenation

The presence of peripheral cyanosis is a late and unreliable method to detect arterial hypoxemia.

Cyanosis usually indicates a significant problem that could result in full cardiovascular collapse. The pulse oximeter has gone from experimental technology in the 1980s to one of the most ubiquitous pieces of equipment in hospitals and offices. To monitor a patient receiving conscious sedation, a pulse oximeter is all that generally will be necessary to assess oxygenation. However, if a patient achieves general anesthesia and ventilation needs to be artificially supported or controlled, a measure of the inspiratory oxygen concentration (FIO_2) also needs to be used. FIO_2 refers to the fraction of inspired oxygen concentration, expressed as a range from 0% to 100%.

Pulse Oximeter

The pulse oximeter has a small noninvasive probe that can be placed on a finger, toe, earlobe, or the forehead (Fig. 11-1). The pulse oximeter probe passes the light of two different wavelengths through the tissue and compares the level of light transmission through hemoglobin and oxyhemoglobin to determine the level of saturation of oxygen in the blood. The physical principles of pulse oximetry are based on the relative difference in which oxygenated and deoxygenated blood transmit and absorb light. The two wavelengths of light used are 660 and 940 nm. Oxygenated hemoglobin absorbs light at 660 nm, whereas deoxygenated hemoglobin absorbs light at 940 nm. When the relative ratio of the transmission of the two wavelengths of light is compared to the standard, a percentage of oxygenated hemoglobin can obtained.

The reported oxygen percentage by the pulse oximeter can be a misleading piece of information, however, unless the examiner understands how to interpret the information. The percentage of oxygen as determined by the pulse oximeter only approximates the oxygen tension in the arterial blood (PaO_2). If the oxygen saturation is 90%, the PaO_2 is approximately 60 mm Hg. This level is usually considered the lowest allowable oxygen level in the body, before the cells in vital organs begin to be starved for oxygen. On further reference to the oxygen-hemoglobin dissociation curve, it becomes apparent that if the PaO_2 is less than 60 mm Hg, the oxygen saturation will decline in a more or less linear fashion (see Fig. 11-1). Moreover, as the PaO_2 increases above 60 mm Hg, the oxygen saturation will rise to 100%, with only a small change in the PaO_2. As long as the oxygen sat-

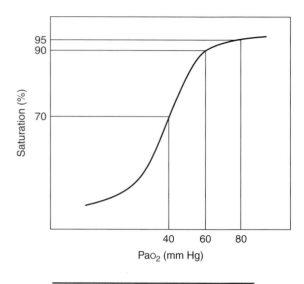

Fig. 11-1 Oxyhemoglobin dissociation curve.

uration remains above 90%, the examiner can be relatively assured that the patient is adequately oxygenated. Occasionally the pulse oximeter provides false information when the probe (on finger or toe), does not detect pulsatile blood flow. Practitioners can be assured that the oximeter is working appropriately if they either hear the rhythmic pulsations in time with the patient's heart rate or see a rhythmic waveform that correlates with the patient's heart rate.

The pulse oximeter should *not* be used as a monitor of ventilation. Ventilation is the process of moving air in and out of the lungs. Oxygenation only represents half of the results of ventilation. Ventilation must be evaluated independently from oxygenation.

Inspired Oxygen

A monitor that measures FIO_2 is usually an integral part of a gas analyzer to detect oxygen, carbon dioxide, and anesthetic gases. Two types of monitors measure FIO_2: in-line and side-stream sampling. Most current monitors are *side-stream sampling devices*. A small piece of tubing is attached to the breathing apparatus near the patient's airway and samples the gas that is inspired and expired. The gas is continuously monitored using infrared technology to provide the anesthetist with a measure of the inspired and expired oxygen concentration (see following discussion). The anesthetist should keep this measured value above 40% to ensure patient safety.

Factors that can interfere with FIO_2 monitoring include the inability to obtain a sample of gas that the patient is breathing due to a loss of patency of either the airway or the sample tubing.

Ventilation

Visual assessment of a patient's respiration is the first and most noninvasive method of monitoring ventilation. Most agents that are considered "anesthetics" decrease the respiratory drive, as evidenced by decreased rate of breathing or a decreased volume of each breath. Opioids tend to produce the most profound effects on ventilation. A considerable amount of information can be obtained, including rate (respiratory rate), depth (tidal volume), and presence of obstruction (as evidenced by wheezing, stridor, or snoring). *Snoring* is a common condition, but snoring during an anesthetic indicates the possibility of impending airway obstruction. *Stridor* is an uncommon, life-threatening condition characterized by a high-pitched whine during inspiration, and it indicates impending airway obstruction due to vocal cord closure.

Visual and auditory assessment, however, can be misleading during general anesthesia. A patient's airway may be completely obstructed, but the patient may continue to attempt to breathe. In this situation, confirmation of airflow in the lungs is necessary, using a precordial stethoscope. The *precordial stethoscope* is a bell-shaped metal device that can be secured to the chest or neck with a piece of double-sided tape. It transmits the patient's breath sounds to the anesthetist's ear through rubber tubing. The earpiece, which is attached to the rubber tubing, is more comfortable when custom-made to fit the anesthetist's ear.

When a patient is under general anesthesia with breathing artificially supported or controlled, an additional monitor of ventilation is required. The *capnograph,* or end-tidal carbon dioxide ($ETCO_2$) monitor, is capable of detecting both the presence and the quality of ventilation by analyzing the concentration of carbon dioxide in the exhaled gasses.

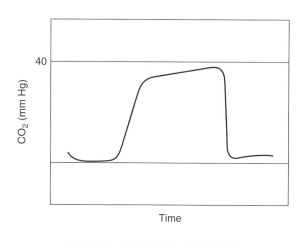

Fig. 11-2 Capnograph (end-tidal CO_2).

Carbon dioxide is the byproduct of cellular metabolism that is exhaled with each breath. The capnograph continuously monitors a small sample of exhaled gas using infrared technology to determine the concentration of carbon dioxide (Fig. 11-2). In the conscious patient or the patient who is not intubated, the sampling line should be placed as close to the mouth or nose as possible to obtain the most accurate reading. In the intubated patient, the sampling line is attached to the anesthesia circuit close to the proximal end of the endotracheal tube. The $ETCO_2$ closely approximates the measured carbon dioxide in arterial blood ($PaCO_2$) but is not exact. The $ETCO_2$ is usually 2 to 5 mm Hg lower than the $PaCO_2$ and has a characteristic waveform (see Fig. 11-2). Different diagnoses can be made based on the shape of the waveform, such as airway obstruction and bronchospasm. Other patient conditions can be inferred, such as inadequate analgesia (low $ETCO_2$), excessive opioid administration, or malignant hyperthermia (elevated $ETCO_2$).

Circulation

A patient's circulation is monitored with two different modalities, the blood pressure (BP) cuff and the electrocardiogram (ECG). It is not possible to identify patients who will demonstrate circulatory abnormalities during general anesthesia, thus all patients who receive general anesthetic medications should be monitored with both the BP cuff and the ECG.

Blood Pressure

All patients receiving anesthetics require frequent evaluation of BP. The deeper the level of sedation, the more frequently BP should be measured. Most guidelines suggest that the anesthetist measure BP at least every 5 minutes. BP can be measured noninvasively with a BP cuff or invasively with an arterial line. Use of an arterial line is not discussed in this chapter because it is considered beyond the scope of office-based anesthesia practice. This is also true for the invasively measured central venous pressure (CVP) or pulmonary artery pressure (PAP). The CVP and PAP are measured with a pulmonary artery catheter, more commonly known as a Swan-Ganz catheter.

The manual measurement of BP by a cuff is a classic assessment method, but recently introduced automated devices have simplified and standardized the measurement of BP. An inflatable BP cuff is applied to the patient using any extremity. The arm is usually selected because it is generally at the same level as the patient's heart.

If an automated device is not available, the auscultatory (hearing) method is typically used. To perform this technique, a stethoscope is placed over the major artery just distal to the BP cuff. The BP cuff is inflated, and the pulsations of blood flow are auscultated over the artery. The sounds of pulsation are called *Korotkoff sounds,* and the first sound of pulsation (first Korotkoff sound) is designated the *systolic* BP (Fig. 11-3). As pressure in the BP cuff declines, the Korotkoff sounds disappear. The pressure at which the Korotkoff sounds completely disappear is designated the *diastolic* BP. The *mean arterial blood pressure* (MAP) is a calculated number from the measured systolic and diastolic pressures. The width of the cuff should be 20% to 30% of the circumference of the arm. If the cuff is too small, the BP measured will be artificially high. If the BP cuff is too small, the BP measured will be artificially low. Fortunately, the majority of cuffs are calibrated to show the range in arm diameters that will be acceptable with a particular cuff size. A variety of cuffs are available and should be stocked according to the patient population treated in a particular office.

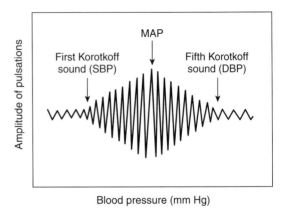

Fig. 11-3 Blood pressure measurement.

Additionally, if the extremity used is above the level of the heart, the BP will also be artificially low. If the extremity used is below the level of the heart, the BP will be artificially high.

The automated devices for measurement of BP use a different form of technology. The BP cuff is applied to the arm, and the cuff inflates automatically. The cuff then deflates slowly and detects the presence and amplitude of pulsations in the arm. The peak amplitude of pulsations in the arm is designated the MAP. The systolic and diastolic blood pressure determinations are calculated from an analysis of the peak amplitude of pulsations and the rate of increase and decline. The automated BP device is more accurate, consistent, and convenient to use.

Cardiac Electrical Activity

Electrocardiogram. The ECG is a device that evaluates the electrical rhythms of the heart. The electrical current detected on the skin surface reflects the spread of electrical impulses through the heart during the excitation/contraction process. Interpretation of the ECG provides useful information on the cardiac status of patients receiving anesthetic medications. The practice of anesthesiologists is to use the ECG at all times, regardless of the depth of anesthesia. Information that can be obtained from the ECG includes heart rate, heart rhythm, myocardial hypertrophy, myocardial ischemia, and myocardial infarction.

The proper application of the ECG leads is to place one lead on the right shoulder, left shoulder, and left thigh area. It is generally acceptable to place the representative lead closer to the hand and foot, but this may result in a greater amount of artifact interference and unreliability. Additionally, a self-adhesive electrode tends to generate better contact with the skin and therefore results in less artifact interference and greater reliability. By placing the leads on the designated extremities, the ECG can monitor the electrical activity of the heart. To obtain a complete evaluation, it is possible to "look at" the heart's electrical activity from different angles. *Lead I* evaluates the electrical activity in the direction from the right arm to the left arm, *lead II* from the right arm to the left leg, and *lead III* from the left arm to the left leg (Fig. 11-4).

In the normal ECG waveform, the first wave is called the *P wave* and indicates electrical activation of the upper chambers of the heart, the atria (Fig. 11-5). The sinoatrial (SA) node is the part of the atria that initiates this activation and is called the heart's "pacemaker." The next waveform is the *QRS complex,* which represents the electrical activation of the two lower chambers of the heart, the ventricles. The last waveform is the *T wave,* which represents the repolarization of the ventricles so that they can be reactivated by an impulse originating in the SA node.

When evaluating the ECG, the anesthetist should first observe the heart rate. The normal heart rate is between 60 and 100 beats/minute. If the heart rate is slower than 60 beats/minute, *bradycardia* is present. If the heart rate is faster than 100 beats/minute, the patient has *tachycardia.* Bradycardia and tachycardia are not necessarily abnormal. Well-conditioned athletes frequently have very slow heart rates, sometimes as low as 40 to 50 beats/minute. When a person engages in strenuous physical activity, the heart rate normally increases above 100 beats/minute. These normal conditions can be identified as *sinus bradycardia* or *sinus tachycardia* by the presence of a P wave in front of each QRS waveform.

Abnormal processes that cause the heart rate to beat too fast or too slow are called *arrhythmias.* In *atrial fibrillation,* the heart rate is usually faster than normal, with irregular QRS complexes and a complete absence of the P wave (Fig. 11-6). If the heart rate is too fast, it may cause the blood pressure to be too low. *Premature contractions* are seen as either extra narrow QRS complexes *(atrial)* or extra wide QRS complexes *(ventricular)* (Fig. 11-7). Both these conditions tend to be caused by long-term heart conditions, and alone generally are not harmful unless

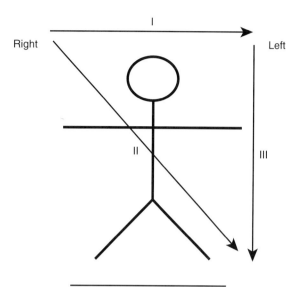

Fig. 11-4 Electrocardiogram leads.

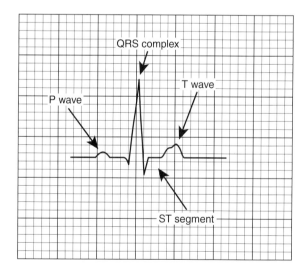

Fig. 11-5 Electrocardiogram (ECG).

they occur more than about 10 times/minute. Occasionally, a patient may have a slow heart rate due to *heart block,* when the normal passage of the electrical impulse through the heart is interrupted. *Complete* heart block means that the impulse is completely blocked from passing from the atria to the

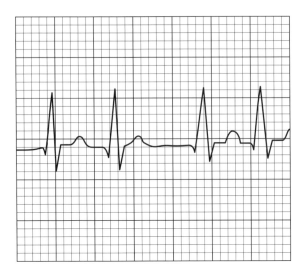

Fig. 11-6 Atrial fibrillation.

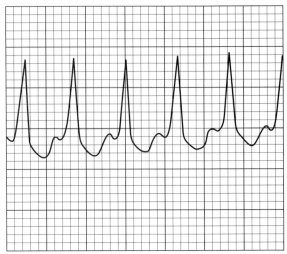

Fig. 11-8 Ventricular tachycardia.

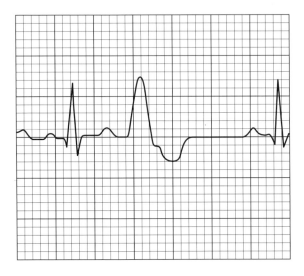

Fig. 11-7 Premature ventricular contractions (PVC).

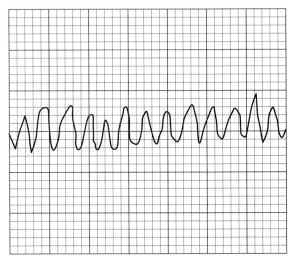

Fig. 11-9 Ventricular fibrillation.

ventricles. This can be identified as QRS complexes that do not always have a P wave in front of them. These patients require a heart specialist (cardiologist) and possibly a pacemaker.

The examiner then looks for unusual but more dangerous heart rhythms, including *supraventricular tachycardia, ventricular tachycardia,* and *ventricular fibrillation.* These arrhythmias are dangerous because they can lead to low BP or indicate the onset of cardiac arrest. A full detailed description of these arrhythmias is beyond the scope of this chapter, but some examples are included to provide a visual representation of abnormal rhythms (Figs. 11-8 and 11-9).

The final consideration is to evaluate the ECG for the presence of *myocardial ischemia* (lack of oxygen) and *myocardial infarction* (actual necrosis of cardiac tissue).

Either is usually only seen with blockages in the coronary arteries (arteries that supply the heart muscle with blood). These conditions can be identified by looking at the part of the ECG between the QRS complex and the T wave. If this normally horizontal line is more than 1 mm below that baseline, myocardial ischemia is present. If the segment is 1 mm or more above the baseline, myocardial infarction is present. To prevent any further damage to the patient's heart, a cardiologist should evaluate the patient.

Automated External Defibrillator. The automated external defibrillator (AED) is a device that is capable of administering an electrical shock to a patient experiencing a life-threatening arrhythmia. The AED is not routinely used on patients; rather, it is reserved for emergency situations. Studies evaluating the effectiveness of cardiopulmonary resuscitation (CPR) and advanced cardiac life support (ACLS) have shown that the most effective way to save a cardiac arrest victim's life is to use a defibrillator as early as possible. The AED is currently not designed for patients weighing less than 70 pounds (31.5 kg). Therefore the pediatric dental practice or office practice with patients weighing less than 70 pounds would require a manual defibrillator. In the typical adult office practice, it is reasonable to consider having an AED available, with training for personnel on operating the device. It is likely that the AED will only be needed in very rare situations and, at a cost of around $3000, can be easily omitted from the office budget. However, for the individual who does require its use, having an AED available could mean the difference between life and death.

Manual Defibrillator. The manual defibrillator is required in offices where deep sedation or general anesthesia is used. This device requires practitioner evaluation of treatable arrhythmias and manual settings of the machine, in addition to manually delivering the shock. Regional regulations determine if an AED can be stocked in place of the traditional manual defibrillator.

Temperature

The patient's temperature should be taken before and after the completion of a surgical or dental procedure involving anesthesia or sedation. The routine use of a temperature monitor during the actual procedure generally is not necessary during conscious sedation. However, when the patient is rendered unconscious (under general anesthesia), the normal thermoregulatory mechanisms are impaired, which warrants continuous temperature monitoring. The temperature can be obtained in many ways; the most convenient but least reliable is on the surface of the skin, such as the forehead. Other sites include oral, rectal, axillary, and at the tympanic membrane.

A temperature monitor is helpful (1) when a patient's normal thermoregulatory mechanisms are impaired under general anesthesia and (2) to identify patients who are experiencing a rare reaction to anesthetic agents known as *malignant hyperthermia*. Children and older adults, especially those with poor circulation or underactive thyroid glands, are the most susceptible to hypothermia. Generally, malignant hyperthermia is a very rare event. Unless the ambient room temperature is profoundly different than comfortable room temperature, and unless the patient is exposed to this cold environment for a considerable period, patients generally will not develop hypothermia.

Level of Awareness

The level of alertness can be easily ascertained if the patient is conscious but is not easily measured if the patient is under general anesthesia. One of the greatest concerns for anesthesiologists administering general anesthesia is to ensure amnesia (lack of conscious recall) but minimize the amount of anesthetic administration to hasten recovery at the conclusion of the surgical or dental procedure.

Two commercially available monitors of anesthetic depth are the Bispectral Index (BIS) monitor (Aspect Medical Systems) and the Patient State Analyzer 4000 (PSA 4000) (Baxter). Both of these monitors evaluate the patient's electroencephalogram (EEG), or brain waves. The BIS evaluates brain waves in one region of the brain, and the PSA 4000 evaluates brain wave activity over four parts of the brain. Both monitors provide a general indication of the depth of anesthesia, but the PSA 4000 seems to experience less interference from other pieces of equipment in the operating room. Both monitors use disposable adhesive probes that are attached to the scalp. To date, little has been published about either monitor, and their cost effectiveness remains in question.

Market Considerations

The different types of monitoring devices may be purchased as separate pieces of equipment or as a single integrated machine. The one exception is the EEG monitor, which currently only comes as a separate device. There are advantages and disadvantages to having separate devices for each monitoring task. The advantages include the ability to upgrade each piece as technologic advancements are made and to make necessary repairs without interfering with other devices. On the other hand, a single integrated piece of equipment has more practical advantages, including lower cost of acquisition, convenience, efficiency, and portability.

SUMMARY

Standards of practice exist for the proper use and documentation of results from current monitoring devices. A piece of monitoring equipment is not capable of replacing an observant and well-trained professional. When monitors are used consistently, operated properly, interpreted correctly, and applied appropriately, both the practitioner and the patient have a greater likelihood of a successful and safe anesthetic experience.

CHAPTER 12

Airway Management

JENNY Z. MITCHELL
JAMES A. ROELOFSE

CHAPTER OUTLINE

Hypoventilation and hypoxemia are associated with significant morbidity and mortality. The ability to manage the airway is a fundamental requirement in basic resuscitation and takes first priority for life support. Knowledge of the anatomy of the airway facilitates recognition of various forms of obstruction. Similarly, familiarity with airway devices facilitates prompt resolution of obstruction and potentially life-threatening hypoxemia. The best resuscitation efforts are futile without adequate oxygenation and ventilation.

Anatomy

The upper airway comprises the nasopharynx, oropharynx, pharynx, and glottis. The *nasopharynx* contains the turbinates, nasal septum, and nasal passages. It is bordered superiorly by the cribriform plate and inferiorly by superior surfaces of the hard and soft palates. The *oropharynx* consists of the teeth, tongue, and adenoids. It is bordered superiorly by the inferior surfaces of the hard and soft palates and inferiorly by the floor of the mouth. The *pharynx* consists of the uvula, tonsils, and epiglottis. It adjoins the nasopharynx and oropharynx and leads to the larynx and hypopharynx (esophagus and gastrointestinal tract). The *glottis* is bordered superiorly by the epiglottis and contains the laryngeal aperture, which is considered the lower airway (Fig. 12-1).

The *larynx* begins at the vocal cords. Its functions include phonation, ventilation, and airway protection. These paired structures are located at the level of the sixth cervical vertebra in the adult. The cords open and close to allow, or impair, movement of air. This area is the narrowest portion of the airway in a normal adult. The larynx itself is composed of nine cartilages, as well as muscles and ligaments. The nine cartilages are either paired (arytenoid, corniculate, cuneiform) or unpaired (thyroid, cricoid, epiglottis).

Inferior to the larynx lies the *cricoid cartilage,* the only complete ring of cartilage in the respiratory tract. The *cricothyroid membrane,* a thin avascular membrane in the cricoid's midline, connects the cricoid cartilage to the thyroid cartilage (Fig. 12-2).

The *trachea* consists of ligaments, muscle, and 20 to 25 horseshoe-shaped cartilages on its anterior surface. It is approximately 20 mm in diameter and 10

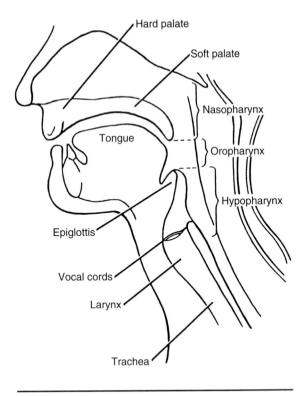

Fig. 12-1 Anatomy of the airway. (From Morgan GE, Mikhail MS: *Clinical anesthesiology,* New York, 1992, Appleton & Lange.)

cm long in the average adult. The *carina* is the bifurcation of the trachea and is typically found at the fourth thoracic vertebra. The bifurcation marks the beginnings of the right and left mainstem bronchus. Each leads to generations of more bifurcations for each lung. The right mainstem bronchus emerges from the trachea at a less acute angle than the left bronchus. This predisposes to placement of an endotracheal tube or blockage by a foreign body in the right bronchus.

The muscles that innervate the larynx may be classified into two groups, intrinsic and extrinsic. The *intrinsic muscles* are the lateral cricoarytenoids (adduction), posterior cricoarytenoids (abduction) and the transverse arytenoids. These muscles function to open and close the glottic opening. The *extrinsic muscles* control tension of the vocal cords and include the cricothyroid, vocalis, and thyroarytenoid muscles.

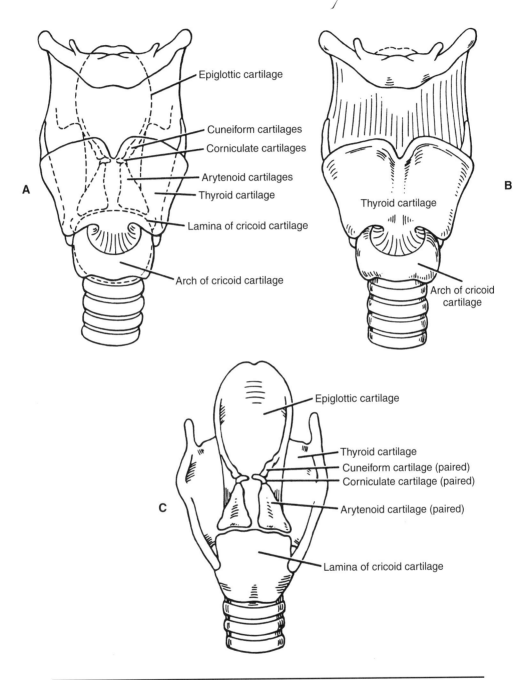

Fig. 12-2 Laryngeal cartilages. **A** and **B,** Anterior views. **C,** Posterior view. (From Rosse C, Gaddum-Rosse P: *Hollinshead's Textbook of anatomy,* ed 5, New York, 1997, Lippincott, Williams & Wilkins.)

Innervation

Sensory innervation to the airway consists mainly of two cranial nerves: the glossopharyngeal (cranial nerve IX) and the vagus (cranial nerve X). The *glossopharyngeal nerve* supplies the posterior third of the tongue, inferior surface of the soft palate, up to and including the superior surface of the epiglottis. The *vagus nerve* branches into the superior laryngeal nerve (SLN) (external and internal branches) and the recurrent laryngeal nerve (RLN). The internal branch of the SLN innervates the inferior surface of the epiglottis up to the vocal cords. The RLN supplies the inferior surface of the vocal cords and the trachea.

Motor function is provided by both the RLN, which innervates the intrinsic muscles of the larynx except the cricothyroid muscle, and the external branch of the SLN, which supplies only the cricothyroid muscle.

Injury to any of these nerves results in specific consequences. Unilateral damage to the RLN results in a vocal cord that is mid position and manifests as hoarseness. Bilateral injury results in paralyzed vocal cords that may cause obstruction and aphonia. SLN damage results in hoarseness and loss of sensation, which may result in aspiration (Table 12-1).

TABLE 12-1

Effects of Laryngeal Nerve Injury on Vocal Cords

Nerve	Effect of Injury
Superior laryngeal nerve	
Unilateral	Minimal effects
Bilateral	Hoarseness, tiring of voice
Recurrent laryngeal nerve	
Unilateral	Hoarseness
Bilateral	
Acute	Stridor, respiratory distress
Chronic	Aphonia
Vagal nerve	
Unilateral	Hoarseness
Bilateral	Aphonia

Evaluation

Evaluation of the airway begins with a thorough history. It is important to note any disease process affecting the airway, the location, and any effects (e.g., tumors, abscesses) that may pose a risk of obstruction. Prior history of head and neck radiation or surgery of the jaw, neck, and face may be the only clue to abnormal anatomy not apparent on physical examination. These patients may have difficulty with manual ventilation, intubation, or both. A prior history of difficult intubation should be thoroughly explored, including the anesthetic record, if available, which may provide valuable information on the event and its management.

Certain medical conditions may also help predict difficulty with intubation, such as arthritis of the neck, with limitation of neck extension; trauma to the neck, resulting in an unstable cervical spine, which may also limit neck mobility; and rheumatoid arthritis. Tumors may result in obstruction (wheezing, stridor) and deviation of the trachea. Infections of the oral cavity may result in edema, and limited mouth opening. Temporomandibular joint disease may limit mouth opening. Radiation may distort anatomy, and resultant friable tissue will predispose to bleeding. Morbid obesity results in an overabundance of soft tissue, large tongue and adenoids leading to obstruction and possibly sleep apnea. Similarly, acromegaly leads to an overabundance of soft tissue, resulting in a large tongue and epiglottis. Congenital diseases such as dwarfism and Down syndrome may be associated with cervical spine instability. Pierre Robin syndrome and Treacher Collins syndrome may present with craniofacial anomalies.

The *Mallampati airway classification* has been used as one tool to predict the difficulty of intubation and ventilation: *class I airway*, complete visualization of uvula, tonsillar pillars, and hard and soft palates; *class II airway*, only partial visualization of uvula; *class III airway*, uvula completely masked by tongue, with only soft palate visible; and *class IV airway*, no structures visible except hard palate. The class IV airway is most likely to present a challenge to intubation. Mallampati class alone does not predict the difficulty of intubation; the entire history and head and neck examination must be taken into consideration (Fig. 12-3).

Examination of the neck should reveal free mobility. Full neck flexion and extension and lateral ro-

Class I

Class II

Class III

Class IV

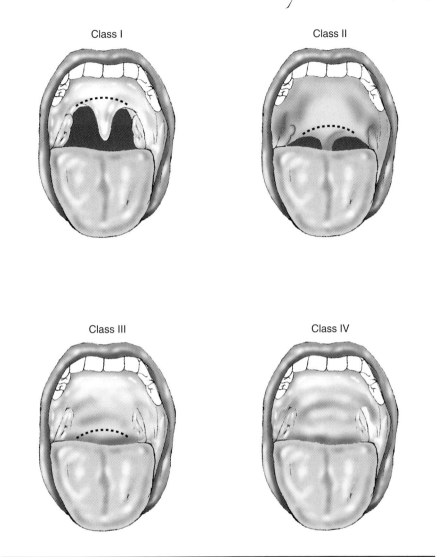

Fig. 12-3 Mallampati airway classification. Increasing Mallampati class correlates with increasing difficulty of intubation. (Redrawn from Frerk CM: *Anaesthesia* 46:1005-1008, 1991.)

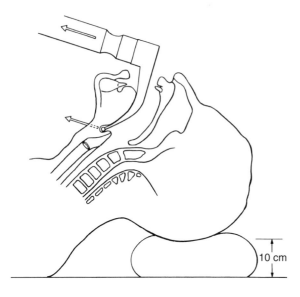

10 cm

Fig. 12-4 Sniffing position and intubation with Macintosh blade. (From Dorsch JA, Dorsch SE: *Understanding anesthesia equipment: construction, care, and complications,* Baltimore, 1984, Williams & Wilkins.)

tation should not produce pain or paresthesia. This may provide clues to potential problems with the patient assuming the sniffing position. The *sniffing position* refers to the alignment of the oropharynx and larynx. When the head is extended at the atlanto-occipital junction and the neck is flexed, both structures are aligned to produce direct visualization of the glottic opening. Inability to assume this position may make visualization of the glottic opening difficult to impossible (Fig. 12-4).

The trachea should also be midline, making palpation of the cricothyroid membrane ideal. The area should be free of scars. If nasal intubation is required, the nares should be examined for evidence of obstruction (polyps, septal deviation) and the most patent nostril elucidated by obstructing each one manually.

The *retropharyngeal space* size is important because it determines relative position of the glottic opening. Adult measurements of thyromental distance (from the thyroid notch to the mental region of the anterior mandible) should ideally reveal a length of greater than 6 cm (approximately three fingerbreadths). A

smaller space may reveal a glottic opening that is anterior in the space and may not align itself in the axis of view.

Inability to open the mouth and achieve an anterior incisal distance of 4 cm may make insertion of the laryngoscope challenging and may predispose to dental trauma. Large protruding teeth and poor dentition can also predispose to dental trauma and bleeding. Dentures should be removed before instrumentation of the airway because replacement may be particularly costly.

A large tongue and adenoids may obscure viewing the laryngeal aperture, may cause upper airway obstruction when the patient is apneic, and may make manual ventilation difficult.

Laboratory studies may be of use in determining difficulty with airway management. Chest radiographs and computed tomography (CT) scans may reveal tracheal deviation or size and location of obstructive lesions, such as mediastinal masses. Arterial blood gases and pulmonary function tests may reveal the degree of functional respiratory compromise. Cervical spine films may reveal C-spine instability.

Equipment

Basic equipment used for airway management includes a variety of devices that facilitate intubation or ventilation. The *face mask,* typically made of soft plastic is placed over the nose and mouth. When fitted properly it provides a tight seal allowing greater tidal volume and accurate oxygen concentration to be delivered. The resuscitation bag when connected to an oxygen source accomplishes the same goal.

An *oral airway* is a curved device made of hard plastic. It is placed into the mouth to relieve obstruction caused by a relaxed tongue. It keeps the tongue from compressing against the posterior pharyngeal wall and serves as a bite block. Several sizes are available. Placement is contraindicated in the semiconscious patient since airway stimulation in this situation may result in patient laryngospasm (Fig. 12-5, *A*). Nasal airways may alternatively be used to accomplish the same goal. These airways are made of soft plastic and are placed in the nares. Several sizes exist. Bleeding may be a complication. The semi-awake patient better tolerates the nasal airway (Fig. 12-5, *B*).

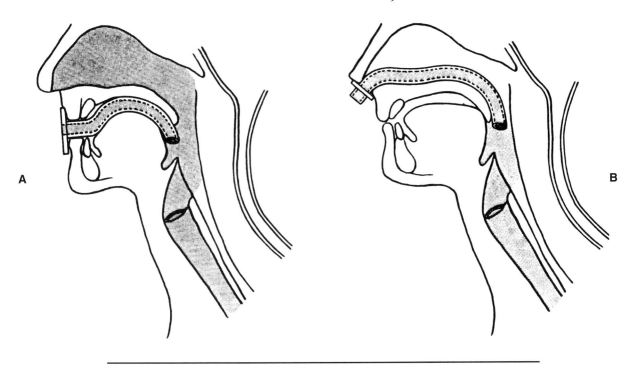

Fig. 12-5 Oropharyngeal and nasopharyngeal airways help to alleviate upper airway obstruction. **A,** Oral airway. **B,** Nasal airway. (From Dorsch JA, Dorsch SE: *Understanding anesthesia equipment: construction, care, and complications,* Baltimore, 1984, Williams & Wilkins.)

The *endotracheal tube* (ETT) is a polyvinyl plastic or latex tube placed into the trachea. The distal portion, which lies in the trachea, contains a cuff that occludes the tracheal lumen when inflated, allowing gas exchange to occur within the lumen of the ETT only. This ensures that adequate tidal volumes are given. This seal also prevents entry of foreign matter into the trachea, such as gastric contents. Uncuffed ETTs are typically used in children to avoid complications of cuff pressure, such as croup (Fig. 12-6).

ETT sizes are classified according to internal diameter. The average adult male trachea can accommodate an 8.0-mm ETT and the female trachea a 7.5-mm tube. Sizes range from 6.0 to 9.0 mm in the adult and 2.5 to 6.0 mm in children. Centimeter markings on the side of the ETT help to ensure correct placement and depth. The distal end should be above the carina (Table 12-2).

Endotracheal intubation is indicated when general anesthesia must be administered and control of ventilation may be technically difficult (morbid obe-

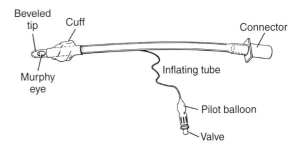

Fig. 12-6 Endotracheal tube consists of connector tube, pilot balloon, cuff, and Murphy eye. (From Morgan GE, Mikhail MS: *Clinical anesthesiology,* New York, 1992, Appleton & Lange.)

sity, head and neck surgery, prone position, lung procedures). Other indications include prevention of aspiration and positive-pressure ventilation.

Most ETTs are straight and made of clear plastic. Tubes reinforced with metal are used to prevent

TABLE 12-2

Airway Measurements at Various Ages for Size and Length of Tracheal Tubes

Age	Internal Diameter (mm)	Distance Inserted from Lips to Place Distal End in Midtrachea (cm)	Diameter of Trachea (mm)	Length of Trachea (cm)	Distance from Lips to Carina (cm)
Premature	2.5	8			
Full term	3.0	10			
1-6 mo	3.5	11	5	6	13
6-12 mo	4.0	12			
2 yr	4.5	13			
4 yr	5.0	14			
6 yr	5.5	15			
8 yr	6.5	16	8	8	18
10 yr	7.0	17-18			
12 yr	7.5	18-20			
≥14 yr	8.0-9.0	20-22	20* 15†	14* 12†	28* 24†

*Males.
†Females.

kinking. Oral and nasal Rae tubes are specifically curved to allow positioning of the breathing system away from the mouth and face and away from the surgical site (Fig. 12-7).

A small syringe filled with air is attached to the pilot balloon. The cuff is inflated after it passes beyond the vocal cords. Ideally the end of the ETT should be halfway between the vocal cords and carina to ensure bilateral ventilation. Markings on the ETT facilitate this goal. The 22-cm marking on the ETT should approximate the lips for females, using 23 cm in males. This minimizes the likelihood of right mainstem intubation.

Laryngoscope

The laryngoscope consists of two components. The base or handle contains a battery, and an interchangeable blade contains a light bulb (Fig. 12-8). The *Macintosh blade* is curved, and the tip is placed into the vallecula. The *Miller blade* is a thin, straight blade placed underneath the epiglottis. Each blade comes in a variety of sizes. Choice of blade is a matter of clinician preference. Benefits of the Macintosh include less dental trauma, less epiglottic trauma, better exposure, and more room to pass the ETT. Advantages of the Miller blade include better exposure of the glottic opening (Fig. 12-9).

Stylets are made in a variety of materials, usually soft metal or vinyl. These thin, pliable tubes are placed into the ETT to provide rigidity, allowing the tube to be bent into a particular shape. An ETT may be bent into an L shape to facilitate navigation of the ETT around an acute angle, especially when the larynx is anterior. The stylet is removed once the ETT is in place. Alternatively, long stylets may be used alone and placed directly into the trachea, with the ETT placed over the stylet (Figure 12-10).

Laryngeal Mask Airway

The laryngeal mask airway (LMA) is a soft plastic device that is inserted into the larynx without the use of a laryngoscope. After insertion the mask is inflated. It covers the glottic opening and allows ventilation to occur. The LMA is indicated for ventilation and administration of general anesthesia when tracheal intubation is undesirable or impossible. It may also be used as an adjunct in a difficult

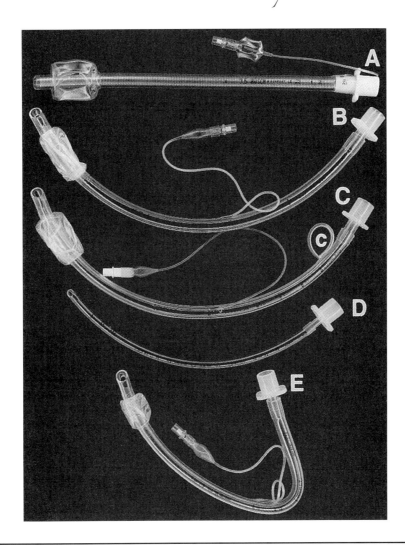

Fig. 12-7 Tracheal tubes. *A,* Reinforced anode endotracheal tube. *B,* Clear polyvinyl chloride endotracheal tube. *C,* Endotracheal tube with tip control ring *(c). D,* Uncuffed endotracheal tube. *E,* Oral RAE tube. (From Stoelting RK, Miller RD: *Basics of anesthesia,* ed 4, New York, 2000, Churchill Livingstone.)

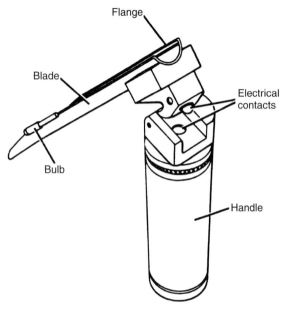

Fig. 12-8 Rigid laryngoscope. Components include handle and blade with light bulb. (From Morgan GE, Mikhail MS: *Clinical anesthesiology,* New York, 1992, Appleton & Lange.)

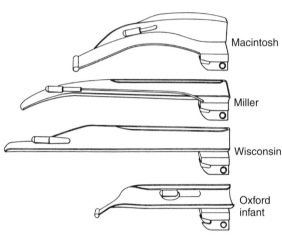

Fig. 12-9 Laryngoscope blades. (From Morgan GE, Mikhail MS: *Clinical anesthesiology,* New York, 1992, Appleton & Lange.)

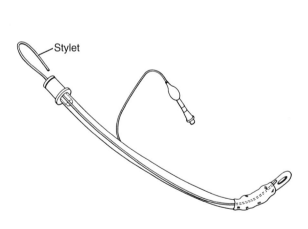

Fig. 12-10 Endotracheal tube with bent stylet. (From Morgan GE, Mikhail MS: *Clinical anesthesiology,* New York, 1992, Appleton & Lange.)

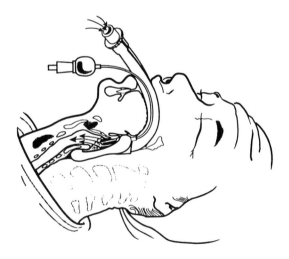

Fig. 12-11 Laryngeal mask airway. Proper positioning requires that the aperture faces the glottic opening. (From Hurford WE, Bailin MT, Davison JK, et al: *Clinical anesthesia procedures of the Massachusetts General Hospital,* ed 5, Philadelphia, 1998, Lippincott-Raven.)

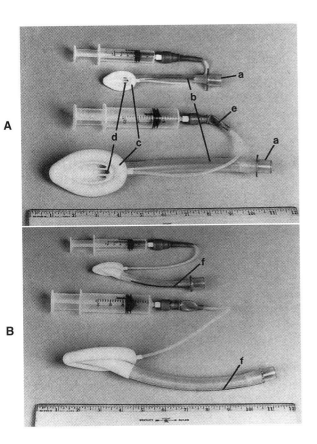

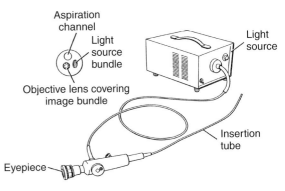

Fig. 12-13 Flexible fiberoptic bronchoscope. (From Morgan GE, Mikhail MS: *Clinical anesthesiology,* New York, 1992, Appleton & Lange.)

Fig. 12-12 Laryngeal mask airway. **A,** Anterior view. Proximal connector *(a)*, shaft *(b)*, cuff *(c)*, opening of shaft *(d)*, and pilot balloon *(e)*. **B,** Lateral view. Black line *(f)* marks reference point to patient. (From Stoelting RK, Miller RD: *Basics of anesthesia,* ed 4, New York, 2000, Churchill Livingstone.)

airway to facilitate ventilation or tracheal intubation. Complications include aspiration and trauma to the soft tissue and laryngeal aperture (Figs. 12-11 and 12-12).

Fiberoptic Intubation

Fiberoptic intubation provides indirect visualization of the larynx using a flexible fiberoptic laryngoscope. It is indicated when apnea is undesirable in a patient who poses a potential for difficult ventilation or intubation (e.g., trauma, altered anatomy) or when neck movement is contraindicated (e.g., unstable cervical spine). Fiberoptic intubation is usually performed in a spontaneously ventilating

patient who may or may not be sedated. Occasionally the patient may be put to sleep if obstruction is not a risk. The fiberoptic laryngoscope may be inserted orally or nasally after appropriate topicalization of the nares or oropharynx is achieved. Once the glottic opening is visualized, the scope is advanced into the trachea and the ETT placed over the scope. The fiberoptic laryngoscope is removed and ETT placement confirmed. The patient is then put to sleep (Fig. 12-13).

Complications of fiberoptic intubation include bleeding (especially from the nares), poor visualization as a result of secretions and combativeness from an inadequately anesthetized patient and damage to the flexible laryngoscope from biting. Most complications can be avoided by adequately preparing the patient. A thoroughly informed patient is less likely to be combative. Carefully titrated midazolam (Versed), or fentanyl/droperidol can provide adequate amnesia and analgesia during the procedure. Administering glycopyrrolate can minimize secretions. Bleeding can be avoided by preparing the nares with phenylephrine (Neo-Synephrine). Further analgesia may be provided by application of local anesthetics to the oropharynx and trachea using topical lidocaine or benzocaine spray and transtracheal and superior laryngeal nerve blocks.

Manual Ventilation

During periods of hypoventilation it may be necessary to assist or completely control the airway and ventilate the patient. Hypoventilation caused by obstruction, most often from the flaccid tongue, may be relieved by a jaw thrust and head tilt. This maneuver pulls the tongue away from the posterior pharyngeal wall. This maneuver can be performed in a semiconscious, spontaneously breathing patient. Alternatively, oropharyngeal and nasopharyngeal airways may be placed to relieve obstruction.

Stridor, snoring, poor chest expansion, and desaturation may characterize obstruction.

Manual ventilation most often occurs when the patient's respiratory effort is inadequate. It is indicated to assist or control ventilation, provide greater oxygen concentration, and deliver inhalational anesthesia.

With the patient in the supine position the face mask is secured over the mouth and nose. The mask is attached to a resuscitation bag or the breathing circuit, which is connected to an oxygen source. The end point of manual ventilation is to maintain oxygenation and ventilation. This is evidenced by good chest excursion, pink mucous membranes, and stable vital signs, including an oxygen saturation of 94% or greater.

Complications

Complications associated with manual ventilation include a *poor mask fit,* usually from a mismatch in the patient's face relative to the size of the mask or from failure of the operator to secure the mask appropriately. This typically occurs around the bridge of the nose and results in air or gas leakage, causing hypoventilation. An improperly placed mask may cause trauma to the bridge of the nose or inappropriate pressure to the eyes.

Laryngospasm usually occurs in the lightly anesthetized or semiconscious patient. It can be precipitated by instrumentation in the airway or by secretions on the vocal cords. This causes partial or complete closure of the glottic opening, resulting in obstruction or stridor. Gentle positive-pressure ventilation may relieve obstruction. Alternatively, a small dose of succinylcholine (10 to 20 mg) will relax the vocal cords so that gas exchange may occur.

Aspiration may occur at any time when the trachea is not secured. Patients at high risk include those who have a full stomach (pregnancy, obesity, ascites, recent meal), those with slow gastric emptying time (diabetics, chronic narcotic use, small bowel obstruction), and those with esophageal dysmotility (reflux, hiatal hernia). This phenomenon can occur in patients without risk factors. Patients with risk factors

should always be intubated for anesthetic techniques that may involve loss of protective airway reflexes and should receive prophylactic treatment with bacitracin, metoclopramide (Reglan), and famotidine (Pepcid) to lessen the severity of aspiration pneumonitis.

Inability to ventilate is a common complication of ventilation by mask. Causes include poor mask fit, soft tissue obstruction (oropharyngeal airway or jaw thrust may help), and chest wall rigidity (e.g., caused by high narcotic dose, severe scoliosis, or muscular dystrophy). In such cases where time is crucial, endotracheal intubation may be necessary.

Endotracheal Intubation

Endotracheal intubation may be indicated to (1) prevent aspiration, (2) maintain patency of the airway for long-term ventilation, (3) manage diseases of the airway, (4) implement frequent suctioning, or (5) facilitate surgery requiring general anesthesia. Intubation is required for procedures involving the airway, lungs, and abdomen. When the anesthesia provider is located far away from the airway (prone position, 180-degree bed turn), intubation is a safe choice for airway management. Mask ventilation for long periods leads to provider fatigue. Intubation allows the anesthetist to attend to other aspects of patient care. In situations where mask ventilation is difficult or impossible, intubation may be necessary.

Orotracheal Intubation

Laryngoscopy and intubation should be preceded by oxygenation with 100% oxygen to minimize the degree of hypoxia associated with apnea. The patient is placed in the supine position. Monitors are applied. General anesthesia is induced. Mask ventilation ensues. The patient is then placed in the sniffing position and the mouth opened wide. The provider places the laryngoscope in the left hand and inserts the blade into the right side of the mouth to sweep the tongue to the left.

The tip of the blade is placed in the vallecula (Macintosh) or under the epiglottis (Miller). Exposure of the glottic opening involves lifting the laryngoscope towards the patient's feet. Once the vocal cords are exposed, the ETT is placed between the cords and the cuff inflated (Figs. 12-14 and Figure 12-15). The presence of symmetric chest expansion, auscultation

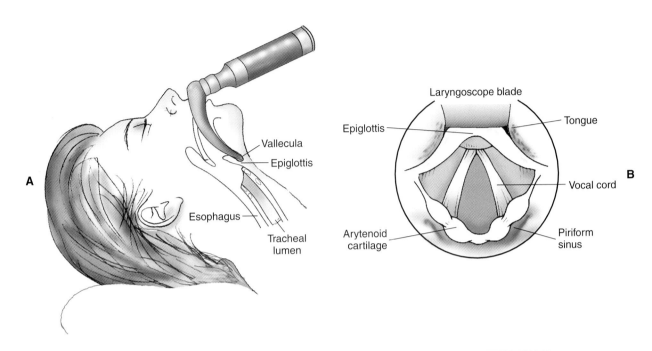

Fig. 12-14 A, Laryngoscope is placed under the epiglottis and lifted toward the patient's feet. It should not be used as a lever. **B,** View of glottic opening. (Redrawn from Hurford WE, Bailin MT, Davison JK, et al: *Clinical anesthesia procedures of the Massachusetts General Hospital,* ed 5, Philadelphia, 1998, Lippincott-Raven.)

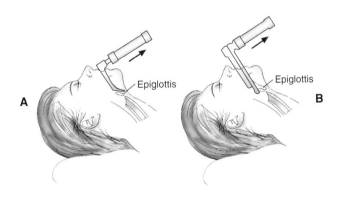

Fig. 12-15 Correct placement of Macintosh and Miller blades. **A,** Macintosh tip is placed into the vallecula. **B,** Miller tip is placed under the epiglottis. (Redrawn from Stoelting RK, Miller RD: *Basics of anesthesia,* ed 4, New York, 2000, Churchill Livingstone.)

of bilateral equal breath sounds, absence of sound in the stomach, and the presence of carbon dioxide on capnography confirm correct ETT placement.

Nasotracheal Intubation

Nasotracheal intubation is indicated for surgery where the ETT may interfere with the operative site (mouth, jaw, teeth). Patients who have poor mouth opening pose a challenge to oral intubation. Nasal ETTs are better tolerated and more comfortable in the awake patient and in those who require prolonged intubation. The nasal tube is less likely to become dislodged by patient movement.

The larger naris is prepared with topical anesthetic (lidocaine jelly, or cocaine when not contraindicated). This is particularly useful in the awake patient. Phenylephrine or cocaine is commonly applied to prevent bleeding. Sequential dilation with progressively larger, lubricated nasal airways facilitates passage of the ETT. Typically, smaller ETT tubes are used (7.0 or 7.5 mm). Laryngoscopy proceeds in standard fashion to expose the vocal cords, assuming there is adequate mouth opening. The ETT tube is placed in the prepared nostril and advanced into the trachea. Magill forceps may be used to grasp the tip of the ETT and guide placement. ETT placement is then confirmed. This technique is contraindicated in the setting of basilar skull fracture.

Blind Nasal Intubation

"Blind" nasal intubation is used when most other attempts at intubation have been unsuccessful or in an extreme emergency. A lubricated ETT is placed in the larger nostril of a spontaneously breathing patient. The provider manipulates the tube to the point of maximal breath sounds and advances the ETT blindly into the trachea.

Awake Intubation

Awake intubations are often performed when the patient has a known or suspected difficult airway or who has a history of difficult intubation or ventilation, in whom loss of protective airway reflexes or frank apnea may have catastrophic effects. Awake intubations are also often performed in situations when blood in the airway may obscure visualization or when neurologic function must be assessed after intubation.

Proper patient preparation is of paramount importance. Intravenous sedation and analgesia should be carefully titrated and administered whenever possible. Amnesia and analgesia facilitate cooperation.

Small does of midazolam, fentanyl, or droperidol are typically used. Apnea and severe hypoventilation must be avoided in the high-risk patient.

Topical analgesia may be administered to the oropharynx (tongue, palate, tonsillar pillars) with lidocaine or benzocaine spray. The nares may be prepared with cocaine, phenylephrine, or lidocaine. Cocaine provides both analgesia and vasoconstriction.

Superior laryngeal nerve blocks may be performed using 3 ml of 1% lidocaine on both sides of the neck. The superior cornu of the hyoid bone is located, and a 25-gauge needle is inserted into the thyrohyoid membrane. The vocal cords, epiglottis, and arytenoids are anesthetized.

A transtracheal injection of 3 ml of 4% lidocaine will anesthetize the glottis and trachea. The cricothyroid membrane is located in the midline and pierced. Aspiration of air confirms correct placement of local anesthetic. Rapid injection ensues. This technique is contraindicated in patients at high risk for aspiration since protective airway reflexes are lost (Fig. 12-16).

Once the objectives of analgesia and sedation are met, laryngoscopy for nasal or oral intubation is performed.

Complications

Orotracheal complications include trauma to the teeth, tongue, and lips. Bleeding from soft tissue can occur with repeated attempts, especially in patients who are anticoagulated or those with a history of radiation therapy. Other complications include damage to the vocal cords and cartilages. Esophageal intubation and right mainstem intubation are common occurrences, and correct ETT placement should always be confirmed. Rarely, tracheal perforation may occur. Any of these problems may occur with nasal intubation, in addition to profuse bleeding from the nasal mucosa.

Emergency Airway Management

The difficult airway algorithm has been established according to recommendations by the American

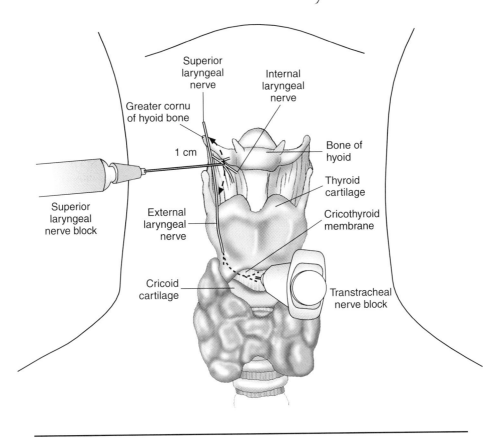

Fig. 12-16 Superior laryngeal nerve block and transtracheal block. (Redrawn from Morgan GE, Mikhail MS: *Clinical anesthesiology,* New York, 1992, Appleton & Lange.)

Association of Anesthesiologists (Fig. 12-17). In the patient who is difficult to intubate, mask ventilation continues until the airway is established.

Cricothyroidotomy

Cricothyroidotomy is an emergency technique performed in situations where it is impossible to ventilate or intubate and when time may be insufficient to establish a surgical airway. It involves placement of a 14-gauge angiocatheter through the cricothyroid membrane. An oxygen source is applied (anesthesia circuit or jet ventilator). It is important to note that oxygenation will occur but not necessarily ventilation. The patient will develop hypercarbia, and a permanent method of securing the airway is necessary. Complications include subcutaneous emphysema,

bleeding, and trauma to the vocal cords if performed incorrectly.

Tracheostomy

A surgical airway often must be established in patients who cannot be intubated or ventilated. This procedure is often performed with local anesthesia. Tracheostomy is a definitive way to control the airway and may be permanent or temporary. Complications are the same as with cricothyroidotomy.

Pediatric Airway

The pediatric airway is significantly different from that of the adult and as such poses some challenges.

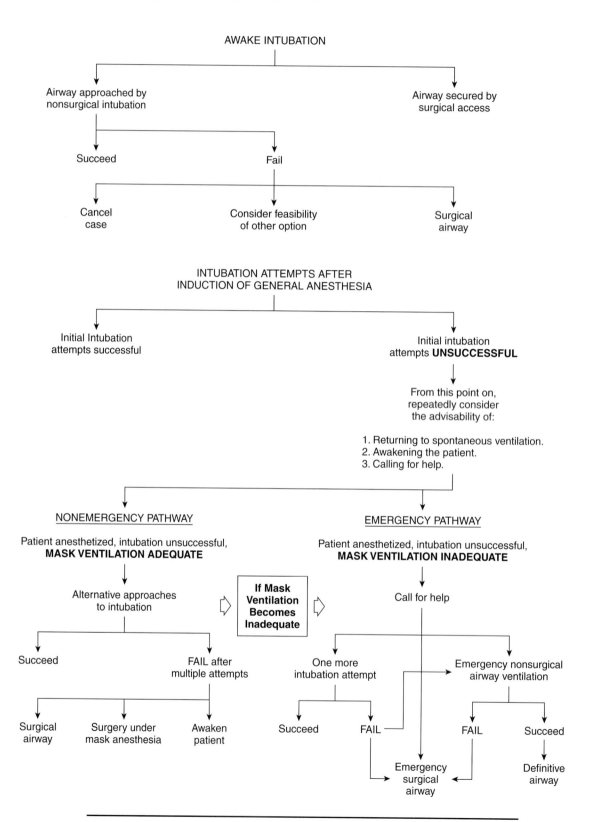

Fig. 12-17 Emergency airway algorithm. (From Hurford WE, Bailin MT, Davison JK, et al: *Clinical anesthesia procedures of the Massachusetts General Hospital*, ed 5, Philadelphia, 1998, Lippincott-Raven.)

Important anatomic differences include a large occiput. This may make positioning the head and obtaining the sniff position difficult. Although children under age 1 year are often edentulous, most will begin to shed dentition by age 5 years. A careful history and oral examination should elucidate any loose teeth.

Infants have large cheeks, which may make mask ventilation difficult. The tongue is large relative to the size of the oral cavity, making obstruction much more likely. The pediatric epiglottis is often long and stiff, making exposure of the vocal cords challenging; this can often be circumvented by use of the Miller blade. The larynx itself is more cephalad than in the adult, usually located at approximately the fourth cervical vertebra. The narrowest part of the airway is at the level of the vocal cords in the adult but at the cricothyroid cartilage in the child.

All these differences often make the child more difficult to intubate. In addition to the anatomic differences, the anesthetist should be aware of any congenital or hereditary anomalies that present in childhood, such as craniofacial abnormalities and Down, Pierre Robin, or Treacher Collins syndrome.

CHAPTER

13

Local Anesthetic Techniques and Adjuncts

J. Mel Hawkins
John Gerard Meechan

CHAPTER OUTLINE

The control of pain in the twenty-first century still presents an old challenge: will there ever be a perfect local anesthetic technique or delivery system? Great strides in air abrasion, laser therapy, hypnosis, electronic dental anesthesia, and audiovisual distractions have helped, but short of general anesthesia, local anesthesia is still the fundamental technique for pain control in dentistry.

Many factors are involved in the successful delivery of local anesthesia. In addition to proper selection of the specific technique, competent patient management is essential to successful anesthetic administration.

Methods and Definitions

Topical anesthesia in dentistry is provided in various formulations, such as sprays, creams, gels, and ointments (Fig. 13-1). Although other agents may be applied topically, drug formulations used topically have been selected to be effective in providing anesthetic to block mucosal nerve endings. Most notably, topical anesthesia is used in diminishing pain perception of needle insertion.

Infiltration anesthesia does not extend beyond the local anesthesia diffusion perimeter because only terminal nerve endings are blocked by the local anesthetic (Fig. 13-2). Infiltration anesthesia is particularly common for single-tooth procedures, hemostasis, and various soft tissue procedures.

In *field block anesthesia* the anesthetic solution is deposited in the area near the larger terminal nerve branches to ensure that areas distal to the injection site are anesthetized (Fig. 13-3). The target point is similar to an infiltration but provides a regional scope of anesthesia.

Nerve block anesthesia refers to the deposition of a local anesthetic solution in proximity to a primary nerve trunk, usually performed with a single injection. It has the advantage of blocking most or all of the hard and soft tissue structures distal to the injection (Fig. 13-4).

Armamentarium

Needles for use with dental syringes are presterilized by the manufacturer and available in various gauges, most often 25, 27, and 30, with a smaller number indicating a needle of greater dimension (Fig. 13-5). Disposable sterile needles must be used for all injections, but the same needle may be used for more than one injection in a patient. One might assume that the smaller needles produce less pain during the

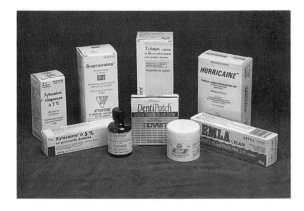

Fig. 13-1 Topical anesthetics.

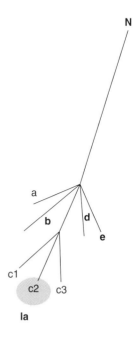

Fig. 13-2 Infiltration anesthesia has limited effect. Deposition of local anesthetic *(la)* at perimeter of a nerve field only affects nerve endings in vicinity of deposition *(c2)*.

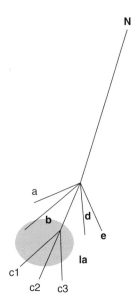

Fig. 13-3 Field block anesthesia produces a greater zone of anesthesia than infiltration. Some larger nerve terminals are affected; *c1, c2,* and *c3,* all branches of nerve terminal *c.* Some terminals from adjacent nerves *(b)* may also be anesthetized.

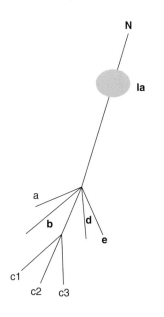

Fig. 13-4 Nerve block anesthesia inhibits transmission in all terminal branches *(a to e)* of nerve trunk *(N).*

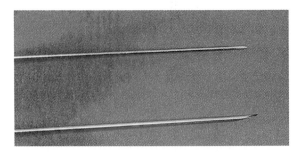

Fig. 13-5 Needles, 27 and 30 gauge, with 30 the narrower gauge.

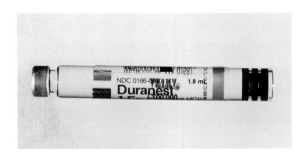

Fig. 13-6 Local anesthetic cartridge, with glass cylinder, rubber plunger, and aluminum ring at needle-penetration end.

injection, but little evidence suggests any variation in discomfort among gauges used in dentistry.[1] All standard dental needles permit aspiration for blood, but those having smaller diameters are more likely to penetrate vessels than their larger counterparts. Therefore in areas where vessel penetration is common, larger diameter needles (no less than 27 gauge) should be used. Furthermore, when deep penetration through tissue is required, there is less deflection with larger needles.[2]

The *cartridge* containing the local anesthetic is prefilled by the manufacturer. The cartridges most often used in North America contain 1.7 and 1.8 ml of solution, although larger cartridges of 2.0 and 2.2 ml are available in other countries. Although the solution within the cartridge is sterile, the external surface in most cases has not been sterilized. Some companies have recently begun to sterilize the entire assembled cartridge[3] (Fig. 13-6).

BOX 13-1

Factors in Selection of Local Anesthesia Cartridge

Contents, including concentration of each agent: allergic reactions, drug interactions, and cardiovascular effects of vasoconstrictors must be considered.
Clarity of solution: cloudy solutions are contaminated and should not be used.
Cracks or breaks in glass: faulty cartridges must not be used.
Large air bubbles and extended plunger: if either is noted, there is probably leakage and thus contamination; do not use.
Expiration date: more of a concern for vasoconstrictors.

BOX 13-2

Composition and Classification of Dental Syringe

Composition
Barrel holds the cartridge.
Hub connects the needle to the syringe.
Plunger is connected to a thumb ring.

Classification
Nonaspirating
Aspirating
Computer-assisted aspirating

BOX 13-3

Assembled Injection System Checklist

Needle-syringe junction: no mobility at needle-syringe contact.
Cartridge stability: cartridge must be seated firmly in the syringe.
Free flow of solution through needle: needle has penetrated cartridge diaphragm.

Cartridges that allow a smooth movement of the plunger without "jerking" are recommended for injection. Plastic cartridges should not be used where significant pressure is involved in the injection (e.g., intraligamentary anesthesia) because they can distort during use, allowing escape of solution through the rubber plunger rather than through the needle.[4]

Some advocate warming the local anesthetic cartridge to body temperature to reduce injection sensation, but this is unnecessary if the cartridge has been allowed to reach room temperature. Patients are unable to determine differences in the temperature of injected solution within the range of 21° to 37° C. Cartridges should not be used directly from refrigerated storage; they should be allowed to reach room temperature. Cartridges should not be stored at 37° C because this temperature increases the chances of bacterial contamination, decreases the efficacy of epinephrine as a vasoconstrictor, and increases the pH of the solution.[5]

Injection of solution of low pH is more uncomfortable than that of a liquid closer to physiologic pH.[6] Physical and chemical factors are both involved in the criteria for cartridge selection (Box 13-1).

A dental *syringe* consists of a barrel, which holds the cartridge; the hub, which connects the needle to the syringe; and the plunger, which has a ring for the thumb. Syringes can be classified as aspirating, nonaspirating, or computer-assisted aspirating (Box 13-2). Nonaspirating syringes are not recommended. Although they do not guarantee extravascular depo-

sition, aspirating systems are invaluable in reducing inadvertent intravascular injections and injection discomfort.[7] When the syringe is assembled, (1) no mobility should exist at the needle-syringe junction, (2) the cartridge must be firmly seated in the syringe barrel, and (3) solution should be free flowing through the needle (Box 13-3). It is generally unacceptable to detect a disruption in the system after the mucosa has been penetrated.

Syringes may be single use or reusable. Reusable syringes must be sterilized by autoclaving for each use.

The dentist can hold a dental local anesthetic syringe in various ways. The technique adopted must allow a steady grasp throughout the injection. The syringe should sit in the dentist's hand with the palm facing upward. The first and second fingers of the dominant hand grip the barrel, and the thumb connects with the thumb rest. Depending on operator preference, either the tip or the base of the thumb may be used to depress the plunger. The third finger may be used as extra support midway along the barrel. The injection hand can be stabilized during the injection by resting on the dentist's nonworking hand or by pressing the forearm against the operator's chest. At all stages the syringe should be held out of the patient's line of vision, either behind the operator's back or handed to the dentist by an assistant below the patient's line of sight.

Dental local anesthetic injections should be delivered by the operator in a seated position. The ideal position for a patient during local anesthetic injections is fully supine. This provides excellent return of blood from the legs to the heart and has the brain at the same level as the heart, thus promoting good cranial perfusion. In addition, this position reduces the chances of syncope during dental local anesthesia. However, many patients (especially children) feel vulnerable in the fully supine position. A compromise is to have the patient reclined at 30 degrees. In fact, this is a useful orientation during the mandibular injections, since the mandibular occlusal plane is approximately parallel to the floor when the mouth is fully open.

Injection Technique

Before applying the topical anesthetic, the mucosa to be injected must be dried with gauze to remove any debris and excess saliva. The topical is applied over a limited area because excess material, which might contact lingual or soft palate mucosa, is unpleasant for the patient and can cause increased salivation. Topical anesthetics must be applied for sufficient time to allow them to act. Application times of a few seconds are rarely useful, but 1 to 2 minutes is ideal. Conventional topical anesthetics will provide sufficient anesthesia of reflected (nonkeratinized) mucosa to allow relatively painless needle penetration to a depth of a few millimeters. Unfortunately, they are not as effective on keratinized mucosa, such as attached gingiva and the mucosa of the hard palate.

The needle should always be inserted through mucosa that is being stretched; this allows the needle to pierce the tissue in a single movement. If the needle is inserted through loose folds of mucosa, the tissue is dragged and torn rather than being pierced.

On needle penetration the patient should be distracted to divert attention from the action of piercing the tissue. This can often be performed with stretching of the tissue. For example, when injecting into the maxillary buccal sulcus, pulling the upper lip and cheek upward and outward stretches the mucosa. The stretched tissue is then pulled down onto the needle, rather than the needle up through the tissues. The area of stimulation by the dentist's fingers is much greater than that stimulated by the tip of the needle, and the patient is often unaware that tissue penetration has occurred.

The local anesthetic solution should be deposited supraperiosteally. Some regional block techniques require the dentist to touch bone with the needle to confirm good approximation to the site of interest. Once bone has been touched, however, the needle should be withdrawn slightly to ensure that the tip is supraperiosteal during injection. Subperiosteal injection should be avoided because it will cause pain at the time of injection and may also produce postinjection discomfort due to stripping of periosteum from bone.

Aspiration before and during injection is mandatory to reduce the chances of accidental intravascular injection of local anesthetic solution. Intravascular injection can have serious consequences. Intraarterial injections are used less often than intravenous injections but can have dramatic sequelae, such as temporary loss of vision if the arterial supply to the eye is affected. Intravenous injection will increase the risk of local anesthetic and vasoconstrictor toxicity and may produce systemic effects such as tachycardia and palpitations. Positive aspiration of blood occurs in more than 10% of some intraoral regional block injections.[8] It is therefore essential to use a syringe that allows aspirations to be performed.

The importance of *slow injection* cannot be overemphasized. Discomfort is decreased both during the injection and postoperatively. Ideally the injection of the cartridge of local anesthetic should take about a minute; a rate less than 30 seconds per cartridge should be discouraged. Similarly, the needle should be removed slowly from the tissues, ensuring that inadvertent tissue damage (e.g., tongue, lip) does not occur on exit from the mouth.

Patient Consent

Reasonable explanation of risk versus benefit should be given to every patient before the administration of local anesthesia. These risks and benefits may vary according to the selected technique. Risks are usually minimal when administering supraperiosteal and field block anesthesia. A portion of the medical history may include the question of the allergies to the local anesthetic chemical groups, which may preclude the patient receiving certain topical anesthetics. When block anesthesia is anticipated, however, certain sequelae must be explained, including the risk of paresthesia, hematoma, trismus, and failure to achieve local anesthesia.

Other complications are generally not accepted to be common enough to divulge to the patient, such as disability and death. According to most legal sources, these need not be discussed with the patient to provide adequate informed consent about the risks of local anesthesia administration.

Maxillary Anesthetic Techniques

The anatomy of the maxilla differs from the mandible in that the thinner cortical plate allows infiltration anesthesia in most situations. This results in greater success for supraperiosteal injection in the maxillary arch than with the mandible, where a mandibular nerve block is generally required.

The second division of the trigeminal nerve arises from the gasserian ganglion in the medial cranial fossa and exits the skull via the foramen rotundum. The nerve then traverses the superior aspect of the pterygopalatine fossa, where it divides into three major branches: the pterygopalatine nerve, the infraorbital nerve, and the zygomatic nerve (Fig. 13-7).

Pterygopalatine Nerve

The main portion of the pterygopalatine nerve passes down the pterygopalatine canal and exits toward the oral cavity at the greater palatine foramen as the anterior palatine nerve. The greater palatine foramen and pterygopalatine canal are traversed to achieve the second division nerve block. The pterygopalatine or sphenopalatine ganglion is attached to the medial side of this nerve, but no fibers of the pterygopalatine nerve have synapses there. The nasal branches are emitted and the medial branches traverse the septum, ending as the *nasopalatine nerve*, which exits at the incisive foramen.

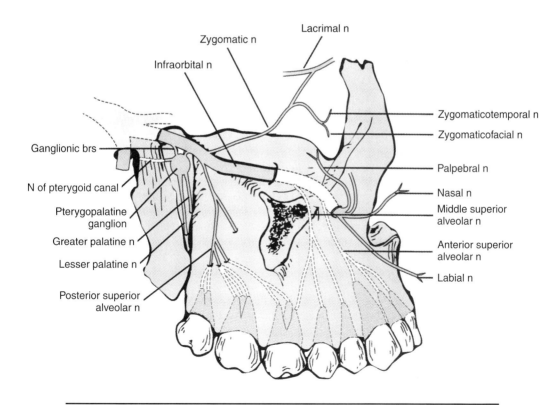

Fig. 13-7 Maxillary nerve. (From Liebgott B: *The anatomical basis of dentistry*, ed 2, St Louis, 2001, Mosby.)

Infraorbital Nerve

The main trunk of the maxillary nerve continues through the pterygopalatine fossa and gives rise to the posterior superior alveolar nerve, which divides into an external gingival branch and the internal dental branch. The main nerve trunk then enters the inferior orbital fissure and travels through the floor of the orbit in the infraorbital canal. While in this canal, it emits the middle superior and anterior superior alveolar nerves, which sometimes exist as a nerve plexus. These nerves travel along the lateral sinus wall to the premolar and anterior teeth, respectively, and send sensory branches to the maxillary sinus mucosa. Approximately 30% of the population do not have the middle superior alveolar nerve, and its areas of innervation are assumed by the posterior and anterior alveolar nerves.[9] The infraorbital nerve exits the maxilla at the infraorbital foramen and divides into three terminal sensory branches: the *superior labial nerve* to the upper lip, the *lateral nasal nerve* to the side of the nose, and the *inferior palpebral nerve* to the lower eyelid.

Zygomatic Nerve

The zygomatic branch emerges from the infraorbital nerve and has two divisions. One branch communicates with the postganglionic parasympathetic fibers from the pterygopalatine ganglion to the lacrimal gland. The other division exits the body of the zygoma and the zygomatic orbital foramen and supplies sensation to the malar eminence.

Anatomically, once the greater palatine foramen is located, the needle tip will approximate a number of structures. As the needle advances, it will transcend the greater palatine fossa and the associated neurovascular bundles. Presumably, damage to these structures can occur, but the incidence of such damage appears to be low. The incidence of positive aspiration has been reported to be only 8% and traumatic injury to the nerve less than 1%.[10]

Posterior Superior Alveolar Nerve Block

The posterior superior alveolar (PSA) nerve is a branch of the maxillary division of the trigeminal nerve. It parts from the main trunk in the pterygopalatine fossa, passes inferiorly along the posterior wall of the maxilla, and enters the bone about 1 cm superior and posterior to the third molar tooth. The PSA nerve supplies the buccal gingivae, periodon-

BOX 13-4

Technique: Posterior Superior Alveolar Nerve Block

1. Use a short or long needle, no less than 27 gauge.
2. Instruct the patient to open the mouth only slightly, and move the lower jaw over to side of injection.
3. Retract the lip and cheek with the thumb or first finger of left hand.
4. Insert the needle at the height of the maxillary buccal sulcus at distal aspect of second molar.
5. Advance the needle posteriorly, superiorly, and medially (at 45-degree angle to each plane) to a depth 15 mm.
6. Perform aspiration.
7. Inject 1.5 ml of solution slowly.
8. If bone is contacted before a depth of 1.5 ml achieved, alter the angle of approach by withdrawing slightly and positioning the syringe medially.

tium, and alveolus associated with the upper molar teeth. It provides innervation to the pulps of all the upper molar teeth with the possible exception of the mesiobuccal pulp of the first molar, which is supplied by the middle superior alveolar (MSA) nerve in approximately 50% of individuals.

Injection for the PSA nerve block is performed in a highly vascular area, and formation of a hematoma is a recognized side effect, especially when the needle is advanced more than 15 mm. Immediate hemorrhage is controlled by pressure, but postinjection trismus may last for weeks. Antibiotic therapy should be prescribed if the hematoma is large (Box 13-4 and Figs. 13-8 and 13-9).

Infraorbital Nerve Block

The infraorbital nerve is one of the terminal branches of the maxillary division of the trigeminal nerve. It innervates the skin of the cheek, skin, and mucosa of the upper lip and part of the nose. The anterior superior alveolar (ASA) nerve separates from the infraorbital nerve within the infraorbital canal about 5 mm before the infraorbital foramen. The ASA nerve supplies sensation to the upper incisor and cuspid teeth and occasionally the bicuspids, buccal periodontium, gingivae, and mucosa, as well as the bone

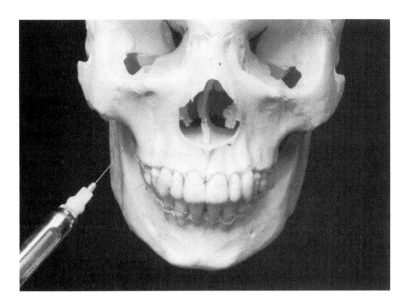

Fig. 13-8 Normal orientation of needle for posterior superior alveolar nerve block. (From Jastak JT, Yagiela JA, Donaldson D: *Local anesthesia of the oral cavity,* Philadelphia, 1995, Saunders.)

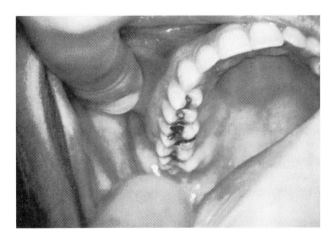

Fig. 13-9 Palpation of zygomatic process in posterior superior alveolar nerve block. Point of needle insertion lies within mucosal pocket posterior to palpating finger. (From Jastak JT, Yagiela JA, Donaldson D: *Local anesthesia of the oral cavity,* Philadelphia, 1995, Saunders.)

associated with these teeth. The MSA nerve supplies the pulps and adjacent tissues of the maxillary bicuspid teeth with the mesiobuccal root of the first molar. The MSA nerve leaves the infraorbital nerve within the infraorbital canal. Either infiltration or regional block techniques can anesthetize the terminal branches of the ASA and MSA nerves. The infraorbital nerve block technique relies on the deposition of local anesthetic close to the infraorbital foramen to allow the solution to diffuse along the infraorbital canal and through surrounding bone to reach the ASA and MSA nerves. The infraorbital foramen is located as a depression in the bone just below the infraorbital branch on the infraorbital margin (Box 13-5 and Figs. 13-10 and 13-11).

BOX 13-5

Technique: Infraorbital Nerve Block

1. Preferably, use a long needle (35 mm) of no less than 27 gauge.
2. Ask the patient to open the mouth slightly.
3. Retract the upper lip with the thumb of the left hand.
4. Use the first finger to palpate the infraorbital foramen extraorally. Keep the first finger in this position throughout injection.
5. Introduce the needle at the height of the maxillary buccal sulcus between the apices of the bicuspid teeth.
6. Advance the needle parallel to the roots of the bicuspids toward the infraorbital foramen until bone is contacted, about 15 to 20 mm.
7. Withdraw the needle slightly, and if aspiration is negative, slowly inject 1.5 ml of solution.

Maxillary Nerve Block

Three techniques are used to block the maxillary nerve, one extraoral approach and two intraoral approaches.[5,11,12] The extraoral approach is not a common or practical procedure in most dental offices.

Intraorally, the two techniques to block the maxillary nerve are the high tuberosity approach (similar to the posterior superior alveolar nerve block) and the greater palatine canal approach. Although less predictable and prone to more complications, the *high tuberosity approach* may be the more comfortable procedure. The goal of this technique is to direct the needle superiorly, medially, and posteriorly along the zygomatic and infratemporal surfaces of the maxilla to enter the pterygopalatine fossa. This depth can be 24 to 44 mm.[13]

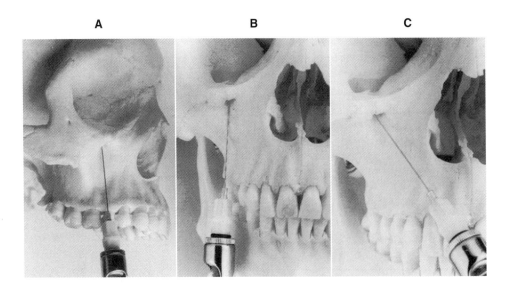

A   B   C

Fig. 13-10 Infraorbital nerve block. Needle tip lies just within infraorbital foramen. **A,** Vertical approach, lateral view. **B,** Vertical approach, frontal view. **C,** Midline approach. (From Jastak JT, Yagiela JA, Donaldson D: *Local anesthesia of the oral cavity,* Philadelphia, 1995, Saunders.)

Complications associated with the high tuberosity technique include the lack of profound anesthesia, caused by either inadequate volume of local anesthetic (it may take more than 1 cartridge of solution to obtain complete anesthesia) or improper positioning and inadequate depth of penetration. The pterygoid plexus of veins is close to the area approached with this technique and there is a relatively high risk of hematoma.

The maxillary nerve block using the *greater palatine canal approach* was first described in 1917 by Mendel.[5] Despite this technique's longevity, it has never become a popular or standard approach. The need to block the hemimaxilla does not arise as frequently as the need to block the mandible. The advantages and indications should be weighed against the disadvantages and possible restrictions (Box 13-6).

Hard and Soft Tissue Landmarks. In most cases the challenge of this maxillary nerve block technique centers on locating the greater palatine canal and being familiar with the anatomy of the palate (Fig. 13-12). With practice, finding the canal entrance and

orienting the needle correctly with respect to the midsagittal plane become easier. Locating the greater palatine canal involves five "landmarking" steps, as follows[13]:

1. The greater palatine canal is located between the middle portion of the third molar and the middle portion of the second molar in 84% of patients. The canal is located mesial to the midportion of the second molar in 10% and distal to the midportion of the third molar in 6% of the population[14] (Fig. 13-13).
2. The greater palatine *foramen* is located anterior to the junction of the hard and soft palate. This junction is seen as a color change; the tissue overlying the soft palate is darker pink than the tissue overlying the hard palate. This border can also be palpated using the dental mirror. The foramen can occur from 1.8 to 12 mm anterior to this border, with an average distance of 7 mm.[14,15]
3. The greater palatine canal is usually located at the junction of the horizontal and vertical bony plates of the hard palate. In patients who have a very deep palatal vault, the canal opening will appear closer to the dentition; in patients with a shallower palatal vault, the foramen will appear closer to the sagittal midline.
4. The greater palatine canal is located along an imaginary line from the ipsilateral hamular process to the ipsilateral cingulum of the lateral incisor (Fig. 13-14).
5. The soft tissue depression that covers the greater palatine canal is a blanched or whitish area

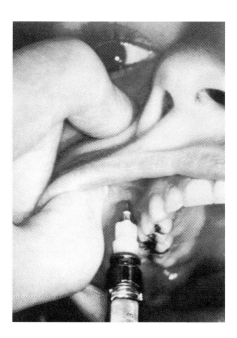

Fig. 13-11 Infraorbital nerve block, vertical approach. Index finger is firmly palpating infraorbital depression while thumb is retracting lip. Needle parallels axis of second maxillary premolar. (From Jastak JT, Yagiela JA, Donaldson D: *Local anesthesia of the oral cavity,* Philadelphia, 1995, Saunders.)

BOX 13-6

Considerations: Maxillary Nerve Block

Advantages
Quadrant dentistry, without need for multiple injections.
Oral infections.
Sinus procedures.
Diagnosis of chronic maxillofacial pain syndromes.
Greater than 95% success rate.

Disadvantages
Hemostasis will not occur.
Infection may occur in area of palatine canal.
Horizontal opening to canal prohibits passage of needle in superior orientation.

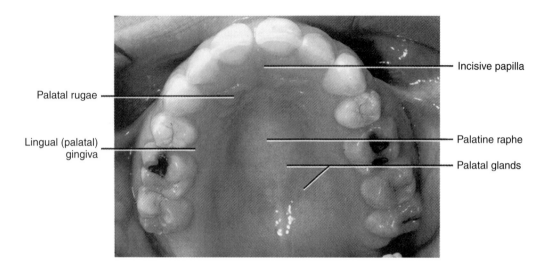

Palatal rugae

Lingual (palatal) gingiva

Incisive papilla

Palatine raphe

Palatal glands

Fig. 13-12 Hard palate of maxilla. (From Liebgott B: *The anatomical basis of dentistry,* ed 2, St Louis, 2001, Mosby.)

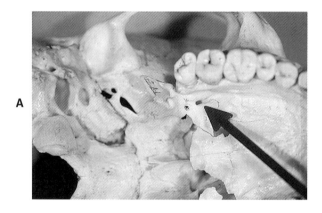

A

Fig. 13-13 A, Greater palatine foramen.
Continued

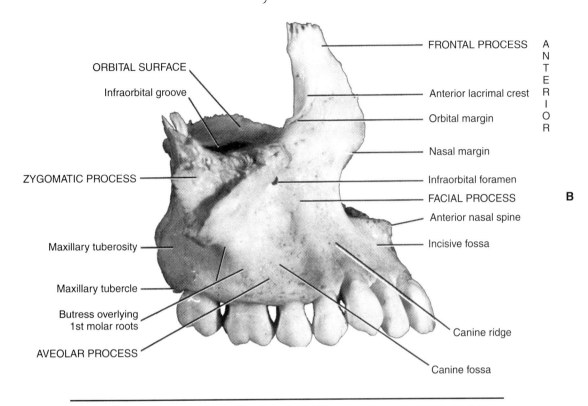

FRONTAL PROCESS

A
N
T
E
R
I
O
R

ORBITAL SURFACE

Infraorbital groove

Anterior lacrimal crest

Orbital margin

Nasal margin

ZYGOMATIC PROCESS

Infraorbital foramen

FACIAL PROCESS

Anterior nasal spine

Maxillary tuberosity

Incisive fossa

Maxillary tubercle

Butress overlying
1st molar roots

Canine ridge

AVEOLAR PROCESS

Canine fossa

B

Fig. 13-13, cont'd **B,** Lateral view of maxilla. (**B** from Liebgott B: *The anatomical basis of dentistry,* ed 2, St Louis, 2001, Mosby.)

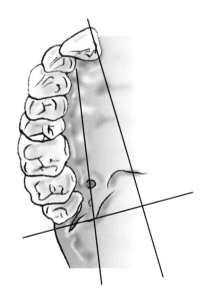

Fig. 13-14 Locating greater palatal foramen.

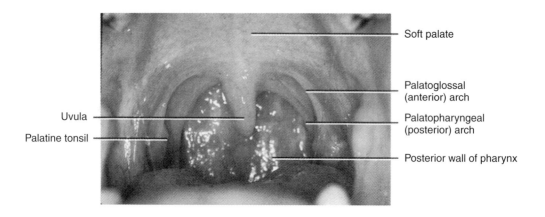

Fig. 13-15 Soft tissue of palate. (From Liebgott B: *The anatomical basis of dentistry,* ed 2, St Louis, 2001, Mosby.)

overlying serous and mucous glands. This lighter colored tissue can also be used to locate the canal (Fig. 13-15).

The *lesser* palatine canal is located posterior to the greater palatine canal on the posterior aspect of the hard palate. This canal is of no clinical significance to this technique because the needle cannot be advanced into the foramen due to its extremely small size.

Armamentarium and Technique Modifications. For patient comfort, preliminary infiltration in the region of the greater palatine foramen is essential. The greater palatine canal approach thus becomes a two-injection technique.

The first syringe is used for the preliminary injection and can be done with a 30-gauge short needle with a solution containing 1:100,000 epinephrine. The rationale for this is twofold. First, the 30-gauge needle tip, having lined up all the landmarks, is very close to the greater palatine foramen and, with its small needle gauge, disallows significant backflow from the small puncture. Second, as vascularity is encountered during the preparatory injection, the 1:100,000 epinephrine solution may minimize extravasation submucosally or onto the surface of the hard palate. The suggested volume is 0.5 ml.

The orientation of the pterygopalatine canal is superior and posterior. The angle that the canal creates with the horizontal hard palate can range from 20 to 70 degrees. However, 75% of the population have

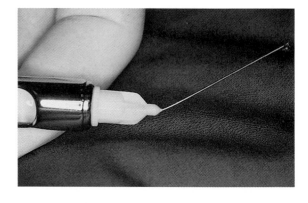

Fig. 13-16 Bent needle offers access to greater palatine canal.

this angle at 37 to 57 degrees.[15] Therefore the second syringe can be prepared with a bend of 45 degrees at the hub, using a 25-gauge or 27-gauge needle with the bevel facing posteriorly, toward the anterior border of the pterygoid plate (Fig. 13-16). In this way the needle bevel can slide along the previously mentioned surface and advance upward through the pterygomaxillary fissure (Fig. 13-17).

Clinical Procedure. The patient must open the mouth wide. Assuming there is no gag reflex, place the mouth mirror at the junction of the hard and soft palate; the greater palatine canal will occur an aver-

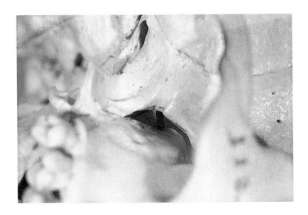

Fig. 13-17 Lateral view of right maxilla.

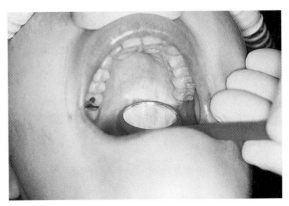

Fig. 13-18 Junction between hard and soft palates.

age of 7 mm anterior to this (Fig. 13-18). If there is a full dental arch present, the foramen will be located between the distal marginal ridge of the second molar and the middle aspect of the third molar in about 85% of patients. Next, line up the ipsilateral hamular process and lateral incisor, and observe the junction of the vertical and horizontal bony plates of the palate. Finally, look for a whiter depression of soft tissue, beneath which lies the opening of the greater palatine canal (see Fig 13-15).

The practitioner can administer the preparatory injection directly into this area, which is essential for a painless maxillary nerve block. To help the patient experience less discomfort from the preparatory injection, a topical anesthetic isolated from the tongue should be used with counterpressure from the mirror. Ensure that this injection is given 3 to 5 mm submucosally so that the local anesthetic solution, in a dose of about 0.5 ml, does not leak back into the oral cavity. Allow 2 to 3 minutes before proceeding with the next injection.

With a 25- or 27-gauge needle bent at 45 degrees and the bevel facing posteriorly, the procedure can begin. The length of the needle should be parallel to the midsagittal plane. Using the needle tip as a probe, locate the foramen (Fig. 13-19). Gently rotate the needle until it falls up into the canal. If bony resistance is encountered, pull back 1 mm and gently try to tease the needle tip around this. Advance in a superior and posterior direction to the final depth, as measured from the gingival crest in

the maxillary bicuspid region to the infraorbital foramen. This depth is almost the same measurement as for the high tuberosity approach. The depth can be 24 to 44 mm, with most adults 25 to 30 mm (Fig. 13-20).

When the final depth has been achieved, aspirate and slowly inject a full cartridge of either a plain local anesthetic solution or a vasoconstrictor concentration of 1:200,000. It should take 30 to 45 seconds to inject the full cartridge; inform the patient that slight pressure will be felt in the middle of the face.

The time of onset for the block to occur is 3 to 10 minutes, and the duration of anesthesia is 1.5 to 2 hours for hard tissue and 2.5 hours for soft tissue with a 1:200,000 epinephrine solution.

Complications. Diplopia of the ipsilateral eye may occur in 35.6% of patients.[16] This results from the local anesthetic diffusing superiorly and medially to bathe the orbital nerve. The patient must be assured that this phenomenon is transient. Permanent diplopia has not been reported.

Depositing anesthetic solution into the nasopharynx can occur if too much pressure is exerted on advancement of the needle. In this case the posterior wall of the canal can be perforated. It is possible to miss the hard palate completely and advance up into the soft palate. Solution is deposited into the nasopharynx, and the patient will complain of a bitter taste and may cough. No block will occur in this situation.

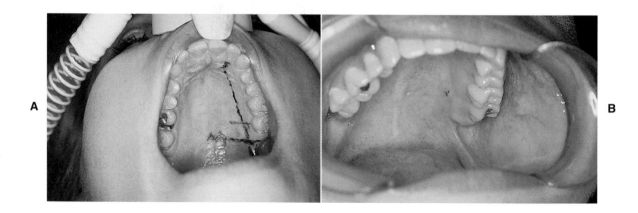

Fig. 13-19 A, Reference grid for location of greater palatine foramen. **B,** Estimated location of foramen.

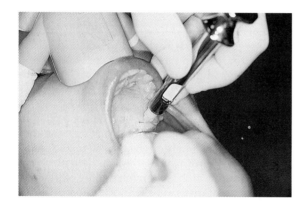

Fig. 13-20 Depth of maxillary nerve block.

Mandibular Anesthetic Techniques

Many difficulties exist clinically in the success rates for maxillary versus mandibular structural anesthesia. The third division of the trigeminal nerve (V3) with its inferior alveolar and associated nerve branches, plus the long buccal and lingual nerve, account for lower success rates with mandibular techniques than for most other anesthetized areas of the intraoral cavity. Success rates of 80% to 85% for the inferior alveolar nerve block attest to this fact. The dense cortical plate of bone normally is a barrier to the diffusion of local anesthesia from the injec-

tion area of the mandibular dentition, with the possible exception of the mandibular incisors. However, a valuable alternative to the conventional inferior alveolar nerve block is the incisive nerve block, commonly misnamed the "mental" nerve block. Other techniques include the anterior condylar neck, Gow-Gates, and Akinosi closed-mouth nerve blocks.

The mandibular division of the trigeminal nerve exits the trigeminal ganglion area through the foramen ovale into the infratemporal fossa. The first branch from the main trunk is the *nervus spinosus* (meningeal branch of mandibular nerve), which runs superiorly through the foramen spinosum to supply the meninges. The next branch is the *first motor nerve*, which supplies the medial pterygoid muscle. The *auriculotemporal nerve* gives sensory perception to the side of the head and scalp. The nerve also sends twigs to the external auditory meatus, tympanic membrane, and temporomandibular joint.

Inferior to the auriculotemporal nerve, the mandibular nerve splits into an anterior trunk and posterior trunk. The anterior trunk is both sensory and motor. The sensory component is the *long buccal nerve,* which supplies the buccal soft tissue distal to the molars. The motor component supplies the masseter, temporal, and lateral pterygoid muscles. The posterior trunk almost immediately divides into the lingual nerve and the inferior alveolar nerve. The *lingual nerve* supplies the anterior two thirds of the tongue and the lingual surface of the mandibular gingiva. The mandibular nerve sends a branch to the mylohyoid muscle and the anterior belly of the digastric, then enters the mandibular canal. This nerve gives sensation to the mandible, buccal gingiva anterior to first molar, mental area, lower lip, and mandibular teeth.

The *inferior alveolar nerve* supplies the pulps of all the teeth and the bone on one side of the mandible. There is a crossover at the midline with the contralateral nerve. The gingivae and periodontium on the buccal side from the second bicuspid anteriorly and the mucosa and skin of the lower lip to the midline also receive sensory supply from this nerve. The lingual nerve supplies sensation to one side of the anterior two thirds of the tongue (with the exception of the circumvallate papillae), floor of the mouth, lingual gingivae, and periodontia adjacent to all the lower teeth on one side.

Inferior Alveolar Nerve Block

The inferior alveolar nerve block is one of the most common forms of local anesthesia used in dentistry. This technique has acceptable reliability but is not 100% successful, especially with inexperienced operators. The aim of the injection is to deposit local anesthetic around the trunk of the inferior alveolar nerve as it enters the mandibular foramen on the lingual aspect of the mandibular ramus. The most common reason for failure is anatomic variation in the position of the mandibular foramen. The height of the foramen in relation to the mandibular occlusal plane varies with age; it is lower in the child compared with the dentate adult. In addition, the anteroposterior position of the foramen varies among individuals. The location of the foramen can be assessed by use of panoramic radiography. This injection may not produce satisfactory dental anesthesia also because of accessory pulpal nerve supply.

Numerous methods, including extraoral approaches, are available for the inferior alveolar nerve block. This section describes the direct and the indirect techniques, as for right-sided blocks by right-handed practitioners and for the "average" dentate adult. As mentioned, however, variations among patients must be expected.

Direct Technique. When performing the direct inferior alveolar nerve block technique in adults, a long needle (35 mm) no smaller than 27 gauge must be used. A long needle is recommended because penetration to 25 mm may be needed, and a needle should not be inserted up to the hub because fracture at that point makes retrieval difficult. Correct

BOX 13-7

Hard Tissue Landmarks: Direct Inferior Alveolar Nerve Block

> Mandibular foramen and lingula
> Anterior posterior borders of mandibular ramus
> Mandibular bicuspid teeth of contralateral side

"landmarking" is essential (Box 13-7 and Fig. 13-21), and the technique follows sequentially (Box 13-8 and Figs. 13-22 to 13-24).

This injection will anesthetize the inferior alveolar nerve and may block the lingual nerve. If anesthesia of the lingual nerve is required, however, the needle is withdrawn halfway and aspiration repeated. If aspiration is negative, the solution remaining in the cartridge is injected at this point, and the needle is then withdrawn.

If bone is contacted after only a few millimeters of penetration, the block will probably fail because the needle will have contacted the internal oblique ridge of the ramus. To overcome this problem, the injection can be reattempted. This involves a second mucosal puncture, however, and similar early contact may recur. The best solution is to attempt the indirect technique, but without removing the needle from the tissues.

Indirect Technique. The indirect inferior alveolar nerve block technique may be employed at the outset or can be used as a salvage maneuver if the direct approach fails. The indirect technique overcomes the problem of contacting the internal oblique ridge of the mandible, but more needle movement is required during correct positioning. Patient orientation, mouth opening, operator's left-hand position, and equipment are the same as for the direct technique. The point of mucosal penetration is also the same, midway between ramus and pterygomandibular raphe at the midpoint of the dentist's thumbnail. The syringe is introduced intraorally along the occlusal plane of the bicuspid and molar teeth of the side to be injected. After mucosal penetration the needle is advanced 10 mm into the tissues. The syringe is then swung across to lie over the bicuspids of the opposite side, and the method then progresses exactly as described for the direct technique.

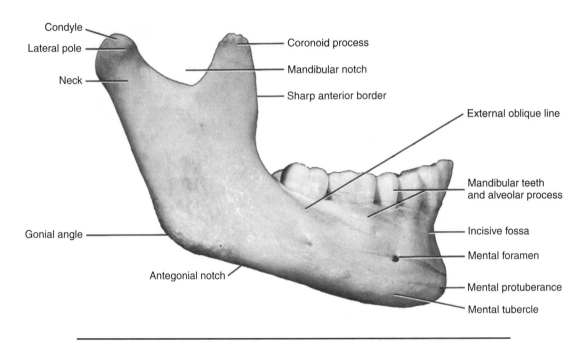

Fig. 13-21 Hard tissue anatomy of mandible. (From Liebgott B: *The anatomical basis of dentistry*, ed 2, St Louis, 2001, Mosby.)

BOX 13-8

Technique: Direct Inferior Alveolar Nerve Block

1. Rest the thumb in a retromolar fossa, palpating the coronoid notch on anterior border of ramus (Fig. 13-22).
2. Rest the first finger on posterior border of ramus at same height as the thumb.
3. Ask the patient to open the mouth widely.
4. Insert the syringe into the oral cavity across the mandibular bicuspids of opposite side parallel to mandibular occlusal plane.
5. Locate the point of penetration by visualizing a V shape composed of the anterior border of ramus of the mandible on the lateral aspect and the pterygomandibular raphe medially. The ramus is palpable and the raphe visible (Fig. 13-23).
6. Penetrate the imaginary V midway between a level halfway up the thumbnail.
7. Advance the needle through tissues until bony contact is made, usually at a depth of 20 to 30 mm (Fig. 13-24).
8. Once the bone is reached, withdraw the needle slightly (supraperiosteal), and aspirate.
9. If aspiration is negative, inject approximately 1.5 ml of solution at the site.

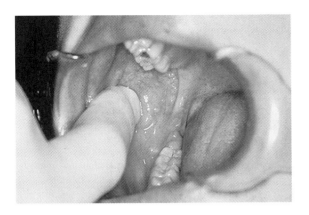

Fig. 13-22 Palpation external oblique ridge (coronoid notch).

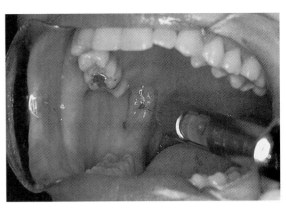

Fig. 13-24 Insertion depth of conventional interior alveolar block.

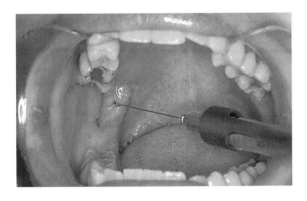

Fig. 13-23 Needle insertion between internal oblique ridge and pterygomandibular raphe.

Common technical problems may result in complications (Box 13-9).

Incisive and Mental Nerve Blocks

The *mental nerve* supplies sensation to the mucosa and skin of the lower lip and the periodontal and gingival tissues from the first lower bicuspid anteriorly on one side of the lower jaw. The *incisive nerve* innervates the pulps of the lower first bicuspid, cuspid and incisor teeth, and their supporting bone.

The incisive nerve block, often inappropriately termed the "mental" block, may be used as an alternative to the inferior alveolar nerve block when treat-

ing the lower bicuspid in some patients. This injection will also anesthetize the soft tissues supplied by the mental nerve. The method relies on deposition of anesthetic solution in the region of the mental foramen, which is located on the buccal side of the body of the mandible (Box 13-10). The exact position of this foramen varies but is usually located between and just below the apices of the premolars. In adults the foramen faces posteriorly; in children it opens anteriorly.

Whereas subjective signs of anesthesia of the mental distribution are a good indication of incisive nerve blockage after inferior alveolar nerve block, such signs are not reliable predictors of incisive anesthesia after an incisive or mental nerve block injection. Although the mental branch is anesthetized readily because it lies in soft tissue close to the injection site, this gives no indication of how much solution has entered the mental foramen and affected the incisive branch.

This injection will not anesthetize the lingual periodontal tissues and must therefore be supplemented with an infiltration of 0.2 to 0.5 ml of solution in the lingually reflected mucosa when appropriate.

Buccal Nerve Block

The long buccal nerve can be anesthetized with an infiltration technique at the anterior ramus or more often in the mucobuccal fold just distal to the posterior mandibular tooth or teeth being treated (Fig. 13-25).

BOX 13-9

Technical Problems: Indirect Inferior Alveolar Nerve Block

Intravascular Injection
More than 10% of aspiration maneuvers actually aspirate blood; it is imperative to aspirate.

Failure to Contact Bone
Passing through mandibular notch between coronoid and condylar processes can miss bone. Avoid this by ensuring syringe is parallel to mandibular occlusal plane.

Neurologic Damage
Nerve trunks (inferior alveolar or lingual). Injury can be caused by physical damage from needle, physical disruption of nerve from solution, and toxic effects of local anesthetic agent. Needle occasionally contacts inferior alveolar or lingual nerve as it is positioned during injection. Patient will be aware of "electric shock" sensation traveling to chin or tip of tongue. Withdraw needle a few millimeters to avoid temporary damage leading to prolonged anesthesia or paresthesia.
Long-lasting anesthesia unrelated to physical damage. This occurs rarely and may be caused by chemical injury from the agent or contaminants.

Hemifacial paralysis. Facial nerve travels within parotid sheath. Injection into substance of parotid gland can lead to conduction blockage in motor facial nerve, causing hemifacial paralysis. Although usually short-lived, this paralysis is embarrassing for dentist and inconvenient or even hazardous for patient. Patient temporarily loses ability to close eyelids and therefore must be provided with protection for affected eye until normal function returns. Also, local anesthesia will not be successful if solution is deposited in parotid gland. To avoid this complication, ensure that bony contact has been established before injection.

Trismus
During administration of block, needle passes through muscle tissue. The buccinator is traversed, and medial pterygoid may be penetrated. If a blood vessel is perforated within substance of medial pterygoid muscle, subsequent bleeding into muscle will produce spasm, resulting in trismus. Injection of local anesthetic solution directly into muscle may also produce trismus. The situation is self-limiting, although it may take 2 to 3 weeks to resolve. If a large hematoma is obvious, antibiotics should be prescribed to prevent secondary infection.

BOX 13-10

Technique: Incisive Nerve Block

1. Ask the patient to half-open the mouth, or they can keep it closed during injection.
2. Preferably, use a long or short needle of 27 or 30 gauge.
3. Direct the needle from behind the second bicuspid apex.
4. Make bony contact, and withdraw the needle slightly.
5. After aspiration, slowly inject 1.5 ml of solution.
6. Do not introduce the needle into mental foramen, since physical damage to the nerve can occur.

Akinosi Closed-Mouth Mandibular Nerve Block

In 1960, Vazirani postulated that local anesthetic, if deposited in the pterygomandibular space, would not require the mouth to be open. Seventeen years later, Akinosi[17] argued the concept of more formal landmarks using primarily maxillary soft tissue anatomy to administer the mandibular

block. This technique has advantages and disadvantages (Box 13-11). This approach to mandibular anesthesia is horizontally parallel to the conventional inferior alveolar block (Fig. 13-26).

The landmarks include the junction of the attached and unattached gingiva on the maxillary mucobuccal fold. These landmarks are reported to be

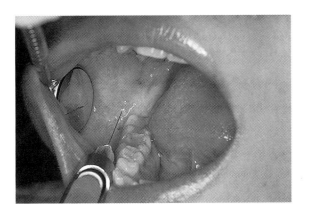

Fig. 13-25 Long buccal nerve block and infiltration.

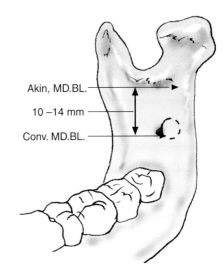

Fig. 13-26 Akinosi block. Height of inferior alveolar nerve block.

BOX 13-11

Considerations: Akinosi Closed-Mouth Mandibular Nerve Block

Advantages	Disadvantages
Macroglossia	Difficult to see mouth if closed
Gag reflex	Difficult to gauge depth
Less trismus	No bony target
Less threatening, greater patient acceptance	Flaring ramus
Decreased incidence of positive aspiration	Zygomatic ridge, as it forms over upper first permanent
Decreased risk of paresthesia	molar; syringe must almost touch maxillary gingiva to
	advance laterally toward ramus

---

about 10 to 14 mm above the conventional inferior alveolar block.[17] The objective is to bypass the internal oblique ridge of the mandible and advance the needle into the lateral plane into the pterygomandibular triangle (Fig. 13-27).

The needle is oriented toward the internal oblique ridge. As the ramus starts to flare superiorly, the needle will pass with less obstruction than the internal oblique ridge would offer in performing the conventional nerve block. This is important because the palpation finger or thumb covering the temporalis tendon will allow the operator to bypass the internal oblique ridge or direct the needle laterally. The initial puncture point is approximately

at the root apices of the maxillary teeth. The bony corridor through which the needle must pass may be different geometrically (Fig. 13-28). Often the syringe barrel will rest on the maxillary soft tissue. Assuming cooperation from the patient, an ipsilateral excursion would increase the space between the maxillary tuberosity and the internal oblique ridge, rendering advancement of the needle more laterally (Fig. 13-29). The bevel of the needle should face the midsagittal plane as opposed to the ramus of the mandible.

The final needle depth in the adult will be approximately 25 to 30 ml. Occasionally, in the heavy-set patient, the buccal fat pad may attempt to surround

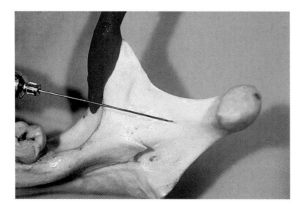

Fig. 13-27 Placement of Akinosi needle.

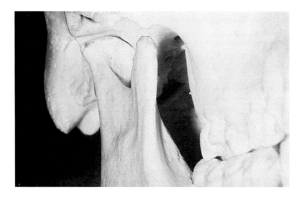

Fig. 13-28 Akinosi block. Bony corridor between internal oblique ridge and maxillary tuberosity.

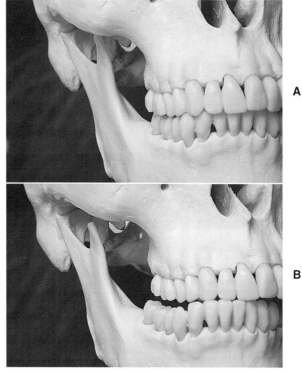

Fig. 13-29 Akinosi block. **A,** Closed in centric. **B,** Right lateral excursion.

the needle hub. This might require the operator physically to displace the buccal fat pad posteriorly to assess the depth of insertion (Figs. 13-30 to 13-32).

This technique carries minimal risk of paresthesia because the lingual and inferior alveolar nerves are not as taut as they are with the mouth wide open and are not bound closely to any tissue, such as the ramus or the medial pterygoid muscle. Needle placement is superior to the parotid gland, and with the mouth closed, trismus of the medial pterygoid muscle is unlikely.

Gow-Gates Mandibular Nerve Block

In the 1960s, Australian Gow-Gates, with the aid of anatomist Watson, assessed the structure of V3 and postulated that the intraoral approach using extraoral landmarks would render mandibular anesthesia more successful. Using the corner of the mouth and tragal notch of the ear as a two-dimensional alignment, they assumed that deposition of solution on the anterior condylar neck would result in an increased success rate for anesthesia.[18] This assumption was based on the favorable histology in this area and the ability to anesthetize any potential accessory nerves and their plexi, which may be emitted from V3 shortly after the nerve pierces the lateral pterygoid muscle. This block has varied advantages and disadvantages (Box 13-12).

The average height of the adult coronoid notch above the occlusal plane (19 mm) is probably inadequate to include the variations in location of the mandibular foramen.[18] The height using extraoral landmarks encompasses most of the anatomic hard tissue variations, however, with minor exception; rarely, two mandibular foramina may occur.[5]

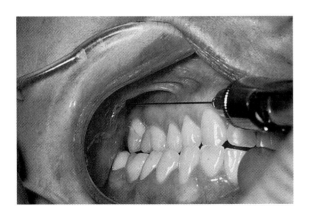

Fig. 13-30 Akinosi block. Maxillary mucogingival junction paralleled.

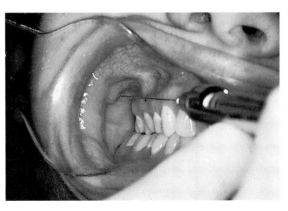

Fig. 13-31 Akinosi block. Needle advancing by passing internal oblique ridge.

Fig. 13-32 Akinosi block. Approaching depth of needle insertion.

BOX 13-12

Considerations: Gow-Gates Mandibular Nerve Block

Advantages
Decreased vascularity
Lower incidence of nerve damage
Loose fatty and connective tissue at injection site
Must infiltrate V3 for hemostatic purposes
Good visibility for procedure
Long-acting anesthesia produced

Disadvantages
Wide-open mouth requires patient cooperation or mouth rest
Use of extraoral landmarks with mouth wide open
Condylar neck closer to nerve when mouth wide open for 2 minutes
Average height of adult coronoid notch not adequate to cover all variations in mandibular foramen

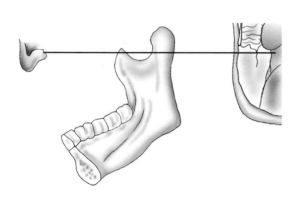

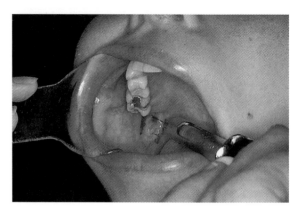

Fig. 13-33 Two-dimensional line from corner of mouth to tragal notch passes through condylar neck.

Fig. 13-34 Gow-Gates mandibular block. Needle contacting condylar neck.

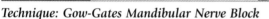

BOX 13-13 ⊕

Technique: Gow-Gates Mandibular Nerve Block

1. Approach target area anteriorly with the mouth wide open.
2. Depth for block in adults is approximately 25 to 27 mm.
3. "Landmarking" teeth is relatively unimportant; the injection point approximates the cusps of the maxillary second molar.
4. Using a line from the tragal notch to the corner of the mouth, guide the needle toward the condylar neck (Fig. 13-33).
5. With the patient's head tilted back and the mouth opened wide, palpate the internal oblique ridge with either finger or thumb.
6. Angulation of the injection will parallel the junction of the two external landmarks.
7. Puncture point will be between the pterygomandibular raphe and internal oblique ridge, approaching the anterior condylar neck from the contralateral premolars (Fig. 13-34).
8. Deposit the entire cartridge of solution.
9. Onset may be slower but is profound for 2 to 3 hours.

Few vessels or nerve branches occur at this level of the pterygomandibular triangle, which minimizes risk for paresthesia, intravascular injection, or absorption of the local anesthesia and vasoconstrictor.[19] If the injection is performed too superiorly to the anterior condylar neck, the condylar capsule may be injured, resulting in pain and spasm. The patient's mouth should remain open for 20 seconds to 2 minutes after injection to allow the solution to diffuse anteriorly into anterior and medial planes[18] (Box 13-13 and Figs. 13-33 and 13-34).

Supplemental Injection Techniques

Supplemental injection techniques, or *site-specific injections,* are indicated for several situations and special circumstances. These techniques can either be used as a sole delivery system for pain control or certain types of dental treatment or as a helpful adjunct when standard supraperiosteal or block anesthesia is contraindicated or to provide adequate pain control. The use of these techniques is most commonly endorsed in the mandible, where the cortical plate is denser and difficulty obtaining block anesthesia well documented. However, their use in maxillary arch is also feasible.

Intrapulpal Anesthesia

Intrapulpal technique is particularly useful during endodontic procedures and involves injecting solution through a small opening into the pulp chamber, allowing pressure to build up within the sensitive endodontic system. Although potentially painful for a brief time, anesthesia is immediate and is usually adequate for successful pulpectomy (Boxes 13-14 and 13-15).

Complications do not usually occur, since the object is to perform the endodontic procedure successfully.

BOX 13-14

Considerations: Intrapulpal Anesthesia

Advantages
Immediate onset
Low volume

Disadvantages
Brief pain
Difficult to assess the canals
Lack of pressure may result in poor anesthesia

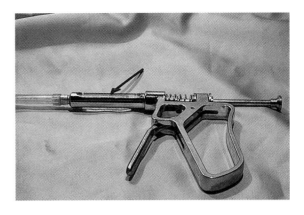

Fig. 13-35 Ligmaject.

BOX 13-15 SUMMARY

Intrapulpal Anesthesia

Narrow-gauge needle is used, such as 30 gauge.
Solution is introduced directly into vital tissue.
Solution must be deposited under pressure in a volume of 0.1 to 0.3 ml, preferably with a bent needle.
Duration and onset are short but adequate to perform pulpal extirpation.

Periodontal Ligament Injection

For procedures other than endodontics, site-specific anesthesia can be obtained by injecting local anesthetic solution in the periodontal ligament (PDL).[20] Suggestions for this technique can be found in local anesthetic textbooks dating from 1912. Advantages and disadvantages must be considered (Box 13-16).

Most recommend 27- or 30-gauge short needles for the PDL technique. Injection may be done with the conventional local anesthetic syringe, although the cartridge may be fractured. The manufactured syringes for this technique usually include circumferential shielding to protect against this potential fracture (Figs. 13-35 and 13-36). Duration of anesthesia varies from 5 to 55 minutes (Box 13-17).

Complications include discomfort, especially if too much anesthetic solution is injected too rapidly. Pain may be decreased with use of topical anesthetic and by keeping the needle close to the tooth structure. It is usually easier to advance the needle deeper into the PDL for periodontally involved patients. Postinjection pain usually involves excessive volume of solution, combined with too high a concentration of vasoconstrictor, which

BOX 13-16

Considerations: Periodontal Ligament Injection

Advantages
Decreased pain and anxiety
Limited area of diffusion of local anesthetic solution
Successful supplement to ineffective block or infiltration anesthesia
Reduced quantity of solution
Lowered incidence of hematoma or trismus
Limited facial and lip anesthesia in children

Disadvantages
Increased postanesthetic sensitivity due to lowered pulpal blood flow
High pressure and effects on periodontium
Difficulty in needle placement
Threatening nature of armamentarium
Special and expensive equipment
Inability to obtain back pressure, with leakage of anesthetic solution into patient's mouth

causes tissue necrosis and compromises the pulpal blood supply.[21]

Intraosseous Anesthesia

Intraosseous injection of local anesthetic has been described since the beginning of the twentieth century, initially using a small round bur to drill a hole through cortical bone, entering the cancellous bone. Once this opening has been made, a needle

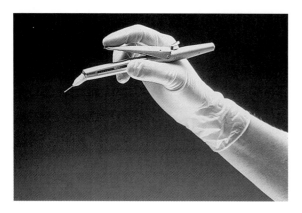

Fig. 13-36 Citoject Athena.

 BOX 13-17 SUMMARY

Periodontal Ligament Injection

> Resistance must be felt during administration.
> Blanching will normally be present.
> Onset of anesthesia is extremely rapid.
> Local anesthetic solution will penetrate the cribriform plate under pressure.
> Area of anesthesia is usually restricted to one tooth surrounding the injection site.
> Advancement of needle is enhanced by orienting bevel of needle toward tooth.
> Molars require injection of both mesial and distal interligamental spaces.
> Injection may be done from buccal or lingual aspect of tooth.

BOX 13-18

Considerations: Intraosseous Anesthesia

> **Advantages**
> Site-specific anesthesia, single or regional teeth without doing block anesthesia
> Atraumatic
> No significant postoperative complications
> Relatively immediate onset
> Very little discomfort on administration, assuming adequate coverage with preoperative anesthesia (minimal attached gingival infiltration or topical anesthetic application)
>
> **Disadvantages**
> Propietary equipment required
> Difficulty in finding predrilled hole
> Cardiovascular implications, especially when vasoconstrictor is used
> May produce a bitter taste of either drug or blood from procedure

of appropriate and lesser diameter is inserted and the local anesthetic solution administered. PDL and intraseptal injections are simply modifications of this intraosseous technique. Recently, a number of new devices have been introduced that enable the dentist to control and simplify the administration of intraosseous anesthesia, with due consideration of advantages and disadvantages (Box 13-18).

The Stabident system (Fairfax Dental) uses a solid perforator in a standard, slow-speed contra-angle handpiece designed to penetrate the cortical plate, followed by an ultrashort, 27-gauge needle through which a small volume of local anesthesia solution is delivered from a standard syringe.[22] This is a two-step procedure, after the site is preanesthetized.

The success of intraosseous technique depends on successful entrance through cortical plate into the cancellous bone (Box 13-19 and Fig. 13-37). Onset occurs within a few seconds,[21] and duration is about 15 to 30 minutes.

Complications include needle breakage, especially in the posterior mandibular area, requiring a bent-needle technique; breakage of the perforator (rarely); and palpitations or tachycardia when vasopressor solutions are used.

Various techniques involve the introduction of a needle into the dental papilla into the intraseptal bone underlying the gingival crest. This technique is used when soft tissue hemostasis is desired and may be useful as an entrance point into the cancellous bone to deliver a variation of intraosseous injection. Although this can be performed with a standard local anesthetic needle, often the resistance to this technique requires a reinforced hubbed needle (Hypoject, Dentsply). Although local anesthetic solution may be introduced into cancellous bone in this format, the needle tip is still some distance from the peripheral anatomy.

Taking intraosseous systems one step further, Weathers introduced the *X-tip* in 1999, for *total, in-*

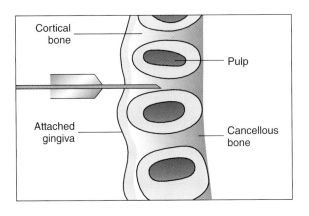

Fig. 13-37 Intraosseous anesthesia. Patient positioning.

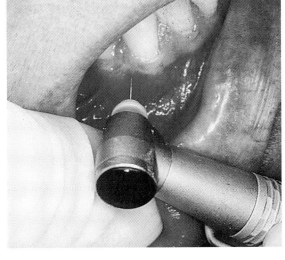

Fig. 13-38 Intraosseous anesthesia. Perforating cortical plate through gingiva and periosteum.

▌ BOX 13-19 ▌ SUMMARY

Technique: Intraosseous Anesthesia

1. Entrance point is 2 to 3 mm apical to gingival margins of teeth.
2. Distal rather than medial site is suggested.
3. Perforation must be on attached gingiva; unattached gingiva will be traumatized by rotation of the perforator.
4. Hole will not be in same location as soft tissue displacement.
5. Topical anesthesia must be applied and injection site infiltrated.
6. Perforation is relatively horizontal in the anterior dentition (Fig. 13-38).
7. An angle of up to 45 degrees from alveolar crest may be necessary in the molar region.
8. Locate the perforation with a 27-gauge, ultrashort needle (Fig. 13-39).
9. Deposit standard local anesthetic solution with a standard syringe.
10. Inject 20% to 50% of the local anesthetic dosage normally used for infiltration anesthesia.
11. Use of vasopressors should be minimized.

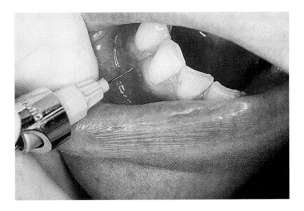

Fig. 13-39 Intraosseous anesthesia. Finding perforation and introducing 27-gauge needle.

---

stant, profound anesthesia (Box 13-20). The attached gingiva must be initially anesthetized by either local infiltration in the buccal fold or direct perforation of the attached gingiva at the site. The *guide sleeve* is the key to this approach. Once the attached gingiva and cortical plate (of bone) is perforated with the contra-angle X-tip system, the guide sleeve will remain in place. The ultrashort 27-gauge needle is introduced into the lumen (Fig. 13-40). Local anesthetic is injected in the volume of 0.04 to 1.0 ml of epinephrine solution of 1:200,000 to 1:100,000 concentration. Postoperative sequelae appear to be rare.

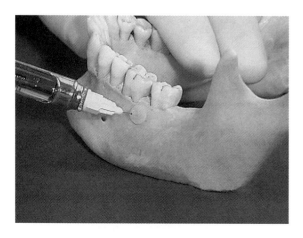

Fig. 13-40 Posterior X-tip technique.

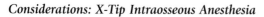

B°X 13-20 ⓐ

Considerations: X-Tip Intraosseous Anesthesia

Advantages
Perforation of cortical plate, easy access
Reentry of site
Postoperative sequelae rare
"Jump-start" longer procedures, added to block
  anesthesia

Disadvantages
Radiographs still required
Longer needle perforator length than Stabident
Difficult to access mandibular molars
Local anesthesia may leak around perforator sleeve,
  requiring "endo" rubber stopper introduced to
  apparatus

The X-tip intraosseous system may be a significant advance for local anesthesia, especially when block anesthesia proves inadequate. Occasionally the apparatus may seem cumbersome or intimidating, but the results seem predictable and reliable.

Computer-Controlled Anesthesia

The *Wand* (Milestone Scientific) represents the first computer-controlled delivery system for dentistry. This device accurately controls both flow rate and pressure,

producing a more comfortable injection experience, as demonstrated in a clinical study performed in the dense gingival tissues of the palate.[23] Dispensing of solution is activated using a foot-controlled rheostat. The system accommodates a dental anesthetic cartridge that is linked by microtubing to a disposable, lightweight, penlike handle with a standard medical Luer-Lok needle attached (Figs. 13-41 and 13-42). The penlike grasp of the handpiece allows the operator to achieve refined tactile control of the needle. Rotation of the handpiece during needle insertion reduces needle deflection for greater accuracy.[24]

The Wand system can be safely used for site-specific anesthesia, including PDL pressure injections.[25] A newly described, *anterior middle superior alveolar* (AMSA) *block* can be produced with a computer-controlled injection of 0.6 to 1.8 ml of solution to the palatal apices of the first and second premolars.[26] This technique relies on the fact that the unpredictable plexi of the anterior and middle superior nerves lie apical and medial to these teeth. A second newly defined injection, *palatal-approach anterior superior alveolar* (P-ASA) *block* has been reported using this device.[27] This technique can produce bilateral anesthesia of the maxillary anterior teeth from a single palatal injection within the nasopalatine canal. Palatal injections can be predictably performed with minimal discomfort when using computer-controlled technology.

The *Comfort Control Syringe* (Dentsply) was introduced to the dental profession in February 2001, invented by Smith from London, Ontario, Canada. It offers a choice of five preprogrammed rates when delivering local anesthetic solution. The programmed rates have been correlated to the standard dental injections (Figs. 13-43 and 13-44). This system uses a hand-activated drive unit that accepts standard dental cartridges and needles. Slightly less expensive than the Wand, the Comfort Control Syringe system has merit and may reinforce the growing trend toward computer-assisted local anesthetic administration.

High-Pressure Needleless Injection

Also frequently called a *jet injection technique,* high-pressure needleless injection has achieved limited popularity despite being available for more than 35 years. Local anesthetic droplets expelled under very high pressure through minute holes in the applicator device permits passage of the solution through the mucosa without the use of a needle. It is mainly

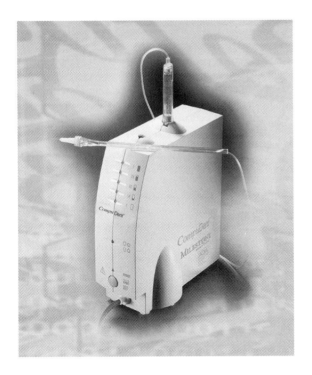

Fig. 13-41 CompuDent computer-controlled local anesthetic delivery system and the Wand handpiece. (Courtesy Milestone Scientific, Livingstone, NJ.)

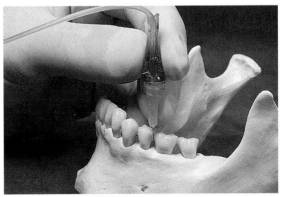

Fig. 13-42 Wand periodontal ligament modified delivery system. (Courtesy Milestone Scientific, Livingstone, NJ.)

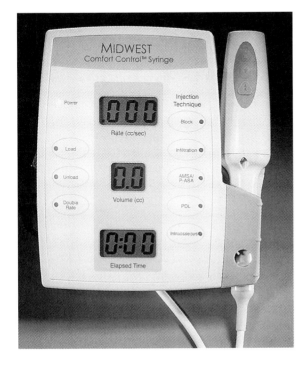

Fig. 13-43 Comfort Control Syringe. (Courtesy Dentsply, Midwest.)

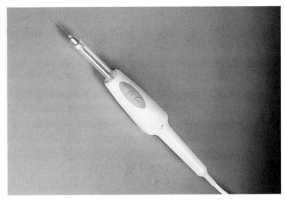

Fig. 13-44 Comfort Control Syringe handpiece, with slow/fast speed and aspiration buttons. (Courtesy Dentsply, Midwest.)

still used for palatal injections. Rendering these injections almost painless, for both the child and the adult, the explosive noise once heard has now been controlled in more recent models (Madajet, MADA Equipment).

References

1. Brownbill JW, Walker PO, Bourcy BD, Keenan KM: Comparison of inferior dental nerve block injections in child patients using 30-gauge and 25-gauge short needles, *Anesth Prog* 34:215-219, 1987.
2. Aldous JA: Needle deflection: a factor in the administration of local anesthetics, *J Am Dent Assoc* 77:602-604, 1968.
3. Septodont: Product monograph for Septocaine.
4. Meechan JG, McCabe JF, Carrick TE: Plastic dental local anesthetic cartridges: a laboratory investigation, *Br Dent J* 169:54-56, 1990.
5. Jastak JT, Yagiela JA, Donaldson D: *Local anesthesia of the oral cavity*, Philadelphia, 1995, Saunders.
6. Oikarinen VJ, Ylipaavalnpemi P, Evers H: Pain and temperature sensations related to local analgesia, *Int J Oral Surg* 4:151-156, 1975.
7. Meechan JG: A comparison of three different automatic aspirating dental cartridge syringes, *J Dent* 16:40-43, 1988.
8. Meechan JG, Blair GS: Clinical experience in oral surgery with two different automatic aspirating syringes, *Int J Oral Maxillofac Surg* 18:87-89, 1989.
9. Malamed SF: *Handbook of local anesthesia*, ed 4, St Louis, 1997, Mosby.
10. Mendel N, Puterbaugh PG: *Conduction, infiltration and general anesthesia in dentistry*, ed 4, New York, 1983, Dental Items of Interest Publishing.
11. Poore TE, Carney FMT: Maxillary nerve block: a useful technique, *J Oral Surg* 31:749-755, 1973.
12. Hawkins JM, Isen DA: Maxillary nerve block . . . pterygopalatine canal approach, *Oral Health* 89(2), 1999.
13. Hawkins JM, Isen DA: Maxillary nerve block . . . pterygopalatine canal approach, *J Calif Dent Assoc* 26:658-664, 1998.
14. Westmoreland EE, Blanton PL: An analysis of the variations in position of the greater palatine foramen in the adult human skull, *Anat Rec* 204:383-388, 1982.
15. Malamed SF, Trieger N: Intraoral maxillary nerve block: an anatomical and clinical study, *Anesth Prog* 30:44-48, 1983.
16. Sved AM, Wong JD, Dunker P: Complications associated with maxillary nerve block via greater palatine canal, *Aust Dent J* 37:340-345, 1992.
17. Akinosi JO: A new approach to the mandibular nerve block, *Br J Oral Surg* 15:83-87, 1977.
18. Gow-Gates GA: Mandibular conduction anesthesia: a new technique using extraoral landmarks, *Oral Surg* 36:321-328, 1973.
19. Gow-Gates GA, Watson JE: The Gow-Gates mandibular block: further understanding, *Anesth Prog* 24:183-189, 1977.
20. Walton RE, Abbott BJ: Periodontal ligament injection: a clinical evaluation, *Oral Health* 7(1):80-84, 1984.
21. Morse DR: *Clinical endontology*, Springfield, Ill, 1974, Thomas.
22. Dillon F: Stabident, London, 1991, Video Insight (video).
23. Hochman MN, Chiarello D, Hochman C, et al: Computerized local anesthesia vs traditional syringe technique: subjective pain response, *NY State Dent J* 63(7):24-29, 1997.
24. Hochman MN, Friedman MJ: In vitro study of needle deflection: a linear insertion technique vs a bidirectional rotation insertion technique, *Quintessence Int* 30:31-39, 2000.
25. Froum SJ, Tarnow DT, Caiazzo A, Hochman MN: Histologic response to intraligament injections using a computerized local anesthetic delivery system: a pilot study in mini-swine, *J Periodont* 71:1453-1459, 2000.
26. Friedman MJ, Hochman MN: The AMSA injection: a new concept for local anesthesia of maxillary teeth using a computer-controlled injection system, *Quintessence Int* 28(5):287-303, 1998.
27. Friedman MJ, Hochman MN: P-ASA block injection: a new palatal technique to anesthetize maxillary anterior teeth, *J Esthetic Dent* 11(2):63-71, 1999.

CHAPTER 14

Nitrous Oxide Sedation

RAYMOND S. GARRISON
STEPHEN R. HOLLIDAY
DAVID P. KRETZSCHMAR

CHAPTER OUTLINE

Nitrous oxide is used in dentistry to allay apprehension and anxiety regarding injections of local anesthetics and treatment in general (Box 14-1). When used properly, nitrous oxide provides sedation and mild analgesia with minimal side effects. In fact, many consider nitrous oxide an inert, benign gas that has little if any influence on vital physiologic functions. This observation is not entirely flawed, since respiratory and cardiovascular functions are minimally influenced, especially when compared with the changes produced by more potent agents. However, this analysis ignores the need to compare agents at equipotent doses and fails to address considerations when nitrous oxide is often combined with other anesthetics, sedatives, or opioids.

Nitrous oxide is an inorganic inhalation agent that is colorless, odorless to sweet smelling, and non-irritating to the tissues. It is nonflammable but will support combustion. Nitrous oxide has low potency but impressive safety and is included in general anesthetic regimens to reduce the amounts of other, more costly and less benign agents. Nitrous oxide alone is incapable of producing general anesthesia reliably, but it is excellent for providing conscious sedation. In emergency departments, ambulatory surgery centers, and dental clinics, nitrous oxide and oxygen administration is a sedation technique with a distinctive place in the spectrum of pain and anxiety control.

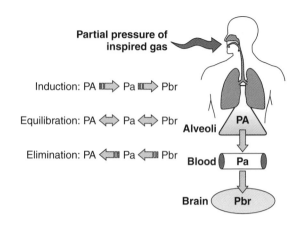

Fig. 14-1 Entry of anesthetic gas into brain depends on pressure gradients attributed to partial pressures of the gas in the alveoli (*PA*), arterial blood (*Pa*), and brain tissues (*Pbr*). Low solubility, reflected as blood:gas coefficient, allows partial pressures to equilibrate rapidly.

BOX 14-1   SUMMARY

Nitrous Oxide

Nitrous oxide is a weak general anesthetic often used with other general anesthetics.

At concentrations of 20% to 50%, nitrous oxide produces sedation and mild analgesia.

Nitrous oxide reliably relieves fear and apprehension in dental patients.

When used alone at sedative concentrations, nitrous oxide has minimal side effects that are readily reversible.

Pharmacokinetics

Uptake, Distribution, and Elimination

The uptake and distribution of an anesthetic gas to brain tissue depends on partial pressure gradients within alveoli, arterial blood, and the brain (Fig. 14-1). After inspiration of an anesthetic gas, an alveolar concentration is achieved, which equilibrates with arterial blood and eventually with brain tissue. The principal factor that determines the speed at which this equilibration occurs is the solubility of the particular gas, expressed as the blood:gas partition coefficient. The lower the solubility, the faster the gas achieves a concentration in blood great enough to drive the gas through the blood-brain barrier into brain tissue. For this reason, nitrous oxide is second only to desflurane in speed of onset (Table 14-1).[1]

Nitrous oxide is transported in blood as free gas (Box 14-2). It does not combine with hemoglobin and does not undergo biotransformation. Elimination is by expiration in a manner that is precisely the reverse of uptake and distribution; the low solubility of nitrous oxide allows rapid elimination.

Transfer to Gas-Filled Spaces

The blood:gas coefficient of nitrous oxide is 0.47, which is approximately 34 times greater than that of nitrogen (0.014). When switching a patient's inspired gas mixture from air containing approximately 78% nitrogen to an anesthetic mixture containing 70% ni-

TABLE 14-1

Comparison of Inhalation Anesthetics

Anesthetic Agent	Blood:Gas Coefficient	Minimum Alveolar Concentration (%)
Nitrous oxide	0.47	104
Desflurane	0.42	6
Isoflurane	1.46	1.15
Enflurane	1.91	1.7
Halothane	2.54	0.77

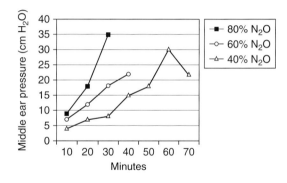

Fig. 14-2 Nitrous oxide (N_2O) enters gas-filled spaces, such as the middle ear and sinuses, much faster than nitrogen can exit. Pressure within the middle ear increases over time according to the concentration administered. Data derived from a healthy volunteer with normal patency of eustachian tube. Clearly, pressure would increase more dramatically with sinus or eustachian blockage. (Modified from Thomsen KA, Terkildsen K, Arnfred I: *Arch Otolaryngol* 82:609, 1965.)

BOX 14-2 SUMMARY

Pharmacokinetics of Nitrous Oxide

Nitrous oxide has a low blood:gas coefficient (solubility), which accounts for rapid onset and elimination.

Nitrous oxide is not metabolized and does not combine with hemoglobin. It is eliminated by expiration.

Nitrous oxide increases pressure in closed gas-filled spaces such as the middle ear.

At concentrations delivered by dental machines, nitrous oxide is unlikely to cause diffusion hypoxia. However, administering 100% oxygen at the conclusion of a procedure is good practice for environmental reasons.

---

trous oxide, the partial pressures of the gases are nearly equal, and the nitrous oxide will enter gas-filled spaces 34 times faster than nitrogen can exit the space. As a result, the volume or pressure within such a space will increase (Fig. 14-2). Although lower concentrations (30% to 50%) of nitrous oxide are used for sedation, and the partial pressure of nitrogen is higher, greater solubility still allows nitrous oxide to enter gas-filled spaces rapidly. Gas volume and pressure can become dangerously high within an obstructed bowel or within the middle ear if patency of the eustachian tube is compromised by inflammation. Rupture of the tympanic membrane is possible during administration of nitrous oxide, and negative pressure may develop after discontinuation, leading to serous otitis media and possibly contributing to postoperative nausea and vomiting.[2,3] Although other anesthetic gases are even more soluble, they are administered in such low concentrations that their partial pressures do not lead to the preferential transfer observed with nitrous oxide.

Diffusion Hypoxia

When inhalation of high concentrations of nitrous oxide is discontinued, the high partial pressure in the blood rapidly transfers the nitrous oxide to the alveoli. The transfer of nitrous oxide dilutes the partial pressure of oxygen in the alveoli and may lead to hypoxemia. For this reason, it is conventional practice to provide the patient with 100% oxygen during the first few minutes after discontinuation of nitrous oxide. However, this concern is more academic than factual. Hypoxemia is significant for only a few minutes and has been documented only when high concentrations (>70%) of nitrous oxide have been delivered by full mask or endotracheal tube. These conditions cannot be met using the conventional dental nitrous oxide machines with nasal masks, and any tendency for diffusion hypoxia is trivial.[4,5] Nevertheless, providing 100% oxygen toward the completion of a dental appointment has other benefits. It allows discontinuation while providing a waning placebo influence, and it allows expired nitrous oxide to enter the scavenging apparatus of the machine.

Pharmacodynamics

Minimum Alveolar Concentration

The dose or concentration at which anesthetic gases produce their effects is expressed as *minimum alveolar concentration* (MAC) (Box 14-3). One MAC is defined as the concentration of gas within the alveoli that will render 50% of patients unresponsive to a surgical stimulus. It is comparable to the effective dose for 50% of patients (ED_{50}) used for other drugs administered by weight (e.g., milligrams). Table 14-1 shows that nitrous oxide is the least potent of all anesthetic gases, and it cannot be used to achieve anesthesia reliably by itself. (The MAC of 104% was extrapolated for normal atmospheric pressure from anesthesia performed on experienced divers in a hyperbaric chamber.) Nevertheless, anesthetic gases demonstrate summation when mixed, and MAC can be achieved by combining one gas with another. For example, nitrous oxide 52% (0.5 MAC) and desflurane 3% (0.5 MAC) will achieve 1 MAC and provide anesthesia for half the population. This regimen would allow the inclusion of 45% oxygen in the mixture.

Although 50% of patients require greater than 1 MAC for surgical anesthesia, some patients are anesthetized at concentrations lower than 1 MAC. Furthermore, the MAC of a particular anesthetic gas is often lower in elderly patients and medically compromised patients. Also, MAC is lowered by the concomitant administration of other central nervous system (CNS) depressants, such as opioids and sedatives. For example, a 20-kg pediatric patient premedicated with a sedative and opioid may only require 60% to 70% nitrous oxide to achieve MAC.

The concentration of nitrous oxide leaving the typical dental unit, and therefore its partial pressure, is not identical to that inspired or that reaching the alveoli. Equipment leakage (e.g., poorly fitted nasal masks), dead space, mouth breathing, and the patient's ventilatory status are among the factors that account for the discrepancy. Although machine settings may indicate up to 70% nitrous oxide, the actual concentration delivered to the alveoli is unlikely to exceed 30% to 50% (Fig. 14-3).[6] In other words, MACs greater than 0.3 to 0.5 probably cannot be achieved using typical dental nitrous oxide units. For this reason, one must use caution when extrapolating data derived from medical studies in which nitrous

---

▍ BoX 14-3   SUMMARY

Pharmacodynamics of Nitrous Oxide

Minimum alveolar concentration (MAC) for nitrous oxide is 104% and cannot be achieved under normal conditions.

MAC for certain patients may be less than 104% and is certainly lower when combined with sedatives or opioids.

Despite the machine settings, it is doubtful that a typical dental unit can deliver more than 0.5 MAC to the patient.

At sedative concentrations (0.3 to 0.5 MAC), nitrous oxide produces a mild analgesic effect; this does not obviate the requirement for local anesthesia.

Nitrous oxide does not depress minute ventilation but does depress ventilatory response to hypercapnia and hypoxemia. If respiratory depression is produced for other reasons, nitrous oxide diminishes a patient's ability to respond.

Cardiovascular function remains stable in patients under nitrous oxide sedation unless sedatives and opioids are added.

Nitrous oxide increases venous tone, which may be helpful during attempts at venipuncture.

Nitrous oxide inhibits the activity of enzymes that function in DNA synthesis. The total dose and duration of exposure required for permanent damage are unknown.

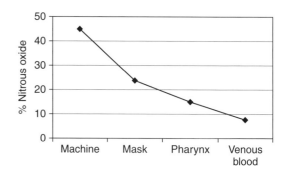

Fig. 14-3 Concentration of nitrous oxide delivered by typical dental machine through concentration that actually reaches the venous blood. (Modified from Sher AM, Braude BM, Cleaton-Jones PE, et al: *Anaesthesia* 39(3):236-239, 1984.)

oxide was delivered by full mask or through the endotracheal tube.

Analgesic and Anesthetic Actions

The mechanism by which anesthetic gases produce general anesthesia is unknown. The leading theory suggests that gases bind to proteins within neuronal membranes and somehow modify ion fluxes and subsequent synaptic transmission.[7]

Unlike other anesthetics, nitrous oxide produces a mild analgesic effect at subanesthetic concentrations. The mechanism for this effect most likely involves an interaction with the endogenous opioid system because it is prevented by administration of the opioid antagonist naloxone. The strongest evidence is that nitrous oxide stimulates release of enkephalins, which bind to opioid receptors that trigger descending noradrenergic pathways.[8] The most common estimate of efficacy suggests that 30% nitrous oxide delivered by full mask is equivalent to morphine 10 to 15 mg.[9]

Respiratory Effects

All anesthetic gases increase respiratory rate and diminish tidal volume. Unlike other agents, however, nitrous oxide causes an increased rate that provides a net increase in minute ventilation[10] (Fig. 14-4). Therefore when used alone for conscious sedation, nitrous oxide does not depress ventilation. When combined with sedatives or opioids that depress ventilation, however, nitrous oxide may be a concern.

Like all anesthetic gases, nitrous oxide produces a dose-dependent depression of ventilatory drive. Its influence is more pronounced on the ventilatory response to hypoxemia than to hypercapnia (Fig. 14-5). As little as 0.1 MAC nitrous oxide can depress hypoxemic drive by 50%.[11,12] That is, if respiratory depression occurs, nitrous oxide obtunds the body's normal response to elevated carbon dioxide tension and lowered oxygen tension. Patients with significant chronic obstructive pulmonary disease (COPD) rely almost entirely on hypoxemic drive, which nitrous oxide depresses most significantly. Some authorities suggest that nitrous oxide should be avoided in these patients, not only for this reason, but also because high oxygen concentrations delivered with nitrous oxide may remove the stimulus for hypoxemic drive. Provided the principles of conscious sedation are followed, however, the patient can always be instructed to breathe deeply.

Cardiovascular Effects

Nitrous oxide mildly depresses myocardial contractility, which is offset by its ability to activate sympathetic

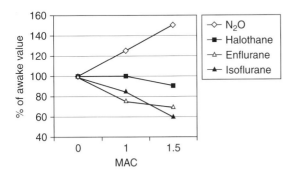

Fig. 14-4 Influence of nitrous oxide on minute ventilation. Nitrous oxide produces a dose-related increase in respiratory rate that more than offsets a mild decrease in tidal volume. Net ventilation is reduced by other anesthetics but actually increases during administration of nitrous oxide. *MAC,* Minimum alveolar concentration. (Modified from Eger EI: *Nitrous oxide,* New York, 1985, Elsevier.)

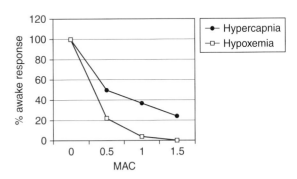

Fig. 14-5 Influence of nitrous oxide on hypercapnic and hypoxemic drives. Nitrous oxide depresses the ventilatory response to elevated carbon dioxide and to low oxygen tensions. It has its greatest effect on ventilation in response to hypoxemia. *MAC,* Minimum alveolar concentration. (Modified from Dahan A, van den Elsen MJ, Berkenbosch A, et al: *Anesthesiology* 80(4):727-738, 1994; and Yacoub O, Doell D, Kryger MH, Anthonisen NR: *Anesthesiology* 45(4):385-389, 1976.)

activity (Fig. 14-6). In both normal patients and those with coronary artery disease, subanesthetic concentrations of nitrous oxide (0.1 to 0.5 MAC) have little influence on cardiac output, stroke volume, and heart rate. At higher concentrations, nitrous oxide increases these variables, whereas volatile agents have the opposite influence.[13] Any depressant influences of nitrous oxide are overshadowed by its augmentation of sympathetic tone. However, opioids depress sympathetic outflow, and when combined with nitrous oxide, depressant effects of nitrous oxide on the myocardium may be revealed.[14,15] This influence may be significant for patients who are compromised by significant degrees of heart failure.

Arterial blood pressure remains stable in patients receiving subanesthetic concentrations of nitrous oxide. As concentrations are increased above 1 MAC, arterial pressure increases due to increased peripheral resistance attributed to sympathetic stimulation[13] (Fig. 14-7). Nitrous oxide increases venous tone, leading to increased venous return to the heart.[13] This effect likely contributes to the stable cardiovascular function observed with nitrous oxide. At times this influence of nitrous oxide on venous tone is exploited to facilitate venous access during difficult venipuncture.

Chronic Toxicity

Chronic exposure to trace amounts of nitrous oxide has been implicated in myriad adversities, including infertility, spontaneous abortion, blood dyscrasias, and neurologic deficits. These concerns pertain only to chronic exposure to health care personnel; it is presumed that healthy surgical patients could receive nitrous oxide for 24 hours without harm.[7]

Nitrous oxide irreversibly oxidizes the cobalt atom of vitamin B_{12} and thereby reduces the activity of B_{12}-dependent enzymes such as methionine and thymidylate synthetases. This appears to be the likely mechanism for toxicity because these enzymes are vital in the synthesis of myelin and nucleic acids. At what minimum concentration and duration of exposure this influence becomes significant, however, is unsettled. Megaloblastic changes in bone marrow are observed after exposure to anesthetic concentrations for 24 hours, and agranulocytosis is apparent after 4 days of exposure.[16] Animal studies using intermittent exposure to trace amounts of various anesthetic gases have failed to reveal any harmful reproductive effects.[17] It is generally accepted that proper

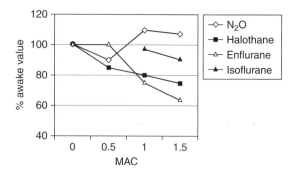

Fig. 14-6 Influence of nitrous oxide on cardiac output. Depressant effect of nitrous oxide on myocardial contractility is more than offset by its stimulation of sympathetic neurons. It has little influence on cardiac output. *MAC,* Minimum alveolar concentration. (Modified from Eger EI: *Nitrous oxide,* New York, 1985, Elsevier.)

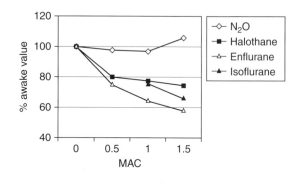

Fig. 14-7 Influence of nitrous oxide on blood pressure. Most general anesthetics decrease arterial pressure, but little influence is observed with nitrous oxide. *MAC,* Minimum alveolar concentration. (Modified from Eger EI: *Nitrous oxide,* New York, 1985, Elsevier.)

use of scavenging devices while providing nitrous oxide to patients in the dental setting eliminates any significant risk (see section on Disinfection and Scavenging Systems).

Equipment

In the United States, nitrous oxide is stored in blue cylinders as a liquid. Unlike oxygen, which exists in

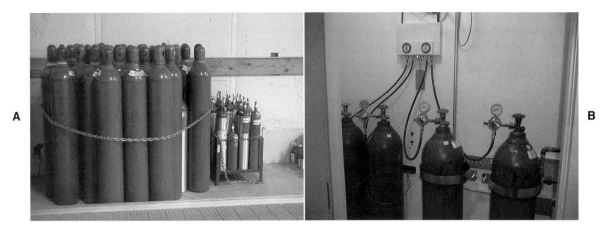

A

B

Fig. 14-8 Medical gases are supplied in cylinders ranging in size designated by letters A to K. **A,** Small E-sized tanks are used with portable units, and large H tanks are for centralized systems **(B).**

TABLE 14-2

Medical Gas Cylinders

	CAPACITY (LITERS)		WEIGHT (POUNDS)	
Cylinder	O_2	N_2O	O_2	N_2O
A	76	189	0.23	0.8
B	196	378	0.6	1.5
D	396	946	1.2	3.8
E	659	1590	1.9	6.4
F	2062	5260	6.0	21.0
M	3000	7570	8.8	30.6
G	5331	13,836	15.5	56.0
H, K	5570-7500	15,899	16-22	64.3

a gaseous state and demonstrates a proportional decrease in tank pressure as it is used, nitrous oxide will maintain a constant pressure of approximately 745 psi at room temperature until all the liquid has evaporated. Therefore the practitioner will not be able to ascertain residual volume unless a scale is used to weigh tank contents.

As with other medical gases, various sizes of storage tanks are available. Generally, E tanks are used for portable delivery units, and G or H tanks are used as central supply storage in offices that require nitrous oxide availability for multiple operatories (Fig. 14-8 and Table 14-2). In contrast to portable, self-contained units, a centralized delivery system requires plumbing and manifolds, which add considerable expense to installation. Offices that use nitrous oxide sedation regularly, however, will realize long-term savings in gas expense and will need to change tanks less frequently.

Nitrous Oxide Machines

Modern nitrous oxide units employ a continuous-flow design that is specific to nitrous oxide delivery

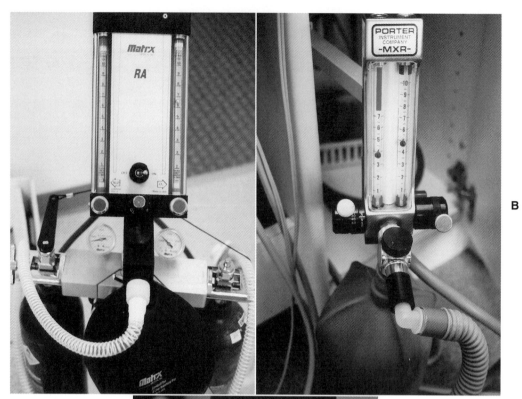

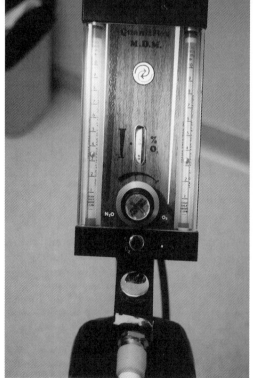

Fig. 14-9 A-C, Nitrous oxide sedation units.

Nitrous Oxide Equipment

> Modern nitrous oxide and oxygen delivery systems feature a continuous-flow design with flowmeters for each gas.
>
> Fail-safe features, such as color coding, adapter size, pin indexing, and minimal oxygen flow settings, make it virtually impossible to set up or deliver improper concentrations.
>
> Alarm systems enhance safety, and locking mechanisms prevent abuse.
>
> Equipment should be regularly inspected for leaks.
>
> A scavenging system is essential in practices where nitrous oxide sedation is used frequently.
>
> Environmental levels of nitrous oxide are significantly reduced in offices that are well ventilated and have appropriate air-handling capabilities.
>
> Monitoring exposure of office personnel should be encouraged.

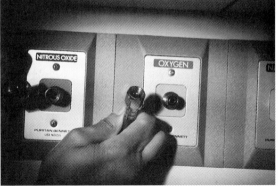

A

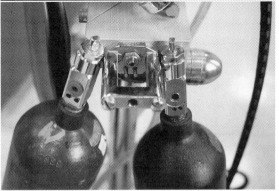

B

Fig. 14-10 A, Diameter-indexed safety system for gas connections. **B,** Pin-indexed safety system.

systems (Box 14-4). Each gas has a flowmeter, which is controlled by either an individual or a common mixing valve. Meters with a common mixing valve allow the clinician to alter the percentages of the two gases without changing the preestablished minute volume (Fig. 14-9). Most units are designed as *open systems;* that is, the machine delivers gases but does not recapture unused or exhaled gases. Recovery of these gases requires a scavenging system, as described later.

The design of modern nitrous oxide and oxygen delivery systems incorporates a number of features to facilitate patient safety. Color coding of valves, supply tubing, connectors, and controls corresponds to the color of the gas cylinders; green designates oxygen and blue is nitrous oxide in the United States. Some countries assign other color schemes to designate the various medical gases.

A *diameter-indexed safety system* (DISS) establishes a specific diameter and thread size for each coupling, which prevents attaching a hose to the wrong outlet (Fig. 14-10, *A*). In addition, a *pin-indexed system* prevents the attachment of a tank to an incorrect yoke of the unit or central supply (Fig. 14-10, *B*). It is important to inspect these attachments routinely to ensure that the pins are intact.

Modern units are designed to deliver a minimum flow of oxygen, thus ensuring the patient cannot receive 100% nitrous oxide. Most devices ensure a minimum of 30% oxygen concentration, although some older units were designed for only 20% to 25%. Fail-safe mechanisms automatically obstruct the flow of nitrous oxide if the flow of oxygen falls below the preestablished minimum. This ensures that nitrous oxide cannot be delivered to the patient if the oxygen supply is depleted. Some units include an alarm system to alert the clinician to low pressure in the oxygen cylinder.

Nitrous oxide machines also contain a high-flow oxygen flush capability. This allows the operator to purge nitrous oxide from the system, including nonrebreathing bag and tubing, and deliver a high oxygen flow to the patient. Although the unit can be used for positive-pressure ventilation, it is difficult. The location of the bag, its non-self-inflating design, and the necessity of replacing the nasal hood with a full-face mask make this practice awkward. It is preferable either to replace the tubing with specially adapted oxygen delivery equipment or to use separate portable oxygen units when managing emergency situations (Fig. 14-11).

Disinfection and Scavenging Systems

Concerns regarding toxicity from chronic exposure have essentially mandated the use of scavenging equipment during nitrous oxide sedation in the den-

tal office. However, proper use of scavenging equipment is only one of several methods for reducing environmental nitrous oxide concentrations. Other considerations include the following:

1. Set maximum vacuum settings per the manufacturer's instructions (Fig. 14-12).
2. Check all fittings for leaks; soapy water is an effective diagnostic agent.
3. Ensure that operatory ventilation and air circulation are adequate; air exchange rates greater than 10 times/hour are recommended.

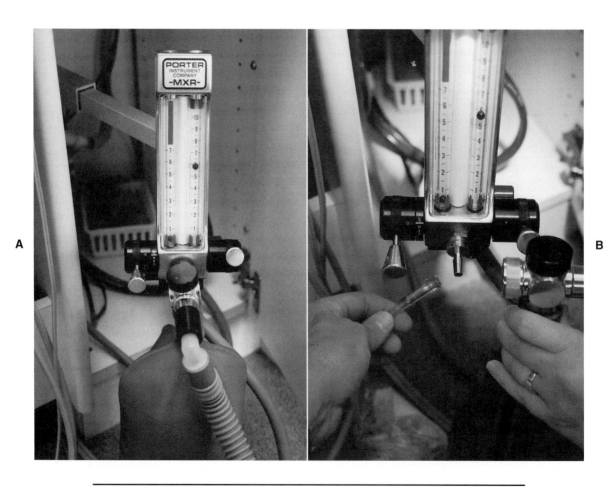

Fig. 14-11 Standard setup is difficult to use for providing positive-pressure oxygen **(A),** but some machines have a detachable housing that reveals an adapter **(B)** for connecting standard oxygen tubing of a rebreathing mask or resuscitation bag.

4. The exhaust system for vacuum suction should vent to the outside of the building.
5. Always use appropriate gas flow, and ensure proper mask fit.
6. Minimize patient conversation.
7. As the procedure nears completion, terminate nitrous oxide flow and administer 100% oxygen for 3 to 5 minutes before removing the nasal hood from the patient.

The Occupational Safety and Health Administration (OSHA) has not established guidelines for limits on environmental exposure to nitrous oxide. In 1990, however, the American Conference of Governmental Industrial Hygienists recommended a threshold value of 50 parts per million (ppm). Other agencies, including the California Occupational and Health Admini-

stration and the American Dental Association, have supported this recommendation in some manner. A limit of 50 ppm is very conservative considering that adverse influences of chronic exposure have been confirmed only at levels well above 1000 ppm.[16,18] Further surveys and human studies are required to develop standards based on reliable data.

Various suppliers have adopted different approaches to facilitate the removal of waste gases through the office vacuum system, such as a "mask within a mask" (Fig. 14-13 and Table 14-3). Whatever the design, most systems reduce exposure levels to 50 ppm, and some have demonstrated even greater reduction if combined with other practices, as mentioned earlier.[9] Some units incorporate an "air sweeper" to aid in the recovery of gases that have either escaped the primary seal of the nasal hood or

Fig. 14-12 To use scavenging devices properly, vacuum settings must be set at appropriate intensity. Floating ball must be aligned with green indicator.

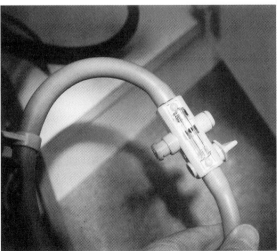
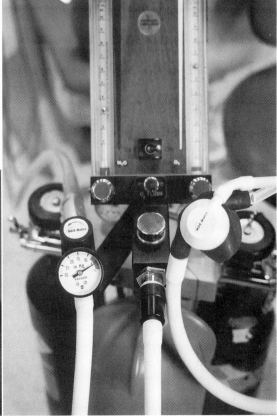

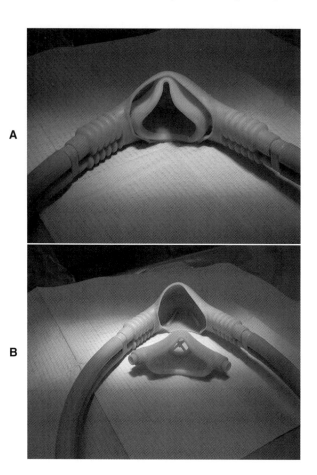

Fig. 14-13 Modified Brown mask **(A)** permits removal and sterilization of mask lining **(B)**.

TABLE 14-3

Comparison of Nasal Masks for Scavenging Adequacy

Tests (*N*)	Mask Type	Mean N_2O (ppm)
35	Brown	43.4
29	Porter	48.2
24	Parkell	54.4
23	Dupaco	61.2
33	Fraser Harlake	62.7
6	Comfort Cushion	34.8
6	McKesson	22.3
6	Dolonox	30.5

been expired through mouth breathing and conversation. Although many of these devices are highly effective, they are cumbersome and hinder access to the oral cavity.

Monitoring

Monitoring of employee exposure levels is not only prudent for offices using nitrous oxide and oxygen sedation on a regular basis, but it may be an implied standard of practice because OSHA mandates the right of employees to know of potential hazards in the workplace.[19] *Passive dosimetry,* such as that used for monitoring radiation exposure, employs badges or vials worn by the worker that absorb nitrous oxide for a predetermined period. They are returned to the manufacturer for analysis and preparation of a time-weighted average exposure report. These services are relatively inexpensive and are available from several companies (e.g., Landauer, Assay Technology, Healthcare Learning Systems).

Infrared spectrophotometry devices use short-radio frequency electromagnetic energy and can detect nitrous oxide levels as low as 1 ppm.[20] These devices are expensive and impractical for continuous use in the private practice setting, but they can be rented for short periods to provide accurate, real-time exposure levels and establish a baseline for office scavenging protocol.

Sterilization

Historically, nitrous oxide delivery systems have presented obstacles to effective sterilization. Concerns regarding hepatitis and human immunodeficiency virus (HIV) have intensified this issue. Under the Spaulding classification of inanimate surfaces, nitrous oxide accessories are considered *semicritical* in terms of infection risk.[21] This classification includes items that contact mucous membranes but are intact and are not contaminated by common bacterial spores.[9] The typical dental office does not harbor nosocomial pathogens, and patients are seldom as infectious or immunologically compromised as those treated in hospitals. Nevertheless, nasal masks and delivery tubing can be contaminated with a variety of human pathogens capable of patient-to-patient transmission (Box 14-5).[22]

In hospitals, all masks and tubing associated with inhalation therapy are sterile and disposable after single use. Although these systems are available for

■ BOX 14-5 ⬛ SUMMARY

Sterilization of Masks and Tubing

> Nitrous oxide masks and tubing are a source of cross-contamination.
> Use of autoclavable or disposable mask and tubing should be encouraged.
> Barrier protection and disinfection are necessary for nonautoclavable surfaces.

■ BOX 14-6 ⬛ SUMMARY

Nitrous Oxide Administration

> Vital signs should be assessed before and after nitrous oxide sedation.
> The desired level of sedation must be achieved by titration.
> Using 100% oxygen, achieve flow rate that accommodates patient's minute volume.
> Initiate titration using 20% to 25% nitrous oxide for 3 to 5 minutes, and increase by 10% increments.
> Faulty mask fit, mouth breathing, and excessive conversation decrease gas delivery to the patient and increase environmental contamination.
> Monitor minute volume throughout procedure, and adjust flow rate accordingly.
> Administer 100% oxygen for 3 to 5 minutes at termination of nitrous oxide delivery.
> Allow 15 to 20 minutes for recovery before patient is discharged.

dental practice and obviate any cross-contamination, they introduce significant expense. Inexpensive, disposable nasal masks are available from several suppliers but do not address contamination of tubing. Glutaraldehyde, iodophors, and other agents have been used as disinfectants, and specialized three-dimensional microwave units have been used for sterilization. All these offer potential alternatives, but each has special limitations and disadvantages.

At present the most viable method of sterilization is the autoclavable mask-tubing units available through most equipment and accessory suppliers. Barrier techniques, along with glutaraldehyde disinfection, should be applied to the surface and connectors of the nitrous oxide unit in the same manner as for chairs, countertops, and other nonautoclavable surfaces.

Administration

As with the administration of any inhalation agent or other sedative regimen, preoperative baseline vital signs must be recorded (Box 14-6). Although adverse physiologic effects of nitrous oxide on the respiratory and cardiovascular system are minimal in the healthy patient, the clinician must have a basis for evaluating untoward responses. Although some patients may reach optimum sedation with as little as 20% to 25% nitrous oxide, other more tolerant subjects may require levels approaching or exceeding 50%. Nitrous oxide must be titrated for optimum sedative effect. This is particularly relevant for administration using nasal masks, since inconsistency in mask fit and mouth breathing leads to unpredictable levels of gas delivery to pulmonary alveoli. Some practitioners advocate the use of rubber dam to minimize mouth breathing, but this may contribute to anxiety and feelings of claustrophobia in selected patients.

After verifying satisfactory levels of cylinder reserves, the clinician should initiate an approximate flow of 6 L/minute of oxygen. This is based on an average tidal volume of 500 ml and a respiratory rate of 12 in the resting, healthy, average-size adult. Children generally demonstrate a higher respiratory rate and a smaller tidal volume; thus it is imperative to adjust the minute volume to suit the individual patient. Next, the clinician places the nasal mask securely on the patient (or allows the patient to seat the mask, as some clinicians prefer) and observes the nonrebreathing bag for verification of gas exchange and adequate minute volume (Fig. 14-14.) If the bag volume diminishes, the oxygen flow should be increased appropriately. A bag that remains distended should not be hastily interpreted as excessive gas delivery but should be thoroughly investigated for improper mask fit and mouth breathing.

After allowing the patient to breathe 100% oxygen for 3 to 5 minutes, a nitrous oxide concentration of 20% to 25% should be initiated. Higher introductory percentages may quickly exceed individual patient comfort levels and produce unpleasant symptoms.

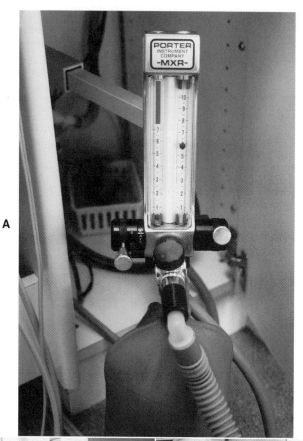

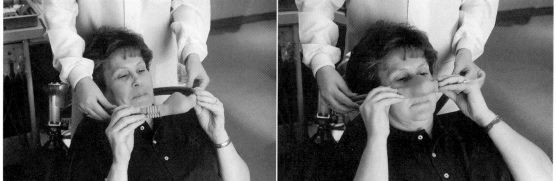

Fig. 14-14 A, Set oxygen flow to 6 L/min, and fill reservoir bag before introducing mask to patient. **B** and **C,** Allow patient to assist in placement of nasal mask. Patient can breathe 100% oxygen until movement of reservoir bag confirms appropriate mask fit and minute volume. Once this is confirmed, titration of nitrous oxide can begin.

During general anesthesia, using a full mask, it requires 3 minutes to achieve initial equilibrium of systemic nitrous oxide gas tension and thus produce peak effects on mental and psychomotor performance.[23] Based on this information, it is reasonable to assume that as much as 5 minutes may be required with a nasal mask.

It is important to evaluate patient responses at the initial induction level, before increasing the percentage of nitrous oxide. The operator should also monitor the nonrebreathing bag throughout the procedure because a patient's minute volume changes during the procedure and requires appropriate adjustment. After the initial induction period, most experienced clinicians will titrate nitrous oxide in 5% to 10% increments from the baseline value until optimum patient comfort levels are achieved. Patients have typical responses to various nitrous oxide concentrations (Table 14-4).

Termination of nitrous oxide should be accomplished at the earliest possible time to purge remaining gas into the scavenging system and reduce further environmental contamination. The clinician should continue 100% oxygen for 3 to 5 minutes after nitrous oxide is terminated. This period is normally sufficient for patients to regain mental and psychomotor skills. A slightly longer period (15 minutes) may be required before patients engage in any activity requiring fine motor skills.[24,25] Vital signs should be recorded at the termination of the procedure.

Contraindications

Nitrous oxide sedation has not been associated with any major adverse effects and can be used safely for almost all patients routinely treated in the ambulatory dental setting. In fact, it could be argued that nitrous oxide is the safest of all the modalities available for sedation in the dental office. As with other pharmacologic agents, however, nitrous oxide may not be suitable for all patients (Box 14-7). It is important to review carefully the medical history of a patient and consider a small number of situations in which nitrous oxide sedation may be contraindicated or at least poses a relative contraindication.

Clearly, inability to use a nasal mask is an absolute contraindication to the use of nitrous oxide. Generally, such patients fall into one of two categories: (1) those who cannot inhale adequately through the nose because of anatomic or disease-induced nasopharyngeal obstructions and (2) those who cannot tolerate and sustain placement of the nasal mask due to psychological or cognitive disturbances. Examples include severely phobic or cognitively impaired patients, as

TABLE   14-4

Typical Effects at Increasing Concentrations of Nitrous Oxide

N₂O Concentration (%)	Symptom/Physiologic Effect
10-20	Body warmth, tingling of hands and feet
20-30	Circumoral numbness
20-40	Numbness of tongue and extremities
	Hearing: distinct but distant, droning sounds
	Analgesia, euphoria, mild sleepiness, heaviness or lightness of body
	Beginning of dissociation
30-50	Sweating, dysphoria
	Amnesia, increased sleepiness
40-60	Dreaming, laughing, giddiness
	Further sleepiness, stupor
	Increased dysphoria
>50	Unconsciousness, light general anesthesia

BOX   14-7

Contraindications to Nitrous Oxide Sedation

Absolute
Inability to use a nasal mask
Upper respiratory infections or sinus blockage
Recent history of middle or inner ear surgery

Relative
Diagnosed personality or psychiatric disorders
Severe chronic obstructive pulmonary disease
Complicated pregnancy

well as those with a deviated septum, nasal polyps, upper respiratory infections, allergic rhinitis, and severe sinusitis. In this latter regard, any compromise in patency of the eustachian tube may lead to pressure increases within the middle ear, as explained previously. In fact, any recent surgery of the ear may present a contraindication for nitrous oxide.[3]

Although nitrous oxide has been used successfully in patients with diagnosed personality and psychiatric disorders, it should be used cautiously when treating those diagnosed with schizophrenia or bipolar disorder. These patients are treated with myriad psychotropic agents, and the use of nitrous oxide may further alter disposition, leading to unpredictable results. Medical consultation is strongly encouraged for these and similar patients.

Nitrous oxide sedation may be contraindicated in patients with COPD, as discussed earlier. The basis for this concern, although academically plausible, carries little substance. Although any CNS depressant might depress ventilation, nitrous oxide is well documented as increasing net ventilation.[10] As with all anesthetic gases, however, nitrous oxide depresses ventilatory effort in response to hypercapnia and hypoxemia.[11,12] In theory, if other factors cause respiratory depression, the patient's response to elevated carbon dioxide and diminished oxygen will be obtunded. This consideration has greatest validity because the COPD patient is naturally tolerant to carbon dioxide tensions and relies almost completely on hypoxemic ventilatory drive. Nitrous oxide not only depresses this mechanism, but it is administered along with high concentrations of oxygen, and the patient may not have adequate stimulus for involuntary breathing. In the conscious patient, any period of apnea is transient and lasts only until oxygen tension drops. Furthermore, the patient retains voluntary control over breathing and merely requires verbal instruction to breathe deeply.

In our experience, COPD patients ill enough to rely completely on hypoxemic drive are rarely treated in the ambulatory dental practice. Clearly, such patients are classified as ASA IV for medical risk status and should be carefully evaluated before any dental treatment. Other CNS depressants should be avoided when using nitrous oxide to sedate any patient with a chronic respiratory disorder, and the use of pulse oximetry should be encouraged.

The question of nitrous oxide use in pregnant patients is complicated by opinions based on concerns related to adverse effects associated with chronic exposure. These issues were addressed previously and warrant the use of scavenging devices to protect the health care provider. The issue under consideration, however, is the use of nitrous oxide sedation during a single appointment. Clearly, all elective dental treatment should be avoided during pregnancy, especially during the first trimester. However, urgent dental care is frequently required for pregnant patients. These patients may be anxious and fearful, and their apprehension should be allayed using the safest agents available, and nitrous oxide fulfills this requirement.[26,27] For ethical reasons, prospective studies cannot address this issue, but retrospective studies of nearly 6000 general anesthetics in pregnant patients failed to reveal any adverse outcome to patient or fetus.[28-30] Virtually all these anesthetics included nitrous oxide.

For the pregnant patient who is apprehensive and requires urgent dental care, nitrous oxide should be regarded as the sedation agent of choice. Any evidence of complication during the pregnancy warrants consultation with the patient's obstetrician.

In summary, few contraindications exist to the use of nitrous oxide. Nitrous oxide can play a major role in reducing the likelihood of stress-related complications when managing most medically compromised patients.

Complications

Nitrous oxide sedation is remarkably safe and is rarely associated with adverse events. Occasionally, a patient within normal psychological parameters will present with a well-documented history of adverse or idiosyncratic reaction to nitrous oxide. Most of these patients probably received excessive concentrations, or the nitrous oxide was titrated too rapidly. Nevertheless, prior adverse events should be investigated and may pose a contraindication to its further use. Patients have reported allergic responses to nitrous oxide, but no reports of nitrous oxide allergy have been confirmed.

All medical gases are produced in an anhydrous state. Therefore the use of a dry gas mixture, particularly for longer procedures, may create problems for contact lens users and for asthmatic patients, in whom drying of bronchial secretions may trigger an acute asthma attack.

Provided nitrous oxide is titrated properly and the dentist monitors the patient's behavior throughout

12. Yacoub O, Doell D, Kryger MH, et al: Depression of hypoxic ventilatory response by nitrous oxide, *Anesthesiology* 45(4):385-389, 1976.
13. Eisele JH: Cardiovascular effects of nitrous oxide. In Eger EI: *Nitrous oxide,* New York, 1985, Elsevier.
14. Stanley TH, Liu WS: Cardiovascular effects of meperidine-N_2O anesthesia before and after pancuronium, *Anesth Analg* 56(5):669-673, 1997.
15. Falk RB Jr, Denlinger JK, Nahrwold ML, et al: Acute vasodilation following induction of anesthesia with intravenous diazepam and nitrous oxide, *Anesthesiology* 49(2):149-150, 1978.
16. Nunn JF: Clinical aspects of the interaction between nitrous oxide and vitamin B_{12}, *Br J Anaesth* 59(1):3-13, 1987.
17. Mazze RI, Fujinaga M, Rice SA, et al: Reproductive and teratogenic effects of nitrous oxide, halothane, isoflurane, and enflurane in Sprague-Dawley rats, *Anesthesiology* 64(3):339-344, 1986.
18. Sweeney B, Bingham RM, Amos RJ, et al: Toxicity of bone marrow in dentists exposed to nitrous oxide, *Br Med J Clin Res Ed* 291(6495):567-569, 1985.
19. National Institute of Occupational Safety and Health: *Criteria for a recommended standard: occupational exposure to waste anesthetic gases and vapors,* DHEW Pub No 77-140, Cincinnati, 1977.
20. Clark MS, Brunick AL: *Handbook of nitrous oxide and oxygen sedation,* St Louis, 1999, Mosby.
21. Favero MS: Chemical disinfection of medical and surgical materials. In Block SS, editor: *Disinfection, sterilization and preservation,* ed 3, Philadelphia, 1985, Lea & Febiger.
22. Hunt LM, Yagiela JA: Bacterial contamination and transmission by nitrous oxide apparatus, *Oral Surg* 44:367-373, 1977.
23. Kortilla K, Ghoniem MM, Jacobs L, et al: Time course of mental and psychomotor effects of 30 percent nitrous oxide during inhalation and recovery, *Anesthesiology* 54:220-236, 1981.
24. McKercher TC, Nelson WJ, Melgaard SA: Recovery and enhancement of reflex reaction time after nitrous oxide analgesia, *J Am Dent Assoc* 101:785-788, 1980.
25. Trieger N, Loskota WJ, Jacobs AW, et al: Nitrous oxide: a study of physiological and psychomotor effects, *J Am Dent Assoc* 82:142-150, 1971.
26. Santos AC, Pederson H, Finster M: Obstetric anesthesia. In Barash PG, Cullen BF, Stoelting RK, editors: *Clinical anesthesia,* ed 3, Philadelphia, 1997, Lippincott-Raven.
27. Rosen MA: Management of anesthesia for the pregnant surgical patient, *Anesthesiology* 91(4):1159-1163, 1999.
28. Mazze RI, Kallen B: Reproductive outcome after anesthesia and operation during pregnancy: a registry study of 5405 cases, *Am J Obstet Gynecol* 161(5):1178-1185, 1989.
29. Aldridge LM, Tunstall ME: Nitrous oxide and the fetus: a review and the results of a retrospective study of 175 cases of anaesthesia for insertion of Shirodkar suture, *Br J Anaesth* 58:1348-1356, 1986.
30. Crawford JS, Lewis M: Nitrous oxide in early human pregnancy, *Anaesthesia* 41:900-905, 1986.

> ## BOX 14-8
>
> ### *Signs of Excessive Nitrous Oxide Concentration*
>
> Rigid mandible
> Repeated mouth closing
> Increasing diaphoresis
> Nausea and vomiting
> Increasing unresponsiveness or unconsciousness
> Increasingly rigid posture and forward movement in dental chair
> Hard, angry look in eyes
> Dizziness with eyes closed

the procedure, an adverse event is unlikely. Signs can warn the dentist that concentrations may be excessive (Box 14-8). If any of these events occurs, the nitrous oxide concentration should be decreased or discontinued.

References

1. Stevens WC, Kingston HGG: Inhalation anesthesia. In Barash PG, Cullen BF, Stoelting RK, editors: *Clinical anesthesia,* ed 3, Philadelphia, 1997, Lippincott-Raven.
2. Thomsen KA, Terkildsen K, Arnfred I: Middle ear variations during anesthesia, *Arch Otolaryngol* 82:609, 1965.
3. Munson ES: Complications of nitrous oxide anesthesia for ear surgery, *Anesth Clin North Am* 11(3):559-572, 1993.
4. Eger EI: Pharmacokinetics. In *Nitrous oxide,* New York, 1985, Elsevier.
5. Quarnstrom FC, Milgrom P, Bishop MJ, et al: Clinical study of diffusion hypoxia after nitrous oxide analgesia, *Anesth Prog* 38(1):21-23, 1991.
6. Sher AM, Braude BM, Cleaton-Jones PE, et al: Nitrous oxide sedation in dentistry: a comparison between Rotameter settings, pharyngeal concentrations, and blood levels of nitrous oxide, *Anaesthesia* 39(3):236-239, 1984.
7. Stoelting RK: *Pharmacology and physiology in anesthetic practice,* ed 3, Philadelphia, 1999, Lippincott-Raven.
8. Zhang C, Davies MF, Guo TZ, et al: The analgesic action of nitrous oxide is dependent on the release of norepinephrine in the dorsal horn of the spinal cord, *Anesthesiology* 91(5):1401-1407, 1999.
9. Jastak JT, Donaldson D: Nitrous oxide, *Anesth Prog* 38(4-5):142-153, 1991.
10. Eger EI: Respiratory effects of nitrous oxide. In *Nitrous oxide,* New York, 1985, Elsevier.
11. Dahan A, van den Elsen MJ, Berkenbosch A, et al: Effects of subanesthetic halothane on the ventilatory responses to hypercapnia and acute hypoxia in healthy volunteers, *Anesthesiology* 80(4):727-738, 1994.

CHAPTER 15

Oral and Rectal Sedation

RAYMOND A. DIONNE
LARRY D. TRAPP

CHAPTER OUTLINE

Most anxious dental patients are still sedated with nitrous oxide or by the oral route of administration due to the limited number of dentists appropriately trained and certified in anesthesia or conscious sedation. Oral sedation with a single drug in the appropriate dose range is generally considered safer than parenteral approaches, but case reports continue to document episodes of serious morbidity and mortality when using the oral route. This chapter reviews the properties of selected drugs used in dental outpatients for oral and rectal sedation and makes therapeutic recommendations for their safe use by dentists without advanced training in conscious sedation or general anesthesia.

Oral Sedation

Oral sedation is probably the most widespread form of sedation in dentistry due to the ease of administration, the ability to provide effective anxiety relief without advanced training beyond dental school, and the presumption of safety (Box 15-1). Patients prefer the oral route over parenteral sedation,[1] presumably because of the pain associated with venipuncture or intramuscular (IM) administration. Limitations to the oral route include delay in onset of drug action, lower ceiling of efficacy than with parenteral administration, inability to titrate the dose based on the patient's response, and difficulty in administering a reversal agent or "emergency" drug in the absence of a patent intravenous (IV) line. Despite

these limitations, oral administration is the most effective and practical form of sedation for practitioners without advanced training in anesthesia or parenteral sedation.

Drug classes historically used for oral sedation in dentistry included the barbiturates, chloral hydrate, opioids (narcotics), antihistamines, phenothiazines, and combinations of these drugs. Some of these agents, such as chloral hydrate, were introduced as sedatives before the adoption of requirements that new drugs show evidence of efficacy in well-controlled clinical trials and demonstrate safety in extensive animal testing and carefully monitored dose-escalation studies in humans. The introduction into clinical practice of drugs that satisfy these criteria and the reevaluation of traditional drugs have led to diminished use of most older drugs in favor of drugs that are more selective for anxiety relief (versus nonspecific sedation) and have a greater margin of safety. The barbiturates have been largely replaced in clinical practice as daytime sedatives, as hypnotics to aid sleep, or as the primary choice for parenteral sedation. Conversely, use of drugs such as chloral hydrate with no apparent advantage over newer drugs has continued for outpatient sedation in dentistry.

This chapter discusses only those drugs commonly used in dentistry, with emphasis on the benzodiazepines as drugs with the most selectivity for anxiety relief and with the greatest margin of safety.

Diazepam

Diazepam (Valium) was introduced in 1963 and quickly became one of the most widely prescribed drugs, often for inappropriate indications or administered for prolonged periods. It has largely displaced the use of barbiturates in dentistry both for oral sedation and parenteral administration. Advantages over barbiturates include a wide margin of safety and the ability to produce anxiety relief at doses that are less likely to lead to loss of consciousness. Limitations to diazepam include the production of active metabolites that can produce residual sedation long beyond the dental procedure and venous irritation when given intravenously.

Diazepam is rapidly absorbed after oral administration, reaching peak concentrations in adults in 60 to 90 minutes and as early as 15 to 30 minutes in children.[2] The rapid absorption of diazepam resulted in a detectable plasma concentration as early as 15 minutes after oral administration, which was half the peak level seen at 60 minutes.[3] The offset of diazepam's sedative effect is mediated initially by redistribution from the brain and bloodstream over a few hours, followed by more prolonged elimination with a half-life of 1.5 days. Diazepam can be eliminated three to four times more slowly in elderly persons, and doses should be adjusted in elderly patients and those with hepatic disease.

The expected side effects of diazepam are extensions of its pharmacologic properties: drowsiness and ataxia. At doses used for oral sedation the most likely adverse effect is continued sedation in the postoperative period. Although overdosage in the general population is relatively common because of its widespread availability, the safety of diazepam given for therapeutic purposes is remarkable.[4] Problems arise when benzodiazepines are combined with other drugs, in particular opioids, to produce deeper levels of sedation. In general, if a dose of 10 to 20 mg of oral diazepam proves ineffective in a normal-sized adult without a history of alcohol or drug abuse, consultation should be sought with a clinician more experienced with parenteral sedation before increasing the diazepam dose or combining it with other drugs.

Diazepam administered orally has been demonstrated to produce significant anxiety relief during dental procedures compared with placebo in adults.[5,6] Recovery rate is similar after oral or parenteral administration, with recovery from psychomotor impairment in 2 to 4 hours.[7] Studies of oral diazepam for pediatric sedation report variable and equivocal results due to variability in dose, outcome end points, and administration in combination with other drugs, which makes it difficult to assess the independent pharmacologic activity of diazepam alone. In general, it appears that diazepam cannot be readily differentiated from placebo based on observer's ratings of behavior or cooperation. One study reported 0.3 to 0.6 mg/kg to be comparable to chloral hydrate in restrained children during a dental procedure, but a lower incidence of sleeping during the procedure suggested a more selective anxiolytic effect.[8] The usual oral dose of diazepam is 5 to 20 mg for adults, given approximately 1 hour before the dental appointment. Recommended pediatric doses are conservative, ranging from 0.04 to 0.2 mg/kg.[9] Much higher doses are used in anesthesia, and 0.6 mg/kg has been reported in some studies, without apparent adverse effects.[8]

Midazolam

The success of diazepam as an anxiolytic agent led to the introduction of other benzodiazepines for both oral and parenteral administration. One such alternative is midazolam (Versed). Its major advantage is availability as a water-soluble salt, which largely eliminates venous irritation associated with IV administration of diazepam's irritating vehicle. Midazolam was associated with numerous incidences of significant morbidity and mortality when first introduced as approximately equipotent with diazepam. Subsequent recognition that it is three to four times more potent than diazepam led to its reformulation in a more dilute concentration and changes in the manufacturer's recommendations for the rate of administration. Although midazolam was not approved initially for oral use due to concern over possible toxicity with repeated administration to laboratory animals, clinicians popularized oral administration of the parenteral formulation in a variety of vehicles, leading to its eventual approval in an elixir for pediatric sedation.

Oral midazolam is rapidly absorbed from the gastrointestinal tract, with peak plasma levels occurring in 30 to 60 minutes. Onset of activity is usually within 30 minutes and extends in most patients for up to 2 hours after oral administration. The effectiveness of oral midazolam for children varies with dose, but most studies report an optimal balance between efficacy and side effect liability when 0.5 mg/kg is administered.[10,11] Higher doses (0.75 to 1.0 mg/kg) produce a higher incidence of side effects and decreased respiration, manifesting as oxygen saturation values below 80% in some children.[12] Few data are available comparing midazolam to other drugs in studies incorporating adequate sample sizes, random allocation of treatments, blinded methodology, or quantifiable patient self-reporting, especially for adults. More problematic is the use of midazolam by other routes of administration, including rectal and nasal administration, where absorption may be more variable.

Most studies evaluating the use of midazolam by the IV and IM routes of administration have been conducted by anesthesiologists in a hospital environment using the drug for preanesthetic medication. The therapeutic goal for this application, eventual loss of consciousness, is distinct from the therapeutic objective in the dental environment, *maintenance of consciousness.* Anesthesiologists have much greater training than dentists in the management of a deeply sedated or unconscious patient, especially airway management or treatment of respiratory depression. An inadvertent overdose due to a higher percentage of absorption than anticipated by one of these alternative routes of administration, combined with poor management of the airway in a outpatient dental environment, could result in significant morbidity and an indefensible medicolegal position for the dentist.

Clinicians popularized oral administration of midazolam despite a lack of U.S. Food and Drug Administration (FDA) approval for this indication and the absence of a commercially available formulation. The approval of midazolam (Versed) syrup now provides a palatable form of oral midazolam for sedation, anxiolysis, and amnesia in pediatric patients before diagnostic, therapeutic, or endoscopic procedures and before induction of anesthesia. This drug formulation provides the potential for greater efficacy and safety than older drugs still inexplicably used in dentistry for sedation, along with FDA approval for use in dental pediatric outpatients, thereby reducing medicolegal liability associated with off-label use of the drug. Midazolam syrup must be used as specified, and warnings highlight the potential for respiratory depression.

Most studies evaluating oral midazolam for preanesthetic sedation were conducted with formulations compounded in a variety of syrups to disguise the drug taste. A direct comparison[1] of several doses of chloral hydrate to midazolam as premedication in children undergoing otolaryngologic surgery revealed comparable efficacy for 50 mg/kg chloral hydrate, the dose usually recommended for pediatric dental patients, and 0.5 mg/kg midazolam, the dose recommended in the package labeling.[1] The taste of chloral hydrate resulted in facial grimaces and struggling in 50% of children younger than 5 years old compared with only 7% of children receiving midazolam. Other measures of efficacy, such as recovery time after anesthesia and surgery, were similar for both drugs at these doses.

Another study comparing oral midazolam (0.25 and 0.50 mg/kg) to diazepam (0.50 mg/kg) and placebo in children for anesthetic premedication found that only the 0.5-mg/kg midazolam dose resulted in a significant reduction in anxiety versus placebo at induction.[13] Similarly, 0.50 mg/kg of midazolam resulted in significantly better anesthetic induction than placebo, with less recall of preoperative events. Conversely, administration of higher midazo-

lam doses (0.75 or 1.0 mg/kg) resulted in a greater incidence of side effects, loss of balance and head control, and blurred vision and dysphoria compared with placebo or 0.50 mg/kg of midazolam.[14] These and similar studies form the basis for recommending 0.50 mg/kg of midazolam for pediatric sedation, especially in an outpatient environment, where loss of head control could result in airway obstruction.

Few studies have evaluated the use of oral midazolam for dental procedures in a dose or formulation similar to the oral midazolam syrup. A crossover study comparing a fixed 7.5-mg midazolam dose to placebo reported significantly less anxiety, greater amnesia, and patient preference for midazolam.[15] A study of anxious children who had failed behavioral approaches showed a significant improvement in patient apprehension and cooperation during the dental procedure after 7.5 mg of oral midazolam versus placebo.[14] Case series and reviews also support the effectiveness and safety of oral midazolam for pediatric dental outpatients.[16,17]

The introduction of oral midazolam (Versed) syrup for pediatric sedation now provides a safer alternative than parenteral sedation, greater selectivity for anxiety over nonspecific central nervous system (CNS) depression, a palatable dose formulation, and reduced medicolegal liability for off-label use of a drug for a high-risk indication. Ironically, the package insert's warning on potential adverse effects and respiratory depression suggests greater risk. These warnings are based on experience gained in millions of patients administered midazolam both orally and parenterally since its introduction and increased recognition of the hazards of administering a CNS depressant drug in a fixed oral dose to a vulnerable patient population. The heightened public awareness of the potential dangers of oral sedation, a continuing medicolegal environment that equates any significant adverse outcome with malpractice, and the specific warning in the package that "Versed Syrup must be used as specified in the label" leave little room for a casual approach to pediatric sedation.

Midazolam syrup should only be administered as a single dose under professional supervision in a dental office equipped for continuous monitoring of respiration and cardiac function, with immediate availability of resuscitative drugs and equipment for ventilation and intubation, if needed. Personnel in the dental office must be trained in the use of these drugs and equipment and skilled in airway management. The recommended dose by patient weight for pediatric patients is 0.25 to 0.50 mg/kg individualized based on patient age (older children need less drug), anxiety, and the level of sedation needed. The availability of the benzodiazepine antagonist flumazenil (Romazicon) is highly recommended. The administration of midazolam syrup in combination with another CNS depressant drug is not recommended, as additive effects may result in oversedation. Also, reducing the midazolam dose to allow for another drug decreases the relatively selective anxiolytic effect of the midazolam in favor of greater nonspecific sedative effects. If treatment fails, the procedure should be abandoned rather than attempting to give additional doses of the midazolam syrup or other drugs with resultant increased risk of morbidity.

The public expectation for safety is illustrated by the comment in a *60 Minutes II* episode, "The issue is simple: each child who walks into a dentist's office should walk out." However, surveys of the general population and special care patients indicate a continuing unmet need for anesthesia and sedation. The ability to provide sedation to help overcome the fear that prevents access to care for many patients also demands steps to ensure safety. The introduction of oral midazolam syrup now provides dentists with an approved, effective, safe drug for this indication but requires strict adherence to the warnings and contraindications in the package label, which define indirectly the medicolegal standards for pediatric sedation in the dental office.

Triazolam

Triazolam (Halcion) is chemically related to diazepam and is used for the short-term treatment of insomnia. Its rapid onset, short duration of action, and lack of active metabolites also makes it a near ideal antianxiety medication for dental patients. When administered by the sublingual route, triazolam produces even greater anxiolytic effects than oral administration of an equivalent dose, but without any detectable increase in side effects or psychomotor impairment. Clinicians are often reluctant to use triazolam for sedation because they are unfamiliar with this application, and the media have issued controversial reports.

Triazolam in a dose of 0.25 mg has proven effective as a preanesthetic medication before general surgery, compared with lorazepam, and before plastic surgery. Administration of triazolam the evening be-

fore surgery improves the onset and duration of sleep without residual impairment[18] and reduces patient reports of anxiety during oral surgery.[19] Comparison of 0.125, 0.25, and 0.5 mg administered an hour before surgery demonstrates significant anxiety reduction with 0.25 and 0.5 mg, but with prolonged postoperative psychomotor impairment after 0.5 mg.[20] Administration of 0.25 mg of triazolam in combination with 40% nitrous oxide resulted in anxiety relief comparable to a mean dose of 19 mg of diazepam but with faster postoperative recovery. These studies indicate that oral triazolam is an anxiolytic comparable in efficacy to IV diazepam, but without the potential toxicity of parenteral drug administration. Oral triazolam has also been demonstrated to be more effective than oral diazepam when administered to anxious patients before an endodontic procedure.[21]

Oral triazolam in doses of 0.25 to 0.5 mg does not produce any adverse changes in respiration, heart rate, or blood pressure despite obvious signs of sedation and psychomotor impairment. In safety studies involving healthy volunteers, even unusually high doses of triazolam (2 to 4 mg) did not depress the respiratory response to carbon dioxide or affect cardiovascular dynamics.[22,23] The absence of any reports of respiratory depression, despite millions of doses administered, indicate that a single dose of triazolam is unlikely to produce respiratory distress in dental patients after a single dose. The most common side effects include drowsiness, lightheadedness, and incoordination. Most adverse effects attributed to triazolam occur at doses higher (0.5 to 1.5 mg) than those recommended for dental outpatients, when given to elderly patients, or when administered chronically with inadequate medical supervision.

Both retrospective and prospective studies indicate that triazolam is remarkably safe when given in doses of 0.125 to 0.25 mg. As with all sedative drugs, triazolam may cause serious adverse effects in a small but finite number of patients. This drug has been deemed safe and effective by the FDA after three reviews over the last decade. Many of the problems attributed to benzodiazepine hypnotics such as triazolam are caused by misuse or inappropriate prescription of the drugs. There is no evidence that a single dose of 0.125 or 0.25 mg of triazolam before a dental procedure will result in drug accumulation or significant adverse effects. Ironically, the same cannot be said for other drugs commonly used by dentists to produce oral sedation.

Hydroxyzine

Hydroxyzine is classified as a sedative agent on the basis of the CNS depressant effects it shares with other antihistamine drugs. This H1-blocking agent is widely used for skin allergies in single doses of 25 mg.[24] Its use as a sedative agent for dental outpatients arose before the advent of the more efficacious benzodiazepines, and hydroxyzine persists because of tradition and familiarity rather than pharmacologic advantage. Hydroxyzine is usually administered orally in a dose of 50 to 100 mg for adults and 0.6 mg/kg for children.[25] As with all sedative drugs, when administered in combination with other CNS depressants such as opioids, the doses of the opioid should be reduced by 50% to avoid excess CNS depression or respiratory depression.

A well-controlled comparison of hydroxyzine to alprazolam for preoperative premedication did not detect any measurable anxiolytic activity for hydroxyzine; alprazolam resulted in a significant decrease in anxiety but with fewer side effects than hydroxyzine.[26] Observer ratings of behavior during a pediatric dental appointment were rated as significantly better for hydroxyzine (50 mg) compared with placebo.[27] IM hydroxyzine in doses of 50, 100, and 150 mg did not have detectable anxiolytic activity as a preanesthetic medication while producing dose-related increases in subjective ratings of sleepiness.[28] Comparison of IM lorazepam (0.05 mg/kg) to IM hydroxyzine (1.5 mg/kg) did demonstrate significantly greater manifestation of sedation for both drugs compared with placebo, but only lorazepam produced significantly greater anxiety relief than placebo.[29] These limited observations suggest that hydroxyzine's ability to relieve anxiety is modest and results from nonspecific CNS depression manifesting as drowsiness.

Hydroxyzine is frequently used in combination with other drugs to produce greater sedation. Such studies are usually flawed in that they fail to demonstrate if the combination has any advantage over increasing the dose of one of the constituents, a long-recognized requirement for evaluating the additive effects of drug combinations. Using two drugs together in subtherapeutic doses often has no advantage over administration of a full therapeutic dose of either agent alone, while increasing the possibility of idiosyncratic and allergic reactions, which are not dose related but increase in direct proportion to the number of drugs administered. For example, a study in 10 patients claimed an advantage to the combination of chloral hydrate, hydroxyzine, and meperidine compared with a combination of chloral hydrate and hydroxyzine in the same doses. Such an experimental design does not demonstrate the independent effects of the individual drugs and does not permit the interpretation that the drug combination provides any advantage that would not result from increasing the dose of either chloral hydrate or hydroxyzine. The paucity of well-controlled studies evaluating hydroxyzine for parenteral sedation, either alone or in combination, and the greater efficacy of the benzodiazepines suggest that hydroxyzine be reserved for use in patients in whom a benzodiazepine is contraindicated.

Chloral Hydrate

Chloral hydrate is one of the oldest sedative-hypnotics used in medicine and dentistry today. Its continued popularity is evidenced by a recent survey of all postgraduate students in pediatric dentistry, in which chloral hydrate's use represented approximately one quarter of all sedative agents administered.[30] Chloral hydrate is used both orally and rectally to produce sedation, generally in 30 to 45 minutes, with a duration of 2 to 5 hours. Chloral hydrate is used alone and in combination with nitrous oxide, hydroxyzine, meperidine, promethazine, diphenhydramine, and diazepam. Chloral hydrate's widespread use is based on its perceived safety. For example, hypnotic doses produce little changes in respiration, blood pressure, or heart rate.

More recent evidence, however, suggests that the use of chloral hydrate as a sedative for children be reexamined in light of evidence that it produces high levels of a known carcinogen at therapeutic doses. Also, chloral hydrate was introduced into clinical practice long before the adoption of federal regulations in 1938 requiring that efficacy and safety be demonstrated for drugs used in humans. This situation is similar to that of other older drugs (e.g., aspirin) for which pharmaceutical firms have not been required to conduct vigorous preclinical and clinical tests to document not only that the drug is effective for its claimed indication but that it is not toxic at therapeutic doses, does not produce birth defects, and is unlikely to be carcinogenic. Rather, chloral hydrate was "grandfathered" under the current regulations and placed into the category "generally recognized as safe."

Chloral hydrate is a product of the hydration of the chloral, a halogenated derivative of acetaldehyde.

Chloral hydrate is rapidly and well absorbed when administered orally and distributes throughout the body with good CNS uptake. It is metabolized rapidly to both trichloroethanol (TCE) and trichloroacetic acid (TCA). The sedative-hypnotic property of chloral hydrate is caused by the activity of TCE, which reaches peak plasma concentrations within 20 to 60 minutes but has a prolonged plasma half-life estimated at 8 hours. Therefore chloral hydrate produces relatively rapid induction of sedation and sleep after oral administration, but its effects are likely to linger long after the patient leaves the treatment facility.

Concern over chloral hydrate's carcinogenic potential were first raised in 1990 with the recognition that chloral hydrate is a metabolite of trichloroethylene, a recognized rodent carcinogen that is also a mutagen and chromosome-damaging agent. Smith[31] calculated that a 60-mg/kg dose of chloral hydrate in a 15-kg child is the equivalent of drinking one liter of water a day contaminated with 5 parts per billion of trichloroethylene, the maximum contaminant level allowed by the Environmental Protection Agency. The other metabolite, TCA, is the major toxic metabolite in humans and an inducer of carcinomas in mice. Both TCE and TCA have long half-lives, even in adults; these metabolites may accumulate to toxic levels with repeated high doses of chloral hydrate. Moreover, chloral hydrate itself has been found to be mutagenic by the Ames test, a standard bacterial model used for screening compounds for the potential as mutagens and carcinogens.[32] Substances that test positive in the Ames test are considered potential human mutagens and carcinogens, given the high correlation between positive results and genetic and carcinogenic effects in mammalian systems. Taken together, these findings suggest that chloral hydrate can induce cancer in humans.

A debatable question is whether these findings in tests involving nonhumans can be extrapolated to patients. Other documented cases of toxicity in humans caused by chloral hydrate include gastric necrosis, esophageal stricture, laryngeal edema, or cardiac arrhythmia. With these two arguments alone, one would question the efficacy of using chloral hydrate, when a recent review of pediatric dental sedatives concluded that it is no more effective than other agents.[33]

The removal of Noctec from the market, a brand of chloral hydrate, indicates there is still concern about the drug's toxicologic potential. Although chloral hydrate is still available generically, the greater efficacy and safety of the benzodiazepines suggest that chloral hydrate may no longer be appropriate for use as a sedative in dental practice.

Therapeutic Recommendations

Not all patients are responsive to oral sedatives and will remain too anxious to permit administration of local anesthesia or performance of the procedure. Administration of a sedative drug may lower inhibitions in very anxious patients, leading to a paradoxical increase in a patient's response to noxious stimulation. Case reports of serious morbidity in the dental office often are based on attempts to manage disruptive behavior with increasing dose or number of drugs, only to produce oversedation, loss of protective airway reflexes, and undetected respiratory depression. If a patient is still anxious and uncooperative after a recommended dose of an oral sedative, and if adequate local anesthesia has been confirmed, the procedure should be terminated and the patient reevaluated for parenteral sedation. Increasing the sedative dose or repeated readministration of local anesthetic, especially in children, could result in CNS depression, leading to respiratory depression or loss of consciousness.

Rectal Sedation

Rectal administration of medications has been used since ancient times. The value of this route of administration has been problematic due to inconsistent bioavailability with resultant decreased effectiveness of suppository drug formulations. The continued interest in the rectal route of administration likely results from the increasing frequency of surgery performed in the office, where advance anesthetic techniques may not be appropriate but safe and effective methods of patient management are still needed.

The usual candidate for rectal sedation is either a child 1 to 7 years of age or an emotionally handicapped older child or adult. Less frequently the dentist encounters a patient who is unable to swallow a tablet and has a needle phobia. Individuals with a severe physical handicap such as cerebral palsy many also be candidates for rectal sedation. Rectal sedation for adults is usually limited to patients who are unable to be optimally sedated by the oral, inhalational, or parenteral routes.

Rectal Physiology

The rectum itself is about 10 to 15 cm long and 15 to 35 cm in diameter, but it is empty and flat most of the time. The main blood supply is from the inferior rectal arteries, which branch from the pudendal and middle rectal arteries. Three veins drain the rectum: the superior, middle, and inferior rectal veins. The superior rectal vein drains the upper (proximal) portion of the rectum and drains into the inferior mesenteric vein and subsequently into the portal vein. The middle and inferior rectal veins drain the remainder of the rectum and eventually join the internal iliac vein, which drains into the internal vena cava.

The blood pattern from the rectum is important because the portion of the rectally administered sedative that is absorbed into the middle and inferior rectal veins does not pass through the liver before entering the systemic circulation. This portion of the absorbed sedative drug does not undergo "first-pass" clearance or elimination in the liver. The fraction of the sedative absorbed via the superior rectal vein passes through the portal circulation and is partially cleared by the liver before entry into the systemic circulation, similar to orally administered sedatives. For drugs that undergo a large first-pass clearance, the physiology of the rectum may allow a higher serum concentration of a rectally administered sedative than for an equivalent oral dose. One factor that reduces predictability is the extensive anastomoses between the inferior, middle, and superior rectal veins; some variability in directional flow has also been reported.

Dosage Form

The most widely used dosage form is the rectal suppository. Pharmacokinetic evidence, however, indicates that a suppository dosage form results in a delayed and much more variable systemic absorption compared with rectally administered solutions. One study demonstrated that peak serum levels of diazepam from a suppository occurred an hour or more after rectal administration but in 20 minutes after administration of a rectal solution.[34,35] Factors affecting absorption of suppositories include particle size, surface properties, drug solubility, and fluid content of the rectum. An additional disadvantage to suppositories is the fixed dosage forms.

In contrast to the slow and variable absorption patterns for suppositories, comparison of rectally administered diazepam to IV administration showed similar peak serum levels, with the time to maximal blood levels occurring only 15 minutes later for rectal administration.[36-38] This rapid systemic uptake after rectal administration of sedative solutions results in quicker onset and less variability than the use of suppositories. An additional advantage to solutions is the ability to titrate the dose rather than administering a fixed dose with a suppository.

Patient Acceptance

In some parts of the world the rectal administration of medications for systemic absorption is not widely accepted or utilized. In the United States, for example, rectal administration of sedative agents is often used to treat young children but much less frequently for adults. An exception is the management of the physically or emotionally handicapped adults, including patients with cerebral palsy, autism, or moderate to severe retardation, as well as those with Down syndrome, Alzheimer's disease, and other disorders where voluntary patient cooperation cannot be expected. These patients may be institutionalized where rectal temperatures are routinely taken, providing an opportunity for rectal administration without special cooperation or even the patient's knowledge. This approach minimizes patient disruption, facilitates treatment, and increases patient and staff safety.

Deep Sedation with Thiopental

The required depth and duration of sedation for a dental outpatient will depend on the extent of patient anxiety and the nature of the procedure to be performed. Based on due considerations (see Chapter 1), deep sedation is indicated for an uncooperative, unpredictable, emotionally labile adult when a short treatment time (e.g., 15 minutes) is anticipated. A prefilled syringe containing a thiopental formulation designed for rectal administration comes with a flared applicator tip, and the desired dose can be set by turning a threaded nut located on the syringe plunger. An effective dose of thiopental for deep sedation is 44 mg/kg, approximately 10 times the IV dose used for general anesthesia.

After a flared applicator tip has been adapted to the syringe barrel, the tip is coated with a water-soluble lubricant. The patient is placed in a non-threatening area and positioned on the left side (assuming that the administrator is right-handed) with the uppermost leg flexed. The clinician stands behind the patient, where access is better and the patient cannot see the syringe. The tip is then inserted into the rectum, the contents injected, and the tip withdrawn. The patient will generally become deeply sedated and fall asleep in 10 minutes.

The appearance of the dentist and equipment usually makes the sedation of an uncooperative patient even more difficult. Elevation of patient anxiety can be minimized if the patient has a responsible attendant or family member who routinely takes rectal temperatures. The attendant or family member can administer the drug after the dose has been set and the tip adapted to the syringe. If the dentist prepares the syringe and explains the procedure to the attendant or family member while out of view of the patient, the dentist can remain out of sight until the patient is sleeping. The patient can be told that they are going to have a temperature taken. This allows for a much smoother and less traumatic induction of sedation. Once adequate sedation has been achieved, an IV infusion should be started, local anesthetic given, and treatment begun. If the treatment cannot be completed in 15 minutes, other sedative drugs can be administered intravenously before the patient becomes awake enough to remove the IV line. Sedation can also be planned as a multidrug approach, with the only goal of rectal thiopental being access to the IV infusion. Sufficient anesthesia training, however, is needed to manage deep sedation for a dentist using rectal sedation with thiopental.

Conscious Sedation with Diazepam

Rectal sedation with a diazepam solution has been accepted outside the United States and is reported to be well accepted and effective for normal adults undergoing outpatient oral surgery when compared to IV sedation with diazepam.[37] The mean rectal dose per kilogram of diazepam is approximately twice that for IV administration. Patients sedated rectally achieve lower peak serum levels (70%) and have greater peak sedative effects, but they also have approximately 50% longer recovery. Both routes of administration result in a similar incidence of amnesia and an equal duration of effect for surgical procedures, approximately 30 minutes. A small percentage of patients receiving rectal diazepam experience rectal pain after administration. The lack of an available formulation for rectal use in the United States make it impractical to recommend rectal sedation with diazepam at this time.

Sedation with Suppositories

Although the use of suppositories is proven effective therapy, lack of widespread use results largely from suppositories' variable bioavailability, consequent variable absorption, and thus lack of dependable clinical effectiveness. The substantial delay to peak effect also reduces their usefulness. If a suppository is used, the dose is selected based on a recommended milligram dose per kilogram body weight. If the commercially available product contains too large a sedative dose, the suppository can be sectioned (i.e., cut in half) to obtain the desired dose. The suppository is inserted without additional lubrication to avoid delays in absorption. A responsible patient, family member, or attendant can do this at home.

Complications

The most common complication of rectal sedation is initiation of a bowel movement and passing part or all of the suppository or drug solution. The incidence of this complication is relatively low, approximately 5% to 10%. The most significant potential complication is overdose from the sedative drug and the unintentional induction of general anesthesia with the potential for airway obstruction by the tongue. Loss of consciousness is not serious if the dentist is well trained in anesthesia and is monitoring closely once the patient has achieved deep sedation (see Chapter 11).

A thorough medical history will prevent the inadvertent administration of thiopental to a patient with a diagnosis of porphyria. Although infrequently encountered, erosion of the rectal or anal mucosa can occur with the uncooperative patient who tightens the anal sphincter during insertion or withdrawal of the syringe tip.

References

1. Phero JC, Dionne RA, McCullagh LM, Gordon SM: Assessment of clinical needs for anesthesia and sedation in the general population. In *Proc Ann Meeting Am Dent Soc Anesth*, Boston, 1994, p 211.
2. Baldessarini R: Drugs and the treatment of psychiatric disorders. In Hardman JG, Limbird LE, Molinoff PB, et al, editors: *Goodman and Gilman's the pharmacological basis of therapeutics*, ed 9, New York, 1990, McGraw-Hill.
3. Finkle BS, McCloskey KL, Goodman LS: Diazepam and drug-associated deaths, *JAMA* 242:429, 1979.

4. Baird ES, Hailey DM: Delayed recovery from a sedative: correlation of the plasma levels of diazepam with clinical effects after oral and intravenous administration, *Br J Anaesth* 44:803, 1972.

5. Baird ES, Curson I: Orally administered diazepam in conservative dentistry, *Br Dent J* 128:25, 1970.

6. Baker PJ, May HJ, Revicki DA, et al: Use of orally administered diazepam in the reduction of dental anxiety, *J Am Dent Assoc* 108:778, 1984.

7. Ghoneim MM, Mewaldt SP, Hinrichs JV: Behavioral effects of oral versus intravenous administration of diazepam, *Pharmacol Biochem Behav* 21:231, 1984.

8. Badalaty MM, Houpt MI, Kownigsberg SR, et al: A comparison of chloral hydrate and diazepam sedation in young children, *Pediatr Dent* 12:33, 1990.

9. Olin BR, editor: *Drug facts and comparisons,* St Louis, 2000, Lippincott.

10. Weldon BC, Watcha MF, White PF: Oral midazolam in children: effect of time and adjunctive therapy, *Anesth Analg* 75:51, 1992.

11. McMillan CO, Spahr-Schopfer IA, Sikich N, et al: Premedication of children with oral midazolam, *Can J Anaesth* 39:545, 1992.

12. Krafft TC, Kramer N, Kunzelmann K-H, Hickel R: Experience with midazolam as sedative in the dental treatment of uncooperative children, *J Dent Child* 60:295, 1993.

13. Parnis SJ, Foate JA, Van Der Walt JH, et al: Oral midazolam is an effective premedication for children having daystay anesthesia, *Anaesth Intensive Care* 20:9-14, 1992.

14. McMillan CO, Spahr-Schopfer IA, Sikich N, et al: Premedication of children with oral midazolam, *Can J Anesth* 39:545-550, 1992.

15. Luyk NH, Whitley B: Efficacy of oral midazolam prior to intravenous sedation for the removal of third molars, *Int J Oral Maxillofac Surg* 20:264-267, 1991.

16. Kraft TC, Kramer N, Kunzelman K-H, et al: Experience with midazolam as sedative in the treatment of uncooperative children, *J Dent Child* 18:123-127, 1994.

17. Hartgraves PM, Primosch RE: An evaluation of oral and nasal midazolam for pediatric dental sedation, *J Dent Child* 61:175-181, 1994.

18. Hughes RRL, Hart DM, Laing M: Lormetazepam or triazolam as night sedation before surgery, *Br J Clin Pract* 40:279, 1986.

19. Lieblich SE, Horswell B: Attenuation of anxiety in ambulatory oral surgery patients with oral triazolam, *J Oral Maxillofac Surg* 49:792,1991.

20. Kaufman E, Hargreaves KM, Dionne RA: Comparison of oral triazolam and nitrous oxide to placebo and intravenous diazepam for outpatient premedication, *Oral Surg Oral Med Oral Pathol* 75:156, 1993.

21. Ehrich D, Lundgren J, Dionne B, et al: Comparison of oral triazolam, diazepam, and placebo as outpatient premedication for endodontic patients, *J Dent Res* 75:267, 1996.

22. Elliott HW, Navarro G, Kikka N, et al: Early phase I evaluation of sedatives, hypnotics or minor tranquilizers. In Kagan F, Harwood T, Rickels K, et al, editors: *Hypnotics: methods of development and evaluation,* New York, 1975, Spectrum.

23. Gottschalk LA, Elliott HW: Effects of triazolam and flurazepam on emotions and intellectual function, *Res Community Psychol Psychiatry Behav* 1:575, 1976.

24. Douglas WW: Histamine and 5-hydroxytryptamine (serotonin) and their antagonists. In Gilman SG, Goodman LS, Rall TW, et al, editors: *Goodman and Gilman's the pharmacological basis of therapeutics,* New York, 1975, McGraw-Hill.

25. Atarax. In *Physicians' desk reference,* Montvale, NJ, 1995, Medical Economics Data.

26. Franssen C, Hans P, Brichant JF, et al: Comparison between alprazolam and hydroxyzine for oral premedication, *Can J Anaesth* 40:13, 1993.

27. Lang L: An evaluation of the efficacy of hydroxyzine (Atarax-Vistaril) in controlling the behavior of child patients, *J Dent Child* 32:253, 1965.

28. Forrest WH, Brown CR, Brown BW: Subjective responses to six common preoperative medications, *Anesthesiology* 47:241, 1977.

29. Wallace G, Mindlin LJ: A controlled double-blind comparison of intramuscular lorazepam and hydroxyzine as surgical premedicants, *Anesth Analg* 63:571, 1984.

30. Houpt M: Report of project USAP: the use of sedative agents in pediatric dentistry, *J Dent Child* 56:302, 1989.

31. Smith MT: Chloral hydrate warning, *Science* 76:339, 1990.

32. Haworth S, Lawlor T, Mortelmans K, et al: Salmonella mutagenicity test results for 250 chemicals, *Environ Mutagen* 1(suppl):3-142, 1983.

33. Moore P, Houpt M: Sedative drug therapy in pediatric dentistry. In Dionne RA, Phero J, editors: *Management of pain and anxiety in dental practice,* New York, 1991, Elsevier.

34. Knudsen F: Plasma diazepam in infants after rectal administration in solution and by suppository, *Acad Pediatr Scand* 66:563-567, 1977.

35. Moolenaar F, Bakker S, Visser J, et al: Comparative biopharmaceutics of diazepam after single rectal, oral, intramuscular, and intravenous administration in man, *Int J Pharmaceutics* 5:127-137, 1980.

36. Lundgren S, Rosenquist J: Comparison of sedation, amnesia, and patient comfort produced by intravenous and rectal diazepam, *J Oral Maxillofac Surg* 42:646-650, 1984.

37. Lundgren S: Serum concentration and drug effect after intravenous and rectal administration of diazepam, *Anesth Prog* 34:128-133, 1987.

38. Rovnborg M, Hasselstrom L, Ostergard D: Premedication with oral and rectal administration of diazepam, *Acad Anesthesiol Scand* 30:132-138, 1986.

Intravenous and Intramuscular Sedation

Daniel E. Becker
C. Richard Bennett

CHAPTER OUTLINE

Previous chapters provide conventional definitions that distinguish conscious sedation, deep sedation, and general anesthesia. Although these descriptions are invaluable for medicolegal and licensure matters, they have limited clinical usefulness for monitoring a patient's status. This chapter addresses intravenous and intramuscular regimens that enable the dentist to produce levels of sedation consistent with the concept of conscious sedation.

In a system for defining sedation levels, *conscious sedation* is descriptive of levels 1 and 2[1] (Box 16-1). Occasional drifting to level 3 must never be an intentional goal but is sometimes unavoidable with light sedation techniques. *Deep sedation* is descriptive of levels 4 and 5 (see Chapter 17). It is not synonymous with general anesthesia because local anesthesia is still required to perform surgery. (If patient does not respond to surgical stimulus, general anesthesia has been achieved.) Because deep sedation introduces a greater degree of risk for respiratory and cardiovascular depression, training to perform deep sedation should be comparable to that for general anesthesia.

Patient fear and anxiety introduce added difficulty while the dentist attempts to provide treatment. Clinicians and researchers continue the search for a "magic potion," operating within the paradigm that an answer lies in the selection of a perfect drug or drug combination. Suggestions have included a staggering number of single-drug and multiple-drug regimens, as well as alternative routes for their administration, including rectal and intranasal. None has achieved universal acceptance because no single drug or combination is suitable for all individuals and clinical situations. Most sedative agents can calm and sedate the anxious patient adequately, provided a sufficient

concentration is achieved within the targeted neural tissues. An understanding of the challenge of achieving an effective but safe drug concentration in the central nervous system (CNS) rests on an appreciation of fundamental principles of pharmacokinetics.

Pharmacokinetics

Pharmacokinetic processes influencing the intensity of a drug's effect include drug absorption, biotransformation (metabolism), distribution, and clearance, or elimination (Box 16-2).

Bioavailability refers to the portion of an administered dose that reaches the systemic circulation in active form, thereby available for distribution to target tissues. Variables that influence drug bioavailability can complicate this process, however, and several questions should be considered (Fig. 16-1). What concentration of drug is required within the targeted tissue (biophase) for a given patient, on a given day, for a given level of anxiety? What serum concentration will provide and sustain this target concentration? Sedative concentrations for midazolam range from 30 to

---

BOX 16-1

Levels of Conscious Sedation

Conscious Sedation
Level 1: awake and calm (no evidence of drowsiness)
Level 2: awake but sedated (slowed or slurred speech)
Level 3: asleep but easily aroused (verbally)

Deep Sedation
Level 4: asleep but difficult to arouse (shake, shout)
Level 5: asleep and unarousable (except by surgical stimulus)

Adapted from Becker DE: *J Am Dent Assoc* 119:153-156, 1989.

BOX 16-2

Pharmacokinetic Processes Influencing Conscious Sedation

Absorption
Process by which drug diffuses from the site of administration and enters the circulation. Final barrier is always capillary endothelium, but depending on route of administration, additional tissue barriers must also be penetrated. Absorption is obviated by IV administration.

Biotransformation
Molecular change of the parent compound. Most often occurs in the liver but may occur in plasma or other tissues. Metabolites may or may not have pharmacologic activity.

Distribution
Equilibration of drug from serum to body tissues. Extent is determined by drug's solubility in and perfusion of the tissue.

Elimination
Clearance of active drug molecules from the body. May be attributed to hepatic conversion to inactive metabolites or renal excretion.

100 ng/ml.[2] What dose must be administered to achieve this precise concentration (Box 16-3)?

Drugs administered by the oral (PO) route are subjected to hepatic metabolism before entering the systemic circulation. This "first-pass" metabolism, along with gastric degradation and varied rate of absorption, makes bioavailability of a PO drug unpredictable. A drug administered by intramuscular (IM) injection is not subjected to degradation or first-pass influences, but varied rates of absorption and elimination preclude any assurance that the peak serum concentration achieved will be adequate.

These issues are obviated when sedatives are titrated intravenously. Because bioavailability after intravenous (IV) administration is 100%, neither total dosages nor precise serum concentrations are germane; increments can be administered repeatedly until sedation is achieved. Such accuracy provides a level of safety and efficacy for this method of drug administration that is unmatched by any other technique, with the exception of inhalation agents. Although IV sedation may be more demanding technically, it is fallacious to consider it less safe than PO or IM regimens. It merely requires insertion of a needle or catheter into a vein, a procedure taught to technical staff having no formal academic training.

Effective levels of sedation are predicated on drug serum concentration, and therefore it is essential to

---

BOX 16-3   SUMMARY

Pharmacokinetics of Intravenous and Intramuscular Sedation

Effective sedation relies more on achieving adequate drug concentration in the blood than selecting the correct drug. The concentration required to produce adequate sedation is highly variable and cannot be achieved reliably by any route of administration that cannot be titrated.

The elimination half-life for sedative drugs has little influence on the actual duration of sedation. Both the time for onset and the duration of clinical effect are influenced more by a drug's lipid solubility. High lipid solubility enhances initial distribution to brain tissues but also accounts for a rapid decline in blood concentration as the drug distributes throughout adipose tissues.

After repeated doses of a sedative, adipose tissues become saturated, and serum concentrations approach steady state, allowing renal and hepatic clearance to play a more significant role in the decline of blood concentration.

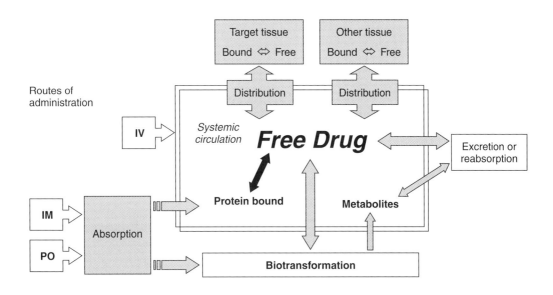

Fig. 16-1 Pharmacokinetics: concentration of drug at target tissue is determined by combined influences of absorption, metabolism, distribution, and elimination (excretion).

appreciate differences in the time-concentration curves for drugs administered by various routes. Stambaugh et al[3] studied meperidine after PO, IM, and IV administration (Fig. 16-2).[3] After IV administration the peak serum concentration is instantaneous and higher than that following either PO or IM administration due to absorption. Time to peak concentration is delayed after PO and IM administration. Furthermore, portions of drug absorbed initially can distribute and undergo clearance before final portions are absorbed, so peak serum concentrations are lower than those after IV administration.

Plasma half-life ($T_{1/2}$) is the time required for plasma concentration to diminish by 50%. After IV injection the decline in serum concentration occurs in two phases. The initial decline is rapid and attributed to drug distribution. This period of decline is regarded as *distribution half-life* ($T_{1/2\alpha}$) and is applicable only to IV drugs. Once distribution is completed, further decline in serum concentration becomes more gradual and is identical to that after PO and IM administration. This rate of decline is attributed to drug clearance and is regarded as *elimination half-life* ($T_{1/2\beta}$). The $T_{1/2\beta}$ for meperidine is approximately 4 hours (see Fig. 16-2) and provides the basis for two clinical correlates: (1) a drug may be considered completely eliminated after four or five half-lives, and (2) steady-state drug concentrations can be achieved after four doses, provided each is administered within one half-life (Fig. 16-3).

A common misconception is that $T_{1/2\beta}$ can be used to predict duration of sedation. Although the drug continues to be present in the blood for several half-lives, this does not identify the point at which the concentration falls below that required to sustain an adequate drug level in the target tissues. After repeated administration leading to steady-state drug concentration, time for elimination may become a more useful correlate. However, this is more often the case during chronic drug therapy, not when a drug is administered during a single dental procedure. If a serum concentration above 40 ng/ml is required to produce sedation, a drug's $T_{1/2\alpha}$ correlates more closely with duration of sedation (Fig. 16-4).

Both onset and duration of conscious sedation more closely parallel a drug's $T_{1/2\alpha}$, which in turn reflects degree of lipid solubility. The greater a drug's lipid solubility, the faster it distributes from the bloodstream through the blood-brain barrier and to peripheral adipose tissues. As serum concentration declines, this same property influences equilibration between body compartments and accounts for redistribution of drug from the brain back into the blood-

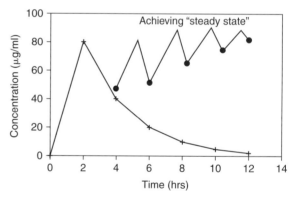

Fig. 16-3 gridded plot: Concentration (µg/ml) vs Time (hrs), labeled "Achieving 'steady state'"

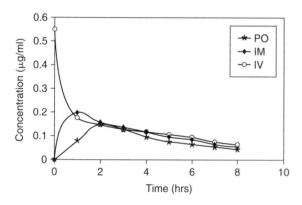

Fig. 16-2 Time-concentration curves for meperidine. Once the processes of absorption and distribution are completed, elimination of drug is identical regardless of the route by which it was administered. Principal differences are peak concentrations and time required to achieve this peak. (Modified from Stambaugh JE et al: *J Clin Pharmacol* 16:245-256, 1976.)

Fig. 16-3 Clinical correlates of elimination half-life. The following table summarizes data for a drug with half-life of 2 hours and peak concentration of 80 µg/ml at 1 PM. By convention the drug is regarded as essentially eliminated after four half-lives. Conversely, serum concentration will achieve steady state after four doses administered every 2 hours.

Time (PM)	Serum Concentration (µg/ml)	Percent Remaining
1	80	100
3	40	50
5	20	25
7	10	12.5
9	5	6.25
11	2.5	3.125

stream and into peripheral tissues. Therefore high lipid solubility provides fast onset but shorter duration. Greenblatt et al[4] have demonstrated this principle using diazepam, which is more lipid-soluble than lorazepam (Fig. 16-5). As expected, onset of sedation is faster for diazepam, but the duration of sedation is shorter, despite the fact that its $T_{\frac{1}{2}\beta}$ is four times that for lorazepam (80 versus 20 hours).

As steady-state serum concentrations are achieved, duration of sedation will generally increase because

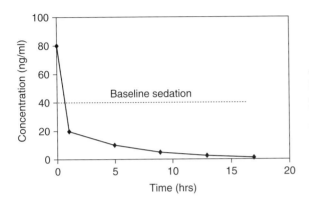

Fig. 16-4 Distribution half-life versus elimination half-life. Drug depicted has distribution half-life of 30 minutes but elimination half-life of 4 hours. Notice that distribution time correlates more closely with serum concentration adequate for sedation.

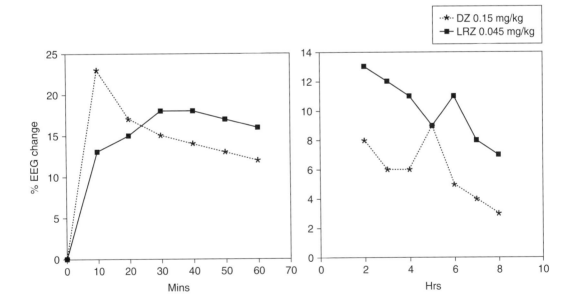

Fig. 16-5 Onset and duration of diazepam versus lorazepam. After IV administration, peak onset for diazepam *(DZ)* is 10 minutes, compared with 30 minutes for lorazepam *(LRZ)*. Although the elimination half-life for lorazepam is shorter than that for diazepam, its duration of effect is longer. This illustrates the influence of lipid solubility on time of onset and duration of effect; lipid solubility speeds onset but decreases duration of clinical effect. Both drugs have considerable lipid solubility, however, which accounts for the rebound effect observed between 4 and 6 hours. A fraction of any lipid-soluble drug can be concentrated in bile and subsequently excreted into the small intestine, where it is reabsorbed. Again, diazepam's greater lipid solubility explains the earlier onset of this phenomenon. (Modified from Greenblatt DJ et al: *J Pharmacol Exp Ther* 250:134, 1989.)

tissue depots become more saturated, and the decline in serum concentration will become more dependent on time for elimination. During IV sedation using midazolam or diazepam, the duration of sedation after the first few increments may last only 15 to 20 minutes, which corresponds to the $T_{1/2\alpha}$ for these drugs. During more lengthy appointments, however, subsequent IV increments may lead to progressively longer durations of sedation, which can be especially problematic during postoperative recovery.

Technical Considerations

Intramuscular Injection

For purposes of conscious sedation, IM injection offers few advantages over PO administration (Box 16-4).[5] Although negative influences of gastric degradation and first-pass metabolism are averted, a fixed dose must still be predetermined, and rates of absorption may vary to such an extent that effective serum concentrations are not attained. Indications for this route are limited essentially to patients uncooperative with oral regimens or circumstances in which IV access has failed. Nevertheless, skill in performing an IM injection may prove useful when administering drugs for other reasons. Examples include IM injection of antihistamines to counter minor allergic reactions or episodes of nausea and administration of depot glucocorticoid preparations to counter postoperative swelling.

Conventional sites for IM injection include mid-deltoid, vastus lateralis, and gluteal muscles. The first two of these are most appropriate in dental practice, with mid-deltoid for adults and vastus lateralis for children. Regardless of the dose selected, the total volume should not exceed 2 ml; use 1 ml if possible. For example, to administer promethazine 50 mg, inject 1 ml of a 50-mg/ml solution rather than 2 ml of a 25-mg/ml solution.

The gauge and length of the needle selected should be based on the viscosity of the solution and the size of the patient's muscle mass. Using the Z-track technique, a 1-inch, 23-gauge needle is adequate for most medications injected in dental practice (Fig. 16-6). The more commonly suggested 1½-inch, 21-gauge needle is required only for gluteal injections or when injecting more viscous solutions, such as procaine penicillin. For obese patients, longer needles are required for any site to obviate risk for subcutaneous administration.

Intravenous Infusion

Drugs can be administered intravenously by direct injection or heparin lock, but for conscious sedation it is preferable to use a continuous infusion. An IV infusion has three components: a physiologic solution, an infusion line or tubing, and a needle or catheter (Fig. 16-7).

Myriad solutions of water, glucose, and electrolytes are available, but the least expensive solutions are 0.9% normal saline (NS) and 5% dextrose in water (D5W). Although NS is less irritating, D5W offers the advantage of countering hypoglycemia during the perioperative period. This is a significant concern for dental patients receiving IV sedation because they are advised against eating solid foods within several hours of the appointment, and they may not eat well after procedures that leave their mouth sensitive. This consideration is also applicable to diabetic patients. A mild elevation in blood sugar produced by D5W 100 to 200 ml is insignificant compared with its protection against hypoglycemia.

BOX 16-4   SUMMARY

Technical Considerations in Intravenous and Intramuscular Sedation

IM sedation offers no advantage over PO administration, except for uncooperative patients. The volume of solution injected should be limited to 1 ml if possible and should never exceed 2 ml in the mid-deltoid and vastus lateralis muscles.

For IV infusions any physiologic solution is acceptable; D5W is preferred for diabetic patients to avoid hypoglycemia.

Ideally minidrip (60 drops/ml) infusion sets should be selected to better control infusion rate.

All supplies should be discarded after a single patient use.

Winged needles or catheters are acceptable for venipuncture and, for routine conscious sedation, do not need to be larger in diameter than 22 or 24 gauge.

When selecting a vein, avoid any arm that is disabled or contains a shunt. Veins located on the dorsum of the hand, forearm, or antecubital area are equally acceptable.

A

B

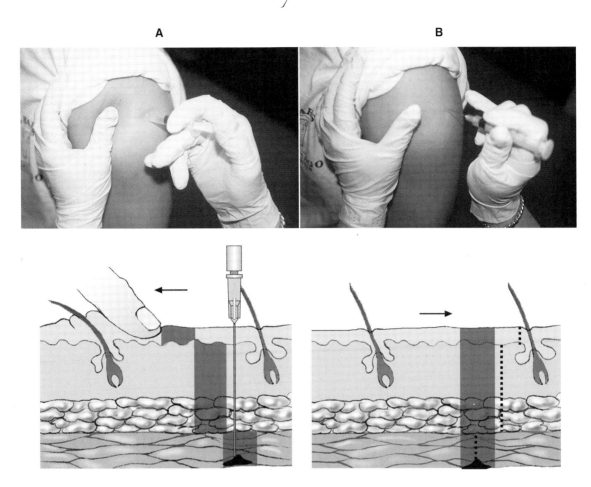

Fig. 16-6 Z-track IM injection technique. **A,** Before needle insertion, skin is drawn to the side. **B,** When needle is withdrawn, tension on skin is simultaneously released, which seals the track left by needle and confines the deposited solution within muscle. (Redrawn from Lambright Eckler JA, Stimmel Fair JM: *Pharmacology essentials,* Philadelphia, 1996, WB Saunders.)

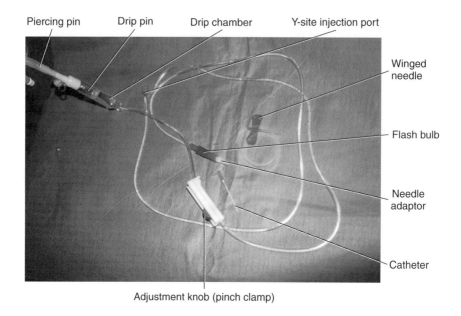

Piercing pin   Drip pin   Drip chamber   Y-site injection port

Winged needle

Flash bulb

Needle adaptor

Catheter

Adjustment knob (pinch clamp)

Fig. 16-7 Intravenous infusion setup.

The proximal end of an infusion set consists of a drip chamber and a piercing pin that inserts into the bag of solution. Fluid in the drip chamber prevents air from entering the remainder of the line, and a drip pin allows the dentist to calculate the amount of solution administered. These drip pins vary in size: 10, 12, 15, 20, and 60 drops/ml. Those delivering 60 drops/ml are called *minidrop* or *microdrop* chambers and are ideal for calculations; allowing an infusion rate of 1 drop/second will deliver 1 ml/minute or 60 ml/hour. At this rate, a 250-ml bag of solution is sufficient for procedures lasting as long as 3 or 4 hours.

The drip chamber is connected to various lengths of IV tubing, most often 72 inches, and has an adjustment clamp that can be positioned any place along the tubing to control the rate of flow. Some infusion lines have a short side port covered with a rubber diaphragm for introducing medications into the infusion line, called *Y sites.* The distal end is a rubber bulb and universal adapter that will connect to any needle or catheter. The bulb serves two purposes: it is an injection port for introducing medications, and it can be squeezed and released to allow flashback of blood to ensure IV patency.

Bags of solutions and infusion lines are disposable items and should not be saved for reuse. Physiologic solutions do not contain paraben or other preservatives to prevent bacterial growth. Furthermore, microbes and serum components can travel "upstream" to contaminate an infusion setup.[6-8] An average setup costs only $5 to $7; common sense, ethics, and medicolegal considerations mandate that disposable items be discarded after each patient.

The most simplistic needle for IV sedation is the *winged needle* or *scalp vein needle,* the most famous of which is the "butterfly" needle (Abbott). These needles are available in various lengths and diameters, ranging from 20 to 27 gauge. All have 1 to 3 inches of tubing attached, which is connected to the IV infusion line before venipuncture. The needle is inserted, secured with tape, and titration of medications can commence (Fig. 16-8). The disadvantage of winged needles is that they are rigid and sharp. After any sudden tension or movement of the arm or hand, the needle can pierce the side of the vein, leading to extravasation. For this reason, the patient's arm must be securely stabilized.

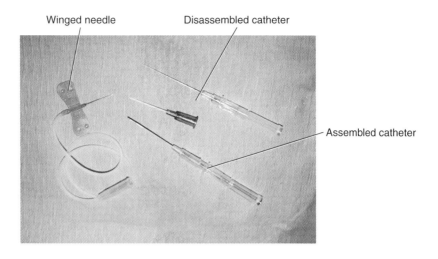

Fig. 16-8 Winged needle and indwelling catheter.

An *indwelling catheter* obviates the previous concern. These devices consist of a needle inside a flexible sleeve (catheter). The needle is inserted into the vein, the catheter is advanced forward over the needle, the needle is removed, and the IV line is attached to the catheter. Although more difficult to use from a technical standpoint, the patient's arm does not need to be stabilized because the catheter is flexible and cannot perforate the side of a vein. Once the infusion is established, extravasation occurs only if the catheter is withdrawn.

Technique. Before seating a patient for intravenous sedation, the operatory must be thoroughly prepared (Fig. 16-9). It is inconsiderate to seat apprehensive patients and allow them to observe final preparations for their procedure. If not ready to commence, the dentist should not seat the patient. Once the patient is seated, reconfirm his or her current medications and allergies, record vital signs, establish the IV infusion, and administer the first increment of medication. Delay excessive conversation until titration of sedation is in progress.

Venipuncture technique cannot be learned from a textbook; it requires hands-on, clinical instruction. The following information addresses only selected highlights for establishing an IV infusion. These suggestions reflect personal preference and should not be viewed contradictory to other methods.

Selection of either a winged needle or indwelling catheter is a matter of choice, as is the gauge and length of needle selected. Most who teach conscious sedation were trained by anesthesiologists in operating rooms where 18- to 20-gauge catheters are standard protocol because they allow for rapid infusion of physiologic solutions and large volumes of medications. These circumstances are unlikely in ambulatory settings during conscious sedation, and the novice will find that 22- and 24-gauge devices will allow adequate infusion rates and are less intimidating to insert.

The vascular anatomy of the upper limb varies considerably from patient to patient. It is more important to appreciate general characteristics of regions for venipuncture than precise names for particular arteries and veins. As with needle selection, selection of a vein is more a matter of operator preference, generally predicated on its size and stability. Veins in the antecubital fossa, forearm, and dorsum of the hand have key features (Fig. 16-10).

A tourniquet is placed proximal to the site selected. If a site is in question, place tourniquets on both upper arms, and allow a couple of minutes for maximal venous distention to aid with selection. A blood pressure cuff can be used in place of a conventional tourniquet and provides the ideal pressure required. Ideally, pressure should approximate diastolic arterial pressure, which will permit arterial flow into the arm

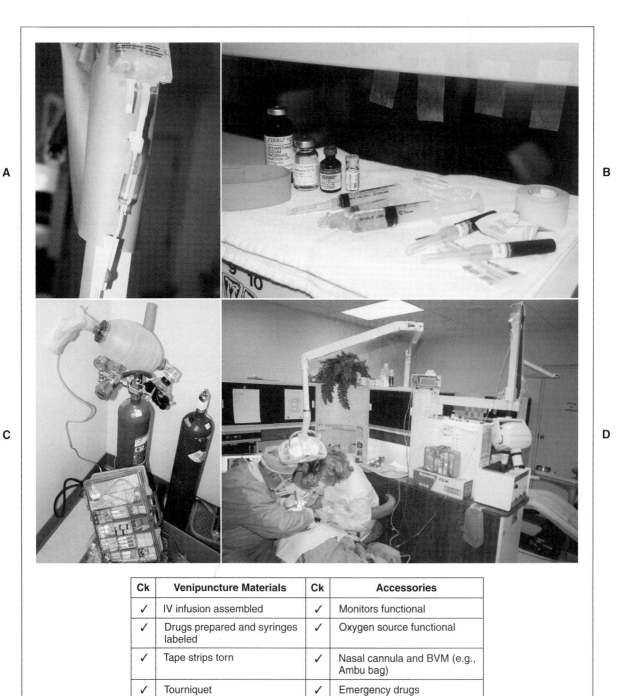

Ck	Venipuncture Materials	Ck	Accessories
✓	IV infusion assembled	✓	Monitors functional
✓	Drugs prepared and syringes labeled	✓	Oxygen source functional
✓	Tape strips torn	✓	Nasal cannula and BVM (e.g., Ambu bag)
✓	Tourniquet	✓	Emergency drugs
✓	Alcohol wipes, Band-Aids	✓	Additional suction tips

Fig. 16-9 A-D, Checklist for operatory preparation. *BVM,* Bag-valve-mask device.

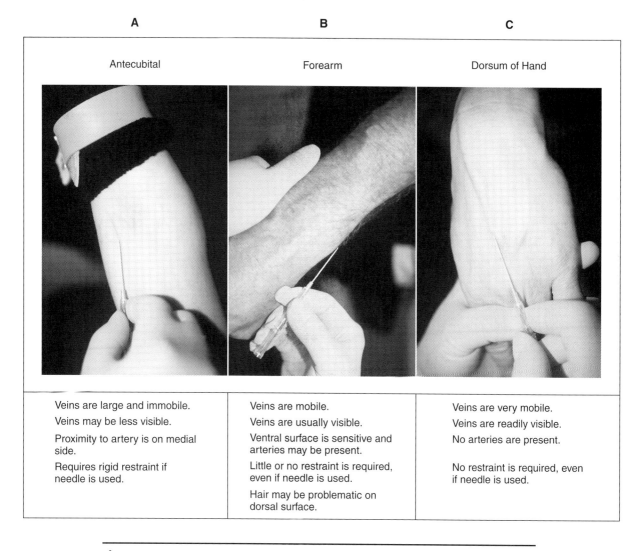

Fig. 16-10 Positive and negative characteristics of three venipuncture sites: **A,** antecubital; **B,** forearm; **C,** dorsum of hand.

but impede venous return. The tourniquet is placed on the forearm when the chosen site is the dorsum of the hand and on the upper arm if the venipuncture is to be in the forearm or antecubital fossa. Once the vein is selected, the site is swabbed with an alcohol wipe and the venipuncture performed (Fig. 16-11). For patients who are especially apprehensive regarding venipuncture, an oral sedative, nitrous oxide sedation, and topical ethyl chloride spray are options to consider.

If venipuncture appears difficult and multiple attempts are anticipated, it is wiser to make the first attempt at a more proximal site and proceed distally. This permits placement of the tourniquet distal to the failed insertion and is unlikely to promote formation of hematomas. A platelet plug forms within 1 or 2 minutes at the failed site, and there is little concern that medication administered at a more distal site will extravasate at the previously injured vessel. Alternating arms may be reasonable as well.

Take control of the arm using the thumb to tighten the skin distal to the anticipated side of entry. The thumb should be distanced so as not to interfere with any subsequent maneuvering of the angiocatheter required during venipuncture.

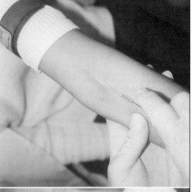

A

Once the vein is entered, back-flash of blood will be seen in the catheter's chamber. *Do not* stop at this point; advance the angiocatheter several millimeters further to assure that the catheter portion is well within the vein. At this point, use your index finger to advance the catheter ahead of the needle and into the vein. (For this to proceed smoothly, tension must be sustained on the skin with the left thumb.) The color of the catheter will darken as blood is able to flow between it and the needle. Once this occurs, the bevel of the needle is fully recessed within the catheter and cannot penetrate or tear the vein. Release the tourniquet and relax; the difficult part is over.

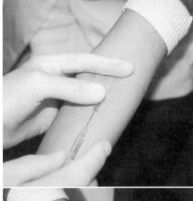

B

Using the index finger of the left hand, palpate the location of the catheter, and depress the vein just proximal to its end. Stabilize the hub of the catheter with the thumb and withdraw the needle. Some prefer to place a 2 x 2 gauze beneath the hub in case of leakage.

C

Connect the infusion line to the catheter, run solution at full flow, and advance catheter completely into vein before securing the site with strips of tape.

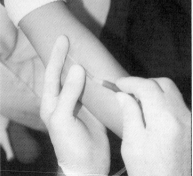

D

Fig. 16-11 Venipuncture using angiocatheter. After applying tourniquet and disinfecting venipuncture site, **A** to **D** sequence is suggested for right-handed operators.

Drug Selection

Many different sedatives, opioids, and adjunctive agents can be used for IV conscious sedation. The general pharmacology and characteristics for each of the categories of drugs should be thoroughly understood; drugs within each category are similar, and only minor differences make each agent unique, such as dosage and patterns of clearance (Box 16-5).

The practitioner first selects the category with the pharmacologic profile that generally fulfills one or more of the objectives (e.g., anxiolytic, sedative, amnesic, analgesic, antiemetic, anticholinergic). For example, the apprehensive patient who becomes sick from anesthesia might be managed with a benzodiazepine and antihistamine combination. The specific agent selected from each of these categories will depend on subtle differences the provider deems an advantage. Duration of action, expense, and pattern of clearance are likely to be considered.

To simplify drug selection, the number of categories of drugs useful for the production of conscious sedation is restricted here to three: sedative-anxiolytics, opioids, and miscellaneous agents. The miscellaneous category includes selected agents that are either unique unto themselves (e.g., ketamine) or are generally considered members of a pharmacologic category not primarily associated with the production of conscious sedation (e.g., droperidol).

When a multiple-drug technique is employed, the sequence of drug administration is largely a matter of personal preference. However, since sedative-anxiolytics are easily titrated to the desired effect, and since they alone may be used to produce conscious sedation, it seems logical to commence with one of these agents.

The titrated end point is reached when the patient is noted to be calm and relaxed. Eyelids droop, mild nystagmus may be seen, and speech may be notably slurred. Many patients will comment on their feelings and describe precisely what they are experiencing. If no remarks are made voluntarily, the patient should be questioned about the effects. Typically, patients may relate losing train of thought or having visual effects, such as double vision, difficulty in focusing the eyes, or a sense that objects in the room are moving.

The principal goal in conscious sedation is to calm and relax the apprehensive patient, which not only benefits the patient but also the doctor and auxiliary personnel. For this reason, the primary category of drug in any regimen should be one having sedative and/or anxiolytic properties. Drug classes within this category include benzodiazepines, barbiturates, and antihistamines. As CNS depressants, they produce several side effects in common, including respiratory depression, hypotension, and a potential for paradoxical excitation. Each of the classes differs in their frequencies for producing these and other effects (Table 16-1).

Benzodiazepines

The most frequently used sedative agents are benzodiazepine derivatives. They are believed to exert their effects by enhancing the chloride channel gating function of gamma-aminobutyric acid (GABA) by facilitating the binding of this inhibitory neurotransmitter to its receptors.[9] This leads to hyperpolarization of the cell membrane, making the neuron resistant to excitation (see Chapter 9).

Principal advantages of this class are their relative safety and ability to produce anterograde amnesia. Benzodiazepines have a high therapeutic index and a

---

BOX 16-5   SUMMARY

Drug Selection in Intravenous and Intramuscular Sedation

A sedative, preferably a benzodiazepine, should be the foundation of any conscious sedation regimen. In most cases a benzodiazepine will be the only drug required.

Opioids may be added to the regimen to potentiate a poor response to conventional doses of a benzodiazepine or to diminish noxious stimulation from local anesthetic injections.

Antihistamines may be added to the regimen to potentiate a poor response to conventional doses of a benzodiazepine or to offset nausea in susceptible patients.

Opioids are the most significant respiratory depressants of all drug classes used for conscious sedation.

TABLE 16-1

Three Principal Classes of Sedative-Anxiolytics

	Benzodiazepines	Barbiturates	Antihistamines
Anxiolytic efficacy	+++	ND	ND
Sedative efficacy	+++	+++	++
Safety	++	+	+++
Anticonvulsant	+++	+++	0
Anticholinergic	0	0	++
Anterograde amnesia	+++	0	0
Antiemetic	0	0	++

0, None; + to +++, least to greatest; *ND*, no data available.

relatively shallow dose-response curve. A high therapeutic index means that the dose of the agent required to produce desired effects is considerably less than that required to produce undesirable ones. Furthermore, the shallow dose-response indicates that a dose required to produce conscious sedation is well below that required to produce hypnosis (unconsciousness). This concept can be illustrated by comparing dose-response curves for midazolam and diazepam (Fig. 16-12).

In addition to the anxiolytic, sedative, and amnestic effects, benzodiazepines may indirectly elevate the patient's threshold for pain. This does not mean that they are analgesics, but the patient appears to reach a state of mental indifference. In this altered state, many patients are less perturbed by mild noxious stimulation that might otherwise be distressing.

Diazepam is conventionally regarded as the prototypic benzodiazepine with which others are compared. Only two other drugs in this category, midazolam and lorazepam, are available for parenteral administration. Lorazepam has very low lipid solubility, which delays its onset to such an extent that titration to sedative end point is difficult. After IV injection, peak onset may require 20 to 30 minutes.[4] Furthermore, lorazepam produces an extended duration of effect that may be troublesome in the ambulatory setting (see Fig. 16-5). For these reasons, diazepam and midazolam are the agents preferred for IV conscious sedation (Table 16-2).

Diazepam frequently causes some pain on IV injection. To reduce this discomfort and patient concern, diazepam should be administered into a rapid

IV infusion at a rate so slow that no discomfort is noted. The largest vein accessible should be selected for venous cannulation. Veins on the dorsum of the hand should be avoided when possible.

Diazepam undergoes hepatic biotransformation to active metabolites, nordiazepam and oxazepam. These products may be concentrated in bile and secreted into the gut, where they are reabsorbed.[4] This resorption may result in a subsequent, although much smaller, peak effect several hours after a single IV dose of diazepam.

Midazolam is water soluble in solution. Unlike diazepam, midazolam is not mixed with propylene glycol and thus is painless on injection. Once injected and exposed to physiologic pH, however, its molecular structure assumes a highly lipid-soluble configuration.[10] Compared with both diazepam and lorazepam, midazolam is not only more lipid soluble but also has shorter distribution and elimination half-lives. These are similar for the parent compound and its only active metabolite, α-hydroxymidazolam.[10,11] Compared with diazepam, midazolam produces a more rapid onset, a shorter duration, and a greater degree of amnesia.[12]

As with all benzodiazepines, midazolam's influence on respiration and circulation is minimal at customary doses, but large doses, such as those employed for anesthetic induction, may reduce systemic blood pressure by approximately 10%.[13,14] After its introduction for general use, however, a significant number of mishaps still were associated with the use of midazolam in conscious sedation.[15] Virtually all these cases can be explained by failure

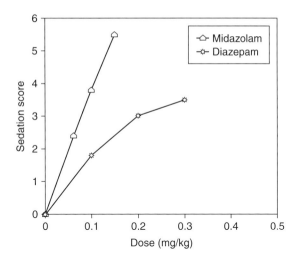

Fig. 16-12 Comparative potencies of midazolam and diazepam. Sedation score: *1,* awake, to *6,* asleep and unarousable verbally. To produce a sedation score of 2, the potency of midazolam is approximately twice that of diazepam (0.05 versus 0.1 mg/kg). At deeper levels of sedation, however, the difference in potency increases. At sedation scores 3 to 4 the potency of midazolam becomes three times that for diazepam (0.1 versus 0.3 mg/kg). This difference would become even greater if dosages of diazepam had been increased enough to produce sedation scores of 4 or 5. (*From White PF et al:* Plast Reconstr Surg *81:703-712, 1988.*)

TABLE 16-2

Midazolam and Diazepam in Conscious Sedation

Characteristics	Midazolam	Diazepam
Pharmacokinetics		
Active metabolites*	No	Yes
Distribution half-life†	6-15 min	30-60 min
Elimination half-life	2-4 hr	24-96 hr
Onset (approx)	30 sec	60 sec
Duration (approx)	20-60 min	30-60 min
Pharmacodynamics		
Unique effects	Mild hypotension	Thrombophlebitis
Potency	1-2 mg	5 mg
Concentration	1 and 5 mg/ml	5 mg/ml
IV increment	1 mg	2.5-5 mg

*Active metabolites of midazolam (1- and 4-hydroxymidazolam) have shorter elimination half-lives than the parent drug. Active metabolite of diazepam (nordazepam, formerly desmethyldiazepam) has a much longer half-life than the parent drug.
†Distribution half-life is more predictive of duration of clinical effect than elimination half-life.

to recognize its potency compared with diazepam, as well as its use in combination with opioids. The manufacturer further complicated matters by marketing the agent initially as a concentration identical to that of diazepam (5 mg/ml), rather than the 1-mg/ml concentration now recommended for IV use. Use of the 5-mg/ml concentration should be reserved for IM administration.

Estimates of midazolam potency vary from two to five times that of diazepam. A comparison of the potencies of diazepam and midazolam found that the dose-response for diazepam was much more gradual.[16] As doses were increased, the difference in their potencies was greater (see Fig. 16-12). This finding provides one explanation for the disagreement regarding equipotent doses reported in the scientific literature. Furthermore, these results confirm present guidelines to carefully titrate this agent in 1-mg increments. This increment should be halved during prolonged cases or when managing geriatric patients and those with significant medical compromise.

The dentist must be particularly careful when administering any drug intravenously to an elderly patient. Benzodiazepines in general, and midazolam in particular, are more likely to produce respiratory and cardiovascular depression in this population. In all probability, age-related reductions in hepatic blood flow and reduced enzyme effectiveness make elderly patients particularly sensitive to midazolam's effects.[17]

Although seldom required, the effects of the benzodiazepines may be reversed within 2 minutes of IV administration by a competitive antagonist.[18] *Flumazenil* (Romazicon) is a selective receptor antagonist that effectively reverses somnolence and respiratory depression attributed to benzodiazepines.[11] It has no affinity for other receptors within the GABA receptor complex, and it will not reverse the actions of drug classes acting at these sites. Flumazenil is prepared as a 0.1 mg/ml concentration in either 5-ml or 10-ml vials. It can be administered intravenously in 0.2-mg increments every 3 to 5 minutes, up to a total dosage of 1 mg. Duration of reversal ranges from 20 to 60 minutes, which could permit resedation if large doses of benzodiazepine have been administered. To manage excessive somnolence or respiratory depression, the dentist first provides standard airway support, including supplemental oxygenation and ventilation. Flumazenil is contraindicated for patients dependent on benzodiazepines and those with a history of panic-anxiety disorders or convulsive seizures.

Barbiturates

In general, barbiturates are less appropriate than benzodiazepines for conscious sedation. The dose-response curve of barbiturates is relatively steep, and without careful administration, unconsciousness is easily produced. This is particularly true for methohexital, which is used more often as an induction agent for general anesthesia. The production of unconsciousness during sedative procedures is fraught with danger and enhances the risk for respiratory arrest, upper airway obstruction, and subsequent anoxia.

Barbiturates lower pain threshold and therefore are regarded as hyperalgesic. When sedated patients experience pain, they frequently become excitable and even combative. Despite the apparent drawbacks, drugs such as methohexital and pentobarbital are useful agents for the production of conscious sedation.

The pharmacology of methohexital and pentobarbital are nearly identical, differing mainly in duration of action. In sedative doses, *methohexital* has a clinical duration of 5 to 7 minutes, whereas that of *pentobarbital* is 1 to 1½ hours. Titration of pentobarbital should proceed using 25- to 50-mg increments.

Methohexital is particularly useful because its short duration permits rapid recovery after its last bolus administration. In addition, its initial effect is seen in one arm-to-brain circulation time (~17 seconds). This attribute permits quick and accurate titration. In a multidrug sedation technique, methohexital should be administered last. Its rapid onset permits "fine tuning" that is more precise than with other agents. Methohexital should be administered in 10-mg increments until sleepiness, slurred speech, and nystagmus are noted. The drug may also be administered via continuous infusion in doses of 25 to 50 µg/kg/min. However, any CNS depressant administered by continuous infusion requires constant vigilance. It should never be attempted by the same clinician who is also providing treatment.

Antihistamines

All traditional antihistamines act as antagonists at H_1 and cholinergic (muscarinic) receptors, which presumably accounts for their sedative and antiemetic influences. At conventional doses, respiratory depression and hemodynamic influences are negligible, but their efficacy as sedatives is also minimal at best. Peripheral anticholinergic side effects and a central anticholinergic syndrome, including delirium, preclude the use of higher doses to achieve greater sedation. The sedative effects of antihistamines, although modest, are additive to those of other CNS depressants.

Antihistamines (H$_1$ blockers) such as *diphenhydramine* (25 to 50 mg) and *promethazine* (25 to 50 mg) are often suggested for preoperative sedation (Table 16-3). Although their sedative efficacy is inferior to that of benzodiazepines and barbiturates, the anticholinergic and antiemetic actions of antihistamines may have prophylactic as well as therapeutic application.

Unlike diphenhydramine, promethazine also has antagonist activity at central dopaminergic receptors. This activity would appear advantageous in terms of antiemetic influences when managing nausea and vomiting associated with the postoperative use of opioid analgesics. However, this action presumably accounts for a higher incidence of agitation and delirium compared with that observed with diphenhydramine. Consistent with other phenothiazine derivatives, promethazine has some ability to block α-adrenergic receptors on vascular smooth muscle, which introduces a risk for postural hypotension.

Two CNS disorders should be considered when using any drug with anticholinergic action. *Parkinson's disease* is a disorder within the basal ganglia attributed to a relative dopamine deficiency and acetylcholine excess. Antihistamines are a desirable component of conscious sedation regimens for patients with Parkin-

son's disease, provided they are not currently receiving other anticholinergic medication. Diphenhydramine has been suggested for this purpose.[19] Promethazine, as with other phenothiazine derivatives, should be avoided because it possesses modest but significant dopaminergic blocking activity. *Alzheimer's disease* is poorly understood but associated with deficient cholinergic transmission. Agents with significant anticholinergic action should be avoided in patients with evidence of significant dementia or Alzheimer's disease.[20]

Opioids

Opioids are typically included in conscious sedation regimens despite a conspicuous lack of scientific studies that confirm any advantage to using sedatives alone. In one of the few studies addressing this issue, Dionne[21] demonstrated a positive effect when managing difficult patients but otherwise found that opioids provided little advantage over single-drug, sedative-anxiolytic regimens. Many putative benefits derived from opioids in conscious sedation regimens are difficult to measure scientifically. Subjectively, they produce a sense of well-being (euphoria) and an unrealistic freedom from fear. Because patients receive local anesthesia, any need for analgesia is usually minimal. During long and difficult appointments, however, dental procedures may result in annoying, noxious stimulation that is attenuated by opioids.

TABLE 16-3

Antihistamines in Conscious Sedation

Characteristics	Diphenhydramine	Promethazine
Pharmacokinetics		
Active metabolites	No	No
Duration	4-6 hr	4-6 hr
Pharmacodynamics		
Muscarinic blockade	+	+
Histaminic blockade	+	+
Dopaminergic blockade	0	+
α-Adrenergic blockade	0	+
Unique effects		Agitation, delirium, hypotension
Concentration	10 and 50 mg/ml	25 and 50 mg/ml
IV increment	25 mg × 2 times	25 mg × 2 times

Sitting motionless for long periods with the mouth open wide can be equally uncomfortable.

Despite some controversy, the use of opioids in anesthesia and conscious sedation is entrenched on an empiric basis, predicated on several confirmed influences. The sedative effect of opioids is synergistic with that of benzodiazepines, and analgesia may diminish the discomfort associated with local anesthetic injections. Furthermore, opioids are viewed as "cardioprotective" because they obtund sympathetic reflexes to noxious stimuli. This influence is beneficial in particular for patients with hypertension, tachyarrhythmias, and ischemic heart disease. Considering the relative safety of conventional doses, it is difficult to contradict their use in carefully titrated conscious sedation regimens.

Opioids mediate sedation at both mu and kappa receptors (see Chapter 8), but this effect is less intense and more unpredictable than that provided by more traditional sedative-anxiolytics. However, drug combinations may result in profound synergism. Vinik et al[22] confirmed a dramatic, dose-dependent reduction in the hypnotic median effective dose (ED_{50}) when combining midazolam with either propofol or alfentanil (Fig. 16-13). Depression of respiratory centers parallels that in other brain regions, providing further insight into the added respiratory depression consistently observed when benzodiazepines and opioids are combined.

Although all opioids have a potential for producing respiratory depression, this concern is overstated for the conservative doses recommended for conscious sedation. *Meperidine* and *fentanyl* are the opioids used most frequently in conscious sedation regimens, but the agonist-antagonist, *nalbuphine*, has gained considerable popularity. At the conventional dosages used for analgesia and conscious sedation, few if any differences exist in their sedative effects.

Compared with meperidine, the principal advantage of fentanyl rests on its brief duration of action (30 to 45 minutes) and lack of histamine release. However, this must be weighted against a steeper dose-response during titration and its potential for producing skeletal muscle rigidity. Fentanyl is extremely potent (25 µg is approximately equipotent to meperidine 25 mg) and must be administered with great care.

Fentanyl (and its derivatives) can produce truncal rigidity of the chest wall in doses as small as 50 µg.[23]

A patient experiencing chest rigidity is unable to breathe, even when conscious, and cannot be ventilated manually. The incidence and severity of muscle rigidity increase after rapid infusion of opioids and by the addition of nitrous oxide. The precise mechanism is unknown but, based on its reversal by naloxone, is believed to be mediated by mu receptors in the caudate nucleus.[24] The appropriate use of naloxone is addressed later.

The agonist-antagonist opioids do not produce euphoria and even provoke dysphoria and delirium in some patients. Agonist-antagonists such as nalbuphine offer several advantages, however, demonstrating a ceiling dose-response curve that diminishes the risk for significant respiratory depression. Furthermore, nalbuphine has little potential for abuse and is not categorized by the U.S. Drug

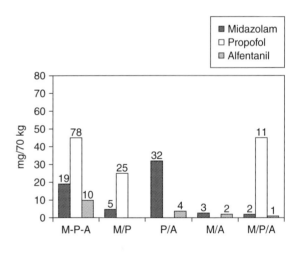

Fig. 16-13 Synergistic effects of central nervous system *(CNS)* depressants. The first group of bars *(M-P-A)* reflects the dosage of midazolam, propofol, and alfentanil required individually to render 50% of patients unconscious (hypnotic ED_{50}). The remaining groups of bars illustrate the dramatic reduction in dosage required when one drug was combined with another. Individually, midazolam (19 mg/70 kg) and alfentanil (10 mg/70 kg) were required to render 50% of patients unconscious. When combined, however, only 3 mg/70 kg of midazolam and 2 mg/70 kg alfentanil were required (see M/A). These dramatic reductions in dosage confirm the synergistic influences of CNS depressants on one another. (Modified from Vinik HR, Bradley EL, Kissin I: *Anesth Analg* 78:354-358, 1994; with dosages modified from mg/kg to mg/70 kg.)

Enforcement Administration (DEA) as a class II narcotic. Nalbuphine is unscheduled and can be purchased without the DEA forms required when ordering meperidine or fentanyl. Because it lacks euphoric influences, nalbuphine is ideal for patients having a prior history of drug abuse. However, nalbuphine must be avoided if a patient has evidence of current opioid dependence, because its action as an antagonist at mu receptors can precipitate symptoms of withdrawal. Like fentanyl, nalbuphine does not mediate histamine release. This eliminates the annoyance of facial flushing and pruritus and reduces the risk for hypotension. In this regard, meperidine triggers greater release of histamine than most conventional opioids.[25]

Whether to administer the opioid before or after the primary sedative in the regimen is a matter of personal preference. Some prefer to administer the opioid after achieving initial sedative end point with a benzodiazepine. The end point when titrating an opioid in this sequence is the production of a feeling of comfort and pleasantness. Others prefer to commence by administering a predetermined increment of opioid for analgesic purposes. In this case the dentist should anticipate little subjective evidence of sedation and euphoria because these influences are unpredictable with opioid titration. The desired end point will follow subsequent titration of the primary sedative agent.

Meperidine, nalbuphine, and fentanyl are the three opioids typically used for conscious sedation (Table 16-4). The degree of sedation they produce is unpredictable, however, and therefore dosage should be limited to two or three increments as a supplement to a carefully titrated sedative-anxiolytic.

Naloxone is the prototypic opioid receptor antagonist. It is capable of reversing the influences of both endogenous (e.g., endorphins) and exogenous opioids. Naloxone effectively reverses all opioid effects, including analgesia, so the dentist must anticipate a sudden onset of pain and associated sympathetic responses if adequate local anesthesia is not present. In such patients, naloxone should be titrated cautiously in 0.1-mg increments until ventilation is restored. Its duration is approximately 30 minutes, and some prefer to follow reversal with a 0.4-mg IM dose that provides subsequent protection.

Although only a matter of curiosity for those using conscious sedation, agonist-antagonists such as nalbuphine can be used to reverse respiratory depression produced by high doses of conventional mu agonists. These agents can reverse the powerful influences mediated at mu receptors while continuing to provide

TABLE 16-4

Opioids in Conscious Sedation

Characteristics	Meperidine	Nalbuphine	Fentanyl
Pharmacokinetics			
Metabolites	Normeperidine	None	Unknown
Elimination half-life	3-8 hr	2-3 hr	3-8 hr
Duration (IM)	3-5 hr	4-6 hr	1-2 hr
Pharmacodynamics			
Mu receptor	++	−	++
Kappa receptor	+	++	+
Unique effects	Anticholinergic, negative inotropic, histamine release	Withdrawal syndrome in opioid-dependent patients	Skeletal muscle rigidity
Relative potency	50 mg	2.5-5 mg	0.05 mg
Concentration	50 and 100 mg/ml	5 mg/ml	0.05 mg/ml
IV increment	25 mg × 4 times	5 mg × 3 times	0.025 mg × 4 times

analgesia at the kappa receptors. This is a major advantage over naloxone after a general anesthetic, when surgical pain could be suddenly unmasked.

Propofol

Propofol (Diprivan) is a relatively new nonbarbiturate hypnotic that may be used, as is methohexital, for the production of conscious sedation or the induction of general anesthesia. Both agents are currently being touted for the maintenance of general anesthesia via continuous infusion in doses four to six times those used for sedative purposes.[26,27] Invariably, other agents (e.g., opioids, muscle relaxants) must accompany these agents for the sustained production of general anesthesia (see Chapter 10). Dosage ranges and serum concentrations for conscious sedation are well below those required for general anesthesia and have been well documented.[27] Unlike methohexital, propofol is antiemetic. Its ability to produce anterograde amnesia is controversial, but a recent study found that propofol produced greater amnestic influences at sedative concentrations than thiopental but less than that produced by midazolam.[28] Propofol is a highly effective agent for conscious sedation, but its most efficient use in this regard, as well as in general anesthesia, requires continuous IV infusion. For this reason, propofol should not be used by those who are simultaneously providing treatment.

Ketamine

Ketamine (Ketalar) is generally considered a dissociative general anesthetic agent in IV doses of 1 to 2 mg/kg or in IM doses of 5 to 10 mg/kg.[29] The state produced is characterized by unconsciousness, amnesia, analgesia, catalepsy, maintenance of protective reflexes, and occasionally, vivid dreams. Ketamine is a derivative of phencyclidine, a known hallucinogen, which accounts for the dreams in 15% to 30% of adults receiving ketamine. These effects are effectively obviated by including a benzodiazepine in the regimen.

A technique using extremely low doses of ketamine produces the state termed *dissociative sedation*.[30] This state is characterized by maintenance of consciousness, mental and physical indifference, analgesia, "robotic" behavior, stable vital signs, and maintenance of protective reflexes. The technique is particularly well suited for obstreperous children and mentally impaired patients of all ages.

IM ketamine injections of 1 to 3 mg/kg produce a dissociative sedative state in 5 to 7 minutes that lasts about 15 to 20 minutes. The preferred alternative is the direct IV injection of a loading dose of 0.5 mg/kg, followed by the continuous IV infusion of doses ranging from 10 to 100 µg/kg/min. Because ketamine stimulates salivary and airway secretions, an antisialogogue should be included in the regimen. Glycopyrrolate, 5 µg/kg up to 0.1 to 0.2 mg, is a common choice.

During the procedure, as with all conscious or dissociative sedation techniques, local anesthesia must be relied on for operative pain control. Patients remain motionless throughout the procedure and generally have no reaction to the administration of the local anesthetic injections.

Patients capable of reason and understanding frequently behave "robotically." Requests to open the mouth, for example, may be followed immediately by exaggerated actions. Often the command being followed will last for an extended time before a reminder is required. Recovery from the dissociative sedative state to conditions suitable for dismissal will be noted in about 1 hour after termination of ketamine infusion.

Droperidol

Droperidol (Inapsine) and haloperidol (Haldol) are butyrophenone derivatives. Along with myriad agents having a phenothiazine structure, such as chlorpromazine (Thorazine), the butyrophenones are most noted for their antipsychotic action. These drugs are useful alone or in combination with other agents for the symptomatic treatment of schizophrenia and other chronic delusional disorders. This influence is mediated through blockade of dopamine receptors within the limbic regions, but this same action in other brain regions, as well as their proclivity for blocking additional receptors, accounts for a disturbing number of side effects (Table 16-5). Although butyrophenones are useful in the management of various psychoses, they cannot relieve situational anxiety. Patients given haloperidol, for example, may appear to be calm and relaxed while in a threatening environment (e.g., operating room, preoperative holding area), but when questioned postoperatively, they will almost uniformly state that the drug did little if anything to relieve anxiety. In conventional doses, 2.5 to 10 mg of IV droperidol or 5 mg of IM haloperidol, these agents are very long-acting.

The butyrophenones are useful in the management of combative patients or those exhibiting acute

TABLE 16-5

Effects of Neuroleptic Drugs

Receptor Blocked	Receptor Location	Resultant Effects
Dopamine	Limbic regions	Antipsychotic
	CTZ	Antiemetic
	Basal ganglia	Extrapyramidal effects
	Hypothalamus	Galactorrhea
Cholinergic	CNS	Sedation, antiemetic
	PNS	Constipation, xerostomia
Histamine	CNS	Sedation, antiemetic
	PNS	Antipruritic
Alpha	CNS	Sedation
	PNS	Postural hypotension

CTZ, Chemoreceptor trigger zone; *CNS,* central nervous system; *PNS,* peripheral nervous system.

hysteria seen frequently in emergency departments. When coupled with potent opioids (e.g., fentanyl), they may also be used to produce a state of mental indifference, termed *neuroleptanalgesia.* These agents may be administered to ventilator-dependent patients in an effort to improve their tolerance of an endotracheal tube and artificial ventilation.

Because of side effects, long duration, and lack of effect on situational anxiety, neuroleptics are not considered suitable for the production of conscious sedation. However, in the armamentarium of conscious sedation administration, these drugs are highly effective antiemetics.[31] At IV doses of 1.25 to 2.5 mg, droperidol is particularly cost-effective as an antiemetic and rarely prolongs recovery times at this low dose.

Complications

Intravenous conscious sedation is predicated on repeated administration of small doses of a drug while observing the patient's reaction to each aliquot. In other words, the drugs are "titrated" to effect. Administration of drugs using this technique nearly precludes any possibility of overdose. Nevertheless, the dentist must always practice standard principles of monitoring and airway support (see Chapters 11 and 12). This section addresses untoward events more uniquely associated with conscious sedation. Chapter 18 details management of other medical complications.

Delirium and Related Syndromes

Agitation, delirium, and combativeness are frequently associated with emergence from general anesthesia. On occasion, however, they appear during or after conscious sedation or on emerging from dissociative sedation. Although any of the drugs used to produce conscious sedation can produce this frustrating syndrome, nonpharmacologic factors are more often the cause and should be given first consideration, especially *pain* attributed to inadequate local anesthesia. Sedated patients may react to noxious stimuli disproportionately to the degree of stimulation, particularly if the sedatives either produce no analgesia (e.g., propofol) or lower the pain threshold (e.g., barbiturates). Adequate local anesthesia is key to the success of conscious sedation.

A second cause for agitation is *hypoxia,* which is very distressing to the conscious patient. Hypoxia may not be detected until cyanosis is observed or a pulse oximeter sounds. The astute observer should not rely on either of these parameters alone; often they are late indicators of a problem. Careful attention to the state of consciousness and observation of respiratory patterns and sounds from the nose and mouth will alert the attentive practitioner to potential hypoxia. Cautious drug titration and patient monitoring should preclude hypoxia of any significance.

Even in the properly sedated patient, however, certain procedures can result in hypoxia. The application of various restraints, such as a "papoose board," can restrict lung movement. Wrapping this device about the chest of a combative or misbehaving patient, such as a child or a developmentally disabled adult or child, can restrict respiration to the point of producing hypoxia. The resulting agitation may be perceived incorrectly as an indication for additional sedation. If care is not taken in these patients, the result will be inadequate ventilation from both chest wall restriction and respiratory depression, a fatal combination in reported cases.

A third reason for agitation is the *urge to urinate*. These patients cannot be properly sedated. Most are too embarrassed to inform the practitioner of their predicament, particularly when a trip to the rest room involves the cumbersome removal of monitors and interruption of dental treatment. To preclude this problem, all patients should be asked to visit the rest room before initiating treatments, and the IV infusion should be maintained at a minimum flow when not administering drugs. There should be little concern regarding any need to administer fluids to offset food and fluid restrictions imposed preoperatively. Hypovolemia and hypoglycemia are extremely rare events. If fluid replacement seems necessary, it can be administered near the end of the procedure, when a trip to the rest room may be more easily accommodated.

The drug most likely to produce delirium, excitation, and perhaps bizarre behavior is *ketamine* (see earlier discussion).[32] The incidence of emergence delirium after general anesthesia produced by ketamine is reportedly as high as 30%. It is seen most often with patients over age 16, when administered in doses of 2 mg/kg or greater. Dreams, often frightening and surrealistic in nature, may accompany overt clinical evidence of dysphoria.[33] The incidence of these reactions is dramatically reduced by preceding ketamine with a benzodiazepine, such as diazepam or midazolam. Personal experience with the use of ketamine alone for the production of dissociative sedation has found negligible incidence of delirium. Patients rarely relate the occurrence of any dreams, and only four cases of agitation accompanied by unusual behavior have been noted. All four episodes occurred in patients with severe mental handicaps, and all were refractory to subsequent administration of benzodiazepines.

Sedative-anxiolytics, opioids, and neuroleptics are all capable of producing dysphoric reactions, even in conservative doses used for conscious sedation. When this event is noted, its treatment is mitigated by the nature of the offending agent. Opioids of the agonist-antagonist variety have the greatest propensity for this side effect, presumably due to their agonist activity at kappa receptors. The operator may elect to administer an increment or two of a benzodiazepine, but delirium attributed to any opioid will most likely require reversal with naloxone administered in 0.1-mg increments. Delirium attributed to benzodiazepines should be managed with flumazenil in increments of 0.1 to 0.2 mg. If necessary, treatment can be repeated at 15- to 20-minute intervals.

Delirium or dysphoria produced by methohexital is not reversible pharmacologically. Barbiturates are noted for their hyperalgesic influence, which means they reduce the patient's ability to tolerate pain. If local anesthesia is inadequate or the procedure is lengthy and produces postural discomfort, patients can become agitated and combative. Such events are generally brief and self-limiting, however, because of the ultrashort duration of action attributed to rapid redistribution. Provided local anesthesia is adequate, an increment or two of an opioid might be useful.

All drugs with anticholinergic actions (e.g., droperidol, diphenhydramine, promethazine) that are lipid soluble and cross the blood-brain barrier are capable of inducing the *central anticholinergic syndrome*. Symptoms range from restlessness and hallucinations to somnolence and unconsciousness. Excessive central cholinergic blockade can be countered with the lipid-soluble cholinesterase inhibitor *physostigmine*. Unfortunately, an increase in cholinergic activity throughout the peripheral nervous system results in parasympathomimetic side effects. This is obviated by pretreatment with glycopyrrolate 0.2 mg, a water-soluble anticholinergic that produces peripheral effects only. After waiting 2 to 3 minutes, physostigmine can be titrated in 0.5-mg increments every 2 minutes.

The *extrapyramidal syndrome* is characterized by involuntary movement of voluntary muscles. The practitioner typically observes uncontrolled yawning, protrusion of the tongue, torticollis, and other dyskinesias, such as twisting or restlessness of the arms and legs. The syndrome is most frequently produced by dopaminergic blocking agents of the phenothiazine or butyrophenone category, including those used for their antiemetic effects, such as droperidol, promethazine, and prochlorperazine. Although extrapyramidal symptoms are bizarre and may frighten the patient and practitioner, they are never fatal. As with Parkinson's disease, the extrapyramidal syndrome reflects not only a defect in dopaminergic pathways but also a relative excess of cholinergic transmission within the basal ganglia. For this reason the anticholinergic actions of diphenhydramine are useful for countering acute episodes.[19]

Local Reactions

Local complications associated with IV injection can be vascular or soft tissue in location and are more bothersome than serious. If ignored or left untreated, however, such sequelae may become problems of major concern.

Pain on IV drug injection is routinely seen with some medications (e.g., diazepam, propofol) and rarely or sporadically noted with others. Pain is more disconcerting than problematic. To prevent pain on IV injection, the following caveats can be useful:

1. Always choose the largest vessels of the arm that are convenient and readily accessible.
2. Be sure to inject medications slowly into a rapidly infusing system.
3. Before administration of agents likely to cause discomfort, consider first administering 2 to 3 ml of a local anesthetic that does not contain paraben or a vasoconstrictor.

Localized vascular *redness* may be noted in opioid-injected vessels due to histamine release, which may be accompanied by *itching*. No specific treatment is required because the condition is self-limiting. Diphenhydramine (25 mg) and lidocaine (10 to 20 mg), as described for pain, may be administered if localized itching persists. Success is variable.

Phlebitis is an inflammatory process of veins that is accompanied by pain, bruiselike discoloration of the vessel, increased local temperature, and ultimately, induration and decannulation of the vessel. Valves of the vein tend to become prominent and a concern to the patient. Generally, phlebitis is not caused by infection but by local irritation due to any foreign body that enters a vein. Phlebitis has been noted after simple needle insertion (e.g., blood sampling) and infusion of solutions or drugs approved for IV administration.

Treatment of phlebitis is palliative because the situation resolves in time. Warm, moist compresses may be applied 20 minutes/hour, a mild nonsteroidal antiinflammatory drug (NSAID) prescribed, and the limb "put to rest" (i.e., no exercise for a few days). If this is not successful, a glucocorticoid such as methylprednisolone is prescribed for 5 or 6 days. The patient should be thoroughly educated regarding phlebitis and its sequelae to prevent false assumptions that can lead to needless and costly visits to an emergency department or attorney's office. Patients must be assured that prominent valves are not foreign bodies on a fatal course to the heart. Although discoloration appears to be "traveling up the arm," it is innocuous and similarly not on a fatal journey. These two concerns have prompted patients to seek medical attention and receive treatment erroneously for cellulitis, with a litigious conclusion.

Infiltration or *extravasation* are terms used to describe the situation in which the IV needle pierces the skin but either does not enter the vein or exits and remains beneath the skin within soft tissue. This allows drug or IV fluids into the soft tissue, producing localized swelling. When this occurs, the needle should be withdrawn and firm pressure applied. The patient should be informed and any fears or concerns dispelled by explaining that fluid in the tissue will be absorbed over time. If discomfort persists, the condition can be managed as described for phlebitis. The same principles for managing infiltration can be applied to cases of hematoma.

On rare occasion, inadvertent *intraarterial needle insertion* may occur, but this can be avoided by palpating the area planned for needle insertion. Arterial puncture is readily apparent by the sudden and pulsating rush of bright-red blood into the catheter or into the tubing of an infusion set when the pinch clamp is released. The needle should be withdrawn and firm pressure applied to the site for 5 minutes.

If the dentist fails to identify that the needle lies within the lumen of an artery, and if inadvertent drug administration occurs, the patient will usually experience intense pain in the arm distal to the injection site. The sequelae include intense arterial spasm accompanied by pain, ischemia, and morbidity up to and including loss of digits or even the entire hand. If a medication is inadvertently injected into an artery, the needle should not be removed. Rather, 2 to 3 ml of a preservative-free local anesthetic should be infused into the vessel, which will help relieve the arterial spasm and reestablish blood flow. The patient should be seen in an emergency department for immediate evaluation and further treatment if required.

Air in the infusion line may be noted in the form of small bubbles and is a concern to many patients. These small amounts of air are harmless because they eventually mix with alveolar air. Relatively large volumes of air (e.g., >1 ml/kg) must enter the vascular system over a short period to cause major problems. Even large volumes may be well tolerated if they enter the system slowly.

If an IV infusion is inadvertently allowed to flow until the fluid bag empties, air will not enter because normal venous pressure will stop the infusion. The only time air in quantities of more than a few milliliters may enter the circulation occurs when one bag of solution is allowed to empty and is replaced with another. Air trapped in the tubing would be forced into the circulation by fluid flowing from the replacement container. Although this small amount of air would in all probability cause no harm, air remaining in the tubing should be removed. This can be accomplished by opening the pinch clamp and aspirating the air with a syringe inserted into an injection port on the IV tubing.

When mixed together in syringes or infusion lines, incompatible drugs may cause clouding of solutions. Drugs that are acidic (e.g., opioids) will precipitate into a milky white substance when combined with alkalis (e.g., barbiturates). It is generally considered inappropriate to inject such a suspension, although for the example mentioned, the drugs return to their original states when buffered by the bloodstream. Other drugs, however, form complexes that are not to be injected under any circumstances. Such incompatibilities are included in the manufacturer's package insert.

Some agents will form a cloudy suspension when mixed with virtually any fluid. Diazepam appears cloudy when injected into the IV tubing but apparently without problem; it becomes cloudy even when mixed with serum.

Preoperative Preparation

Preoperative preparation of the patient to receive conscious sedation should be distinguished from preoperative assessment or evaluation of medical status, including physical and psychological conditions, needs, and abilities to undergo conscious sedation (see Chapter 5). Patient preparation commences after this assessment process, ideally at an appointment preceding the one at which conscious sedation will be administered. Based on the medical assessment, the operator chooses the drug or drug combination to be used, the need for any premedication, and the administration route for conscious sedation.

Patient Education

Preoperative preparation can be initiated by explaining in lay terms the nature of conscious sedation and how it will benefit the patient. Fears of "losing control" and "not waking up" should be dispelled. Many patients want to "go to sleep" and "not know anything" about the procedure. These patients should be told that conscious sedation is a safe alternative to general anesthesia and that they will be pleasantly relaxed throughout, will have little recall, and will experience no discomfort. Patients who insist on general anesthesia usually relent when told that the reason conscious sedation is being employed rather than general anesthesia is because it is necessary for them to hold their mouth open.

Preoperative preparation continues by telling the patient to wear comfortable, loose-fitting garments, preferably with short sleeves. They must be told not to operate a motor vehicle or engage in other hazardous activities for 24 hours, and they must be escorted from the office by a responsible adult. Normal medications can generally be continued unless there is significant risk for interactions.

Dietary Restrictions: NPO Issues

Since drugs used for the production of conscious sedation are not emetics, and since protective reflexes will remain intact throughout the procedure, nausea and vomiting are not the concerns they once were. Historically, general anesthetics were notorious not only for the production of postoperative nausea and vomiting, but also for aspiration of vomitus during the course of the anesthetic. It was not unusual for the stomach of an adult to contain an average 60 to 65 ml of gastric acid at a pH of 1.0.

A logical preventive measure routinely taken was to make sure that the patient took no food or drink by mouth for 8 or more hours. In many cases, however, this protocol merely provided a false sense of security for the anesthetist. Nausea and vomiting are not necessarily precluded by dietary restriction. Many studies have found that patients are in a safer state when solid food is restricted but unlimited consumption of clear liquid is permitted for up to 2 to 3 hours before general anesthesia.[34]

The same or more lenient restrictions can be permitted when using agents with little propensity for inducing nausea and vomiting, and the patient maintains protective reflexes. This diet appears to be safe because clear liquids, particularly cold ones, promote gastric emptying and elevate the pH of gastric acid. The clear-liquid recommendation reduces gastric acid to approximately 25 ml at a pH of about 2.5. The reduction in volume and increase in pH preclude the development of pulmonary complications should aspiration occur.[35] Vomiting may be unpleasant but probably is not hazardous.

Informed Consent

Assuming that the suggested or similar preoperative patient preparation has been followed and that the patient understands and agrees to this protocol, the patient will have given informed consent. The patient has not been asked to sign anything at any time during the preparation process. Contrary to popular thought, informed consent need not be in writing. Similarly, asking a patient to sign a "consent form" does not, of itself, constitute "informed" consent. Patients may sign forms without reading or understanding the document they signed. Practitioners should not be lulled to a false sense of security by thinking that a signed form provides immunity or "protection" from legal action.

The dentist might ask patients if they have any unanswered questions, understand the procedure planned, and realize that certain complications, although unlikely, may occur. From a medicolegal standpoint, if the dentist always follows a particular protocol or presents information in a consistent fashion, the information need not be documented in writing. In most courts, rules of evidence permit evidence of a "habitual" or "routine practice" as admissible. Practitioners might want to keep a list of such habits and routine practices on file, however, in the event such information became an issue in court.

Discharge Criteria

Drugs for conscious sedation may produce sustained effects for 24 hours or more after completion of the procedure. At dismissal, patients may appear clinically "normal" but may have slight impairment in judgment, perception of depth and speed, or various motor skills. In this regard, the concepts of standards and guidelines must be distinguished. *Standards* reflect procedures that should be followed if the dentist is to avoid medicolegal consequences; variance from these standards would suggest an inferior standard of care. There are no "standards" for discharge of patients. In contrast, many *guidelines* have been published for discharge of surgical patients receiving sedation or gen-

---

BOX 16-6

Discharge Criteria after Conscious Sedation

At termination of procedure, the following criteria should follow in sequence:
- Record vital signs with patient fully upright in chair.
- If vital signs acceptable, discontinue IV infusion; apply pressure and bandage.
- Address all verbal instructions to patient's escort and provide a written copy, including avoidance of alcoholic beverages, operation of a motor vehicle or dangerous tools and appliances, and important decision making for the next 24 hours.
- Discharge to escort based on the following:
  1. Patient is awake or awake on command.
  2. Patient can breathe deeply and cough on command.
  3. Oxygen saturation is greater than 92% breathing room air.
  4. Blood pressure is 20% of baseline.
  5. Patient can ambulate with minimal assistance to vehicle.
  6. Patient has no postoperative nausea or vomiting.
  7. Patient has no pain.
  8. Bleeding is controlled.

Modified from Aldrete JA: *J Clin Anesth* 7:89-91, 1995; Marshall S, Chung F: *Curr Opin Anesthesiol* 10:445-450, 1997; and Kortila K: *Anaesthesia* 50S:22-28,1995.

---

eral anesthesia. Virtually all these guidelines, however, address procedures performed in hospitals and presume patients are discharged by means of a wheelchair to their awaiting vehicle.[36] A modified composite of these scales is suggested for discharge from the dental office (Box 16-6).

References

1. Becker DE: The respiratory effects of drugs used for conscious sedation and general anesthesia, *J Am Dent Assoc* 119:153-156, 1989.
2. Park GR, Gempeler F: *Critical care management: sedation and analgesia*, Philadelphia, 1993, WB Saunders.
3. Stambaugh JE et al: The clinical pharmacology of meperidine: comparison of routes of administration, *J Clin Pharmacol* 16:245-256, 1976.

4. Greenblatt DJ et al: Kinetic and dynamic study of intravenous lorazepam: comparison with intravenous diazepam, *J Pharmacol Exp Ther* 250:134-140, 1989.

5. Nicolson SC, Betts EK: Comparison of oral and intramuscular preanesthetic medication for pediatric inpatient surgery, *Anesthesiology* 71:8-10, 1989.

6. Kempen PM: Contamination of syringes, *Can J Anaesth* 37:730-731, 1990.

7. Parlow JL: Blood contamination of drug syringes used in anaesthesia, *Can J Anaesth* 36:S61-S62, 1989.

8. Trepanier CA et al: Risk of cross-infection related to the multiple use of disposable syringes, *Can J Anaesth* 37:156-159, 1990.

9. Richter JJ: Current theories about the mechanisms of benzodiazepines and neuroleptic drugs, *Anesthesiology* 54:66-72, 1981.

10. Reves JG et al: Midazolam: pharmacology and uses, *Anesthesiology* 62:310-324, 1985.

11. Olin BR, Hebel SK, Dombek CE, editors: *Drug facts and comparisons,* St Louis, 1998, Facts and Comparisons.

12. Wright SW et al: Comparison of midazolam and diazepam for conscious sedation in the emergency department, *Ann Emerg Med* 22:201-205, 1993.

13. Hemelrijck JV, White PF: Nonopioid intravenous anesthesia. In Barash PG, Cullen BF, Stoelting RK, editors: *Clinical anesthesia,* ed 3, Philadelphia, 1997, JB Lippincott.

14. Samuelson PN et al: Hemodynamic responses to anesthetic induction with midazolam or diazepam in patients with ischemic heart disease, *Anesth Analg* 60:802-809, 1981.

15. Bailey PL et al: Frequent hypoxemia and apnea after sedation with midazolam and fentanyl, *Anesthesiology* 73:826-830, 1990.

16. White PF et al: Comparison of midazolam and diazepam for sedation during plastic surgery, *Plast Reconstr Surg* 81:703-712, 1988.

17. Greenblatt DJ et al: Effect of age, gender, and obesity on midazolam kinetics, *Anesthesiology* 61:27-35, 1984.

18. Haefely W: The preclinical pharmacology of flumazenil, *Eur J Anesthesiol* 2:25-36, 1988.

19. Stone DJ, DiFazio CA: Sedation for patients with Parkinson's disease undergoing ophthalmologic surgery, *Anesthesiology* 68:821, 1988.

20. Dierdorf SF: Rare co-existing diseases. In Barash PG, Cullen BF, Stoelting RK, editors: *Clinical anesthesia,* ed 2, Philadelphia, 1992, JB Lippincott.

21. Dionne RA: Differential pharmacology of drugs used for intravenous premedication, *J Dent Res* 63:842-847, 1984.

22. Vinik HR, Bradley EL, Kissin I: Triple anesthetic combination: propofol-midazolam-alfentanil, *Anesth Analg* 78:354-358, 1994.

23. Vaughn RL, Bennett CR: Fentanyl chest wall rigidity syndrome: a case report, *Anesth Prog* 28:50-51, 1981.

24. Murphy MR: Opioids. In Barash PG, Cullen BF, Stoelting RK, editors: *Clinical anesthesia,* ed 2, Philadelphia, 1992, JB Lippincott.

25. Flacke JW et al: Histamine release by four narcotics: a double-blind study in humans, *Anesth Analg* 66:723-730, 1987.

26. Spelina KR et al: Dose requirements of propofol by infusion during nitrous oxide anesthesia in man. I. Patients premedicated with morphine sulfate, *Br J Anaesth* 58:1080-1084, 1986.

27. Shafer SL: Advances in propofol pharmacokinetics and pharmacodynamics, *J Clin Anesth* 5:14S-21S, 1993.

28. Veselis RA et al: The comparative amnestic effects of midazolam, propofol, thiopental, and fentanyl at equisedative concentrations, *Anesthesiology* 87:749-764, 1997.

29. Stoelting RK: *Pharmacology and physiology in anesthetic practice,* ed 2, Philadelphia, 1991, JB Lippincott.

30. Bennett CR: Ketamine. In Paris PM, Stewart RD, editors: *Pain management in emergency medicine,* East Norwalk, Conn, 1988, Appleton & Lange.

31. Santos A, Datta S: Prophylactic use of droperidol for control of anesthesia for cesarean section, *Anesth Analg* 63:85-87, 1984.

32. Reich DL, Silway G: Ketamine: an update on the first twenty-five years of clinical experience, *Can J Anesth* 36:186-197, 1989.

33. White PF, Way WL, Trevor A: Ketamine: its pharmacology and therapeutic uses, *Anesthesiology* 56:119-136, 1982.

34. Gilbert SS, Easy WR, Fitch WW: The effect of pre-operative oral fluids on morbidity following anesthesia for minor surgery, *Anesthesia* 50:79-81, 1995.

35. Haines MM: AANA journal course: update for nurse anesthetists—pulmonary aspiration revisited: changing attitudes toward preoperative fasting, *AANA J* 63:389-396, 1995.

36. Chung FC: Discharge requirements. In White PF: *Ambulatory anesthesia and surgery,* Philadelphia, 1997, WB Saunders.

CHAPTER 17

Deep Sedation and General Anesthesia

Morton B. Rosenberg

Leonard J. Lind

CHAPTER OUTLINE

After the first public demonstration of general anesthesia in 1846, anesthesia administered by dentists rapidly became an essential part of dental care for extremely apprehensive children and adults, patients with special needs and medical conditions that prevented access to routine dental care, and those requiring extensive surgical procedures. By definition, general anesthesia—a controlled state of unconsciousness accompanied by partial or complete loss of protective reflexes, including the inability to independently maintain a patent airway and respond purposefully to physical stimulation or verbal command—is dramatically different from conscious sedation. The depth of central nervous system (CNS) depression and the potential for respiratory and cardiovascular complications occurring during the administration of general anesthesia and deep sedation dictates meticulous monitoring, specialized equipment, comprehensive training of personnel, and specific patient selection criteria and preparation.

In 1985 the National Institutes of Health Consensus Conference on Sedation and Anesthesia in the Dental Office reaffirmed the necessity and the safety of office-based general anesthesia for dentistry.[1] The American Dental Association's Policy Statement on Sedation, Deep Sedation, and General Anesthesia in 1986 recognized the right of qualified dentists to provide anesthesia services for dental procedures. To emphasize the importance, complexity, and need for special competency in this area, guidelines for the administration of general anesthesia for dentistry have been developed by a number of dental specialty groups (American Dental Society of Anesthesiology, American Association of Oral and Maxillofacial Surgeons, American Academy of Pediatric Dentistry, American Association of Periodontology) and interested medical groups (American Society of Anesthesiologists, Academy of Pediatrics). Most importantly, state boards of dental registration and state legislatures have promulgated rules and statutes to regulate this unique area of dental practice.[2-5] Virtually all of these guidelines, rules, and statutes consider deep sedation and general anesthesia as medicolegally equivalent.

Anesthesia for dental procedures is most often performed in an office setting. Only in the last two decades have medical colleagues recognized the advantages of ambulatory surgery, and its acceptance by patients and physicians has been extraordinary, with more than 60% of all surgical procedures performed in the United States on an outpatient basis. This explosive growth has resulted primarily from decreased cost and resource utilization, as well as from fewer nosocomial infections, recovery in the more relaxed atmosphere of home, and decreased separation anxiety for children associated with overnight admissions. The development of anesthetic agents with rapid onset, shorter duration, and superior recovery profiles has aided in this growth. A further stimulus for growth has been the dramatic increase in dental and medical cosmetic procedures, in which the patients directly assume much of the cost. This trend shows no signs of abating, with medically compromised patients accepted as candidates and more extensive surgeries being contemplated.[6-8]

This chapter reviews deep sedation and ambulatory anesthesia in the dental office and topics in hospital-based anesthesiology. Mastery of general anesthesia is predicated on a solid foundation of related basic sciences (e.g., physiology, physics, pharmacology, anatomy) and clinical training with emphasis on patient evaluation, monitoring, and diagnosis and management of perioperative complications.

Preoperative Management

Patient Evaluation

The adage "never treat a stranger" is never more important than in a dental practice employing general anesthesia. A thorough preoperative evaluation is mandatory for each patient and consists of (1) complete past medical/surgical and drug use history, (2) focused physical examination, (3) psychological evaluation, (4) appropriate laboratory testing and consultations, and (5) determination of physical status and risk assessment. The medical history must include a review of systems with special emphasis on cardiovascular and respiratory symptoms, previous illnesses and hospitalizations, previous surgeries and anesthetics, determination of familial problems with anesthetics, allergies, current medications, smoking history, possibility of pregnancy, and "nothing by mouth" (NPO) status. A well-planned patient questionnaire is an excellent method for the initial gathering of information. This history must be reviewed by the dentist and positive findings explored in depth with the patient.

The history and focused physical examination complement one another. The physical examination helps detect abnormalities not readily apparent from the history, whereas the past medical history helps focus on the organ systems that need special attention. The main focus of the physical examination before anesthesia is on examination of the heart and lungs. Observation of cyanosis, clubbing of the fingers, dyspnea, body habitus, and airway abnormalities are of particular importance to determine suitability for office-based anesthesia. The importance of examining and evaluating the airway cannot be overemphasized. A brief psychological evaluation will alert the dentist to the need of preoperative medication and in developing an acceptable pain and anxiety control plan. Finally, consultation with the patient's physician to ensure that the medically compromised patient is stable and in optimal physical condition for the procedure planned is an important step in risk reduction.[9]

Routine preprocedural laboratory testing is costly, and the results obtained may not alter anesthesia or surgical plans. In recent years it has become evident that a minimum of preoperative screening is indicated for healthy patients scheduled for general anesthesia. Patients with significant medical disease (e.g., hypertension, coronary artery disease, diabetes) will need testing specific for their condition.[9,10] To be of value, the ordering of a preoperative test implies increased risk when an abnormality is detected and reduced risk when it is corrected. Controversy still surrounds the routine testing of fertile women for undiagnosed pregnancies to avoid exposure to the possible teratogenic effects of anesthetics on the fetus. Any woman who is unsure of her pregnancy status should be tested before anesthesia for elective procedures[10,11] (Box 17-1).

B°X 17-1

Anesthesia Preoperative Preparation

Patient History	Cardiovascular
Statement of current problem	Renal
Other known medical problems	Gastrointestinal
Medication history	Neurologic
Allergies/drug intolerance	Endocrine
Present drug therapy	Hematologic
Prescription	Psychiatric
Nonprescription	
Substance abuse	**Focused Physical Examination**
Tobacco, alcohol, illicit drugs	Vital signs
	Airway evaluation
Anesthetic/Surgical Review	Heart
Previous anesthetics, surgery, obstetric deliveries	Lungs
Family medical history	Neurologic
Familial anesthetic difficulties	Indicated laboratory testing
	ASA physical classification
Review of Organ Systems	
General: activity level and limitations	
Respiratory	

Physical Status Classification

The American Society of Anesthesiologists (ASA) physical status classification is the universally accepted standard for assessment of the operative patient. The classes generally correlate with perioperative mortality rates and are useful in planning anesthetic techniques, determining the degree of monitoring, and performing outcome studies (Box 17-2).

Once all preoperative data are collected and reviewed, a specific anesthesia plan can be developed and discussed with the patient. Written, informed consent can then be obtained after all questions have been answered, risks have been explained, and alternatives have been discussed. All this information must be included in a written preoperative note, including the results of the complete medical history, physical examination, appropriate laboratory tests, physical status, NPO status, consultations, anesthetic plan, and any potential complicating factors.

Generally only healthy (ASA I) patients or those with mild systemic disease (ASA II) are candidates for general anesthesia in the dental office. With the advent of improved monitoring and preoperative evaluation, selected ASA III patients (systemic diseases well controlled preoperatively) appear to be at no greater risk for perioperative complications than ASA I or II patients.[8]

Mortality and Morbidity

The risks of anesthesia are most often related to a combination of factors, including general health status and age of the patient, extent of the surgical procedure planned, anesthetic management, and experience of the surgeon and anesthetist.[9] Over the past two decades, there has been a steady decline in perioperative mortality and morbidity attributable to anesthetic causes, in both large dental and in-hospital studies (Table 17-1). This decline is a result of development and utilization of new monitoring techniques (especially oximetry and capnography), safer agents, and general improvement in anesthesia training and certification.[12]

Bⓞ**X 17-2** ⓦ

ASA Physical Status Classification*

Class I: normal, healthy patient
Class II: patient with mild systemic disease and with no functional limitations
Class III: patient with moderate to severe systemic disease that results in some functional limitations
Class IV: patient with severe systemic disease that is a constant threat to life; functionally incapacitated
Class V: moribund patient not expected to live 24 hours with or without surgery

*If the procedure is an emergency, the letter "E" follows the physical status class number.

TABLE 17-1 🖻

Mortality Rates in Outpatient Dental Sedation and Anesthesia

Author	Year	Deaths	Mortality Rate
Tomlin (UK)	1974	29/7,956,000	1/274,000
Driscoll (USA)	1974	11/5,285,570	1/480,500
Coplans (UK)	1982	63/14,473,000	1/229,730
Lytle (USA)	1989	7/4,711,900	1/673,000
D'Eramo (USA)	1992	2/2,082,805	1/1 million
D'Eramo (USA)	1994	0/1,500,000	0/1.5 million

After removing patient and surgical variables from mortality and morbidity data, attention has been directed toward studying anesthetic complications, which may be categorized as either preventable or nonpreventable. Of the preventable incidents, most involve human error, with the most serious anesthetic complications associated with adverse respiratory events (Box 17-3). Many critical anesthesia incidents only occur after a series of coincidental events, misjudgments, and technical errors. Strategies to reduce the incidence of these serious preventable anesthesia complications include the application of better and more specific monitoring, the introduction of improved anesthetic techniques and preoperative evaluation algorithms, and the adherence to more comprehensive treatment protocols and standards of practice.[13,14]

Fasting Guidelines

Preoperative fasting will reduce the risk of pulmonary aspiration of gastric contents during the induction and maintenance of anesthesia. Fasting guidelines have been in a state of flux in recent years because studies have reported that small amounts of clear fluid ingested 2 hours before surgery may *increase* gastric emptying. It is still a conservative recommendation that patients older than 5 years of age have no solid food for 8 hours before a procedure, but they may be allowed clear fluids up to 3 hours before surgery. Children ages 6 months to 5 years may have clear fluids up to 3 hours before anesthesia and no solid foods 6 hours before surgery.[15]

Patients should be instructed to continue essential maintenance medications, including β-blockers, calcium channel blockers, antiarrhythmics, steroids, and antibiotics. These medications can be safely given with small amounts of oral fluids.[9]

Aspiration Prophylaxis

Patients "at risk" for aspiration have been defined as having a minimum of 25 ml of gastric fluid of a pH less than 2.5. A number of clinical conditions place patients at risk for the pulmonary aspiration of gastric contents during anesthesia, including hiatal hernia, obesity, diabetes, gastric or duodenal ulcer, pain, narcotic analgesics, and esophageal reflux. Routine acid aspiration prophylaxis should be strongly considered for any patients who have any of these conditions before the induction of general anesthesia. The use of oral antacids, such as sodium citrate, oral and intramuscular (IM) or intravenous (IV) H_2-receptor antagonists (ranitidine or cimetidine), and metoclopramide, a gastrokinetic agent, have been advocated to reduce the risk of aspiration. Metoclopramide is an excellent choice in many cases because it not only increases gastroesophageal sphincter tone and accelerates gastric emptying but also has antiemetic properties and does not appear to prolong recovery.[16]

Several studies have suggested that outpatients are more at risk than inpatients. Prophylaxis against acid aspiration remains an area of intense controversy in outpatient anesthesia, with some authorities even advocating routine administration of oral antacids or H_2-receptor antagonists to all outpatients, especially for cases not using endotracheal intubation. Others, however, question the efficacy and cost/benefit ratio aspects of routine prophylaxis.[17]

Prophylactic Antiemetics

The many causes of nausea and vomiting in the postoperative period include preexisting medical conditions (e.g., diabetes, pregnancy), positive-pressure ventilation (e.g., air in stomach), drugs (e.g., nitrous oxide, narcotics, etomidate, isoflurane), specific procedures (e.g., head and neck), and other variables (e.g., history of motion sickness, time in menstrual cycle). *Droperidol* (0.625 mg intravenously) is an effective antiemetic if

---

BOX 17-3

Preventable Anesthesia Complications

Equipment Malfunction
Breathing circuit
Monitoring devices
Ventilator
Anesthesia machine

Human Error
Drug administration (syringe swap, dose)
Airway management
Unrecognized circuit disconnection
Fluid management

Associated Factors
Inadequate preparation
Inadequate training
Poor communication
Fatigue

TABLE 17-2

Benzodiazepine Premedicants: Diazepam and Midazolam

	Diazepam (Valium)	Midazolam (Versed)
Structure	1,4-Benzodiazepine	Imidazole ring
Solubility in water	Poor	Excellent
Organic solvent	Propylene glycol	None
Distribution half-life	30-60 minutes	15-30 minutes
Elimination half-life	20-40 hours	1-5 hours
Metabolites	Active	Active
Cardiovascular effects	Slight decrease in blood pressure	Decrease in blood pressure / Increase in heart rate
Thrombophlebitis at injection site	5%-30%	1%-5%
Pain on injection	23%	1%
Routes of administration	Oral, rectal, intravenous	Oral, intramuscular, intranasal, intravenous

administered preoperatively or intraoperatively, and it does not prolong recovery. The application of transdermal *scopolamine* 24 hours before anesthesia has received attention for patients at particularly high risk for nausea and vomiting. The serotonin (5-HT3) receptor antagonists (dolasetron, granisetron, ondansetron) are also very effective in decreasing nausea and vomiting but are very expensive.[18]

Monitoring

The basic elements of monitoring are reviewed in Chapter 11. All patients undergoing general anesthesia require a precordial, pretracheal, or esophageal stethoscope, blood pressure monitor, continuous electrocardiogram (ECG), pulse oximeter, and time-interval anesthetic record. Capnography (detection of end-tidal carbon dioxide) is mandated to confirm placement in all patients needing a tracheal tube. The ability to monitor temperature must be readily available. Monitoring standards are the cornerstone of all dental and medical specialty guidelines for deep sedation/general anesthesia.

Premedication

Premedication is often administered to reduce apprehension, anxiety, fear, pain, and oral secretions. In the past the use of premedication for ambulatory patients was not routinely recommended because of concerns about prolonged recovery. However, studies involving the preoperative use of oral diazepam (0.25 mg/kg), IM meperidine (1 mg/kg), IV fentanyl (1 to 2 µg/kg), IV midazolam, and oral midazolam for the pediatric patient (0.50 mg/kg) have not found delayed recovery after general anesthesia, supporting the judicious use of premedicants in ambulatory anesthesia.[19,20] IV midazolam has become the drug of choice in most situations because of its lack of venous irritation, predictable calming effect, and superior amnestic qualities (Table 17-2). Opioids may be indicated to treat preprocedural pain or musculoskeletal discomfort and to reduce the hemodynamic stimulation observed after laryngoscopy and tracheal intubation. When anticholinergic medication is required, *glycopyrrolate* (Robinul) can be given intravenously instead of atropine, without concern for postprocedural confusion or sedation, since it does not cross the blood-brain barrier due to its quaternary amine structure.

General Anesthesia Techniques

For dental procedures, general anesthesia can be provided with or without endotracheal intubation. In children, a mask induction may be preferred, with placement of an IV catheter after induction. For the adult patient, both techniques necessitate the placement of an indwelling peripheral venous catheter, and generally the induction of anesthesia is by this route. The choice for maintenance of anesthesia depends on the duration and complexity of the procedure, patient medical history and physical evaluation, and training of the dentist.

Nonendotracheal techniques are usually performed for procedures of relatively short duration, with oxygen or nitrous oxide and oxygen delivered through a nasal hood or nasal prongs in office-based practices. A dedicated anesthesia assistant is present to provide support of the head and maintain a patent airway. Care must be taken to avoid entrance of fluids (e.g., blood, saliva) into the hypopharynx to prevent laryngospasm.

An endotracheal tube provides an uninterrupted conduit for oxygen and anesthetic gases to enter the lungs while protecting the airway from the aspiration of foreign material. An evaluation of the airway is mandatory to ascertain possible difficulties in airway management and intubation.

Airway Evaluation

Prognostic signs of potential difficulties in airway management and intubation include prognathism and micrognathia; short massive neck; protruding maxillary incisors; limitation of temporomandibular joint from trismus, arthritis, trauma, or infection; long, high, arched palate associated with a long, narrow mouth; and limited mobility of the neck, especially extension at the atlantooccipital joint. A simple airway evaluation technique is determining the distance between the lower border of the mandible and the thyroid notch. If this distance is less than 6.5 cm in the adult, or equal to 6.5 cm with any of the predisposing factors just mentioned, difficult visualization and intubation of the larynx and trachea may be anticipated. Intubation scoring systems, such as those proposed by Mallampati, Cormack and Lehane, and Wilson, provide useful clinical information on the potential for difficulties in airway management.[21,22]

Head and neck position are important for intubation. The classic *sniffing position* (flexion of cervical spine and extension of head at the atlantooccipital joint) facilitates alignment of the long axes of the pharynx and larynx, improving visualization during laryngoscopy. When the larynx lies in a more anterior position, pressure on the cricoid or thyroid cartilage directed posteriorly may provide a better view of the larynx.[23]

Nasotracheal Intubation

Many dental procedures require the placement of a nasotracheal tube to provide unobstructed access to the oral cavity. The application of a vasoconstrictor to the nasal mucosa will reduce the likelihood of bleeding during tracheal tube insertion. Although dilute solutions of cocaine were used for this purpose in the past, most practitioners currently use a mixture of lidocaine and phenylephrine for topical anesthesia and vasoconstriction.

The method of choice for placing a nasotracheal tube involves passing the tube through the nares into the hypopharynx, then performing a laryngoscopy and directing the tube into the larynx under direct vision. Distal guidance of the tube can be done with either manipulation of the exposed proximal end of the tube, in addition to the extension or flexion of the neck or side-to-side movement of the larynx. Magill forceps (used to manipulate objects in the hypopharynx) often allow the operator to place the tip of the endotracheal tube into the larynx while the tube is advanced from above. Care must be taken not to damage the endotracheal tube cuff with these forceps. Often the tip of the tube can be inserted through the vocal cords, but it cannot be advanced because of the upward bend of the tube angling toward the anterior aspect of the trachea. Rotating the tube 180 degrees will often change the direction of the tube, allowing easy passage into the trachea if this situation is encountered.

For the patient spontaneously breathing, auscultation of breath sounds through the tube will allow "blind" insertion. This can be accomplished by placing the ear close to the proximal end of the endotracheal tube or attaching IV tubing to the proximal end and connecting it to a stethoscope or ear piece to listen to breath sounds. Using this technique, breath sounds increase as the nasotracheal tube is advanced towards the trachea and diminish as it enters the esophagus. Connecting the proximal end of the tracheal tube to a capnograph can also indicate when the tube is close to the larynx. End-tidal carbon dioxide concentration will increase as the tube approaches the glottic area.

When a difficult airway is anticipated, patient preparation and management must be carefully planned. Patients do not generally suffer adverse consequences from an inability to intubate but rather from a failure of oxygenation during attempted intubation. The practitioner should never administer an induction agent when there is a question of whether the patient can be adequately ventilated. The administration of a muscle relaxant to a patient who cannot be ventilated and who may not be able to be intubated in the event of anticipated airway difficulties is a serious and potentially fatal mistake. Patient injury or death from hypoxia or anoxia usually results from continued failed attempts at intubation.

Placement of a tracheal tube in an awake or mildly sedated patient is the method of choice in patients with a potentially difficult airway. The fiberoptic bronchoscope has made the intubation of these patients easier and safer. Fiberoptic intubation is a skill that should be mastered by providers who routinely use endotracheal intubation to secure the airway.[24] The ASA has devised an important algorithm regarding management of the difficult airway, and practitioners who administer drugs that may produce airway obstruction must be familiar with these recommendations and be facile at alternative methods of airway manipulation.[25] Unfortunately, oral or nasotracheal intubation may be impossible, and equipment needed to perform an emergency cricothyrotomy, or in some situations an emergency tracheostomy, must be available at all anesthetizing locations.[26]

Confirmation of correct tracheal tube placement can be accomplished in a number of ways. Auscultation of the lungs, lung and chest wall compliance as evidenced by the "feel" of the reservoir bag, auscultation of the stomach, and direct visualization entering the larynx all have been used to confirm placement. The use of end-tidal carbon dioxide concentrations through capnography, however, is the most reliable method of conformation. This method is not totally foolproof, and carbon dioxide levels may transiently be recorded when the tube is in the esophagus, further confusing the clinical picture during a difficult intubation. In times of uncertainty (e.g., difficulty discerning breath sounds, equipment malfunction, emergency situations when capnography may be unavailable), checking tube placement through direct laryngoscopy can be lifesaving.[27]

Complications can occur during intubation (e.g., trauma to dentition, bleeding, mediastinal emphysema, retropharyngeal dissection, cervical fracture or subluxation), after intubation (e.g., obstruction outside or inside tube, kinking of tube, blockage within tube from secretions or other materials), and after extubation. Postextubation complications are divided into three categories: early, up to 24 hours (e.g., sore throat, vocal cord damage or paralysis, damage to lingual nerve, glottic edema); intermediate, 24 to 72 hours (e.g., infections); and late, after 72 hours (e.g.,

laryngeal ulcer, granuloma, laryngotracheal membranes and webs, laryngotracheal fibrosis, stricture of nostril).

General Anesthesia Agents

Many IV and inhalation agents are available for the induction and maintenance of general anesthesia. The desirable characteristics of outpatient anesthetic agents include a rapid and smooth onset of action, intraoperative amnesia and analgesia, and a short recovery period without side effects. Unfortunately, the "ideal" agent does not exist. In practice, combinations of medications are used to provide rapid induction, muscle relaxation, intraoperative anesthesia and analgesia, amnesia, rapid recovery, and postoperative analgesia.

In adult patients, induction is typically accomplished with an IV agent, most often ultrashort-acting barbiturates (thiopental and methohexital), imidazoles (etomidate), arylcyclohexylamines (ketamine), and alkylphenols (propofol) (Tables 17-3 to 17-6).

Benzodiazepines

Benzodiazepines (diazepam, midazolam, and lorazepam) are rarely used as the primary induction agent for the outpatient due to prolonged recovery. However, they remain the most widely used agents for preoperative sedation.[28,29] A specific benzodiazepine antagonist, *flumazenil*, can reverse benzodiazepine-induced sedation; however, due to its short terminal elimination half-life (0.83 to 1.5 hours) compared with the benzodiazepine agonists, the routine reversal of large doses of benzodiazepines is not advocated. Flumazenil can antagonize the respiratory depression, apnea, and unconsciousness observed in benzodiazepine overdose, as well as the desired sedation, anxiolysis, skeletal muscle relaxation, and amnesia. The onset time of IV flumazenil is 1 to 5 minutes.[30]

Barbiturates

The ultrashort-acting barbiturates (thiopental and methohexital) are highly lipid soluble and easily cross the blood-brain barrier, resulting in a rapid loss of consciousness. The barbiturates produce a dose-dependent depression of the CNS, with short distribution and elimination half-lives. *Methohexital* pro-

TABLE 17-3

Pharmacologic Profiles of Intravenous Anesthetic Agents

Agent	Onset	Duration	Analgesia	Amnesia
Barbiturates				
Thiopental	Rapid	Ultrashort	Anti*	Yes
Methohexital	Rapid	Ultrashort	Anti*	Yes
Benzodiazepines				
Diazepam	Slow	Long	None	Yes
Midazolam	Intermediate	Intermediate	None	Yes
Opioids				
Morphine	Slow	Long	Yes	No
Meperidine	Slow	Long	Yes	No
Fentanyl	Intermediate	Intermediate	Yes	No
Sufentanil	Intermediate	Intermediate	Yes	No
Alfentanil	Rapid	Short	Yes	No
Remifentanil	Rapid	Short	Yes	No
Miscellaneous Agents				
Ketamine	Rapid	Short	Yes	Yes
Etomidate	Rapid	Short	No	Yes
Propofol	Rapid	Ultrashort	No	Yes

*Pain perception may be increased.

TABLE 17-4

Respiratory and Cardiovascular Effects of Intravenous Agents

Drug	Blood Pressure	Heart Rate	Cardiac Output	Venous Dilatation	Minute Ventilation
Thiopental	↓	↑	↓	↑	↓
Methohexital	↓	↑	↓	↑	↓
Propofol	↓↓	↓	↓	↑	↓↓
Etomidate	0	0	0	0	↓
Ketamine	↑	↑	↑	0	0
Midazolam	↓	0	↓	↑	0

duces a more rapid recovery than thiopental due to its high clearance rate, three to four times that of thiopental (Table 17-7). For this reason, methohexital is the most popular IV anesthetic for oral and maxillofacial surgery. Unfortunately, methohexital is also associated with excitatory phenomena (e.g., hiccoughs, involuntary movements), and cumulative effects of repeated small doses may prolong recovery as body storage sites become saturated.

Both methohexital and thiopental are well suited for continuous infusions techniques, which may decrease the total dose given, providing a more rapid recovery and decreasing the potential for adverse respiratory and cardiovascular events. Intraarterial injection of barbiturates can result in severe vasospasm distal to the site of injection, leading to severe tissue ischemia. Therefore careful injection of these medications into a free-flowing IV infusion line is

TABLE 17-5

Speed of Onset of Intravenous Anesthetic Agents

Drug	Time to Peak Effect (Seconds)
Midazolam	180-480
Diazepam	60-180
Fentanyl	180-300
Remifentanil	60-90
Methohexital	90-120
Propofol	120-150
Ketamine	60-180

TABLE 17-6

Recovery Characteristics of Intravenous Agents

Drug	Emergence	Risk of Emesis
Barbiturates	Moderate impairment	Low to moderate
Propofol	Minimal impairment, euphoria	Antiemetic
Etomidate	Mild impairment	Very high
Ketamine	Possible delirium	Moderate to high
Midazolam	Mild impairment, amnesia	Minimal
Diazepam	Prolonged impairment, amnesia	Minimal

TABLE 17-7

Pharmacokinetics of Methohexital and Thiopental

Drug	Volume of Distribution (L/kg)	Clearance (ml/kg/min)	Elimination Half-Life (hr)	Hepatic Extraction
Thiopental	2.5	3.4	11.6	0.15
Methohexital	2.2	10.9	3.9	0.5

recommended. Barbiturates are contraindicated in patients with *acute intermittent porphyria*, an inborn metabolic disorder characterized by the inability to metabolize porphyrin.[31,32]

Imidazoles

The induction of anesthesia with *etomidate* is characterized by a rapid onset of action without cardiovascular depression or histamine release. Recovery of psychomotor function after etomidate is intermediate between thiopental and methohexital. Despite these attributes, etomidate has a limited role as an induction agent for outpatient general anesthesia because of associated pain on injection, high incidence of postoperative nausea and vomiting, and involuntary body movements.[33]

Acylcyclohexylamines

Ketamine produces a "dissociative" anesthetic state characterized by catalepsy, analgesia, and amnesia. Cardiovascular stimulation, mediated by the sympathetic nervous system, occurs after injection of ketamine, with only mild respiratory depressant effects. Relaxation of the bronchial smooth muscle, with decreased airway resistance and a reduction of bronchospasm, can be helpful in patients with severe asthma. Ketamine does not maintain laryngeal reflexes, and aspiration of gastric contents has been reported in at-risk patients when airways have not been protected by a tracheal tube.[34]

An antisialagogue (atropine or scopolamine) is recommended when the use of ketamine is contemplated, to reduce the incidence of laryngospasm caused by ketamine-induced secretions. Emergence

TABLE 17-8

Comparative Pharmacokinetics of Inhalation Anesthetics

Agent	Blood:Gas Coefficient	Onset of Action	Recovery Time	Metabolism (%)
Desflurane	0.42	Very rapid	Very rapid	0.02
Enflurane	1.91	Rapid	Rapid	2.4 (fluoride ions)
Halothane	2.5	Rapid	Slow	Up to 20
Isoflurane	1.43	Rapid	Rapid	0.17
Nitrous oxide	0.47	Very rapid	Very rapid	0
Sevoflurane	0.69	Rapid	Rapid	5 (fluoride ions)

and postoperative *delirium* has limited the use of ketamine as an induction agent. Although a significant reduction in the incidence of this disturbing side effect can be seen with concomitant use of a benzodiazepine, delirium is a troubling side effect. Ketamine is a unique drug that continues to be a important agent in many situations.[35]

Alkylphenols

Propofol is an extremely rapid-acting and potent agent for the induction and maintenance of conscious sedation, deep sedation, and general anesthesia. Its advantages include a reduction in residual postoperative sedation and psychomotor impairment compared with barbiturates and a low incidence of nausea and vomiting. Propofol produces dose-dependent cardiovascular and respiratory depression, with a pharmacodynamic profile similar to methohexital. Side effects include pain on injection, involuntary muscle movements, coughing, and hiccoughing. Propofol is best administered for maintenance of anesthesia using a variable-infusion pump.[36,37]

Nitrous Oxide

Nitrous oxide is routinely used in conjunction with IV agents and volatile anesthetic gases for maintenance of anesthesia, with a predictable reduction of doses of coadministered medication needed to achieve suitable anesthetic depth. The disadvantages of nitrous oxide use include increasing the pressure in air-containing closed body spaces, diffusion hypoxia at emergence, and association with higher-than-predicted incidence of nausea and vomiting. As with all the inhalation anesthetic gases, it is mandatory to scavenge nitrous oxide from the operating room environment to reduce the incidence of reproductive problems and other medical considerations related to the chronic exposure of trace amounts of inhalation agents by health care personnel.

Volatile Agents

Generally, volatile anesthetic agents (halothane, enflurane, isoflurane, desflurane, and sevoflurane) are used in combination with nitrous oxide and oxygen or oxygen alone for the maintenance of anesthesia in the adult patient and for the induction of anesthesia in the pediatric patient. Halothane, isoflurane, and enflurane can be thought of as one group with similar pharmacologic activity in the healthy outpatient and the newer agents desflurane and sevoflurane as another group (Table 17-8).

Halothane is the least pungent of the first group, providing a smooth anesthetic course. Halothane administration is typically associated with bradycardia, moderate depression of cardiac output, and decreased blood pressure. Ventricular arrhythmias, particularly during light planes of anesthesia, in the presence of hypercarbia, and when large amounts of exogenous epinephrine are administered, are often observed. A limit of 1 μg/kg of exogenous epinephrine in the presence of halothane is recommended. Fulminant hepatic failure after halothane administration was reported shortly after introduction of this halogenated agent. Although the mechanism is unclear, an immune-mediated process is suggested by the propensity for hepatic dysfunction after repeated exposure. As with all the potent inhalation anesthetics, halothane can act as a trigger of malignant hyperthermia, especially when used in conjunction with the depolarizing skeletal muscle relaxant succinylcholine.

Enflurane and *isoflurane* are significantly less arrhythmogenic than halothane. The maximum dose of epinephrine solution that can be injected during anesthesia with enflurane is 2 µg/kg and 3 µg/kg with isoflurane. In the clinical setting the induction and recovery times of these three agents are very similar, with enflurane demonstrating a slightly more rapid recovery than halothane or isoflurane.

Two newer potent inhalation agents offer significant advantages for outpatient anesthesia. *Desflurane* has a very low blood:gas solubility coefficient (0.42, similar to nitrous oxide), producing rapid induction and recovery from anesthesia. It is less potent than the older volatile agents, with a minimum alveolar concentration (MAC) of 5% to 7%, but undergoes little or no biotransformation. Desflurane has a pungent odor and may cause a stormy inhalation induction. *Sevoflurane* also has a low blood:gas solubility (0.6 to 0.7), with a potency (MAC of 1.7%) similar to enflurane. Sevoflurane's lack of pungency allows for smooth inhalation induction in children and adults. Sevoflurane does not appear to sensitize the myocardium to exogenous epinephrine. Approximately 2% of sevoflurane is metabolized, yielding free fluoride ions, which can lead to renal dysfunction after prolonged anesthesia. Sevoflurane has become extremely popular in ambulatory anesthesia because of its rapid recovery profile.[38-40]

Opioid and Nonopioid Analgesic Agents

Opioids are often administered with volatile agents or used in combination with nitrous oxide to allow maintenance of anesthesia at lower inhaled gas concentrations, resulting in a more rapid emergence, pain-free awakening, and uneventful recovery. For ambulatory anesthesia, the "ideal" opioid analgesic should have rapid onset, short duration of action, potent analgesic effect, minimal cardiovascular effects, and no emetic effect. All opioids act on central receptors, and the pharmacologic properties of specific drugs depend on the degree of affinity and activity at the receptor site[41] (Tables 17-9 and 17-10).

Opiate analgesics produce well-described dose-dependent depression of the CNS and respiratory drive, delay in gastric emptying, and potentiation of

TABLE 17-9

Effects of Opioid Receptors

Opioid Receptor	Effect
Mu-1	Supraspinal analgesia
	Euphoria/dependence
	Nausea and vomiting
	Urinary retention
	Pruritus
Mu-2	Spinal analgesia
	Sedation
	Respiratory depression
	Hypotension/bradycardia
	Ileus
Kappa	Sedation
	Psychomimetic reactions
	Analgesia
Delta	Moderate mu activity
	Supraspinal and spinal anesthesia

postoperative nausea and vomiting. Truncal or chest wall rigidity may result from rapid administration of large doses of opioids but rarely results from small doses. Rigidity may be treated with small doses of succinylcholine (10 to 20 mg) and is one reason why only practitioners with advanced anesthesia training should administer these opioids. Naloxone may also be effective in reversing this chest wall stiffness, but it also reverses analgesia and euphoria.

Morphine and *meperidine* are most often used for inpatient perioperative analgesia. However, the long duration of action and side effect profiles of these opioids are not well suited for most ambulatory care procedures. Meperidine administration is associated with tachycardia, hyperactive reflexes, and muscle tremors. Morphine can cause profound hypotension, related in part to histamine release.[42]

The synthetic opioid analgesics *fentanyl* and its newer derivatives do not induce histamine release. They are excellent adjunctive agents for ambulatory anesthesia. As with all opioids, fentanyl can produce severe respiratory depression. A recurrence of this depression has been reported up to 4 hours after administration, especially in elderly patients. *Sufentanil* is an extremely potent opioid, 500 to 1000 times more potent than morphine. Sufentanil has a more rapid onset and may be associated with a more rapid

TABLE 17-10

Affinity and Activity at Mu and Kappa Receptors

| | MU | | KAPPA | |
Agent	Affinity	Activity	Affinity	Activity
Morphine	High	High	Low	Low
Meperidine	Moderate	Moderate	Low	Low
Fentanyl	Very high	Very high	—	—
Nalbuphine	Moderate	—	High	High

recovery than fentanyl due to its shorter elimination half-life. *Alfentanil* is a rapid-onset, short-acting opioid with approximately one-fifth to one-tenth the potency of fentanyl. Alfentanil has an elimination half-life that is significantly shorter than for fentanyl because of alfentanil's small volume of distribution. This translates clinically into a compound that can be used for the induction and maintenance of anesthesia without producing prolonged postoperative sedation and respiratory depression. *Remifentanil*, the newest synthetic opioid agonist, is more potent than alfentanil and is proving to be an excellent drug for ambulatory anesthesia due to its extremely short duration of action.[43]

Many IV anesthetics can be delivered more efficiently and controllably through the use of *continuous variable-rate infusion*. This technique is of special interest to drugs with rapid metabolism and small volumes of distribution, such as methohexital, propofol, alfentanil, and remifentanil. The traditional intermittent bolus injection of drugs leads to "peaks and valleys" in blood concentrations. Continuous variable-rate infusions can decrease the total amount of drug delivered, improve anesthetic conditions, and shorten recovery times considerably.[44]

Opioid Antagonist

The use of *naloxone*, an opioid antagonist, is occasionally necessary to reverse profound opioid-induced sedation and respiratory depression. It should never be used as a "routine" drug administered at the end of anesthesia to speed recovery, since naloxone administration also will reverse the analgesic effects of opioids and can cause pulmonary edema, hypertension, and ventricular arrhythmias.[45]

Opioid Agonist-Antagonists

Agonist-antagonist analgesics such as butorphanol, nalbuphine, and pentazocine have been recommended by some practitioners to replace pure agonists. Less nausea and vomiting are seen than with their true opioid counterparts. Concerns surround their long duration, however, as well as the difficulty of concomitant or subsequent administration of pure agonist opioids. A common characteristic of this class of drugs is a "ceiling" on the analgesia and sedation produced with increasing doses, which limits their usefulness as true anesthetic agents.

Butorphanol has less psychomimetic and cardiodepressant effects than pentazocine. In doses of 2 to 3 mg, butorphanol is equianalgesic to morphine sulfate 10 mg. In larger doses, hypertension and prolonged recovery have been reported. *Nalbuphine* has the least psychomimetic and cardiodepressant side effects, and on a milligram-for-milligram basis, it is equipotent to morphine. Nalbuphine is probably the most clinically valuable of these drugs as an adjunctive analgesic in the outpatient setting.

Muscle Relaxants

For dental procedures, muscle relaxants are indicated for facilitating intubation of the trachea and allowing a lighter level of anesthesia to be maintained (Table 17-11).

Succinylcholine, a depolarizing muscle relaxant with rapid onset and short duration, has been the standard drug for intubation. The short duration of action (5 to 10 minutes) is related to its rapid breakdown by plasma cholinesterase. A familial or anesthetic history of difficulty in metabolizing succinylcholine should

TABLE 17-11

Neuromuscular Blocking Drugs

Drug	Onset (min)	Duration (min)	Primary Route of Elimination
Atracurium	2-2.5	35-45	Plasma
Metocurine	1-4	60-120	Kidneys
Mivacurium	2-2.5	15-20	Plasma
Pancuronium	2-3	60-120	Kidneys/liver
Rapacuronium	1	15-20	Kidneys/liver
Rocuronium	1-1.5	20-30	Kidneys/liver
Succinylcholine	0.5-1	4-10	Plasma
Tubocurarine	1-2	60-120	Kidneys/liver
Vecuronium	2.5-3	25-40	Kidneys/liver

alert the dentist to either deficiencies in quality or quantity of plasmacholinesterase. Interactions with anticholinesterase drugs (e.g., for glaucoma) can decrease the activity of plasmacholinesterase, thus prolonging the activity of succinylcholine. In patients with myopathies (especially Duchenne's), paraplegia, and prolonged immobility, succinylcholine should not be used; it may cause hyperkalemia and subsequent cardiac arrest. Succinylcholine administration is also associated with elevations of intracranial, intraocular, and intragastric pressures. Young, healthy patients often experience postoperative myalgias after succinylcholine administration, which can be severe and outlast the discomfort at the surgical site. A number of strategies have been suggested to decrease the incidence and severity of the myalgias, including pretreatment with small doses of nondepolarizing muscle relaxants, diazepam, and even with small aliquots of succinylcholine itself ("self-taming" dose). Despite the problems associated with succinylcholine use, many anesthetists continue to prefer this relaxant for its unmatched speed of onset and ability to provide excellent intubating conditions, especially for patients with "full stomachs" who require a rapid sequence intubation.

Malignant hyperthermia, a hypermetabolic crisis triggered by some anesthetic agents, is most likely to occur when triggering agents such as volatile inhalation anesthetics and succinylcholine are used. IV sedative-anesthetic agents and local anesthetics used for dental outpatient procedures are considered to be nontriggering agents. Malignant hyperthermia is usu-

ally manifested as an elevation in end-tidal carbon dioxide levels and an unexplained, progressive tachycardia. Masseter muscle spasm after administration of succinylcholine may also signal the onset of malignant hyperthermia. Muscle rigidity, cyanosis, dysrhythmias, and elevated temperature appear soon after the initial signs. Definitive treatment depends on early diagnosis and immediate use of IV sodium dantrolene (1 to 10 mg/kg), as well as ventilation with 100% oxygen, changing the anesthetic circuit, and cooling the patient.[46]

In the past the only available nondepolarizing muscle relaxants had a slow onset and a relatively long duration of action (e.g., *d*-tubocurarine, pancuronium bromide). The introduction of nondepolarizing muscle relaxants both with intermediate onset and duration (e.g., atracurium, vecuronium) and more recently with rapid onset and short duration (e.g., rocuronium, rapacuronium) has provided nondepolarizing drugs that have clinical utility for most needs. They may even replace the routine use of succinylcholine.[47,48]

Related Anesthetic Considerations

The administration of local anesthetics with concentrations of epinephrine as high as 1:50,000 for hemostasis during periodontal procedures, as well as the use of gingival retraction cords impregnated with racemic epinephrine to provide hemostasis for impression of crown preparations, can produce dysrhythmias in the presence of halogenated hydrocarbons, especially halothane. It is imperative to keep track of doses of exogenous catecholamines and stay well below suggested levels. In addition, epinephrine use may be contraindicated in patients with severe coronary artery disease, mitral stenosis, or cerebral aneurysm.[49]

Acute fulminating infections of the face and neck become life threatening by impinging on the airway or by leading to the development of septicemia. Ludwig's angina, for example, presents as a massive, rapidly spreading inflammatory process involving the submandibular, submental, and sublingual spaces bilaterally. The resulting edema enlarges and elevates the tongue so that it presses on the hard and soft palates and projects the tongue back into hypopharynx, creating acute respiratory obstruction. Initial treatment centers around securing the airway by endotracheal intubation or in some patients, tracheostomy. Even with a fiberoptic laryngoscope, intubation can be extremely difficult because of cellulitis and edema of the tongue, pharynx, and glottis.[50]

The use of air-driven dental instruments has been implicated in the occurrence of iatrogenic *emphysema* of the facial and cervical tissues. The cervical spread of such emphysema has been reported to cause respiratory obstruction. Recently, several cases of subcutaneous emphysema and air embolism have been reported during the insertion of dental implants under general anesthesia.[51,52]

The increasing popularity of major *orthognathic surgery* to improve appearance and correct malocclusion by osteotomies of the maxilla, mandible, or both has created some unique intraoperative problems. During the down-fracture of the maxilla in a LeFort I osteotomy, it is possible to sever the nasotracheal tube or damage the pilot tube connected to the inflatable cuff. A major air leak, aspiration of blood into the trachea, or inability to ventilate the patient's lungs may result. Attempting to change a nasotracheal tube during the procedure may be extremely difficult.[53]

Controlled or deliberate *hypotension* is often requested by the surgical team during orthognathic surgery to reduce blood loss and improve operating conditions in the surgical field. Although controlled hypotension is relatively safe when the mean arterial pressure is slowly reduced to 55 to 60 mg Hg, the potential for reduced coronary, cerebral, and renal perfusion may lead to increased morbidity and mortality. Many agents and adjuncts have been employed electively to lower blood pressure. A common technique uses a deep level of anesthesia with potent volatile agents (halothane, enflurane, and isoflurane), but this approach may prolong recovery and produce severe myocardial depression. The use of *sodium nitroprusside* provides excellent control of blood pressure but necessitates placement of an indwelling arterial line. It also can cause cyanide toxicity and rebound hypertension on its cessation. IV *nitroglycerin* can effectively lower blood pressure, but high doses may result in methemoglobinemia and may increase pulmonary shunting. Combined α- and β-receptor antagonists (e.g., labetalol) and a β-receptor antagonist (esmolol) have been used to control blood pressure during orthognathic surgery without serious untoward effects.[54-57]

Equipment and Emergency Drugs

A properly equipped ambulatory anesthesia facility is essential to ensure patient safety during anesthesia for dental procedures. Anesthesia equipment may be categorized as special, optional, or basic. *Special equipment* includes (1) a blockade monitor if nondepolarizing muscle relaxants are used, (2) a fiberoptic bronchoscope if patients with anticipated difficult airways are considered candidates for general anesthesia, or (3) infusion pumps for anesthetic techniques that incorporate a continuously titrated IV infusion for maintenance of general anesthesia. The selection of special techniques is unique to the needs of each facility and practitioner.

Optional equipment includes items generally considered "desirable" or possibly "an emerging standard" but not yet universally recognized as mandatory. Examples include specific volatile agent monitors and depth of anesthesia monitors.

Basic equipment includes items that are necessary and fundamental to provide safe outpatient general anesthesia, such as the following:

1. Adequate lighting and portable battery backup light source
2. Adequate suction and portable, self-contained backup (Venturi or battery powered)
3. Manifold (reserve oxygen supply) system with alarms if central gas supply is used
4. Functional anesthesia machine checked out to current Food Drug Administration (FDA) specifications and a separate, portable source of

oxygen and a bag-mask device that can deliver positive pressure through an endotracheal tube or mask
5. Oxygen analyzer with alarm for machines capable of delivering less than 25% oxygen (for machines lacking "fail-safe" devices, "flow safe" devices, or both)
6. Assortment of oral and nasopharyngeal airways, endotracheal tubes, and laryngoscope blades consistent with age and size of patients treated
7. Laryngoscope handle and backup with spare batteries and bulbs
8. Intubating (Magill) forceps
9. Intravenous infusion equipment: catheters, syringes, infusion tubing, IV fluids, tourniquets
10. Emergency surgical airway equipment for cricothyrotomy
11. Appropriate emergency anesthetic adjunctive drugs, including but not limited to nitroglycerin, epinephrine, skeletal muscle relaxants, anticonvulsants, vagolytics, vasopressors, bronchodilators, antiarrhythmics, glucocorticosteroids, antihistamines, dextrose, and a readily available source of sodium dantrolene if the routine use of volatile agents or succinylcholine is contemplated
12. Basic monitoring equipment, including ECG/defibrillator, blood pressure monitoring equipment, stethoscopes, pulse oximeter, capnograph if endotracheal intubation is routine, and thermometer
13. Well-trained surgical/anesthesia team certified in advanced cardiac life support (ACLS)

Anesthetic Emergencies

A carefully reviewed past medical history and focused physical examination are critical in reducing the incidence of anesthetic emergencies. Anesthetic drugs and equipment must be readily available and organized so that the dentist and auxiliaries can manage emergencies effectively. Patients must be continuously monitored to facilitate early recognition of problems before they become true anesthetic emergencies.

Airway and Ventilation Problems

Problems with the airway and ventilation are the most common causes of anesthetic mortality and morbidity. Intraoperative emergencies often begin as mild respiratory obstruction or depression, progress to hypoxia and hypercarbia, and then to cardiovascular collapse. The pulse oximeter and capnograph, as well as better-trained anesthesia providers, have improved respiratory monitoring, and there has been a marked reduction in adverse respiratory event claims and mortality.[58] Mechanical obstruction of the airway by the tongue and soft tissues of the hypopharynx is common, especially during the induction of anesthesia, and is easily recognized and managed. Enlarged tonsils, airway edema, pharyngeal gauze partitions, and foreign bodies may also cause airway obstruction. Repositioning the head, inserting oropharyngeal or nasopharyngeal airways, performing a direct laryngoscopy, intubating the trachea, or establishing a surgical airway through a cricothyrotomy may be necessary to alleviate mechanical obstruction.

Laryngospasm

Laryngospasm is an involuntary closure of the vocal cords and glottis in an attempt by the body to protect the airway. Secretions, irrigating solutions, blood, surgical debris, insufficient level of anesthesia, irritating gases, and pain may all initiate laryngospasm. A laryngospasm is a protective reflex, which may lead to either partial or complete airway obstruction. During a partial or incomplete laryngospasm, high-pitched "crowing" sounds are produced on inspiration; no sounds, however, are produced during a total or complete laryngospasm. Suctioning into the hypopharynx and gentle application of oxygen under positive pressure are initial treatments. Anesthesia may also be deepened to decrease laryngeal irritability. If these initial attempts at treating laryngospasm are not successful, the administration of a small IV dose of succinylcholine to relax the laryngeal musculature may be necessary. Early diagnosis and aggressive treatment of laryngospasm are imperative, since succinylcholine administration in the face of hypoxia and hypercarbia may result in profound bradycardia and asystole.

Bronchospasm

Bronchospasm, the involuntary contraction of the smooth musculature of the small airway of the tracheobronchial tree, must be included in any differential diagnosis of ventilatory difficulties during general anesthesia. Whether caused by acute asthma, histamine release related to drugs, anaphylaxis, surgical stimulation with light planes of anesthesia, or aspiration, bronchospasm must be recognized early and vigorously treated. Unlike laryngospasm, bronchospasm is not protective and is the underlying cause of many cases of anesthetic-related hypoxemia and hypercarbia. Therapy is directed at alleviating smooth muscle constriction, ensuring oxygenation, and removing the noxious stimuli. Inhalation of a β_2-adrenergic drug, such as albuterol, metaproterenol, isoproterenol, or epinephrine, is recommended. Subcutaneous injection of a β_2-adrenergic drug (e.g., terbutaline) can also be useful. For severe and life-threatening bronchospasm, the drug of choice is IV epinephrine. Patients must be closely monitored for major changes in blood pressure, heart rate, and cardiac rhythm. Glucocorticosteroids are useful adjuncts to β-agonist drug therapy, but their slow onset times render them ineffective as initial emergency drugs. Aminophylline is not a direct-acting bronchodilator and is associated with hypotension when administered rapidly. Anesthetic drugs with bronchodilating properties, including halothane and ketamine, are indicated for patients at risk.[58,59]

Aspiration

Aspiration of gastric contents during general anesthesia can occur during procedures not using an endotracheal tube but also at times of intubation and extubation. Initial management includes vigorous suctioning of the hypopharynx while ensuring ventilation and oxygenation. The lung fields are then auscultated, and bronchospasm, if present, is treated. Endotracheal intubation, positive-pressure ventilation, direct tracheal suctioning with rigid bronchoscopy, and institution of positive end-expiratory pressure (PEEP) may be necessary to overcome hypoxia and hypercarbia. Hospitalization is indicated for symptomatic patients (dyspnea, fever, cough) or when supplemented oxygen is required to maintain oxygenation. Except in patients with massive aspiration, radiographic abnormalities can be subtle on initial chest examinations.[60]

Pulmonary Edema

Pulmonary edema may arise from a variety of causes, most notably acute congestive heart failure, myocardial infarction, and as a consequence of airway obstruction. Signs include low oxygen saturation, pres-

ence of rales on auscultation, and evidence of pink, frothy sputum in the airway. Treatment is symptomatic and depends partly on etiology. Oxygen, diuretics, and morphine combined with sublingual nitroglycerin or nifedipine are helpful before transfer to an acute care facility.

Hypotensive and Hypertensive Crises

Hypotensive and hypertensive crises are likewise managed symptomatically and guided by physiologic monitoring. Many hypotensive episodes respond to decreasing the anesthetic depth and increasing intravascular fluid volume. IV atropine in 0.5-mg increments should be considered in patients with hypotension accompanied by bradycardia. α-Agonists and β-agonists may be indicated to increase peripheral vascular resistance, heart rate, and myocardial contractility.

Hypertensive urgencies and emergencies are often short-lived, particularly if initiated by vascular uptake of local anesthetic vasoconstrictor solutions. Sublingual administration of nitroglycerin or nifedipine generally produces a moderate reduction in blood pressure without producing profound hypotension. IV agents used in hypertensive emergencies include labetalol, esmolol, and hydralazine. The use of IV nitroglycerin and sodium nitroprusside to treat hypertension should be limited to the hospital setting, where intraarterial blood pressure monitoring can guide therapy of these potent vasodilators. It is also important to remember that chronic hypertensive patients with elevated peripheral vascular tone may be volume constricted and may readily become profoundly hypotensive when treated with anesthetics or other vasodilating drugs.

Myocardial Infarction

The diagnosis of myocardial infarction during general anesthesia is rare, and the interpretation of an intraoperative ECG (e.g., ST-segment elevation or depression) can be difficult. Patients with histories of unstable angina or recent myocardial infarction need comprehensive cardiac evaluation before anesthesia. The awake patient with substernal chest pain or other anginal pain variants should be treated immediately with oxygen and sublingual nitroglycerin. If the pain is not totally relieved after these doses, the patient must be immediately transferred for advanced medical therapy.

Cardiac Dysrhythmias

Cardiac dysrhythmias frequently occur during surgical procedures as a result of anxiety, pain, reflex stimulation, exogenous catecholamines, hypoxia, hypercarbia, and drug interactions. The dentist must react quickly to their presence and attempt to identify their etiology, as well as discern relatively harmless rhythm disturbances from malignant, life-threatening interactions. Treatment is indicated when cardiac electrical disturbances depress cardiac output and jeopardize perfusion. The guidelines developed by the American Heart Association's Advanced Cardiac Life Support Committee are an important step in standardizing treatment of alterations in the normal cardiac rhythm.

Drug Interactions

Adverse effects of drugs and interactions between drugs may occur predictably or infrequently. This problem is more common in elderly patients, who may take 5 to 10 maintenance medications daily.[61] Since many drug interactions are dose dependent, early recognition may prevent progression to more serious sequelae. Of special concern to anesthetists are interactions of monoamine oxidase inhibitors, tricyclic antidepressants, or catecholamines with anesthetic agents.

Recovery

Transport to the recovery area should occur after recovery of airway reflexes, uncompromised airway patency, and a stable blood pressure and pulse rate are observed in the anesthetizing location. Transient hypoxia after anesthesia is always possible, and supplemental oxygen must be available during patient transport and in the recovery area. The recovery area must be appropriately staffed and well lighted and must have adequate suction and monitoring capability with equipment to deliver oxygen under positive pressure.

Rather than using specific time intervals, patients should be carefully considered ready for discharge when they demonstrate "street fitness" and meet specific, documented discharge criteria. Discharge criteria should include (1) stable vital signs with a return to preoperative baseline values, (2) return to usual state of alertness and ambulatory status, (3) acceptable surgical site, and (4) presence of a responsible adult escort who can assist the patient at home.

Before discharge, written and verbal instructions must be given to the patient and escort regarding surgery- and anesthesia-related aspects of recovery. Clear instructions of whom to contact in case of unanticipated problems should be included in these instructions. A note detailing the intraoperative and postoperative course should describe any untoward events, type of anesthesia administered, and condition at discharge.[61-63]

SUMMARY

Ambulatory anesthesia for dental procedures has a long history of safety, cost-effectiveness, and patient acceptance and satisfaction when performed by qualified dentists in properly equipped and staffed practices. Continued development of dental anesthesia residency programs; involvement of dentists in anesthesia research, drug development, and clinical trials; and support of anesthesia education by all dental specialties will help ensure quality of care and a successful future of anesthesia and pain control in dentistry.

1. Dionne RA, Laskin DM, editors: *Anesthesia and sedation in the dental office,* New York, 1986, Elsevier.
2. American Academy of Pediatric Dentistry: Guidelines for the elective use of conscious sedation, deep sedation, and general anesthesia in pediatric patients, *Pediatr Dent* 7:334-337, 1985.
3. American Association of Oral and Maxillofacial Surgeons: *Office evaluation manual,* ed 3, 1986.
4. Rosenberg MB, Campbell RL: Guidelines for intraoperative monitoring of dental patients undergoing conscious sedation, deep sedation and general anesthesia, *Oral Surg Oral Med Oral Pathol* 71:2-8, 1991.
5. Task Force on Sedation and Analgesia by Non-Anesthesiologists: Practice guidelines for sedation and analgesia by non-anesthesiologists, *Anesthesiology* 84:459-471, 1996.
6. Welcher BV, editor: *Anesthesia for ambulatory surgery,* Philadelphia, 1995, JB Lippincott.
7. Natof HE: Ambulatory surgery: patients with pre-existing medical problems, *Ill Med J* 166:101-104, 1996.
8. Lind LJ, Mushlin PS, Schnitman PA: Monitored anesthesia care for dental implant surgery, *J Oral Implantol* 16:106-113, 1990.
9. Lind LJ: Anesthetic management, *Oral Maxillofac Surg Clin North Am* 8:235-244, 1996.
10. Roizen MF: Routine preoperative testing. In Miller RD, editor: *Anesthesia,* ed 2, New York, 1986, Churchill Livingstone.

11. Kaplan EB, Sheier LB, Boeckmann MS, et al: The usefulness of preoperative laboratory screening, *JAMA* 253:3576-3581, 1985.

12. Rosenberg M: Monitoring in the dental office, *Oral Maxillofac Surg Clin North Am* 4:751-758, 1992.

13. Cooper JB, Newbower RS, Long CD, et al: Preventable anesthesia mishaps: a study of human factors, *Anesthesiology* 49(6):399-406, 1978.

14. Cheney FW: ASA closed claims project progress report: the effect of pulse oximetry and end-tidal CO_2 monitoring on adverse respiratory effects, *ASA Newslett* 56:6-10, 1992.

15. Hutchinson A, Malby JR, Reid CRG: Gastric fluid volume and pH in elective inpatients. Part I. Coffee or orange juice versus overnight fast, *Can J Anaesth* 35:12-15, 1988.

16. Manchikanti L, Canella MG, Hohlbein LJ, et al: Assessment of effect of various modes of premedication on aspiration risk factors in outpatient surgery, *Anesth Analg* 66(1):81-84, 1987.

17. Ong BY, Palahniuk RJ, Cumming M: Gastric volume in outpatients, *Can Anaesth Soc J* 66:81-84, 1987.

18. Cohen SE, Woods WA, Wyner J: Antiemetic effects of droperidol and metoclopramide, *Anesthesiology* 60:67-69, 1984.

19. Jackson H, Hertz JB, Johansen JR, et al: Premedication before day of surgery, *Br J Anaesth* 57:300-305, 1985.

20. Clark AJM, Hurtig JB: Predmedication with meperidine and atropine does not prolong recovery to stress fitness after outpatient anesthesia, *Can Anaesth Soc J* 28:390-393, 1981.

21. Mallampati SR, Gatt SP, Gugino LD, et al: A clinical sign to predict difficult tracheal intubation: a prospective study, *Can Anaesth Soc J* 32:429-434, 1985.

22. Wilson ME, Spiegelhalter D, Robertson JA, et al: Predicting difficult intubation, *Br J Anaesth* 61:211-216, 1988.

23. Benumof J: Management of the difficult or impossible airway, *Anesthesiology* 75:1087-1110, 1991.

24. Dellinger RP: Fiberoptic bronchoscopy in adult airway management, *Crit Care Med* 18:882-887, 1990.

25. Practice guidelines for management of the difficult airway: a report by the ASA Task Force on Management of the Difficult Airway, *Anesthesiology* 78:597-602, 1993.

26. Mill RL: Invasive methods for securing an airway, *Int Anesthesiol Clin* 28:115-118, 1990.

27. Murray IP, Modell JH: Early detection of endotracheal tube accidents by monitoring carbon dioxide concentration in respiratory gas, *Anesthesiology* 59:344-346, 1983.

28. Reves JG, Fragen RJ, Vinik HR, et al: Midazolam: pharmacology and uses, *Anesthesiology* 62:310-324, 1985.

29. Stoelting RK: Benzodiazepines. In *Pharmacology and physiology in anesthetic practice*, ed 2, Philadelphia, 1991, JB Lippincott.

30. Klotz U, Kanto J: Pharmacokinetics and clinical use of flumazenil, *J Anaesthesiol Suppl* 20:491-505, 1988.

31. Fragen RJ, Avram MJ: Barbiturates. In Miller RD, editor: *Anesthesia*, ed 4, New York, 1994, Churchill-Livingstone.

32. Allen GD, Kennedy WF, Everett G, et al: A comparison of the cardiorespiratory effects of methohexital and thiopental supplementation for outpatient dental anesthesia, *Anesth Analg* 48:730-737, 1969.

33. Doenicke A, Ostwald P: Etomidate. In White PF, editor: *Textbook of intravenous anesthesia*, Baltimore, 1997, Williams & Wilkins.

34. White PF, Way WL, Trevor AJ: Ketamine: its pharmacology and therapeutic uses, *Anesthesiology* 56(2):119-136, 1982.

35. Recih DL, Silvayh G: Ketamine: an update on the first twenty-five years of clinical experience, *Can J Anaesth* 36:186-194, 1989.

36. Sebel PS, Lowdon JD: Propofol: a new intravenous anesthetic, *Anesthesiology* 71:260-277, 1989.

37. Smith I et al: Propofol: an update on its use, *Anesthesiology* 81:1005-1021, 1994.

38. Marshall BE, Longnecker DE: General anesthetics. In *Goodman and Gilman's the pharmacologic basis of therapeutics*, ed 8, New York, 1990, Pergamon.

39. Eger EI: *Nitrous oxide*, ed 2, London, 1984, Elsevier.

40. Eger I: New inhaled anesthetics, *Anesthesiology* 80:906-923, 1994.

41. Estafanow FG, editor: *Opioids in anesthesia*, London, 1990, Butterworth-Heinemann.

42. Foldes FF, Swerdlow M, Siker ES, editors: *Narcotics and narcotic antagonists: chemistry, pharmacology, and applications in anesthesia and obstetrics*, Springfield, Ill, 1964, Thomas.

43. Shafer SL, Varvel JR: Pharmacokinetics, pharmacodynamics, and rational opioid selection, *Anesthesiology* 74:53-63, 1991.

44. Hughes MA, Glass PSA, Jacobs JR: Context-sensitive half-time in multicompartment pharmacokinetic models for intravenous anesthetic drugs, *Anesthesiology* 76:334-341, 1992.

45. Azar O, Turndorf H: Severe hypertension and multiple atrial premature contractions following naloxone administration, *Anesth Analg* 58:524-527, 1979.

46. Rosenberg H: Malignant hyperthermia. In ASA Annual Meeting Refresher Course Lectures, No 124, 2000.

47. Savarese JJ: Some considerations on the new muscle relaxants, *Anesth Analg Suppl*, 1998, pp 119-127.

48. Eger EI: *Desflurane (Suprane): a compendium and reference*, Rutherford, NJ, 1993, Healthpress.

49. Hilley MD, Milam SB, Gieschke AH, et al: Fatality associated with the combined use of halothane and gingival retraction cord, *Anesthesiology* 60:587-588, 1984.

50. Gutman D, Laufer D, Neder A: Ludwig's angina: report of two cases, *J Oral Surg* 23:277-280, 1965.

51. Rosenberg MB, Wunderlich BW, Reynolds RN: Iatrogenic subcutaneous emphysema during dental anesthesia, *Anesthesiology* 51:80-81, 1979.

52. Davies JM, Campbell LA: Fatal air embolism during dental implant surgery: a report of three cases, *Can J Anaesth* 37:112-121, 1990.

53. Fagraeus L, Angelillo JC, Dolan EA: A serious anesthetic hazard during orthognathic surgery, *Anesth Analg* 59:150-153, 1980.

54. Fromme GA, MacKenzie RA, Gould AB, et al: Controlled hypotension for orthognathic surgery, *Anesth Analg* 65:683-686, 1986.

55. Gallagher DM, Milliken RA: Induced hypotension for orthognathic surgery, *J Oral Surg* 37:47-51, 1979.

56. Tinker JH, Michenfelder JD: Sodium nitroprusside: pharmacology, toxicology, and therapeutics, *Anesthesiology* 45:340-354, 1976.

57. Golia JK, Woo R, Farole A, et al: Nitroglycerin-controlled circulation in orthognathic surgery, *J Oral Maxillofac Surg* 43:342-345, 1985.

58. Cheney FW: The American Society of Anesthesiologists Closed Claims Project, *Anesthesiology* 91:552-556, 1999.

59. Gal TJ: Bronchospasm: clinical perspectives for anesthesiologists. In IARS Review Course Lectures Supplement to *Anesth Analg*, 1999, pp 37-48.

60. Lindahl SGE: Current treatment of adult respiratory distress syndrome. In IARS Review Course Lectures Supplement to *Anesth Analg*, 1999, pp 58-63.

61. Marshall SI et al: Discharge criteria and complication after outpatient surgery, *Anesth Analg* 88:508-517, 1999.

62. Davis GA, Chandler MH: Drug therapy and drug interactions, *Oral Maxillofac Surg Clin North Am* 8:245-263, 1996.

63. Welcher BV: Problem solving in the postanesthetic care unit. In Welcher BV, editor: *Anesthesia for ambulatory surgery,* New York, 1985, JB Lippincott.

CHAPTER 18

Management of Complications and Emergencies

DANIEL E. BECKER
JAMES C. PHERO

CHAPTER OUTLINE

General Considerations

The risk for medical complications in dental practice is greatest when caring for patients already medically compromised. It is reassuring that significant untoward events can generally be prevented by careful preoperative assessment, along with attentive intraoperative monitoring and support. Nevertheless, dentists must be prepared to manage adverse events should they arise. Conscious sedation does not increase the risk for the medical urgencies and emergencies discussed here, except respiratory depression and perhaps hypotension. In fact, by reducing fear and anxiety regarding dental treatment, the use of conscious sedation most likely lowers the incidence of most adverse events.

Primary Assessment

The management of any medical urgency or emergency should commence with patient assessment predicated on the airway, breathing, and circulation protocols (ABCs) taught during all courses in basic life support (BLS). Airway patency is the first priority; there is little use in assessing breathing or circulation if any degree of obstruction is present. Lift the head and chin, and examine the mouth and throat for any foreign material. Once patency is ensured, direct attention to breathing or ventilation. Ask a conscious patient to take a slow, deep breath. If the patient is unconscious, "look, listen, and feel" for ventilatory effort. A useful caveat is to place your hand on the patient's diaphragm; the chest does not always rise noticeably during quiet breathing. The carotid pulse can be palpated either simultaneously or after this assessment. Assuming that the patient is breathing and has a pulse, blood pressure should be recorded. During this assessment, other personnel should provide supplemental oxygenation. An enriched oxygen concentration is indicated for patients who are spontaneously breathing, regardless of their level of consciousness.

Oxygenation

The equipment required to provide supplemental oxygen includes a 100% oxygen source, a regulator, tubing, and either a nasal cannula or mask. The *nasal cannula* is ideal for administering supplemental oxygen to conscious patients who may be frightened by a mask. Furthermore, the fractional inspiratory oxygen concentration (FIO_2) delivered to a patient can be estimated using a simple formula: $FIO_2 = 20 + 4 \times O_2$ flow (L/min).[1] This information is useful when providing oxygen to patients with any form of chronic obstructive pulmonary disease (COPD). In these patients, FIO_2 should not exceed 40% to avoid suppressing peripheral hypoxemic drive. This formula approximates oxygen concentration delivered by nasal cannula only and is not applicable to masks.

The *mask with reservoir* should not be used for patients with a history of COPD but may be appropriate to deliver high oxygen concentrations to other unconscious, breathing patients. When using any mask, the flow rate should be at least 6 L/min to avoid feelings of suffocation. Provided the mask has a reservoir, this flow rate will deliver an oxygen concentration of 60%, and each additional L/min will increase FIO_2 by approximately 10%. An oxygen concentration approximating 100% can be delivered if the flow rate is 10 L/min.

The apneic patient will lose consciousness and requires positive-pressure ventilation. Mouth-to-mouth ventilation is the simplest method but provides only 16% expired oxygen concentration, and it runs the risk of disease transmission. The *pocket mask* is a more hygienic alternative to mouth-to-mouth ventilation and, supplemented with a 100% oxygen source, can deliver oxygen at concentrations of 50% to 60%. Correct use of a pocket mask requires practice, which can be readily attained during BLS courses for health care providers.

Bag-valve-mask (BVM) *devices* with reservoirs can provide 90% to 100% oxygen concentrations, but their proper use requires considerable operator skill. Proper head position, effective mask seal, and bag compression are skills that must be developed if BVM devices are to be used effectively. In certain cases, training may be offered on manikins during BLS courses. Skill for airway management is addressed in much greater detail during advanced cardiac life support (ACLS) training and includes instruction in the proper use of oropharyngeal airways. This particular airway adjunct improves airway patency by keeping the mouth open and preventing the base of the tongue from sagging against the posterior pharyngeal wall. The Guedel style of airway is hollow and facilitates insertion of a suction catheter to clear the pharynx of secretions.

Oxygen-powered, manually triggered devices *(demand valves)* consist of high-pressure tubing and a valve that is activated by a lever or push button. These devices deliver 100% oxygen, but many deliver flow rates that are unacceptably high (e.g., 50 L/min). Pressure generated by these flow rates can open the esophagus and produce gastric distention during positive-pressure ventilation. Also, when used in the demand mode, these devices have unac-

ceptably high triggering pressures, requiring considerable inspiratory effort when used to supplement spontaneously breathing patients. Use of oxygen-powered devices is contraindicated in pediatric patients (Fig. 18-1).

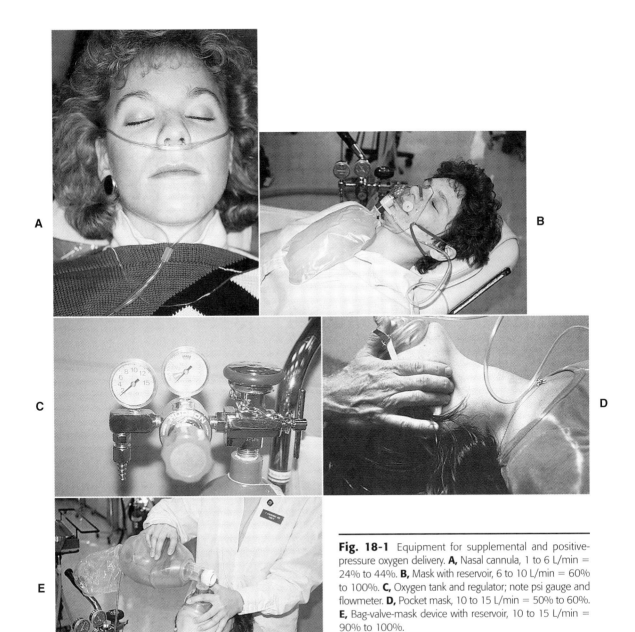

Fig. 18-1 Equipment for supplemental and positive-pressure oxygen delivery. **A,** Nasal cannula, 1 to 6 L/min = 24% to 44%. **B,** Mask with reservoir, 6 to 10 L/min = 60% to 100%. **C,** Oxygen tank and regulator; note psi gauge and flowmeter. **D,** Pocket mask, 10 to 15 L/min = 50% to 60%. **E,** Bag-valve-mask device with reservoir, 10 to 15 L/min = 90% to 100%.

Cardiovascular Considerations

Syncope

Fainting, or syncope, is the most common medical complication in dental practice. It is attributed to inadequate delivery of oxygen or glucose to brain tissues. In most patients, altered cardiovascular function is central in the pathogenesis and may be the result of primary cardiac disorders or, more often, vasovagal reactions triggered by fear or pain. In some patients, vagal influences are severe enough to induce transient periods of asystole that persist for 30 to 40 seconds. Furthermore, patients often exhibit brief episodes of convulsive activity that can be mistakenly viewed as a primary seizure.[2,3] Regardless of the cause or severity, vasovagal events will generally subside during implementation of primary measures for assessment and airway support. Subsequently, attention must be directed toward abnormalities in blood pressure and heart rate, which may or may not require pharmacologic intervention.

Hypotension

Despite the complexity of cardiovascular physiology, the purpose of this system is rather simplistic; it must perfuse tissues with oxygenated blood. The blood pressure required to perfuse tissues adequately varies from patient to patient and is influenced by medical status and posture at the time of assessment. Numeric values that change significantly from baseline should alert the clinician, but evaluation of *tissue perfusion* is the most significant component of cardiovascular assessment.

To assess perfusion of peripheral tissues, apply finger pressure to nail beds or oral mucosa. Color should return within 3 seconds, assuming normal room temperature. Perfusion within the central nervous system (CNS) can be evaluated by the patient's response to verbal and painful stimuli or by the pupil reflex when unconscious or heavily sedated. If perfusion is considered inadequate, the clinician may elect to increase systolic blood pressure, diastolic blood pressure, or both. In each case a separate set of physiologic determinants should be considered.

Systolic blood pressure (SBP) is determined by cardiac output, which is the volume of blood ejected by the left ventricle each minute. It follows that cardiac output is the product of heart rate and stroke volume, the latter being most significant. Heart rate acts merely to compensate for changes in stroke volume. Slow rates are common in well-trained athletes, whereas rapid rates are required to sustain a comparable cardiac output and thus SBP in the patient with heart failure or other conditions associated with low ejection fractions.

Stroke volume is influenced directly by myocardial contractility, which is augmented by sympathetic stimulation and by venous return (preload). According to the Frank-Starling law, preload is directly related to stroke volume, although this relationship is limited. If a critical volume is exceeded, congestion occurs. This volume is lower for patients with compromised cardiac function and should be considered when positioning a patient. Although cited most often as the preferred position for patients experiencing medical emergencies, the Trendelenburg position may allow excessive venous return (preload) and may compromise patients with cardiac or respiratory conditions. In fact, this position may offer few advantages.[4,5] A semi-reclined, or *semi-Fowler*, position is more appropriate when managing most medical complications.

For the heart to eject a stroke volume, ventricular systole must generate a pressure that exceeds peripheral resistance. In other words, ventricular pressure must exceed diastolic blood pressure (DBP). This resistance to ventricular ejection is described as *afterload*, and for compromised patients, elevated DBP may prevent ejection of an adequate stroke volume. For this reason, administration of vasopressors to elevate DBP could result in a negative influence on cardiac function. Although peripheral resistance is credited with coronary perfusion during diastole, a DBP as low as 40 mm/Hg is adequate.

In general, an SBP of 90 mm Hg will sustain mean arterial pressure sufficiently to perfuse tissues in the recumbent patient. (SBP is used as a reference point because DBP may be difficult to ascertain in the hypotensive patient.) If SBP or DBP drops 15 to 20 mm Hg below baseline, however, tissue perfusion should be assessed.

For hypotensive patients with syncopal signs and symptoms, a *syncope protocol* consists of assessing the ABCs, placing the patient in semi-Fowler position, and providing supplemental oxygen (Fig. 18-2). This should be the initial procedure when managing any medical complication. If an intravenous (IV) line is in place or can be established readily, 250 to 500 ml of physiologic solution should be administered rapidly. Generally, this will increase preload sufficiently

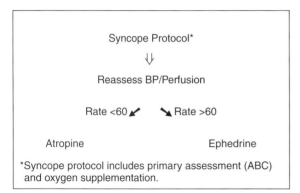

Fig. 18-2 Algorithm for hypotensive patient.

Drugs for Hypotension

Atropine
Action: anticholinergic; blocks vagal slowing of heart rate
Preparation: 1 mg/ml, SDV or ampules
Dose: IV or sublingual, 0.5 mg every 3 to 5 minutes up to 4 doses

Ephedrine
Action: mixed-acting α/β-receptor agonist; increases systolic/diastolic blood pressures
Preparation: 50 mg/ml, ampules or SDV
Dose: sublingual, 25 mg every 3 to 5 minutes up to two doses; IV, 10 mg every 3 to 5 minutes up to five doses

SDV, Single-dose vial; *IV,* intravenous.

to improve stroke volume and raise SBP. When this maneuver cannot be accomplished or proves unsuccessful, the patient's heart rate should guide further treatment. If bradycardia is present (<60 beats/minute), atropine (0.5 mg every 3 to 5 minutes up to four doses, by IV or submucosal injection) is administered until the rate is within normal limits. If the rate is greater than 60 beats/minute and pressure remains low, increasing the rate further will do little to improve SBP. This merely reduces the time allocated for diastolic filling, and each subsequent stroke volume will decline. Alternatively, attention should be directed to increasing stroke volume, peripheral resistance, or both.

Although several adrenergic drugs may be acceptable, *ephedrine* is an ideal choice for several reasons. Hypotension encountered during dental practice is attributed to either vasovagal episodes or use of sedatives and anesthetics that depress sympathetic outflow to the cardiovascular system. In either case, ephedrine specifically counters these influences indirectly by stimulating norepinephrine release from sympathetic nerve endings. Also, ephedrine acts directly on α-adrenergic and β-adrenergic receptors, leading to vasoconstriction and increased cardiac output. However, ephedrine constricts veins to a greater extent than arteries, which enables it to increase preload more than afterload.[6] This results in less myocardial oxygen demand than with other vasopressors. Finally, unlike epinephrine and other catecholamines with brief durations of action (5 to 10 minutes), the cardiovascular effects of ephedrine continue for 60 to 90 minutes. Ephedrine

should be administered intravenously in 10-mg increments every 3 to 5 minutes or by sublingual injection, 20 to 25 mg. Total dose should not exceed 50 mg (Box 18-1).

Hypertension

Sudden elevations in blood pressure are fairly common in dental practice but generally pass unnoticed because continuous monitoring is not routine practice. A "significant elevation" has not been defined, but *hypertensive crisis* is the conventional term for sudden elevations in DBP of 120 mm Hg or higher.[7,8] Unfortunately, this term is "alarming" and does not take into account the patient's baseline pressure. In patients with chronic hypertension, autoregulation of cerebral blood flow is reset to a higher level, and abruptly lowering pressure can lead to ischemia, particularly in elderly patients.[7] An acute hypertensive episode is regarded as an *urgency* if the patient remains asymptomatic and as an *emergency* if symptoms are present, including chest pain or tightness, headache, or visual disturbances.

If a patient's blood pressure increases suddenly, consider hypoxia, pain, and anxiety, which are the most likely causes for this reflex response. In our experience, these episodes occur most often during lengthy surgical procedures and reflect onset of pain

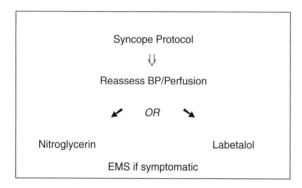

Fig. 18-3 Algorithm for hypertensive patient.

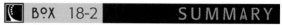

Drugs for Hypertensive Crisis

Labetalol (Normodyne, Trandate)
Action: blocks α- and β-adrenergic receptors, leading to vasodilation and decreased cardiac output, which decreases blood pressure
Preparation: 5 mg/ml, MDV
Dose: IV, 10 to 20 mg every 10 minutes, up to 100 mg total

Nitroglycerin
See Box 18-4.

MDV, Multidose vial; *IV,* intravenous.

due to waning influences of the local anesthetic. If additional local anesthetic fails to improve the episode, any need for additional pharmacologic intervention should be based on signs and symptoms of end-organ damage. Most significant in this regard are chest pain, indicative of increased myocardial workload, and CNS symptoms such as headache and mental clouding.

Nitroglycerin is available in most emergency kits and is a logical choice as a vasodilator. It can be administered in the same manner as for treating anginal episodes (see later discussion). Alternatively, *labetalol* (Normodyne, Trandate) is available for IV use. Unlike other IV vasodilators (e.g., hydralazine, diazoxide), labetalol also produces β-blocking activity that prevents reflex tachycardia. Labetalol should be carefully titrated in 10-mg to 20-mg increments every 10 minutes, and supine blood pressure should be recorded before adding each additional increment[7] (Fig. 18-3). The same contraindications and precautions described for propranolol and other β-blockers should be followed, including continuous electrocardiography (ECG) monitoring (see following section). The use of nifedipine (Procardia) capsules is no longer recommended. Absorption is unpredictable, and episodes of severe hypotension have been reported after nifedipine's use for acute hypertensive events[7-9] (Box 18-2).

Abnormal Rate and Rhythm

Episodes of *bradycardia* may accompany vasovagal syncope or the use of any of the CNS depressants used for conscious sedation and anesthesia. Treat-

ment is not required unless heart rate is insufficient to sustain blood pressure or the pulse becomes irregular due to ventricular escape or premature ventricular contractions (PVCs). In either case, 0.5-mg increments of atropine should be administered, up to 2.0 mg. Provided blood pressure and pulse rhythm are acceptable, a slow heart rate is beneficial in terms of myocardial oxygen demand. For patients with a history of ischemic heart disease, increasing heart rate indiscriminately could prove detrimental.

Transient episodes of *tachycardia* are triggered most often by pain, stress, and vasopressors included in local anesthetic solutions. However, tachycardia is also a reflex response to hypoxia or hypotension, and these should be considered during patient assessment. Once these possibilities have been attended, persistent tachycardia may cause the patient to complain of palpitations. In this case, initiate the syncope protocol and the fluid challenge portion of the hypotensive protocol described earlier. This will rule out the possibility that the rapid heart rate is sustaining blood pressure or is a reflex response to hypoxia. If the episode continues, a β-receptor antagonist such as propranolol (Inderal) can be titrated intravenously in 0.5-mg increments to gradually decrease sympathetic stimulation to the heart.

Beta blockers are relatively safe but should only be used when ECG monitoring is in place. β-blockers are contraindicated in heart failure or any degree of atrioventricular block. Patients having a history of atopy, asthma, or COPD have an added risk for bronchospasm after β-blockade, but this can be managed using any standard bronchodilator. Under no circumstances should β-blockers be used to correct a tachycardia that is compensating for hypotension or heart failure. It is also significant that β-blockers potentiate the hypertensive effects of epinephrine, even the low doses contained in local anesthetic solutions. If a local anesthetic with vasopressor has been administered within the previous 30 minutes, propranolol should not be administered. Issues regarding interactions with vasopressors, as well as risk for bronchospasm, are virtually eliminated by using a cardioselective β-blocker such as metoprolol. These drugs are much more expensive, however, and their β₁-adrenergic specificity is not absolute, especially at high doses (Box 18-3).

Angina and Myocardial Infarction

Ischemic heart disease is a condition whereby coronary perfusion is inadequate for myocardial oxygen requirements. If atherosclerosis is significant, the clinician can do little to improve coronary blood flow. In acute care settings the practitioner should devote complete attention to reducing myocardial oxygen requirements, rendering the compromised coronary perfusion adequate.

Angina is chest pain attributed to ischemic heart disease. An acute event may reflect either a compromise in coronary perfusion, generally attributable to sudden increases in cardiac effort, or a complete thrombotic obstruction, during which myocardial cells undergo necrosis. In dental practice the onset of angina is generally the result of a sudden increase in cardiac effort and greater myocardial oxygen demand. Nevertheless, chest pain of cardiac origin may represent a significant event (e.g., heart failure, dysrhythmia, myocardial infarction), and prompt intervention may avert progression to complete cardiac arrest.

When a patient experiences chest pain, initiate a typical syncope protocol and direct attention to reducing myocardial oxygen demand (Fig. 18-4). Comforting the patient will reduce stress-induced increases in heart rate and blood pressure. At low serum concentrations, such as after sublingual administration, *nitroglycerin* dilates systemic veins and reduces venous return (preload). This reduction in diastolic wall tension may also allow improved coronary perfusion, especially in the subendocardial regions. Nitroglycerin can be repeated every 5 minutes until symptoms improve or side effects occur, such as hypotension and reflex tachycardia. Hypotension is particularly troublesome because it could compromise coronary perfusion further, and reflex tachycardia increases myocardial oxygen demand. Although re-

clining patients are not likely to experience these problems, blood pressure and pulse should be assessed before administering each dose of nitroglycerin. When symptoms subside, the clinician must use personal judgment regarding subsequent action. For example, a patient who responds to a single dose of nitroglycerin may be sent home after the dental treatment is completed. In contrast, the patient with no prior history of angina or who requires several doses to relieve symptoms should be transported to an emergency treatment center for further evaluation.

BOX 18-3   **SUMMARY**

Drugs for Bradycardia and Tachycardia

Atropine
See Box 18-1.

Propranolol (Inderal)
Action: blocks β₁- and β₂-adrenergic receptors; β₁-blockade counters sympathetic stimulation to heart and decreases heart rate
Preparation: 1 mg/ml, ampules
Dose: IV, 0.5 mg every 5 minutes up to four doses

Metoprolol (Lopressor)
Action: selectively blocks β₁-receptors; counters sympathetic stimulation to heart and decreases heart rate
Preparation: 1 mg/ml, in 5-ml ampules
Dose: IV, 1 mg every 3 minutes up to five doses

IV, Intravenous.

Syncope Protocol

⇓

Nitroglycerin q5min × 3

⇓

Assume MI/Call EMS
NTG q5min if SBP >90
[Prepare for cardiac arrest]

Fig. 18-4 Algorithm for angina and myocardial infarction *(MI)*. *EMS,* Emergency medial services; *NTG,* nitroglycerin; *SBP,* systolic blood pressure.

In all cases, the patient's physician should be consulted when possible.

If three doses of nitroglycerin over 15 to 20 minutes fail to relieve symptoms, the clinician should assume that a *myocardial infarction* (MI) is evolving and summon emergency medical services (EMS) transport. While awaiting EMS, the clinician should administer a standard 300-mg tablet of aspirin. Platelet aggregation is a key factor during coronary thrombosis, and the maximum antiplatelet influence of aspirin is achieved within 1 hour of administration.[10] Nitroglycerin can be continued every 5 minutes, provided SBP is at least 90 to 100 mm Hg and heart rate is within normal limits. Alternatively, if pain and anxiety are persistent, an opioid (narcotic) can be administered. Opioids not only relieve pain and anxiety but also reduce peripheral resistance (afterload) and venous capacitance (preload). This reduces myocardial oxygen demand, a nitroglycerin-like effect. Because opioids are more likely to produce hypotension if nitroglycerin has been administered, the clinician should monitor blood pressure carefully (Box 18-4).

The most common sequela to MI is a lethal ventricular arrhythmia, such as tachycardia or fibrillation. The dentist should be familiar with local EMS response times to aid decisions regarding the need to monitor and deliver more advanced care. If IV access and ECG monitoring are available, significant ventricular ectopy (e.g., >6 PVCs/min, multiforme PVCs, couplets, R-on-T complexes) should be managed with lidocaine, 1.0 to 1.5 mg/kg. Half this amount can be repeated every 10 minutes until EMS arrival. While awaiting EMS, the office team should quietly prepare to administer cardiopulmonary resuscitation (CPR) in the event of cardiac arrest.

Cardiac Arrest

Cardiac arrest is a clinical term used to describe the absence of pulse. In dental practice, cardiac arrest is most likely to follow prolonged hypoxia, hypotension, or an acute ischemic event. If the preceding recommendations regarding preoperative assessment and management are followed closely, such an event is unlikely. The most common arrhythmias that accompany early cardiac arrest are ventricular tachycardia and fibrillation. Regardless of the specific ECG status, however, the initial treatment protocol is the same: CPR and epinephrine administration.

Ventilation should be performed using a positive-pressure device with a 100% oxygen source. This may

BOX 18-4   SUMMARY

Drugs for Angina and Myocardial Infarction

Nitroglycerin
Action: relaxes vascular smooth muscle; more venodilation than arteriodilation, thus reducing preload more than afterload, with both decreasing myocardial oxygen consumption
Preparation: 0.4-mg tablets
Dose: sublingual, 1 tablet every 5 minutes up to three doses

Aspirin
Action: inhibits synthesis of thromboxane A_2, which promotes platelet aggregation
Preparation: 300-mg tablets
Dose: PO, 1 tablet

Morphine*
Action: useful effects include analgesia, sedation, and reduction in preload and afterload; lowers myocardial oxygen consumption
Preparation: 5 mg/ml, in 2-ml ampules
Dose: IV, 2.5 mg every 3 minutes up to four doses

PO, Oral (by mouth); *IV,* intravenous.
*Meperidine (Demerol) and Nalbuphine (Nubain) are alternatives: morphine 2.5 mg = nalbuphine 2.5 mg = meperidine 25 mg.

be accomplished using a pocket mask with oxygen inlet or a BVM device (e.g., Ambu bag). Chest compressions must be rapid, 80 to 100/minute, with pauses after 15 compressions to allow for two ventilations. According to the 2001 American Heart Association guidelines, this 15:2 ratio should be followed for both one- and two-person CPR. The entire office staff should be certified in BLS annually.

Because early cardiac arrest is caused by ventricular tachycardia or fibrillation, definitive treatment requires electrical defibrillation as soon as it is available. The beneficial role of CPR likely rests in its modest influence on coronary perfusion, which may sustain electrical activity until defibrillation is available. This concept is supported by data illustrating greatest success when CPR is initiated immediately and is followed by ACLS within 8 to 10 minutes of cardiac arrest.

Coronary perfusion is essential to sustain myocardial viability, and the protocol for cardiac arrest includes attempts to improve peripheral resistance to facilitate this effort. For this reason, epinephrine is indicated in all cases of cardiac arrest, and this actually precludes an absolute requirement for ECG classification. Current ACLS standards recommend a 1-mg dose repeated every 5 minutes as necessary during CPR. This can be accomplished by injecting either 10 ml of a 1:10,000 solution or 1 ml of a 1:1000 solution into an antecubital vein. If an IV line is not in place at the time of arrest, access should not be attempted unless a vein is readily accessible and the dentist is skilled at venipuncture. For those skilled in tracheal intubation (accomplished within 30 seconds), this maneuver not only allows superior ventilation but also provides access for instillation of epinephrine, with 2 to 3 mg in normal saline 20 ml. An alternative is to inject 1 or 2 ml of a 1:1000 solution sublingually, although data are limited regarding absorption and distribution during cardiac arrest.

Respiratory Considerations

Respiratory Depression

In general, use of conscious sedation has a positive influence on patients undergoing dental procedures. Reducing fear and anxiety decreases stress on the cardiovascular system, and vasovagal reactions are less likely. Compared with local anesthesia alone, the most significant negative variable introduced by conscious sedation, as well as deep sedation and general anesthesia, is the added risk for respiratory depression. All sedatives, opioids, and inhalation agents have the potential to depress central hypercapnic and peripheral hypoxemic drives. This risk is minimal, however, provided the practitioner uses conventional doses and monitors the patient according to guidelines presented in this text. Nevertheless, the clinician must be thoroughly skilled in managing respiratory depression.

As with any complication, management of respiratory depression should commence with standard airway support. Pharmacologic intervention is indicated only when a patient is apneic or fails to respond adequately to oxygen supplementation. Among the drug classes used for sedation and anesthesia, *opioids* are the most powerful respiratory depressants. If an opioid has been included in the regimen, naloxone (Narcan) should be the first drug administered. It can

---

BOX 18-5   SUMMARY
Drugs for Respiratory Depression

Naloxone (Narcan)
Action: blocks mu and kappa opioid receptors, reversing analgesia, sedation, and respiratory depression
Preparation: 0.4 mg/ml, SDV or ampule
Dose: IV, 0.1 to 0.4 mg every 3 minutes, up to 0.8 mg; sublingual, 0.4 mg every 5 minutes up to two doses

Flumazenil (Romazicon)
Action: selectively blocks benzodiazepine receptors, reversing sedation and respiratory depression
Preparation: 0.1 mg/ml, in 5-ml and 10-ml MDV
Dose: IV or sublingual, 0.2 mg every 3 minutes up to five doses

SDV, Single-dose vial; *IV,* intravenous; *MDV,* multidose vial.

---

be titrated intravenously in 0.1-mg to 0.4-mg increments every 3 to 5 minutes, up to 0.8 mg. The higher doses in this range should be reserved for patients who are apneic. Alternatively, naloxone (0.4 mg) can be injected sublingually and repeated after 5 minutes if necessary. Naloxone should not be administered to a patient with a current history of opioid dependence unless the event is life threatening and other interventions have been futile.

Respiratory depression mediated by benzodiazepines can be reversed using the specific antagonist *flumazenil* (Romazicon). It can be titrated intravenously or injected sublingually in 0.2-mg increments every 2 to 3 minutes, up to 1 mg. Flumazenil should not be administered to patients with a history of seizure disorder or dependence on benzodiazepines (Box 18-5).

Upper Airway Obstruction

Upper airway obstruction may result from a foreign body or pathologic conditions such as laryngospasm or laryngeal edema. It is essential to distinguish laryngeal edema, laryngospasm, and bronchospasm. The hallmark of asthmatic and anaphylactoid reactions is contraction or spasm of bronchial smooth muscle. This muscle is under autonomic nervous control and requires β_2-sympathomimetics for relaxation. Swelling of laryngeal mucosa (laryngeal edema) accompanies anaphylactoid reactions and requires administration of agents with decongestant influences, such as epinephrine. In contrast, the vocal cords are abducted by skeletal muscle that is innervated by somatic efferents. Spasm of laryngeal muscles can be triggered during emergence from general anesthesia or by irritation from secretory or foreign debris.

Management of upper airway obstruction should commence with proper head positioning and oropharyngeal suctioning. If these interventions fail to correct the obstruction and a foreign body is suspected, abdominal thrusts should be performed according to BLS protocol. Laryngospasm will generally respond to positive-pressure oxygenation using a standard BVM device. To be successful, the mask must seal tightly against the patient's face, with gentle continuous pressure applied to the bag until the spasm relaxes. In the rare event that the cords fail to relax, pharmacologic intervention requires neuromuscular blockers such as succinylcholine. Generally a small dose (0.1 mg/kg) is sufficient and should only supplement the continued application of positive-pressure oxygenation.

Regardless of the cause, inability to ventilate an apneic, unconscious patient presents a sobering dilemma for even the most trained clinician. When suctioning, abdominal thrusts, and further attempts to ventilate and/or intubate the patient fail, *transtracheal oxygenation* should be attempted. This intervention is not surgical and must not be confused with cricothyrotomy or the more sophisticated tracheotomy.

Many techniques and devices have been described in the literature for emergency airway access, but the simplest approach employs a 12- or 14-gauge IV catheter attached to a standard 3-ml syringe. This device is used to puncture the cricothyroid membrane, thus entering the trachea, and the plunger of the syringe is removed. The plunger is replaced with the adapter from a standard 7.5-mm endotracheal tube, and a bag-valve device (e.g., Ambu bag) is attached. Alternatively, an adapter from a 3.0-mm or 3.5-mm endotracheal tube can be connected directly to the catheter, obviating the syringe. The bag is connected to a 100% oxygen source, and positive-pressure oxygen is delivered into the trachea (Fig. 18-5). This technique oxygenates the patient but does not provide effective ventilation; hypercarbia and acidosis are not prevented.[11] However, the goal of transtracheal oxygenation is to sustain an acceptable arterial oxygen tension. Despite elevated arterial carbon dioxide tension and acidosis, this procedure can maintain reasonable cardiovascular stability until EMS transport.

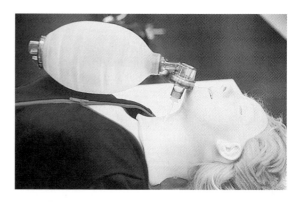

Fig. 18-5 Equipment for transtracheal oxygenation. Using adapter from 3.0 pediatric endotracheal tube connected to bag-valve-mask device, oxygenation can be delivered through 14- to 16-gauge angiocatheter inserted through cricothyroid membrane.

Bronchospasm

In asthma the tracheobronchial tree is overly responsive to a variety of stimuli. The principal features of an acute asthmatic attack are mucus secretion and acute bronchospasm. Dyspnea and wheezing herald the onset of an acute asthmatic attack and demand immediate intervention. Patients with chronic forms of respiratory disease (e.g., COPD) are also at risk for bronchospasm, which is a primary concern during their emergency management as well. Primary treatment should consist of oxygen supplementation and administration of a bronchodilator. Antiinflammatory steroids and mucolytic agents are essential components of chronic therapy, but they have little efficacy during acute intervention.

Oxygen supplementation may consist of 4 to 6 L/min via nasal cannula or 10 L/min by mask. The nasal cannula is less frightening and ideal for COPD patients, for whom oxygen concentration should not exceed 40%. Cannulas also allow simultaneous inhalation of albuterol (Proventil, Ventolin), the preferred bronchodilator for managing acute episodes of bronchospasm. Selective β_2-agonists such as albuterol are ideal because they are less likely to produce positive cardiotonic side effects than nonselective agents with β_1-adrenergic activity.

Patients must cooperate if inhalants are to be administered effectively. Spacer chambers can be attached to inhalers and minimize the need for a coordinated effort from the patient. If a patient becomes hysterical or for other reasons cannot be administered an inhalant, 0.3 to 0.5 mg of epinephrine (1:1000) can be injected subcutaneously or sublingually. Aminophylline, often cited in dental literature for emergency management, has limited efficacy as a single agent for acute intervention and requires a sophisticated dosage regimen.[12,13] Similarly, anticholinergics such as ipratropium (Atrovent) are useful in chronic management but have not proven useful during acute events.

Allergic Reactions

Immediate allergic reactions are attributed to immunoglobulin E (IgE)-mediated release of several mediators from mast cells and basophils. These, along with additional autacoids, can also be synthesized and released by non-IgE mechanisms, producing a similar clinical syndrome. Because an IgE mechanism cannot always be confirmed, it has become conventional to use the terms *pseudoallergic* and *anaphylactoid* when describing these reactions.

Minor allergic or pseudoallergic reactions involve only the skin, presenting as pruritus, maculopapular rash, and urticaria. Cutaneous reactions are mediated primarily by histamine and can be counteracted by antihistamines such as diphenhydramine.

Anaphylactoid reactions may also present cutaneous signs but can be distinguished by a syndrome of systemic complications that include acute bronchospasm, laryngeal edema, and hypotension. In addition to histamine, other autacoids contribute to the pathogenesis of anaphylactoid reactions. These include prostaglandins, leukotrienes, and a variety of proteases for which no specific antagonists exist. Glucocorticoids produce a more generalized inhibitory effect on inflammatory autacoids, but this influence is not appreciated for several hours after administration and limits their value for managing the acute event. Any patient who experiences an anaphylactoid event will require EMS transport to an emergency department; steroid administration may be delayed until that time or at least until the acute syndrome is stabilized.

Management of an acute anaphylactoid event requires oxygen supplementation and administration of epinephrine (Box 18-6). Stimulation of both α-adrenergic and β-adrenergic receptors is required to reverse physiologically the anaphylactoid syndrome. α-Receptor-induced vasoconstriction reduces laryngeal edema and increases blood pressure. β-Receptor stimulation relieves bronchospasm and improves cardiac output (Fig. 18-6).

▨ B◌X 18-6   **SUMMARY**

Drugs for Asthmatic and Allergic Reactions

Albuterol (Ventolin, Proventil)
Action: selective β_2-receptor agonist; relaxes bronchial smooth muscle
Preparation: metered-dose inhaler
Dose: 1 or 2 inhalations every 3 minutes

Diphenhydramine (Benadryl)
Action: selectively blocks histamine receptors; counteracts cutaneous reactions, including pruritus, rash, and urticaria
Preparation: 50 mg/ml, SDV, ampules, prefilled syringes
Dose: IV, 25 mg every 5 minutes up to two doses; IM, 50 mg

Epinephrine
Action: α/β-receptor agonist; increases cardiac output, bronchodilates and decongests edematous mucosa
Preparation: 1 mg/ml, ampules and prefilled syringes
Dose: subcutaneous, 0.3 to 0.5 mg every 5 minutes up to two doses; IV, 0.1 mg every 3 minutes up to five doses

SDV, Single-vial dose; *IV,* intravenous; *IM,* intramuscular.

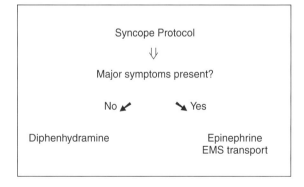

Fig. 18-6 Algorithm for allergic reaction.

Many doses and administration routes for epinephrine have been suggested in the literature, but subcutaneous or IV doses of 0.3 to 0.5 mg are recommended most consistently. A 1:1000 concentration (0.3 to 0.5 ml) is preferred for subcutaneous and a 1:10,000 concentration (3 to 5 ml) for IV epinephrine. Duration of effect may be as brief as 5 to 10 minutes, and additional doses may be required before EMS arrival at the office. If IV access is available, hypotension should also be managed with fluid challenge to correct hypovolemia accompanying increased permeability of the vascular bed.[14]

Other Complications

Diabetic Complications

Diabetes mellitus is a disorder of carbohydrate metabolism that results from defects in insulin secretion, insulin action, or both.[15] The type 1 diabetic has absolute insulin deficiency, whereas type 2 diabetics produce inadequate amounts of insulin and exhibit tissue resistance. Type 2 diabetics are generally managed with diet or oral hypoglycemic agents but may require insulin replacement. Only type 1 diabetics experience acute diabetic coma, which manifests not only as hyperglycemia with subsequent hyperosmolar coma but also as ketoacidosis from lack of insulin's inhibitory influence on lipolysis. This complication is highly unlikely, generally presenting in the undiagnosed patient.

Regardless of classification, *hypoglycemia* is the most common acute event in diabetic patients and can be attributed to excessive medication or inadequate carbohydrate intake. As serum glucose dips below 60 mg/dl, compensatory hormones are released, including epinephrine, which accounts for the early warning signs of tachycardia, shakiness, and diaphoresis. As the concentration drops further, generally to less than 50 mg/dl, cognitive and additional CNS functions become impaired. Hypoglycemic reactions must be taken seriously because brain tissue relies on glucose exclusively as an energy substrate. In addition to the standard syncope protocol, the patient must be given concentrated glucose. Provided they retain consciousness, patients can be permitted to drink a sweetened beverage, but a viscous glucose concentrate should be available for more severe episodes. The concentrate should be placed in the buccal mucosa and permitted to dissolve and seep down the esophagus and into the stomach. Contrary to popular belief, glucose cannot diffuse through oral mucosa.[16] If an IV line is in place, 25 to 50 ml of a 50% dextrose solution can be infused slowly, keeping in mind that its osmolarity leads to venous irritation. Glucagon is a less attractive alternative. After IM administration, glucagon elevates blood glucose by stimulation of glycogenolysis. This action requires 10 to 20 minutes and can be ineffective in patients having limited stores of glycogen, such as poorly nourished or dieting patients.

Convulsive Seizures

Convulsive seizures are attributable to excessive, synchronous discharge of large numbers of cortical neurons and may be caused by drug toxicity or a variety of injuries and diseases. They are designated as *epileptic seizures* only if they have a chronic pattern of recurrence. The typical *grand mal seizures* last a minute or less and require only that the patient is protected from physical harm. After a seizure, patients are tired and require the supportive measures included in a standard syncope protocol. The patient's physician will appreciate notification and will generally want to obtain a serum level for the anticonvulsant medication. Although EMS transport is not indicated, the patient should be discharged only to a responsible adult.

Status seizures are those that continue unabated for 20 to 30 minutes or repeat without full recovery. This definition is based on the length of time required until injury to CNS neurons occurs and is impractical for clinical practice. A more operational definition is a seizure that continues for 5 minutes unabated or that repeats without complete recovery.[17] Despite brief periods of apnea and cyanosis, most patients breathe adequately, provided their airway patency is maintained.

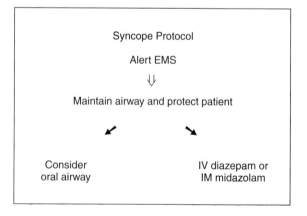

Fig. 18-7 Algorithm for status seizures.

Benzodiazepines are the preferred agents for terminating seizure activity. If IV access is available, diazepam (10 to 20 mg) or lorazepam (4 to 8 mg) is the usual choice. Alternatively, midazolam (0.2 to 0.3 mg/kg) can be administered intramuscularly and generally takes effect in approximately 10 minutes (Fig. 18-7).[17]

SUMMARY

Preoperative assessment and intraoperative assessment of cardiovascular and respiratory status are essential for patient care and for effective management of adverse events. Instructions for managing each specific event can be prepared in algorithmic format and placed in a plastic "baggie" along with specific medications and syringes. During the chaos of medical urgencies and emergencies, the clinician cannot be expected to precisely recall the algorithms and drug dosages explained throughout this chapter. However, fundamental principles of physiology and patient assessment should be familiar if the clinician is to assess properly the patient's status and select the appropriate treatment protocol. This familiarity distinguishes cognitive from technical ability and ensures optimal care for the patient.

References

1. American Thoracic Society: Standards for the diagnosis and care of patients with chronic obstructive pulmonary disease (COPD), *Am J Respir Crit Care Med* 152:S77-S120, 1995.
2. Deihl RR, Linden D: Images in clinical medicine: neurocardiogenic syncope, *N Engl J Med* 339:312, 1998.
3. Thrush DN, Downs JB: Vagotonia and cardiac arrest during spinal anesthesia, *Anesthesiology* 91:1171-1173, 1999.
4. Sibbald WJ et al: The Trendelenburg position: hemodynamic effects in hypotensive and normotensive patients, *Crit Care Med* 7:218-224, 1979.
5. Coonan TJ, Hope CE: Cardiorespiratory effects of change of body position, *Can Anaesth Soc J* 30:424-437, 1983.
6. Lawson NW, Meyer DJ: Autonomic nervous system: physiology and pharmacology. In Barash PG, Cullen BF, Stoelting RK, editors: *Clinical anesthesia*, ed 3, Philadelphia, 1997, Lippincott-Raven.
7. Varon J, Marik PE: The diagnosis and management of hypertensive crisis, *Chest* 118:214-227, 2000.
8. Thach AM, Schultz PJ: Nonemergent hypertension: new perspectives for the emergency medicine physician, *Emerg Med Clin North Am* 13:1009-1035, 1995.
9. Grossman E et al: Should a moratorium be placed on sublingual nifedipine capsules given for hypertensive emergencies and pseudoemergencies? *JAMA* 276:1328-1331, 1342-1343, 1996 (editorial).
10. Collins R et al: Drug therapy: aspirin, heparin, and fibrinolytic therapy in suspected acute myocardial infarction, *N Engl J Med* 336:847-860, 1997.
11. Yealy DM, Stewart RD, Kaplan RM: Myths and pitfalls in emergency translaryngeal ventilation: correcting misimpressions, *Ann Emerg Med* 17:690-692, 1988.
12. Littenberg B: Aminophylline treatment in severe, acute asthma: a meta-analysis, *JAMA* 259:1678-1684, 1988.
13. Fitzgerald JM, Hargreave FE: The assessment and management of acute life-threatening asthma, *Chest* 95:888-894, 1989.
14. Weiss ME, Adkinson NF, Hirshman CA: Evaluation of allergic drug reactions in the perioperative period, *Anesthesiology* 71:483-486, 1989.
15. American Diabetes Association: Report of the Expert Committee on the Diagnosis and Classification of Diabetes Mellitus, *Diabetes Care* 20:1183-1197, 1997.
16. Gunning RR, Garber AJ: Bioactivity of instant glucose: failure of absorption through oral mucosa, *JAMA* 240:1611-1612, 1978.
17. Lowenstein DH, Alldredge BK: Status epilepticus, *N Engl J Med* 338:970-976, 1998.

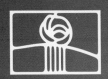

MANAGEMENT OF PATIENTS
WITH SPECIAL REQUIREMENTS

CHAPTER 19

Pediatric Sedation

Milton I. Houpt
Joseph A. Giovannitti, Jr.

CHAPTER OUTLINE

Children are the building blocks of a general dental practice. Parents frequently send children to a new dentist before they themselves present for treatment. Furthermore, children grow up to become future adult patients. Consequently, it is wise for a practitioner to treat children in a family practice. Although most children like to visit the dentist, some occasionally are fearful and have behavioral problems.

Children may come to the dental office with general anxieties or specific fears. *General anxieties* are related to basic personality traits influenced by parents, siblings, or peers, whereas *specific fears* may result from previous painful dental procedures or reports from others of unpleasant experiences. Coping skills are either underdeveloped or nonexistent, and the child has no incentive to cooperate. Unlike adults, children do not understand or care that cooperation during treatment may produce a favorable cosmetic or functional result. General anxieties or specific fears lead children to display different behaviors depending on their developmental stage. Children may be cooperative, apprehensive, fearful, or defiant. Children may be emotionally immature and unable to communicate properly. Children also may be physically, mentally, or emotionally handicapped, which may influence their behavior.

Nonpharmacologic techniques, including "tell-show-do" and voice control, are used to manage child behavior, and the vast majority of children receiving dental care are treated with these techniques. Occasionally, *pharmacologic techniques*, including conscious sedation, deep sedation, and general anesthesia, are required. A recent survey of pediatric dentists[1] provides evidence of the occasional need for pharmacologic techniques: 47% indicated that they used nitrous oxide less than 10% of the time, and only 17% used other types of sedatives for more than 10% of their patients. Most children (78%) receiving sedative agents other than nitrous oxide were under 5 years of age.

Pharmacologic techniques are indicated for patients with extreme anxiety and those with whom it is difficult to communicate, such as children under 2 years of age, developmentally disabled children, or extremely fearful children. Deep sedation and general anesthesia are reserved for children who require extensive treatment or those for whom nonpharmacologic techniques and conscious sedation might be unsuccessful. The goal of pediatric sedation is to accomplish treatment on a comfortable and cooperative child. Unfortunately, in the uncooperative child, the two are not always synonymous. Comfort is directly related to fear and anxiety control, which can be achieved with or without drugs. Although cooperation may be achieved in the same fashion, a comfortable child is not always a cooperative one. Often, cooperation will be gained only when levels of sedation deepen and the child becomes unconscious.

Drug responses vary and are unpredictable, and sedatives do not necessarily induce cooperation. Overdosage may occur, especially when opioids are used, when redosing occurs, or when drug combinations are used. Only properly trained individuals with appropriate monitoring and resuscitation equipment readily available should attempt sedation and general anesthesia. Guidelines developed by the American Academy of Pediatric Dentistry should be observed whenever sedation is used with pediatric patients[2] (Box 19-1).

Pediatric Anatomy and Physiology

Significant anatomic and physiologic differences exist between pediatric and adult patients that influence anesthetic management. Pediatric patients have large heads, short necks, relatively large tongues and soft tissue, and narrow nasal passages, which are readily blocked by secretion or edema. The larynx is more cephalad and anterior in a child, with the glottis at the level of the third and fourth cervical vertebrae (C3-4), versus level C4-5 in the adult. The epiglottis is long and stiff and protrudes posteriorly at a 45-degree angle. The narrowest portion of the upper airway is at the cricoid ring, and the trachea is 4 to 5.7 cm from the glottis to the carina, versus 6 to 8 cm in the adult. The angles of the right and left mainstem bronchi with the trachea are equal. Pediatric patients have fewer lung alveoli, the 20 million present at birth increase to 300 million by age 8. These anatomic traits combine to make the pediatric patient an airway management challenge.

A higher metabolic rate in infants and children results in a proportionally greater alveolar ventilation (100 to 150 ml/kg/min) than in adults (60 ml/kg/min). The functional residual capacity (FRC), which is the sum of the expiratory reserve volume (ERV) and the residual volume (RV), acts as a buffer to maintain arterial oxygenation during inspiration and expiration. In an adult the ratio of alveolar ventilation to FRC is 1.5:1. In the infant the ratio is 5:1, making the pediatric patient much more susceptible to the development of arterial hypoxemia. The

Text continued on p. 306

BOX 19-1

Guidelines for the Elective Use of Conscious Sedation, Deep Sedation and General Anesthesia In Pediatric Dental Patients

The American Academy of Pediatric Dentistry's *Guidelines for the Elective Use of Pharmacological Conscious Sedation and Deep Sedation in Pediatric Dental Patients* were revised and published in 1996. At that time, no attempt was made to address the issue of general anesthesia for pediatric dental patients. However, some children and developmentally disabled patients require general anesthesia services in order to receive comprehensive dental care in a humane fashion. Access to hospital based general anesthesia may be limited for a variety of reasons including restriction of coverage by certain insurance companies. Many pediatric dentists (and others who treat children) have sought to provide general anesthesia in their office or other facilities (e.g., outpatient care clinics).

Therefore we have included general anesthesia in the guidelines to help facilitate safe anesthesia services for pediatric dental patients.

In 1985, the American Academy of Pediatric Dentistry established the *Guidelines for the Elective Use of Conscious Sedation, Deep Sedation and General Anesthesia in Pediatric Patients*. To be consistent with all aspects of delivery of care using pharmacologic interventions, it is appropriate and timely to expand and institute guidelines that address general anesthesia as well as sedation for those practitioners who provide care to pediatric dental patients. General anesthesia may be used when indicated for the delivery of oral health care to pediatric patients. It must be provided only by qualified and appropriately trained individuals and in accordance with state regulation. Such providers may include pediatric dentists who have completed advanced education in anesthesiology, dental or medical anesthesiologists, oral surgeons or certified registered nurse anesthetists.

The 1998 AAPD guidelines revision reflects the current understanding of appropriate monitoring needs and further, provides definitions and characteristics of five functional levels of sedation and general anesthesia involving pediatric patients in the context of recognized sedation terminology (i.e., "conscious" and "deep"). Table I provides a descriptive template for recognizing that sedation is a continuum; however, the practitioner's expected clinical outcomes in sedating the "average" patient can be targeted with the targeting being dependent on his/her training and experience in the use of sedative agents. The template shows five levels of sedation each with its own goals, characteristics, and requirements.

The pediatric dentist must be responsible for evaluating the qualifications of the general anesthesia provider and establishing a safe environment that complies with state rules and regulations as well as these guidelines for the protection of the patient. Educational qualifications for general anesthesia providers are outlined in these guidelines.

Educational preparation, while necessary, is only one aspect of safe general anesthesia care. As outlined in the Guidelines, the following are all essential in order to minimize the risk for the patient:

- facilities and equipment;
- selection of pharmacologic agents and dosages;
- monitoring and documentation;
- patient selection utilizing physical status and indication for anesthetic management;
- operative evaluation;
- appropriately trained support personnel;
- and emergency medications, equipment and protocols.

The use of conscious sedation, deep sedation, and general anesthesia will be affected by advances in pain and anxiety control, pharmacologic development, and monitoring and patient safety techniques. As research defines safer and more effective techniques, the Guidelines will be revised accordingly.

Definition of Terms
For the purpose of this document, the following definitions shall apply:

Guideline: Guidelines are systematically developed recommendations to assist practitioner and patient decisions about appropriate health care for specific clinical circumstances. These recommendations may be adopted, modified, or rejected according to clinical needs and constraints. Guidelines are not intended as standards or absolute requirements and their use cannot guarantee any specific outcome.

Like a recommendation, it originates in an organization with acknowledged professional stature. Although it may be unsolicited, it usually is developed following a stated request or perceived need for such advice or instruction.

From The American Academy of Pediatric Dentistry, revised May, 1998.

BOX 19-1

Guidelines for the Elective Use of Conscious Sedation, Deep Sedation and General Anesthesia In Pediatric Dental Patients—cont'd

Pediatric dental patients: Includes all patients who are infants, children, and adolescents less than age of majority.

Must or shall: Indicates an imperative need and/or duty; as essential or indispensable; mandatory.

Should: Indicates the recommended need and/or duty; highly desirable.

May or could: Indicates freedom or liberty to follow a suggested or reasonable alternative.

Conscious sedation: Conscious sedation (Table I, levels 1, 2, and 3) is a controlled, pharmacologically induced, minimally depressed level of consciousness that retains the patient's ability to maintain a patent airway independently and continuously and respond appropriately to physical stimulation and/or verbal command. The drugs, dosages, and techniques used should carry a margin of safety which is unlikely to render the child non-interactive and non-arousable (Table I, levels 4 and 5).

Deep sedation: Deep sedation (Table I, level 4) is a controlled, pharmacologically-induced state of depressed consciousness from which the patient is not easily aroused and which may be accompanied by a partial loss of protective reflexes, including the ability to maintain a patent airway independently and/or respond purposefully to physical stimulation or verbal command.

General anesthesia: General anesthesia (Table I, level 5) is an induced state of unconsciousness accompanied by partial or complete loss of protective reflexes, including the ability to independently maintain an airway and respond purposefully to physical stimulation or verbal command.

General Considerations

Goals of sedation and general anesthesia

The sedation of children for the delivery of oral health care is recognized as and represents a unique clinical challenge. Consideration must be given to such factors as patient's age and corresponding levels of cognitive and coping skills. Because of patient extremes in responsiveness and acceptability of treatment modalities, the intended goals and outcome of sedations will vary depending on a host of factors. These guidelines should aid clinicians in achieving the benefits of sedation while minimizing associated risks and adverse outcomes for the patient.

The goals of sedation in the pediatric dental patient are to: (1) facilitate the provision of quality care; (2) minimize the extremes of disruptive behavior; (3) promote a positive psychologic response to treatment; (4) promote patient welfare and safety; (5) return the patient to a physiologic state in which safe discharge, as determined by recognized criteria, is possible (Appendix I).

The goals of general anesthesia in the pediatric dental patient are to eliminate cognitive, sensory and skeletal motor activity in order to facilitate the delivery of quality comprehensive diagnostic and restorative dental services.

Indication for sedation and general anesthesia

The indications for conscious sedation include:

- Preschool children who cannot understand or cooperate for definitive treatment
- Patients requiring dental care who cannot cooperate due to lack of psychological or emotional maturity
- Patients requiring dental treatment who cannot cooperate due to a cognitive, physical and medical disability
- Patients who require dental care but are fearful and anxious and cannot cooperate for treatment

The indications for deep sedation and general anesthesia in pediatric dental patients include:

- Patients with certain physical, mental or medically compromising conditions
- Patients with dental restorative or surgical needs for whom local anesthesia in ineffective
- The extremely uncooperative, fearful, anxious, or physically resistant child or adolescent with substantial dental needs and no expectation that the behavior will improve soon
- Patients who have sustained extensive orofacial or dental trauma
- Patients with dental needs who otherwise would not receive comprehensive dental care

Local Anesthesia Considerations during Sedation

All local anesthetic agents can become cardiac and CNS depressants when administered in excessive doses. There is a potential interaction between local anesthetic

Continued

Guidelines for the Elective Use of Conscious Sedation, Deep Sedation and General Anesthesia In Pediatric Dental Patients—cont'd

and sedatives used in pediatric dentistry which can result in enhanced sedative effects and/or untoward events; therefore, particular attention should be paid to doses used in children. For the patient who is going to be sedated, to avoid excessive doses, a maximum recommended dose in mg/kg or mg/lb should be calculated and the dose administered should be recorded for each patient prior to administration for all sedatives and local anesthetics.

Candidates

Patients who are ASA (American Society of Anesthesiologists) Class I or II (Appendix II) may be considered candidates for conscious sedation (Table I, levels 1, 2, or 3) or deep sedation (Table I, level 4) or general anesthesia (Table I, level 5). Patients in ASA Class III or IV present special problems and treatment in a hospital setting should be considered.

Responsible adult

The pediatric patient shall be accompanied to and from the treatment facility by a parent, legal guardian or other responsible adult who shall be required to remain at the facility for the entire treatment period.

Facilities

The practitioner who utilizes any type of sedative or local anesthetic in a pediatric patient shall possess appropriate training and skills and have available the proper facilities, personnel, and equipment to manage any reasonably foreseeable emergency situation that might be experienced. All newly installed facilities for delivering nitrous oxide and oxygen must be checked for proper gas delivery and fail-safe function prior to use. Where equipment and facilities are mandated by state law, such statutes shall supersede these guidelines.

Equipment

A positive-pressure oxygen delivery system that is capable of administering greater than 90% oxygen at a 10 L/min flow for at least 60 minutes (650 liter, "E" cylinder) must be available. When a self-inflating bag valve mask device is used for delivering positive pressure oxygen, a 15 L/min flow is recommended. All equipment must be able to accommodate children of all ages and sizes. A functional suction apparatus with appropriate suc-

tion catheters must be immediately available. A sphygmomanometer with cuffs of appropriate size for pediatric patients shall be immediately available.

Inhalation sedation equipment must have the capacity for delivering 100%, and never less than 25%, oxygen concentration at a flow rate appropriate to the child's size, and must have a fail-safe system that is checked and calibrated annually. If nitrous oxide and oxygen delivery equipment capable of delivering more than 75% nitrous oxide and less than 25% oxygen is used, an in-line oxygen analyzer must be used. The equipment must have an appropriate scavenging system.

Equipment that is appropriate for the technique used and capable of monitoring the physiologic state of the patient before, during, and after the procedure must be present.

Specific equipment monitoring and recommendations are listed in the sections on conscious sedation, deep sedation and general anesthesia and in the template of these guidelines (Table I).

An emergency cart or kit must be readily accessible and should include the necessary drugs and age- and size-appropriate equipment to resuscitate a nonbreathing and unconscious pediatric patient and provide continuous support while the patient is being transported to a medical facility. There should be documentation that all emergency equipment and drugs are checked and maintained on a regularly scheduled basis (e.g., monthly) (see Appendix III for suggested drugs).

Back-up emergency services

Back-up emergency services should be identified. A protocol outlining necessary procedures for their immediate employment should be developed and operational for each facility. For non-hospital facilities, an emergency assist system should be established with the nearest hospital emergency facility and ready access to ambulance service must be assured.

Documentation

The practitioner must document each sedation or general anesthesia procedure in the patient's record. Documentation shall include the following:

Informed consent. Each patient, parent, or other responsible individual is entitled to be informed regarding

From The American Academy of Pediatric Dentistry, revised May, 1998.

BOX 19-1

Guidelines for the Elective Use of Conscious Sedation, Deep Sedation and General Anesthesia In Pediatric Dental Patients—cont'd

benefits, risks, and alternatives to sedation or general anesthesia and to give consent. The patient record shall document that appropriate informed consent was obtained according to the procedures outlined by individual state laws and/or institutional requirements.

Instructions to parents or responsible individual. The practitioner shall provide verbal and written instructions to the parents or responsible individual. Instructions should be explicit and include an explanation of pre- and post-sedation dietary precautions, potential or anticipated post-operative behavior, and limitation of activities. A 24-hr contact number for the practitioner should be provided to all patients

Dietary precautions. The administration of sedative drugs or general anesthetic agents shall be preceded by an evaluation of the patient's food and liquid intake. Intake of food and liquids should be as follows: (a) no milk or solids for 6 hours for children 6-36 months and 6-8 hours for children 36 months and older; (b) clear liquids up to 3 hours before procedure for children ages 6 months and older.

Preoperative health evaluation. Prior to the administration of sedatives, the practitioner shall obtain and document information about the patient's current health status. The health status evaluation should include:

Health history including:

- Allergies and previous allergic or adverse drug reactions
- Current medications including dose, time, route, and site of administration
- Diseases, disorders, or physical abnormalities and pregnancy status
- Previous hospitalization to include the date, purpose, and hospital course
- History of general anesthesia or sedation and any associated complications
- Family history of diseases or disorders
- Review of systems
- Age in years and months and weight in kilograms of pounds

Physical evaluation including:

- Vital signs, including heart and respiratory rates and blood pressure
- Evaluation of airway patency

- Risk assessment, e.g., ASA classification (see Appendix II)

Hospitalized patients. The current hospital records may suffice for adequate documentation of pre-sedation health. A brief note shall be written documenting that the record was reviewed, positive findings were noted, and there were no contraindications to the planned procedure(s).

Child's physician. Name, address, and telephone number of the child's physician or family physician should be recorded in the patient's record.

Rationale for sedation of general anesthesia. The practitioner shall briefly document the reason for the need for sedation or general anesthesia.

Baseline vital signs. Before administration of sedatives or general anesthesia, a baseline determination of vital signs (heart and respiratory rates and blood pressure) should be documented in the patient's record. If determination of baseline vital signs is prevented by the patient's resistance or emotional condition, the reason(s) should be documented.

Preprocedural prescriptions. The only classification of drugs for sedation to be administered enterally by a responsible adult pre-procedurally outside the treatment facility is minor tranquilizers. Minor tranquilizers (e.g., hydroxyzine or diazepam) do not include chloral hydrate or narcotics. A copy of a note describing the content of the prescription should be documented in the patient's record, along with a description of the instructions given to the responsible individual.

Vital signs. The patient's record shall contain documentation of intermittent quantitative monitoring and recording of oxygen saturation (pulse oximetry) and heart and respiratory rates and blood pressure, as recommended for specific sedation techniques. It should be documented that the responsiveness of the patient was monitored at specific intervals before and during the procedure and until the patient was discharged.

Drugs. The patient's record shall document the name, dose and route, site, and time of administration of all drugs administered. The maximum recommended dose per kilogram or pound should be calculated and the actual dose given shall be documented in milligrams. The concentrations, flow rate, and duration of administration of oxygen and nitrous oxide shall be documented.

Continued

BOX 19-1

Guidelines for the Elective Use of Conscious Sedation, Deep Sedation and General Anesthesia In Pediatric Dental Patients—cont'd

Recovery

The condition of the child and the time of discharge from the treatment facility should be documented in the record. Documentation shall include that appropriate discharge criteria have been met (see Appendix II). The record should also identify the responsible adult to whose care the patient was discharged.

Conscious Sedation (Levels 1, 2, 3)

Personnel

The practitioner responsible for the treatment of the patient and/or the administration of drugs for conscious sedation (levels 1, 2, and 3) shall be appropriately trained in the use of such drugs and techniques, and shall provide appropriate monitoring, and shall be capable of managing any reasonable foreseeable complications.

Drugs, other than minor tranquilizers, used for the purpose of conscious sedation (levels 1, 2, and 3) shall be administered in the treatment facility and shall be prescribed, dispensed, or administered only by appropriately licensed individuals, or under the direct supervision thereof, according to state law.

In addition to the operating practitioner, an individual trained to monitor appropriate physiologic parameters and to assist in any supportive or resuscitative measures required shall be present. Both individuals must have training in basic life support, shall have specific assignments, and shall have familiarity of the emergency cart (kit) inventory.

The practitioner and all treatment facility personnel should participate in periodic reviews of the office's emergency protocol, the emergency drug kit, and simulated exercises, to assure proper emergency management response.

Operating facility and equipment

The operating facility used for the administration of conscious sedation, (levels 1, 2, or 3), shall have available all facilities and equipment previously recommended. With the possible exception of conscious sedation, (level 1), mediated by minor tranquilizers administered enterally and/or nitrous oxide and oxygen inhalation sedation at 50% nitrous oxide concentration or less, minimum monitoring equipment for conscious sedation (levels 2, 3) shall be a pulse oximeter. Capnography is desirable for level 3.

A sphygmomanometer shall be immediately available. A precordial/pretracheal stethoscope is required for level 3.

Monitoring procedures
(before and during treatment)

Whenever drugs for conscious sedation, (levels 1, 2, or 3), are administered, the patient should be monitored continuously for patient responsiveness and airway patency. With the possible exception of conscious sedation (level 1), mediated by minor tranquilizers administered enterally and/or nitrous oxide and oxygen inhalation sedation at 50% nitrous oxide concentration or less, there shall be continual monitoring of oxygen saturation and heart and respiratory rates. Oxygen saturation and heart and respiratory rates shall be recorded at specific intervals throughout the procedure until the child has met documented discharge criteria. A precordial/pretracheal stethoscope shall be used for obtaining additional information on heart and respiratory rates and for monitoring airway patency during level 3 sedations. Clinical observation should accompany all levels of sedation. Treatment immobilization devices should be checked periodically to prevent airway obstruction or check restriction and insure limb perfusion. The child's head position shall be checked frequently to ensure airway patency. A sedated patient shall be observed continuously by a trained individual.

Recovery

After completion of the treatment procedures, vital signs should be recorded at specific intervals. The practitioner shall assess the patient's responsiveness and discharge the patient only when the appropriate discharge criteria have been met (Appendix I).

Deep Sedation (Level 4)

Personnel

The techniques of deep sedation (level 4) require the following three individuals: (1) the treating practitioner who may direct the sedation; (2) a qualified individual to assist with observation and monitoring the patient and who may administer drugs if appropriately licensed; and (3) other personnel to assist the operator as necessary. Of the three individuals, one shall be currently certified in Advanced Cardiac Life Support or

From The American Academy of Pediatric Dentistry, revised May, 1998.

BOX 19-1

Guidelines for the Elective Use of Conscious Sedation, Deep Sedation and General Anesthesia
In Pediatric Dental Patients—cont'd

Pediatric Advanced Life Support and the other two shall be currently certified in basic life support.

Operating facility and equipment

In addition to the facilities and equipment previously recommended for conscious sedation (levels 1, 2, and 3), deep sedation requires an ECG and a capnograph in conjunction with pulse oximetry. The availability of a defibrillator for pediatric patients is desirable.

Intravenous access

Patients receiving deep sedation (level 4) should have an intravenous line in place or have immediately available an individual skilled in establishing vascular access in pediatric patients.

Monitoring procedures
(before and during treatment)

The sedated patient shall be continuously monitored by an appropriately trained individual. There shall be continual monitoring of oxygen saturation by oximetry and expired carbon dioxide concentration via capnography, heart and respiratory rates, and blood pressure, all of which shall be recorded minimally every 5 minutes. A pulse oximeter and capnograph, precordial/pretracheal stethoscope, ECG, and blood pressure cuff are required. Temperature monitoring is desirable. The child's head position must be checked frequently to ensure airway patency. The operator should be observing the patient as well as the monitors and observing trends in the data obtained from the monitors. At no time shall a sedated patient be left unobserved by an appropriately trained individual.

Recovery

After treatment has been completed the patient must be observed in a suitably equipped recovery facility. This facility must have functioning suction apparatus and suction catheters of appropriate size, as well as the capacity to deliver greater than 90% oxygen and provide positive pressure ventilation for pediatric patients. An individual experienced in recovery care must be in attendance at all times in order to assess and record vital signs, observe the patient and ensure airway patency until the patient is stable. The patient must remain in the recovery facility until cardiovascular and respiratory stability are ensured and appropriate discharge criteria have been met (see Appendix I).

General Anesthesia (Level 5)
Personnel

The provision of general anesthesia requires the following three individuals: (1) a physician or dentist who has completed an advanced training program in anesthesia or oral and maxillofacial surgery and related subjects beyond the undergraduate medical or dental curriculum, who is responsible for anesthesia and monitoring of the patient, (2) a treating dentist, responsible for the provision of dental services, (3) other personnel to assist the operator as necessary. Of these individuals, the anesthetist shall be currently certified in Advanced Cardiac Life Support or Pediatric Advanced Life Support and the others shall be certified currently in basic life support. When a Certified Registered Nurse Anesthetist is permitted to function under the supervision of a dentist, the dentist is required to have completed training in general anesthesia, as specified above.

Operating facility and equipment

In addition to the facilities and equipment previously recommended for conscious sedation and deep sedation (level 4), i.e., pulse oximeter, capnograph, precordial stethoscope, blood pressure monitor and electrocardiograph, a temperature monitor and defibrillator are also required.

Monitoring procedures

The anesthetized patient shall be continuously monitored by the anesthesia provider. There shall be continual monitoring of oxygen saturation by pulse oximetry and expired carbon dioxide concentration via capnography, heart and respiratory rates, and blood pressure, all of which shall be recorded minimally every 5 minutes. The anesthesia provider should be visualizing the patient as well as the monitors and observing trends in the data obtained from the monitors. At no time should the patient be unobserved by trained personnel until discharge criteria have been met.

Recovery

After treatment has been completed, the patient must be observed continuously and monitored appropriately in a suitably equipped recovery facility until the patient becomes stable. This facility must have functioning suction apparatus and suction catheters of appropriate size,

Continued

BOX 19-1

Guidelines for the Elective Use of Conscious Sedation, Deep Sedation and General Anesthesia In Pediatric Dental Patients—cont'd

as well as the capacity to deliver greater than 90% oxygen and provide positive pressure ventilation for pediatric patients. An individual experienced in recovery care must be in attendance at all times in order to assess and record vital signs, observe the patient, and ensure airway patency. The patient must remain in the recovery facility until cardiovascular and respiratory parameters and function are stable and appropriate discharge criteria have been met (see Appendix I).

Appendix I

Recommended discharge criteria

1. Cardiovascular function satisfactory and stable
2. Airway patency uncompromised and satisfactory
3. Patient easily arousable and protective reflexes intact
4. State of hydration adequate
5. Patient can talk, if applicable
6. Patient can sit unaided, if applicable
7. Patient can ambulate, if applicable, with minimal assistance
8. For the child who is very young or disabled, and incapable of the usually expected responses, the pre-sedation level of responsiveness or the level as close as possible for that child should be achieved.
9. Responsible individual is available.

Appendix II

American Society of Anesthesiologists Classification (modified)

Class I.   A normally healthy patient with no organic, physiologic, biochemical, or psychiatric disturbance or disease.

Class II.   A patient with mild-to-moderate systemic disturbance or disease.

Class III.   A patient with severe systemic disturbance or disease.

Class IV.   A patient with severe and life-threatening systemic disease or disorder.

Class V.   A moribund patient who is unlikely to survive without the planned procedure.

Appendix III

Appropriate emergency equipment should be available whenever sedative drugs, capable of causing cardiorespiratory and central nervous system depression, are administered. The table below should be used as a guide, which should be modified depending upon the individual practice circumstances.

Emergency medications
Oxygen
Ammonia spirits
Glucose (50%)
Atropine
Diazepam
Lidocaine (cardiac)
Diphenhydramine hydrochloride
Hydrocortisone
Pharmacologic antagonists
Naloxone hydrochloride
Flumazenil
Basic airway management equipment
Nasal and oral airways of different sizes
Portable oxygen delivery system capable of delivering bag and mask ventilation greater than 90% at 10 L/min flow for at least 60 minutes (e.g., "E" cylinder) and resuscitation bag with masks that will accommodate children of all sizes.

Intravenous equipment (level 4 sedations)
Gloves
Alcohol wipes
Tourniquets
Sterile gauze pads
Tape
Intravenous solutions and equipment for administration appropriate to the patient population being treated.

From The American Academy of Pediatric Dentistry, revised May, 1998.

TABLE 1

Template of Definitions And Characteristics For Levels of Sedation And General Anesthesia

	Conscious Sedation			Deep Sedation	General Anesthesia
Functional Level of Sedation					
Mild (anxiolysis)	Interactive	Noninteractive/ arousable with mild/ moderate stimulus		Noninteractive/non-arousable except with intense stimulus	General
Goal					
Level 1 Decrease anxiety; facilitate coping skills	**Level 2** Decrease or eliminate anxiety; facilitate coping skills	**Level 3** Decrease or eliminate anxiety; facilitate coping skills; promote noninteraction sleep		**Level 4** Eliminate anxiety; coping skills overridden.	**Level 5** Eliminate cognitive, sensory, and skeletal motor activity; some autonomic activity depressed
Responsiveness					
Uninterrupted interactive ability; totally awake	Minimally depressed LOC; eyes open or temporarily closed; responds appropriately to verbal commands	Moderately depressed LOC; mimics sleep (vitals not different from that of sleep); eyes closed most of time; may respond to verbal prompts alone; responds to mild/ moderate stimuli (e.g., repeated trapezius pinching or needle insertion in oral tissues elicits reflex withdrawal and appropriate verbalization [complaint, moan, crying]); airway occasionally may require readjustment via chin thrust.		Deeply depressed LOC; sleep-like state, but vitals may be slightly depressed compared to sleep; eyes closed; does not respond to verbal prompts alone; reflex withdrawal with no verbalization when intense stimuli occurs (e.g., repeated, prolonged, and intense pinching of the trapezius); airway requires constant monitoring and frequent management	Unconscious and unresponsive to surgical stimuli. Partial or complete loss of protective reflexes, including airway; does not respond purposefully to physical and verbal command.
Personnel Monitoring Equipment					
2: Clinical observation*	2: PO; precordial recommended†	2: PO, precordial, BP; capno desirable†		3: PO and Capno, ECG, precordial, BP, defibrillator desirable†	3: PO, Capno, precordial, BP, ECG, temp, and defibrillator required
Monitoring Info					
None	HR, RR, O$_2$ pre-; during (q 15 min); post, as needed	HR, RR, O$_2$ BP; CO$_2$ if available pre-; during (q 10 min); post till stable/Discharge Criteria		HR, RR, O$_2$, CO$_2$, BP, ECG pre-; during (q 5 min); post till stable/Discharge Criteria	HR, RR, O$_2$, CO$_2$, BP, ECG, temp pre-; during (q 5 min minimum); post till stable/ Discharge Criteria

LOC, Level of consciousness; *PO,* pulse oximetry; *Capno,* capnography; *BP,* blood pressure cuff; *ECG,* electrocardiogram; *HR,* heart rate; *RR,* respiratory rate

*It should be noted that clinical observation should accompany any level of sedation and general anesthesia.

†"Recommended" and "Desirable" should be interpreted as not a necessity, but as an adjunct in assessing patient status.

supine position required for dental treatment further decreases the FRC by 20% to 30%. Since the metabolic demand for oxygen is 60% greater than in the adult, and the alveolar ventilation to FRC ratio is so high, hypoxemia develops rapidly in the pediatric patient. Bradycardia is always the initial response to hypoxemia, so an unexplained bradycardia should be treated with 100% oxygen.

Routes and Doses of Administration

Various routes are used to administer drugs for sedation in pediatric dentistry. Common routes include inhalation, oral, intravenous (IV), and intramuscular (IM). Other administration routes, such as rectal, submucosal, and intranasal, are used less frequently. Each route of administration has advantages and disadvantages (Table 19-1). Factors such as convenience, safety, economy, ease of administration, rapid onset, quick recovery, minimal side effects, and patient acceptance all contribute to advantages of specific routes of administration. In contrast, factors such as prolonged onset, inability to titrate dosage, variable effect, prolonged recovery, difficult administration, and frequency of side effects contribute to the disadvantages of specific routes of administration.

Some routes of administration (e.g., IV) are restricted in various jurisdictions to personnel with specialized training, and these routes may also require increased cost for malpractice liability insurance. In addition, whereas venipuncture might be desirable in providing IV access in case of emergency, many practitioners are reluctant to use the IV route because of a lack of experience. Some drugs can only be administered with one route of administration (e.g., nitrous oxide by inhalation), whereas others might be used with more than one route (e.g., oral and IV meperidine and diazepam). Generally, the same drug administered intravenously will produce a greater sedative effect than when administered orally. The same drug also will produce a more profound effect when it is used in combination with other drugs than when used as a sole agent.

When sedative drugs are used with adults, drug dosages usually have been determined after extensive clinical study. Dose-response studies to substantiate dosage recommendations for use of sedative doses in children are lacking. Children usually require increased dosages of drugs (on a mg/kg ba-

sis) because of their higher basal metabolic rate. Various rules used to determine drug dosages include those based on body weight, those based on body surface area, and fixed dosages determined by age or behavioral state of the child. Currently, the most accepted practice is to determine dose by body weight. Nevertheless, even dose-by-weight recommendations in the literature vary. For example, although the standard recommended dose for chloral hydrate is 50 mg/kg, dosages of 60 or 70 mg/kg or greater have appeared in the literature.[3] Practitioners should be guided by usual customary dosage recommendations (Table 19-2), recognizing that no drug is 100% successful for conscious sedation. When a drug has not produced expected results, increasing the dosage above recommended levels may not necessarily improve the result but will increase the incidence of undesirable side effects.

Sedation Methods for Pediatric Dentistry

Conscious sedation is defined as "a controlled, pharmacologically induced, minimally depressed level of consciousness that retains the patient's ability to maintain a patent airway independently and continuously, and to respond appropriately to physical stimulation and/or verbal command."[2] The effect of the drug is determined by the type of drug, dose of drug, route of administration, behavior of the child, and psychological development of the child.

Inhalation Sedation

Nitrous oxide is the most frequently used drug to sedate children for dental treatment. This sweet-smelling, colorless gas is administered by inhalation, producing an altered state of consciousness in which fear and anxiety are reduced (see Chapter 14). In the various levels of conscious sedation defined by the American Academy of Pediatric Dentistry,[2] nitrous oxide produces mild sedation, or level 1 of conscious sedation. Although the gas does have analgesic properties, it is usually not used as a substitute for local anesthesia. Nitrous oxide use for children is similar to its use with adults, in that it can be used as a sole agent or as an adjunct to other sedative drugs. Dosage levels with children usually range between 30% and 50% nitrous oxide for optimal effect. When used with children, minimal side effects (e.g., nau-

TABLE 19-1

Advantages and Disadvantages of Drug Administration Routes for Children

Route	Advantages	Disadvantages
Oral	Convenient Safe Economical Easy administration	Slow onset time Variable effect Not titratable Slow recovery time Sometimes difficult to administer Side effects
Inhalation nitrous oxide, oxygen	Rapid onset Titratable Rapid recovery No serious side effects Patient acceptance	Relatively weak agent Needs patient cooperation Inconvenient Major equipment required Occupational hazard
Intramuscular	Dependable absorption Economical Easy administration	Slow onset time Variable effect Not titratable Slow recovery time Side effects Liability insurance costs Regulatory restrictions
Intravenous	Rapid onset Test dose possible Titratable Rapid recovery Intravenous access	Venipuncture required Potency Side effects Liability insurance costs Regulatory restrictions

TABLE 19-2

Dosages of Drugs Used for Sedation in Pediatric Dentistry

Drug	Route	Dosage
Nitrous oxide	Inhalation	30%-50%
Chloral hydrate	Oral	50 mg/kg
Hydroxyzine	Oral	—
	Intramuscular	1-2 mg/kg
Promethazine	Oral	—
	Intramuscular	—
	Intravenous	1-2 mg/kg
Diazepam	Oral	0.3-0.6 mg/kg
Midazolam	Intravenous	0.05-0.1 mg/kg
	Intramuscular	0.15-0.2 mg/kg
	Intranasal	0.2-0.3 mg/kg
	Oral	0.3-0.75 mg/kg
Meperidine	Oral	1-2 mg/kg
	Intramuscular	0.5-2.0 mg/kg
Ketamine	Intramuscular	2-4 mg/kg
	Intravenous infusion	50 μg/kg/min 4-8 mg/kg
Propofol	Intravenous infusion	25-100 μg/kg/min

sea, vomiting) may occur. Numerous clinical studies have established that nitrous oxide is safe and effective when used to control mild anxiety in children.[4]

Nitrous oxide inhalation sedation has the distinct advantage of quick onset of action and quick peak clinical effect. Depth of sedation is titratable and because reversibility is extremely quick, the duration of action is controllable and recovery time is extremely short. Few side effects are experienced in children, and some degree of analgesia is produced.[5] Most children react positively to nitrous oxide sedation. The major disadvantage of using nitrous oxide with children is that it might be relatively ineffective if a crying child is breathing mainly through the mouth rather than the nose during dental treatment, thus not receiving the administered dose of the inhaled gas.

Administration of nitrous oxide to children is similar to the administration with adults. The correct-size scavenger nasal mask is selected and placed comfortably on the child's face with 100% oxygen flowing. Nitrous oxide concentration is then increased in increments of 10% until the patient begins to feel symptoms, such as a tingling sensation in the extremities. These symptoms usually occur at a concentration of 30% to 50% nitrous oxide, with a total liter flow of about 6 L. For young children, many practitioners arbitrarily use a fixed concentration of 40% or 50%. The general rule is to use the minimum concentration of nitrous oxide to achieve the desired effect; however, not all children show a benefit from nitrous oxide administration.

Oral Sedation

Chloral Hydrate. Chloral hydrate is one of the oldest sedative-hypnotic drugs. In solution it has a bitter taste and usually is mixed with a flavoring agent for oral administration. Chloral hydrate is often used for the treatment of insomnia in adults and has been extensively used for sedation of young children for medical or dental procedures. The pharmacologic action of chloral hydrate is similar to the action of alcohol in that it depresses the central nervous system (CNS) to induce sleep. It is administered orally or rectally. After absorption, chloral hydrate is rapidly metabolized to trichloroethanol, which is thought to be responsible for the CNS depressant effects.

The typical effect of chloral hydrate is to produce drowsiness or a rousable sleep after 30 to 45 minutes, which lasts 2 to 5 hours. Occasionally, the child might become hyperexcited 15 to 30 minutes after drug administration and before onset of sleep. This sleep is referred to as a "rousable" sleep because the patient can be aroused easily when stimulated. Usually, no changes in vital signs follow chloral hydrate administration, although nausea and vomiting may occur because of its gastric irritant properties.

Chloral hydrate is available in capsules (250 or 500 mg) and as a syrup (500 mg/5 ml). The usual dose is 50 mg/kg (or about 25 mg/lb) of body weight, to a maximum of 1000 mg, although higher doses have been used. Many practitioners use the drug as a sole agent, although others administer the drug together with other agents or use inhalation nitrous oxide to supplement the drug effect.

Numerous clinical studies have reported the safety and effectiveness of chloral hydrate. In general the drug seems to be effective when used with younger children at appropriate doses and does not appear to be effective either with low doses or with older handicapped individuals. Common problems encountered with the use of chloral hydrate are difficulty with oral administration, occasional nausea or vomiting, and undersedation with some children. Therapeutic doses of chloral hydrate are thought to have minimal effects on the respiratory and cardiovascular systems. However, high doses of chloral hydrate are associated with a significant incidence of cardiac dysrhythmias.[6] Respiratory depression and death have been reported after overdose. An additive effect may occur when chloral hydrate is used with other agents, and reduction of drug dosage may be required.

When chloral hydrate is administered, it is best to have the patient drink the agent. If the patient refuses to do so, oral administration can be forced by placing the drug at the back of the throat with the aid of a needleless syringe; however, caution must be used so that the drug is not forced into the trachea, producing a laryngeal spasm.[6]

Hydroxyzine and Promethazine. Hydroxyzine and promethazine are used to provide mild sedation for the mild to moderately fearful pediatric dental patient. The agents have a wide margin of safety and can be administered orally. The drugs also have antiemetic properties and are frequently used in combination with chloral hydrate or meperidine to decrease the incidence of nausea or vomiting.

Hydroxyzine (Atarax, Vistaril) is an antihistaminic drug administered orally or intramuscularly; it is too irritating for IV or submucosal use. Although fixed-dosage recommendations appear in the literature, the dose of 1 to 2 mg/kg is recommended, whether hydroxyzine is used as a sole agent or in combination with other drugs. Clinical effects begin 30 to 60 minutes after administration and last 1 to 2 hours.

Promethazine (Phenergan) is a phenothiazine derivative administered orally, intravenously, or intramuscularly, but it is contraindicated for submucosal administration. It is considered to be an extremely safe drug, although reported side effects include hyperexcitability and hallucinations. Dosage recommendations for promethazine are 1 to 2 mg/kg when the drug is used as a sole agent or administered in combination with other sedative agents. A fixed dose of 25 mg also has been used. Onset of sedation effects is within 20 minutes of oral or IM administration and 3 to 5 minutes after IV injection. Sedative effects may last 2 to 8 hours, depending on dose and route of administration.

Benzodiazepines. The benzodiazepine group of drugs is widely used to control anxiety in adults. The two drugs most often used to sedate children are diazepam and midazolam.

Diazepam (Valium) is available as a tablet (2.5 or 10 mg) and as a liquid suspension for oral administration (l mg/ml). A parenteral preparation (5 mg/ml) is available for IM and IV use. After administration the effect of the drug is on the brainstem, reticular system, limbic system, thalamus, and hypothalamus. When properly administered, there is little change in cardiac output, blood pressure, or respiration rate in healthy children. The drug is metabolized in the liver, and most of the metabolites are excreted in the urine, with a small amount appearing in the feces.

Diazepam is administered orally and parenterally, both as a sole agent and in combination with other drugs, including nitrous oxide. When used orally, the usual dose for diazepam is 0.3 to 0.6 mg/kg. Sedative effects occur after 30 minutes, with peak effects in 2 hours. The elimination half-life of diazepam is 1 to 2 days. The typical effect is drowsiness and a general calming of the child. Sleep occurs much less frequently than with chloral hydrate. When used with children, diazepam is considered to be a very safe drug, with drowsiness as the major side effect. Although the drug has not been formally approved for use in children, extensive clinical studies have demonstrated both safety and effectiveness

in pediatric dentistry. Some amnesic affect has been reported.

In recent years the more potent benzodiazepine *midazolam* (Versed) has been used for conscious sedation in pediatric dentistry. Midazolam is a short-acting, water-soluble benzodiazepine with anxiolytic, sedative, hypnotic, anticonvulsant, muscle relaxant, and anterograde amnesic effects. The drug is oxidized by the liver much more rapidly than other benzodiazepines and has a short duration of action. Peak serum concentrations are reached at different times depending on the route of administration. IM and rectal routes produce peak serum concentrations at 15 and 30 minutes after administration, whereas the oral route results in peak serum concentration in less than 1 hour. Elimination half-life is approximately 45 to 60 minutes in a child, compared with 2 to 6 hours in an adult. Midazolam is eliminated significantly faster than diazepam, which has an elimination half-life of 24 to 57 hours.

Although midazolam was approved only for parenteral administration, it has been used orally at doses of 0.3 to 0.75 mg/kg. Clinical studies of oral midazolam have given conflicting results. However, most studies indicate that the oral dose should be approximately double or triple the IV dose to achieve similar effects. Onset of action for oral midazolam is 20 to 30 minutes.

Midazolam has been used intranasally for more than 10 years at doses of 0.2 to 0.3 mg/kg. A reduced repeat dose could be administered after 10 minutes if needed. Children sedated with intranasal midazolam become moderately drowsy but usually do not fall completely asleep. Peak serum concentration usually occurs within 10 minutes, and recovery time is approximately 30 minutes. No significant respiratory depression, emesis, or oversedation has been reported, and all vital signs, including oxygen saturation, remain stable during sedation. Midazolam is relatively free of any side effects; the major risks associated with high doses are hypoventilation and associated hypoxia. Intranasal administration may be considered parenteral in some jurisdictions, and this route of administration might be limited to practitioners with special sedation permits.

The relative safety of midazolam and lack of adverse effects may be attributed to its selective rather than generalized CNS depressant action. The drug effect can be reversed by IV administration of flumazenil, which should be reserved only for emergency situations. Midazolam produces antero-grade amnesia more reliably and for a longer dura-tion than diazepam and is an ideal agent for short procedures in pediatric dentistry.

The oral benzodiazepine *triazolam* offers the ad-vantage of rapid absorption from the gut and a short elimination half-life (2.3 hours). Although used mainly as a sleep aid and as an adult oral premed-icant, triazolam holds promise as a pediatric seda-tive. The safety and efficacy of triazolam at a dose of 0.02 mg/kg in children have been demonstrated. As with midazolam, more research is needed to evaluate triazolam as a primary sedative in the pediatric den-tal population.

Opioids. Opioid agonists exert their primary action on the CNS and the bowel.[1] In the CNS, opioids produce analgesia without loss of consciousness, drowsiness, or mood alteration. Opioids lower both sensory intensity of nociceptive stimuli and the associated affective com-ponent of pain. Opioids are respiratory depressants that affect both respiratory rate and tidal volume by de-creasing the responsiveness of the medullary respira-tory centers to increasing concentrations of carbon dioxide. The stimulus to breathe is obtunded in a dose-related fashion as carbon dioxide levels rise. Thus the ventilatory status must be closely monitored. Opioids at therapeutic doses have minimal cardiovascular ef-fects, producing minimal changes in blood pressure, heart rate, or heart rhythm in the recumbent patient.[1] Peripheral vasodilation may result from histamine re-lease when agents such as morphine or meperidine are used. Thus postural hypotension and syncope may oc-cur when patients are returned to an upright position. Opioids may cause delays in gastric emptying and slow gastrointestinal (GI) motility, leading to constipation. Opioids also increase smooth muscle tone in the ureter and bladder, which may result in urinary retention.

The desirable pharmacologic effects of analgesia and sedation produced by opioids make them use-ful for oral, IM, or IV sedation. However, opioids are poorly absorbed orally and may vary greatly in seda-tive activity. When administered alone and in the ab-sence of pain, opioids may produce dysphoria in-stead of the desired sedation or tranquilization. Opioids may produce GI disturbances such as nausea and vomiting, which increase with dose and in am-bulatory patients.

Opioids are used in pediatric sedation either orally, intramuscularly, submucosally, or intra-venously. Short-acting agents such as meperidine and *fentanyl* are used most often. *Meperidine* is the opioid most frequently used orally in pediatric sedation. It is often used in combination with promethazine or hy-droxyzine. When young or uncooperative children are sedated, the oral or IM route is most often used. When older children or adolescents are sedated, opi-oids are used as an adjunct to IV conscious sedation.

Pediatric mortality and morbidity are more preva-lent when opioids are used as part of a combination drug sedation regimen. This may be caused in part by severe respiratory depression and local anesthetic drug interactions, leading to toxicity.[2] Local anes-thetic doses should be reduced by half when used with opioid sedation in pediatric patients. Also, the common pediatric cocktail of meperidine and promethazine has also been associated with in-creases in pediatric mortality.[3]

The ultrashort-acting opioids, such as *alfentanil* and *remifentanil*, have provided a new degree of con-trol over the level of sedation. These drugs are ad-ministered intravenously by continuous infusion and have an immediate onset. When the infusion is dis-continued, there is rapid redistribution and plasma hydrolysis with remifentanil.[4] This rapid onset and elimination permit more precise control of the anal-gesic and sedative effects. These properties have the potential to reduce significantly the liabilities of opi-oid sedation. Alfentanil and remifentanil may be used alone or in combination with benzodiazepines, ketamine, or propofol to produce safe, reliable, and controlled sedation.

Intramuscular Sedation

The IM injection sites of choice in pediatric patients are the deltoid and vastus lateralis. In infants and young children the vastus lateralis muscle is more developed and is the preferred site. The deltoid is pre-ferred in older children because of the ease of access and the high vascularity. One of the first techniques used the combination of meperidine, promethazine, and chlorpromazine for anesthetic premedication and pediatric sedation. Also known as DPT, or the "lytic cocktail," this drug combination produced var-ied successes and failures. Although still in use today, it has been relegated primarily to the management of unruly pediatric patients in the hospital emer-gency department environment. Other popular tech-niques use meperidine in combination with either promethazine or hydroxyzine in doses similar to those used for oral premedication.

As with oral medications, the benzodiazepines make the most sense for IM sedation in pediatric patients. Diazepam itself is not well suited for IM administration because of its water insolubility, poor absorption, and pain during injection. Midazolam, however, is ideal for IM administration. Although clinical IM experience in pediatric dental patients is limited, midazolam appears to offer great promise as a pediatric sedative.

IM barbiturates such as secobarbital, pentobarbital, and methohexital are of questionable value in pediatrics and generally are no longer used.

Alternative Routes of Administration

Many new and ingenious ways have been suggested to administer sedative medications to an unsuspecting child. Many are effective and show promise, whereas others are problematic.

With *rectal sedation*, a typical technique is to administer 20 to 30 mg/kg of a 10% methohexital solution rectally using a catheter-tipped syringe. Alternatively, diazepam (0.3 to 0.6 mg/kg) or midazolam (0.2 mg/kg) may be used. Ketamine is also administered by this route. Sedation through the rectal route usually occurs rapidly, but blood levels of the drug may be unpredictable from patient to patient. Because drug distribution is between the veins leading to the systemic circulation and those leading to the portal circulation, it is difficult to predict precise blood levels. Bioavailability is decreased significantly if a large portion of the drug undergoes first-pass metabolism in the liver. Also, the distribution and absorption of the drug may be impeded by the presence of feces or mucus in the rectum, and there is a 5% to 15% incidence of defecation. Despite these draw-backs, rectal sedation has been shown to be safe and effective in both preschool-age children and developmentally disabled adults.

The most controversial alternative route of administration is *submucosal injection* of opioid analgesics because of possible serious morbidity or death. Despite being associated with increased pediatric morbidity and mortality, opioids continue to be used because of the perceived ineffectiveness of other sedation modalities. The dosages used are relatively high, and the sedation that results is different from that of the benzodiazepines. Although opioids may control some behavior and decrease movement, this apparent cooperation often comes at the expense of oversedation. Also, local anesthetic toxicity may be enhanced by opioids. Given the potential toxicity of opioids administered submucosally, it is prudent for dentists to abandon the use of opioids via this route in favor of other sedative techniques with a higher margin of safety.

Another alternative drug route being used for pediatric sedation is *intranasal instillation*. Opioids such as fentanyl, remifentanil, alfentanil, sufentanil, and butorphanol have been used with success in both adults and children. Although midazolam has been given intranasally, experience and studies are lacking. Controlled studies are needed to permit evaluation of the safety and efficacy of intranasal drug administration for pediatric sedation in an outpatient setting.

Deep Sedation

Since conscious sedation may have limited effect, deep sedation is indicated when more complete patient cooperation and stress control are required or as an alternative to treatment with general anesthesia. Deep sedation is defined as "a controlled, pharmacologically induced state of depressed consciousness from which the patient is not easily aroused which may be accompanied by a partial loss of protective reflexes, including the ability to maintain a patent airway independently and/or respond purposely to physical stimulation or verbal command."[2]

Deep sedation may be produced by the type and dose of drug used, the route of drug administration, and by drugs used in combination. Generally, IV drugs and combination drugs have the potential to produce deep sedation. A form of deep sedation referred to as *dissociative sedation* is produced with ketamine and has been described as a safe and reliable alternative to general anesthesia.

Ketamine

Ketamine is a derivative of the hallucinogen phencyclidine, which was first synthesized in 1963. Ketamine is used to produce deep sedation with cooperation, occasional robotic behavior, amnesia, and analgesia. Because of its high degree of lipid solubility, ketamine enters the CNS rapidly and is thought to produce its unique clinical state by inducing dissociation between the thalamoneocortical and limbic systems, thus preventing the higher centers from perceiving visual, auditory, and painful stimuli. This produces a catatonic-like patient with a vacant stare, glassy eyes, and horizontal nystagmus. Patients may appear to be removed or detached from their physical being but may still respond to commands when ketamine has been administered in a low dose.

Ketamine is an extremely rapid-acting agent when administered intravenously or intramuscularly. Peak plasma concentrations are achieved about 1 minute after IV administration or about 5 minutes after IM administration. The clinical effects of ketamine begin to wane about 15 minutes after IV administration and 30 to 120 minutes after IM injection. The elimination half-life of ketamine is 2 to 3 hours in adults, but since children metabolize the drug more rapidly than adults, the elimination half-life is only 1 to 2 hours in children. The drug is first metabolized in the liver to norketamine, an active metabolite with one third of the dissociative potency of ketamine itself. The concomitant administration of other drugs metabolized in the liver may extend the half-life of ketamine and prolong recovery time.

Patients generally are able to maintain their own airways because ketamine preserves spontaneous respiration and enhances the muscular tone of the upper airways. Blood oxygen saturation levels are maintained, and protective reflexes also remain intact. Ketamine stimulates salivary and tracheobronchial secretions, which may lead to laryngospasm. The effects can be adequately controlled by the concomitant administration of an antisialagogue. Although laryngospasm is a possible side effect of ketamine administration and can be life threatening, it rarely occurs. Also, since upper airway protective reflexes remain intact, there appears to be minimal risk of aspiration of gastric contents. Thirty years of use have demonstrated the safety of ketamine. Only two cases of aspiration and two cases of laryngospasm were reported in 11,589 administrations to children.

Ketamine has a stimulatory effect on the cardiovascular system that results in mild to moderate increases in blood pressure, heart rate, and cardiac output. It may produce skeletal muscle hypertonicity and rigidity, which may interfere with dental procedures due to inability to open the mouth. This reaction appears to be a dose-related phenomenon, and increasing the ketamine dose or the addition of other sedative agents will alleviate this problem. Random movement unrelated to surgical or painful stimuli often occurs with ketamine administration. This random movement may be mistaken for an inadequate

sedation level but is unrelated to the dental procedure. Myoclonus with twitching and jerking movements is common after ketamine administration, and it has been mistaken for seizure activity when extensive. However, ketamine has been shown to have anticonvulsive properties and has been used without complication in patients with seizure problems.

Emergence phenomena after ketamine administration include ataxia and dizziness, which may persist for up to 4 hours. Rapid independent ambulation is not recommended after drug administration. Psychic phenomena has been reported at 0% to 10% in children. These experiences have been described as detachment, floating or bodily suspension, out-of-body experiences, and strange thoughts or dreams. Another emergence phenomena of concern is nausea and vomiting, which may occur in up to 10% of pediatric patients. Vomiting often occurs late in the recovery phase, when the patient is alert and the airway can be cleared without assistance.

Dissociative sedation may be induced with IV or IM ketamine. If IV catheter placement is used, ketamine 0.25 mg/kg is administered. IM induction may be with ketamine 2 to 4 mg/kg mixed with glycopyrrolate 5 μg/kg for salivation control. Maintenance may be with either a continuous infusion at a rate of 50 μg/kg/min or by intermittent 5-mg to 10-mg boluses as needed. Other drugs may be used in combination to augment sedation and minimize side effects. Ketamine was used in 112 child patients at a dose of 4 mg/kg for emergency treatment with a 97% success rate. Parental acceptance was high, particularly because separation anxiety was eliminated, and physical restraint, hospitalization, and preoperative testing were unnecessary. Nightmares were not reported. A review of 97 reports covering 17,550 administrations, including 11,598 with children, demonstrated the safety and efficacy of ketamine for pediatric sedation. Recent clinical research has demonstrated the safety and effectiveness of oral administration of ketamine in pediatric dentistry. Nevertheless, ketamine administration should be performed by an individual experienced with its use and proficient in treating airway complications.

Propofol

A more recent drug for deep sedation is *propofol,* an IV diisoprophylphenol agent that appears as a white oil in water emulsion. Because it is free of preservatives and contains vehicles capable of supporting rapid growth of microorganisms, strict aseptic technique is necessary in its preparation, and the unused drug is discarded the same day as the vial is opened to avoid contamination. Pharmacokinetically, propofol has two distribution phases, a rapid phase with a distribution half-life of 1.8 to 8.3 minutes and a slower distribution phase with a half-life of 34 to 64 minutes. The terminal elimination half-life of propofol is 300 to 700 minutes, which occurs through rapid redistribution from the CNS through peripheral tissues. Although propofol has a high metabolic clearance, the termination of activity does not depend on the elimination half-life. Patients are usually responsive within 8 minutes after cessation of propofol infusion. The dose requirement is increased in children by 1½ times compared with adults due to the shorter elimination half-life and more rapid metabolism in pediatric patients.

Cardiorespiratory effects of propofol may include systemic hypotension, apnea, airway obstruction, and respiratory depression. These effects occur in a dose-dependent fashion and are more likely after a rapid IV bolus injection. Propofol has been used with ketamine. In patients unwilling or unable to cooperate with IV catheter placement, IM induction with ketamine is performed, followed by placement of an IV catheter. Propofol may then be given in 10-mg to 20-mg intermittent boluses, as needed, or as a continuous infusion at a rate of 50 to 150 μg/kg/min for maintenance of sedation. Arousal occurs within 10 minutes after the infusion has been discontinued. This technique provides excellent behavior management. Spontaneous ventilation and oxygen saturation are maintained. Propofol may be used with other drugs, including ketamine, midazolam, or ultrashort-acting opioids such as alfentanil and remifentanil.

Balancing Therapeutic Success and Patient Safety

The effect of a drug is determined by type and dose, route of administration, and most importantly, the child's preoperative behavior. The success of a sedation procedure is more difficult to determine and depends on who is judging the procedure. Patients, parents, practitioners, third-party payers, state board agencies, and malpractice insurers all have different criteria to define success of a sedation procedure (Box 19-2). Variables include safety of the procedure; anxiety of the patient, parent, or practitioner; amount of treatment rendered; comfort of the patient before, during, and after the procedure; and relative cost of the procedure compared with alternative approaches. For the pediatric patient, anxiety reduction and comfort are paramount. For all others, safety of the procedure is presumed. Parents are concerned about the child's comfort and their own anxiety regarding the procedure. The practitioner is concerned about the relative competence and subsequent confidence with a particular sedation technique. A third-party payer is concerned primarily about the relative cost of the procedure. Finally, state board agencies and malpractice insurers become involved only if procedures are determined to be unsafe or if complaints are registered against the practitioner.

Although articles on sedation in pediatric dentistry have appeared in the scientific literature since the early 1950s, no consensus has been reached regarding the definition of "success of sedation." Some authors report their procedures as either successful or not, whereas others report procedures as being excellent, good, fair, or poor. Sedation is not general anesthesia, and young children often cry or move during the dental procedure. Consequently, success

---

BOX 19-2

Parameters of Success for Conscious Sedation

Patient
Anxiety
Comfort (before, during, after)
Parent separation
Treatment rendered

Parent
Parent anxiety
Safety
Patient comfort
Treatment rendered
Cost

Practitioner
Safety
Treatment rendered

Patient discomfort
Own anxiety
Third parties

State Board
Safety
Patient complaint

Payer
Treatment rendered
Cost
Safety
Patient satisfaction

Malpractice Insurer
Safety
Patient complaint

of sedation could be operationally defined to consider the degree of crying or movement that interfered with treatment[7] (Box 19-3). Crying could range from intermittent whimpering to continuous, hysterical screaming. Movement could range from slight movement at the time of mouth prop insertion or local anesthesia to continuous struggling necessitating the use of external restraints (e.g., Papoose board) to complete all procedures. However, no consensus exists on how much crying or movement is considered acceptable. Some practitioners accept some crying or movement as long as treatment can be accomplished. They might choose to perform a partially successful conscious sedation procedure rather than use deep sedation or general anesthesia. Other practitioners are uncomfortable with any crying and with use of external restraints for a child. They believe that the child might be traumatized unnecessarily, and they modify their procedures so that deep sedation or general anesthesia can be used as an alternative to conscious sedation. Consequently, all treatment can be performed in one atraumatic appointment. In addition, quality of treatment might be improved because the dentist does not have to rush or cope with disruptive behavior.

Practitioner bias depends on many factors, including the prior training and experience of a practitioner with a particular technique. Cost and availability of treatment options also influence approaches to sedation. Whether a pediatric patient is administered conscious sedation or is treated with deep sedation or general anesthesia seems to depend less on the needs of the patient and more on the particular bias of the practitioner.

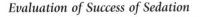

BOX 19-3

Evaluation of Success of Sedation

Excellent: no crying or movement
Very good: some limited crying or movement (e.g., during local anesthesia or mouth prop insertion)
Good: difficult, but all treatment performed
Fair: treatment interrupted but eventually all completed
Poor: treatment interrupted, only partial treatment completed
Aborted: no treatment performed

References

1. Houpt MI: Project USAP 2000: a 15-year update of the use of sedative agents by pediatric dentists (unpublished data).
2. Guidelines for the Elective Use of Conscious Sedation, Deep Sedation, and General Anesthesia in Pediatric Patients, Revised May, 1998. AAPD Reference Manual, *Ped Dent* 22(7):73-78, 2000 (special issue).
3. Houpt MI: Report of Project USAP: The use of sedative agents by pediatric dentists, *J Dent Child* 56(4):302-309, 1989.
4. Duncan G, Moore P: Nitrous oxide and the dental patient: a review of adverse reactions, *J Am Dent Assoc* 108(2):213-219, 1984.
5. Hogue D, Ternisky M, Iranpour B: The responses of nitrous oxide analgesia in children, *J Dent Child* 38(2):129-133, 1971.
6. Granoff DM, McDaniel DB, Berkowf SP: Cardiorespiratory arrest following aspiration of chloral hydrate, *Am J Dis Child* 122:170-171, 1971.
7. Houpt MI, Koenigsberg SR, Weiss NJ, et al: Comparison of chloral hydrate with and without promethazine in the sedation of young children, *Ped Dent* 7(1):41-46, 1985.

20

Anesthesia for the Developmentally Disabled Patient

Jeffrey D. Bennett
John W. Leyman

CHAPTER OUTLINE

Management of the developmentally disabled patient requires special training, including knowledge of the medical conditions that influence the anesthetic care necessary to provide optimal treatment. Whereas in the past these patients were routinely treated in tertiary care centers, the present health care shift toward cost containment places new emphasis on providing primary care in a community setting. This presents unique challenges in the provision of dental care, including the need to provide sedation or general anesthesia because of the developmentally disabled patient's inability to cooperate fully during dental therapy.

Mental impairment can range from mild to severe. The degree of impairment contributes to the patient's ability to tolerate routine dental treatment and to perform self-care at home, which helps guide both anesthetic and dental treatment decisions. Some patients with mild mental impairment can receive dental treatment similar to that of other dental outpatients, whereas others require sedation or general anesthesia.[1] The complexity of the treatment plan also affects the decision on the type of anesthesia provided. Postoperatively, residual effects of sedation or general anesthesia can further disorient the patient. Uncooperative and even aggressive behavior is occasionally seen during the recovery phase.

Mental impairment can also be associated with various congenital and acquired syndromes. These syndromes are often associated with physiologic and anatomic abnormalities, which can further complicate both the dental treatment and the anesthetic management of this patient. Additional physiologic and anatomic abnormalities must be ruled out by physical examination before the onset of treatment. Alternatively, physical disabilities (e.g., cerebral palsy) are not always associated with mental impairment. These individuals, however, are frequently treated as if they are mentally impaired because of their inability to communicate normally.

A complete medical history and review of systems are mandatory. The physical examination at least must include cardiovascular and pulmonary examinations. This testing should be of sufficient detail to identify significant physiologic or anatomic abnormalities that would adversely effect the patient's dental or anesthetic care. The decision to subject the patient to a more comprehensive examination and laboratory testing is guided by the initial findings, since many of these patients also have significant systemic disease, which requires a modification of the anesthetic technique. Cardiovascular, respiratory, renal, hepatic, endocrine, neurologic, and muscular abnormalities all can have a significant impact on the anesthetic treatment.

This chapter provides an introduction to the anesthetic management of the patient with mental or physical impairments undergoing dental treatment. The intent is to identify the physiologic and anatomic features associated with the developmentally disabled patient that are significant and require a modification in the patient's anesthetic management. Anesthetic techniques and pharmacologic agents addressed in other chapters also are discussed here in the context of the developmentally disabled patient.

Primary Assessment

General Considerations

The goal in treating any patient is to establish a satisfactory level of comfort and cooperation to allow the safe completion of the dental treatment. *Discomfort* associated with a dental procedure may place the patient in a frightened or agitated emotional state. *Physical impairment* may prevent patients from comfortably positioning themselves in the dental chair. Both these factors may result in an inability for the patient to cooperate for completely different reasons. Sedation or general anesthesia may be a suitable solution for both these problems. Additionally, the physically impaired patient who normally receives treatment under local anesthesia may desire anesthesia for select procedures (e.g., extraction of wisdom teeth), similar to the delivery of care for the non–physically impaired patient.

The goal of the primary anesthetic assessment is to determine the anesthetic level that the patient will require: conscious sedation, deep sedation, or general anesthesia. The anesthetic agents are then chosen to provide an optimal blend of anxiolysis, amnesia, sedation, and analgesia, as well as local effects such as salivary drying.

The patient who is comfortable during conscious sedation will not necessarily be cooperative during treatment. Deep sedation and general anesthesia are often necessary to complete the dental treatment if the patient's developmental or physical status results in distracting behavior or treatment-compromising movements. Because the patient is more susceptible to hemodynamic and airway changes, deep sedation and general anesthesia should only be administered in a properly equipped facility by individuals who have received additional training in the anesthetic management of special care patients.

Respiratory Assessment

Many developmentally disabled patients have syndromes with anatomic abnormalities in the head and neck region, including macroglossia, micrognathia, limited mouth opening, kyphosis, scoliosis, or cervical spine abnormalities. These patients also may have had a previous tracheostomy with associated tracheal stenosis. Physiologic abnormalities may include hypersalivation, decreased lung volume, or decreased respiratory reserve secondary to muscular, neurologic, or anatomic components of their disease.

The spontaneously ventilating patients with limited pulmonary reserve may desaturate very quickly under anesthesia, even with anesthetic doses that would not cause respiratory depression in most other patients. In patients with physical abnormalities, keeping an airway patent may be difficult, and intubation may be difficult or impossible. These patients are best treated with a spontaneous ventilation technique, but they may still be susceptible to rapid respiratory depression.

Cardiovascular Assessment

Many developmentally disabled patients also have significant cardiovascular disease associated with their syndrome (Table 20-1). Common acquired diseases, such as hypertension and atherosclerosis, occur in this population as well.

TABLE 20-1

Cardiovascular Disease Associated with Developmental Disorders

Anomaly	Syndrome
Ischemic heart disease	Ehlers-Danlos
Congenital heart disease	Apert's
	Down
	Marfan
	Noonan's
	Tetralogy of Fallot
Autonomic dysfunction	Shy-Drager
	Wolff-Parkinson-White
Cardiomyopathy dystrophy	Duchenne's muscular

Consultation with the patient's physician before treatment is usually required for patients with a history of acquired or congenital heart disease. Occasionally, a patient with significant cardiovascular impairment may have drifted away from routine medical care. It is critically important that the patient be referred to the appropriate physician specialist for evaluation before the consideration of any dental treatment, with or without anesthesia.

Neurologic Assessment

Neurologic disorders occur frequently in developmentally disabled patients. Clinical manifestations may include extrapyramidal symptoms, motor neuron degeneration (e.g., swallowing and speech abnormalities), and seizures. Patients frequently are taking various medications to control these symptoms. The clinician must be cognizant of the effect of the patient's medications on both the systemic health and the potential interaction with the anesthetic agents.

Many anesthetic medications exacerbate extrapyramidal symptoms. These include droperidol, metoclopramide, compazine, and phenothiazines. Patients with motor neuron degeneration or demyelinating disease may be more susceptible to neuromuscular blocking agents. Succinylcholine should be avoided because of possible hyperkalemia in these patients.[2]

Additionally, patients taking anticonvulsant medications have altered hematologic states; therefore hematologic testing is often appropriate. Hepatic enzyme induction by the anticonvulsant may also alter the dose of anesthetic medication required to achieve a specific effect.

Many anesthetic agents have both proconvulsant and anticonvulsant effects. Benzodiazepines and opioids are generally safe. The use of ketamine and methohexital has been associated with seizures.[3] However, seizures are rare and should not preclude the use of these agents in patients with a seizure history unless specifically contraindicated.

Specific Diseases

Down Syndrome

Down syndrome, or *trisomy 21*, is a common chromosomal disorder occurring at a rate of 1.5 per 1000 live births.[3] It is usually characterized by mild to moderate mental retardation, cardiovascular abnormalities, and craniofacial abnormalities. The anesthetic management of the patient with Down syndrome depends on the severity of these three conditions. The practitioner must fully understand the cardiovascular and craniofacial abnormalities to avoid potential complications.

Craniofacial abnormalities that have an impact on the anesthetic management of these patients include macroglossia, micrognathia, short neck, and possible atlantoaxial instability. Persistent snoring and mouth breathing are secondary to macroglossia and the resulting diminished nasopharyngeal space. Patients exhibiting these tendencies are at increased risk for airway obstruction during sedation. Other airway problems include subglottic stenosis and generalized joint laxity. The latter may be associated with subluxation of the temporomandibular joint during airway manipulation.

Atlantoaxial instability occurs in approximately 20% of patients with Down syndrome.[3] Significant instances are usually characterized by significant symptoms or declining neurologic function without other neurologic disorder. Specific symptoms may include positive Babinski's sign, hyperactive deep tendon reflexes, ankle clonus, neck discomfort, and gait abnormalities. This cervical spine instability is a contraindication for routine treatment until both the patient and the treatment risks are fully evaluated. Airway maneuvers, such as neck positioning during anesthesia for airway opening or intubation, may induce a serious cervical injury (C1-2 subluxation). Neurologic symptoms suggestive of an injury include neck pain, arm pain, extremity weakness, and torticollis.

Approximately 40% of the patients born with Down syndrome have congenital heart disease.[4] Abnormalities include endocardial cushion defect, tetralogy of Fallot, patent ductus arteriosus, and atrial septal defect. Care of the patient with these significant cardiovascular problems should be in conjunction with the patient's physician.

Cerebral Palsy

Cerebral palsy is characterized by motor dysfunction and varying degrees of mental retardation secondary to a hypoxic cerebral injury, usually at birth. The motor dysfunction includes skeletal muscle spasticity, athetosis/choreoathetosis, and ataxia. The severity of the lesions may be progressive, from monoplegia to quadriplegia. Other manifestations of the disorder include gastroesophageal reflux, swallowing abnormalities, speech abnormalities, and seizures.[4]

Neuromuscular dysfunction can contribute to the patient's dental disease and the overall difficulty in treating the patient. Severe contractures may make positioning the patient in the dental chair difficult. Stabilizing the patient's head may be necessary due to poor muscle tone. The patient may also experience dyskinetic movements, manifested by jerky and irregular movements of the jaws and tongue. Neuromuscular dysfunction complicates dental treatment of patients with cerebral palsy.

Anesthetic management of these patients must consider the severity and individual characteristics of the patient's neuromuscular dysfunction, the severity of mental retardation, and the severity of associated conditions. Anesthetic management can vary from sedation to general anesthesia. Neuromuscular manifestations may be intensified by stress and anxiety. Anesthetic techniques that decrease stress and anxiety will therefore facilitate dental treatment. The anesthetic requirements of these patients may be influenced by a number of factors, including the use of antiepileptic drugs.

Patients with cerebral palsy may also have compromised pharyngolaryngeal reflexes.[3] If the patient has a history of frequent emesis, advanced airway protection measures should be used during general anesthesia.

Cystic Fibrosis

Cystic fibrosis is an autosomal recessive disorder with an incidence of 1 in 2500 live births.[5] Life expectancy is improving due to better medical care and often extends into the adult years. In this complex multisystem disease, the pulmonary component is the primary factor. Respiratory complications are characterized by excessive bronchial secretions, patchy atelectasis, gas trapping and hyperinflation, and recurrent lower respiratory infections.[3] All these factors contribute to ventilation-perfusion abnormalities, a tendency toward pneumothorax, and hypoxemia. Treatment includes chest physiotherapy, antibiotic therapy, and the use of bronchodilators. The majority of patients with cystic fibrosis have chronic sinusitis and multiple nasal polyps, which can result in nasal obstruction.

These patients also have nonrespiratory components of the disease. Pancreatic insufficiency (causing diabetes mellitus) may occur in patients with cystic fibrosis.[5] Microangiopathic complications associated with diabetes can further compromise the health of these patients.

Hepatobiliary disease is also common and can result in portal hypertension. Intermittent bowel obstruction occurs in up to 20% of adult patients with cystic fibrosis. Opioids should be avoided because of the potential for postoperative constipation. Bowel obstruction, which is a medical emergency, can result in abdominal distention, which can compromise an already-marginal pulmonary reserve. Patients with bowel obstruction also have a greatly increased risk of emesis and aspiration pneumonitis.[5]

Since the most common cause of death in cystic fibrosis is respiratory failure,[6] significant attention is given to a careful and complete assessment of the factors that can contribute to perioperative respiratory failure. The patient must be in optimal physical condition before treatment to ensure the best possible outcome.

The decision to provide parenteral anesthesia to the cystic fibrosis patient depends on the severity of the disease. These patients present a significant challenge for anesthesia and are at an increased risk for respiratory failure during the perioperative period. It is most appropriate that the care be directed to an institution experienced in the treatment of patients with cystic fibrosis.

Multiple Sclerosis

Multiple sclerosis is a progressive disease of the central and peripheral nervous systems characterized by demyelination of neurons. The patient frequently goes through periods of exacerbation and remission.[1] Each exacerbation period results in a progression of the disease. Manifestations of multiple sclerosis include spasticity, ataxia, depression, bladder dysfunction,[3] and pain symptoms mimicking trigeminal neuralgia. Treatment is usually symptomatic (i.e., controls the intensity of the manifestations). Medications include corticosteroids, immunosuppresive agents, carbamazepine, tricyclic antidepressants, and benzodiazepines. Modifications in the anesthetic management of these patients depend on the patient's medications.

Muscular Dystrophy

The muscular dystrophy patient is characterized by progressive muscle degeneration and weakness.[1] The most common form, Duchenne's muscular dystro-phy, is inherited as an X-linked recessive characteristic.[7] Medical concerns in these patients include cardiac abnormalities, poor respiratory function, adrenal suppression (secondary to prescribed steroids), gastroparesis, risk of hyperkalemic arrest with succinylcholine, and potential malignant hyperthermia.[3] Although more than 50% of the patients with muscular dystrophy can have cardiac abnormalities (manifested as dysrhythmias), impaired cardiac function is clinically significant in only 10%.[8] Avoidance of medications that can depress cardiac contractility should be considered in these patients.

The most frequent concern is usually the potential of impaired respiratory function. The perioperative severity of this potential complication frequently mirrors the patient's preexisting condition. There have been reports of adverse events secondary to muscle weakness that were not evident in the preoperative evaluation. Anesthetic medications should be titrated slowly, with the knowledge that the patient may require respiratory assistance. Conscious sedation may therefore be an unwise management technique unless administered by an experienced clinician.

Spinal Cord Injuries

Anesthetic management of a patient with a spinal cord injury raises several problems. Patients with a high spinal cord injury may have a history of multiple respiratory infections and limited respiratory reserve, which makes them more susceptible to the respiratory depressant effects of anesthetic agents. Lack of afferent stimulation below the injury may make the patient susceptible to orthostatic hypotension because of the lack of regulatory control. Autonomic hyperreflexia can also result from sympathetic spinal reflex activity, which is separate from the central nervous system (CNS) inhibitory control.[3] This may be the most significant sequela of chronic spinal cord transection on anesthetic management. Symptoms of autonomic hyperreflexia include bradycardia, dysrhythmias, hypertension, and seizures.

Renal failure may result secondarily from chronic urinary tract infections. Electrolyte abnormalities, anemia, and altered elimination of pharmacologic agents may result from the renal failure. Succinylcholine is contraindicated in patients with a spinal cord injury, since the denervated muscles may release massive amounts of potassium, leading to cardiac arrest.[3]

Spina Bifida

Spina bifida is a congenital malformation associated with failure of the vertebral arches to fuse.[3] Deficits are determined by the level of the defect. Many complications in providing anesthetic care for the patient with spina bifida depend on the level of the deficit. Although the defect is most frequently found in the lumbosacral area, more extensive involvement and failure of closure of the neural crest may occur at any level. Other associated anomalies, such as congenital heart defects, may be associated with spina bifida.

These patients may require multiple surgical procedures. The latter point is significant because it may contribute toward the high incidence of latex allergy in spina bifida patients.[3] Recurrent genitourinary tract instrumentation and frequent use of indwelling catheters may also be contributing factors. Anaphylactic reactions and death have been reported. Compliance with universal precautions has undoubtedly contributed to the increased incidence of latex allergy. If the patient demonstrates latex sensitization, a latex-free environment must be established before rendering care. All products must be evaluated for their latex content. Potential items include latex gloves, medication syringes, local anesthesia cartridges, rubber dams, prophylaxis cups, and nitrous oxide administration devices. Latex proteins carried in the cornstarch of latex gloves also should be controlled to avoid respiratory problems.

Treatment of the latex-sensitive patient can be safely provided. In addition to avoiding latex-containing items, scheduling the patient as the first appointment will minimize the potential for airborne latex proteins contaminating the dental operatory.

Anesthetic Techniques

Preoperative Care

Patients with mental impairment often may be frightened. Their fear of the unknown and lack of understanding may be manifested in aggressive behavior. Large body size and physical strength may make them difficult to manage, which may be problematic during both anesthetic induction and recovery. These patients may not readily accept intravenous (IV) placement, oral sedation, or intramuscular (IM) injections. Recovery from anesthesia can be associated with dizziness, visual disturbances, dysphoria, and hallucinations, all of which may also lead to aggressive behavior.

Physically impaired or systemically compromised patients frequently are fully cognizant of their increased perioperative anesthetic risk. These patients may depend on the clinician to move and care for them. They may have had numerous medical procedures under anesthesia, a situation that can also lead to further preoperative anxiety.

Physiologically, these patients may have multiple systemic complicating factors. The severity of these complex conditions may mandate referral to tertiary centers. Many healthy-appearing patients may present significant problems when medically challenged. The dentist must realize that many of these patients can sustain significant complications secondary to the slightest alteration in their homeostatic state. The most important point is to *know the patient*, including a thorough knowledge of the presenting medical conditions. The patient should be in optimal physical condition before the procedure.

General Management

Anesthetic management of these patients varies from conscious sedation to general anesthesia. The anesthetic technique chosen depends on both the patient's ability to cooperate and the clinical manifestations of the disease or condition. The ability to cooperate is often associated with the patient's degree of mental impairment, including his or her recollection of past dental or surgical treatment. Mildly mentally impaired patients can frequently be managed with conscious sedation. This sedation can be achieved with nitrous oxide, oral sedation, or a simple IV anesthetic. Moderate to severe mental impairment will usually mandate the use of deep sedation or general anesthesia.

Management of the anxious physically impaired patient depends on the clinical manifestations of the systemic disease. Spasticity in the patient with cerebral palsy potentially may be managed with nitrous oxide or an IV benzodiazepine. These agents decrease both the incidence of spasticity and the patient's anxiety. If conscious sedation is unsuccessful, deepening the anesthetic can be complicated by the symptoms of the disease. Swallowing abnormalities, compromised pharyngolaryngeal reflexes, and gastroesophageal reflux may increase the risk in the deeply sedated patient. General anesthesia managed by an experienced individual may be the most appropriate anesthetic option.

Many anesthetic agents can be used for the management of the developmentally disabled patient, including nitrous oxide, benzodiazepines, narcotics, ketamine, and propofol. Although different agents will require varying levels of training, both nitrous oxide and benzodiazepines are appropriate agents for the dentist trained in conscious sedation. However, the dentist must choose the appropriate patient situation in which to use these agents. It is always appropriate to interrupt a procedure and reschedule if a planned sedation is not achieving the desired effect (Table 20-2).

Postoperative Care

The final stage of the anesthetic management is the postanesthetic recovery and discharge of the patient. During this phase the patient must be continuously monitored by a trained individual. The length and nature of recovery primarily depend on three factors: type of surgery, nature of the anesthetic administered, and the patient's medical history.

Disorientation or dysphoria may complicate and prolong the recovery from anesthesia, often due to postoperative pain but also caused by hypercarbia (respiratory insufficiency). The patient must be fully evaluated before any pharmacologic intervention. Administering an opioid, for example, would be inappropriate if the patient was experiencing hypercarbia from hypoventilation.

Occasionally a patient requires physical or pharmacologic restraint to prevent self-injury or injury to personnel during recovery. Use of restraints in medicine is controversial. Soft restraints, secured so as not to compromise limb circulation, should be used to secure the patient in a safe position. Situations warranting restraints include the self-abusive patient, the aggressive patient, and the active patient who tries to change position (in an attempt to leave the area prematurely) before being hemodynamically stable.

Anesthetic medications or gastric irritability (secondary to swallowed blood) can also result in nausea or vomiting, which naturally compromises the patient's ability to resume normal dietary intake. The patient's inability to communicate distress may confound the diagnosis and delay appropriate treatment.

Care must also be taken to assess the severity and duration of the anticipated postoperative pain. Opioid analgesics administered in the recovery period can prolong and exacerbate existing respiratory difficulties and therefore may not be appropriate. Additionally, mentally impaired patients may not be able to communicate their level of postoperative

TABLE 20-2

Potential Interactions with Select Anesthetic Agents for Patients with Neurologic Disorders

Anesthetic Agent	Interaction or Adverse Outcome
Phenothiazines (e.g., droperidol)	May exacerbate existing extrapyramidal symptoms
Neuromuscular blocking agents	Increased sensitivity of patient
Succinylcholine	Hyperkalemia

pain. It becomes the clinician's responsibility to ensure that the patient remains comfortable. The clinician must anticipate postoperative pain and prescribe analgesic medication on a time-based contingency (as opposed to "as required" [prn]) to ensure that the noncommunicative patient remains comfortable. Explicit instructions must be given to the guardian who cares for the patient.

Anesthetic Agents

Ketamine

Ketamine has unique properties that make it a good drug in the mentally impaired patient. Ketamine is a dissociative anesthetic with analgesic and amnestic effects.[9] It creates a cataleptic-like state in which the patient's eyes may remain open while under general anesthesia. Varying the dose and route can alter the degree of "dissociation" achieved.

Ketamine is associated with a 5% to 30% occurrence of *emergence phenomena* (dysphoria), which may manifest as hallucinations or bad dreams. The incidence of dysphoria is infrequent in children; it first appears in the teen years and increases with age. Dysphoria also occurs in patients with psychiatric illness, in females, with higher doses, and with more rapid IV administration. The addition of a benzodiazepine to ketamine decreases the necessary dose of ketamine and also tends to minimize or prevent the likelihood of emergence phenomena.[9]

The most important side effect of ketamine, however, is the *hypersalivation* associated with its use. Therefore an anticholinergic agent should be administered simultaneously. Of the anticholinergic agents available, *glycopyrrolate* (Robinul, a quaternary amine) effectively blocks the hypersecretion even though it does not act as rapidly as ketamine. Glycopyrrolate does not cross the blood-brain barrier and therefore does not potentiate the CNS effects of ketamine. It also has less cardiovascular effects and does not contribute to the increased cardiac output and increased heart rate that occur with ketamine.

Ketamine is water soluble and can be administered orally, intranasally, intramuscularly, or intravenously. It has a high therapeutic index. Onset is rapid and predictable regardless of route of administration. In the uncooperative patient who will not allow the placement of an IV catheter, ketamine can be administered orally, intranasally, or intramuscularly. The IM route is frequently used because it does not depend on patient compliance. Although oral administration is less traumatic, the bitter taste of ketamine precludes its use in noncompliant patients.

It may be impossible to physically restrain some developmentally disabled patients to minimize the risk of injuring either the patient or a health care provider. In these patients the oral administration of ketamine is effective. The unique dissociative effect of the medication establishes a controllable environment in which an IV catheter can be inserted and additional medication administered to achieve induction and maintenance of anesthesia. Because of the potential to induce general anesthesia with even a small dose, ketamine should be administered only by individuals trained in general anesthesia.

Ketamine increases cardiac output, heart rate, and blood pressure secondary to sympathetic stimulation. Cautious use of ketamine is the rule in patients with cardiac disease.

Nitrous Oxide

Nitrous oxide is a nonirritating, sweet-smelling, minimally potent inhalant agent shown to alter both the attitude to pain and the perception of pain. The low blood:gas solubility allows rapid and easy titration of a sedative state. Cardiovascular and respiratory effects in developmentally impaired patients include mild myocardial depression, decreased baroreceptor reflex, depressed ventilatory response to hypoxia and hypercarbia, and mildly depressed pharyngolaryngeal reflexes secondary to decreased electromyographic activity, which may be of some benefit in patients with dyskinetic movements. Nitrous oxide

can cause nausea and vomiting. Although no specific "nothing by mouth" (NPO) guidelines are suggested for nitrous oxide, the physically impaired (and restrained) patient may be at an increased risk for aspiration.

Once thought to be inert, nitrous oxide undergoes metabolic transformation at a very low rate within the body.[10,11] It interferes significantly with the formation of the enzyme methionine synthetase after brief surgical exposure or chronic periods of low exposure. Because methionine synthetase is essential for the formation of vitamin B_{12}, exposure to nitrous oxide in patients with pernicious anemia may result in acute neurologic deterioration.[12] Therefore any patient with a history of neurologic sequelae after nitrous oxide administration should not receive nitrous oxide because of the high incidence of recurrence of neurologic symptoms.

SUMMARY

Management of the mentally or physically impaired patient can be very rewarding. Each patient must be individually assessed and a specific treatment plan developed. The provision of anesthesia allows for the routine dental treatment of an entire class of patients who have not routinely received dental treatment in past years. Preanesthetic planning is especially important because complications can arise during the anesthetic management of these patients.

References

1. Quinn CL: The physically compromised patient. In Malamed SF, editor: *Sedation: a guide to patient management*, ed 3, St Louis, 1995, Mosby.
2. Martz DG, Schreibman DL, Matjasko MJ: Neurologic diseases. In Katz J, Benumof JL, Kadis LB, editors: *Anesthesia and uncommon diseases*, ed 3, Philadelphia, 1990, WB Saunders.
3. Stoelting RK, Dierdorf SF: *Anesthesia and co-existing disease*, ed 3, New York, 1993, Churchill Livingstone.
4. Leyman JW, Mashni M, Trapp LD, et al: Anesthesia for the elderly and special needs patient, *Dent Clin North Am* 43(2):301-319, 1999.
5. Pavlin EG: Respiratory diseases. In Katz J, Benumof JL, Kadis LB, editors: *Anesthesia and uncommon diseases*, ed 3, Philadelphia, 1990, WB Saunders.
6. Rubin E, Farber JL: Developmental and genetic diseases. In Rubin E, Farber JL, editors: *Pathology*, ed 2, Philadelphia, 1994, JB Lippincott.
7. Armbrustmacher VW: Skeletal muscle. In Rubin E, Farber JL, editors: *Pathology*, ed 2, Philadelphia, 1994, JB Lippincott.

8. Miller JD, Lee CL: Muscle diseases. In Katz J, Benumof JL, Kadis LB, editors. *Anesthesia and uncommon diseases,* ed 3, Philadelphia, 1990, WB Saunders.

9. Jeffers G, Dembo J: Deep sedation. In Dionne RA, Phero JC, editors: *Management of pain and anxiety in dental practice,* New York, 1991, Elsevier.

10. Royston BD, Bottiglieri T, Nunn JF: Short term effects of nitrous oxide on methionine and *s*-adenosyl methionine concentrations, *Br J Anaesth* 62:419-424, 1989.

11. Sharer NM, Nunn JF, Royston JP, et al: Effect of chronic exposure to nitrous oxide on methionine synthase activity, *Br J Anaesth* 55:693-701, 1983.

12. Schilling RF: Is nitrous oxide a dangerous anesthetic for vitamin B_{12}-deficient subjects? *JAMA* 255(12):1605-1606, 1986.

DIAGNOSIS AND MANAGEMENT
OF CHRONIC OROFACIAL PAIN

Behavioral Management in Patients with Temporomandibular Disorders

KATE M. HATHAWAY
GEORGE E. PARSONS

CHAPTER OUTLINE

Behavioral and Psychosocial Factors in Temporomandibular Disorders

Behavioral and psychological interventions have been used since the 1960s for craniomandibular disorders, such as headaches, neck pain, temporomandibular disorders (TMD), and orofacial pain conditions. These treatments have been designed to (1) reduce oral habits, (2) change maladaptive health behaviors (e.g., low general exercise, poor diet, poor sleep habits), (3) address stress management (e.g., relaxation, hypnosis), and (4) help patients improve general coping mechanisms to deal with life's challenges in general and with pain in particular. Similar treatments have been successfully used with patients experiencing chronic neck and back pain, anxiety difficulties, and long-standing and debilitating diseases, such as diabetes, rheumatoid arthritis, and cancer.

Patients with TMD have varying physical signs and clinical symptoms, but the predominant treatment goal for clinicians is to alleviate pain and improve jaw function. The vast majority of patients seen in general practice with TMD have relatively "simple" pain problems, such as muscle pain in the masseter or temporalis area, tooth pain, or preauricular pain. Most often, patients cope well with these discomforts and are merely looking for a way to reduce the frequency, duration, or intensity of pain. A combination of splint therapy, physical therapy home exercises, instruction in jaw relaxation, and oral habit change techniques will be successful for most patients. Emotional difficulties may be present for some TMD patients, however, especially for those experiencing more chronic pain and dysfunction. It is critical to address these emotional issues as well.

Role of Behavioral Factors

As with many musculoskeletal difficulties, the major factors contributing to the onset, maintenance, or exacerbation of facial pain and headaches may involve maladaptive behaviors. These behaviors may result in specific *microtrauma* to the involved muscles and joints, such as clenching of teeth resulting in masseter and temporalis pain. Other behaviors may influence muscle and joint function indirectly, such as general physical deconditioning resulting in muscle fatigue. These behaviors are among the primary contributors to TMD and should be the primary target for behavioral assessment and intervention. Behavioral treatments include habit-reversal training, lifestyle counseling, and relaxation training.

Role of Psychosocial Factors

Scientists do not know the degree to which psychosocial factors contribute to the patient's experience of TMD. Current knowledge regarding the etiology of facial pain does not offer overwhelming support for the hypothesis that a "functional" component is involved. Orofacial pain problems are probably no more prevalent among mental health patients than among "normal" patients. Similarly, there appears to be no greater incidence of anxiety, depression, or major mental illness among TMD patients than among general medical patients.[1] On the other hand, depression, psychosocial dysfunction, somatization, and defensiveness may occur more often in chronic and acute TMD patients than in the general, *nonmedical* population.[2] As such, these factors must be evaluated as part of the general assessment of patients with chronic facial pain.

Understanding and treating the biobehavioral factors in combination with the physical pathology are considered the best hope for alleviation of TMD difficulties. The involvement of mental health professionals in the early assessment of TMD and orofacial pain may be beneficial.

This chapter focuses on general assessment techniques for TMD patients and offers an overview of diagnostic models for assessing the biobehavioral elements in facial pain and headaches. Various patient evaluation inventories are available for assessing the psychological factors related to TMD. Behavioral-psychologic treatment options include stress and pain management, hypnosis, relaxation, and psychotherapy.

Pretreatment Evaluation

The importance of a thorough pretreatment evaluation cannot be overemphasized. A number of protocols for assessment of TMD have been suggested. Research diagnostic criteria for TMD combine an axis I physical assessment in three categories—(1) muscular disorders, (2) disk displacement, and (3) arthralgia, arthritis, and arthrosis—with an axis II assessment of behavioral and psychosocial factors.[3] This discussion focuses on different aspects of the axis II assessment.

During the pretreatment evaluation, the clinician must dedicate time to gathering information about behavior and coping. In orofacial pain patients the physical examination may yield a tentative physical diagnosis; generating a list of factors contributing to the experience of pain or dysfunction is also critical.

Ability to predict treatment outcomes on the basis of physical diagnosis alone is not particularly good.[4] A biopsychosocial treatment protocol incorporates both physical diagnoses and relevant contributing factors.[5] The initial assessment is not complete until it includes a list of contributing factors, such as oral habits, stress management concerns, lifestyle issues (e.g., excessive caffeine or alcohol use), emotional issues, depression, and malocclusion. Although additional time is needed to gather information on contributing factors, this is often the most important part of the assessment.

A thorough pretreatment evaluation should include the following:

1. Assessment of oral habits
2. Assessment of general lifestyle habits
3. Assessment of pain management skills
4. Assessment of stress management skills
5. Prediction of likely compliance with self-management instructions (e.g., splint use, home exercises, relaxation)
6. Assessment of general physical health
7. General emotional screening, including a chemical dependency assessment
8. An understanding of the patient's hypothesis regarding the pain and the patient's motivation and preferences for treatment
9. Assessment of possible obstacles to successful completion of treatment (e.g., time, money, inability to tolerate the oral appliance)

Oral Habits. Oral habit assessment should include specific questioning to assess the presence of behaviors such as clenching the teeth together, jaw muscle tightening without tooth contact (jaw rigidity habits), bruxism (grinding teeth, diurnal and nocturnal), nail biting, gum chewing (or chronic use of hard or chewy candy), object chewing (e.g., pencils, pens), tongue or jaw thrust habits, incorrect tongue position, or chronic overuse of the jaw for other activities (e.g., musical instrument playing, tobacco chewing). These habits are extremely prevalent in the general population, with estimates for bruxism alone ranging from 5% to 80% in various studies.[6] The high prevalence of oral habits demands that clinicians screen for them routinely in dental patients, especially orofacial pain patients. These habits result in masticatory muscle contraction, overloading the temporomandibular joints. This in turn contributes directly to the muscle and joint strain often seen in patients with major craniofacial diagnoses.

General Lifestyle Habits. General lifestyle habit assessment should include information gathering about possible contributors to poor general health status. Low levels of exercise and poor eating habits may result in muscle deconditioning, contributing to a poor prognosis for specific muscle rehabilitation treatments, such as those required for improvement in TMD. Poor general health habits may further decrease resistance to the effects of life's stressors. The practitioner should ask questions about general nutritional habits (meals per day, nutritional value of food consumed, binge/purge habits, use of caffeine, tobacco, alcohol), general exercise, and activity level. On occasion, effective treatment might involve simply prescribing a decrease in caffeine use, a change in over-the-counter (OTC) medication use, or alteration in eating patterns.

Sleep behaviors are a specific area of concern for patients with long-standing craniofacial pain. A poor sleeping pattern often predicts decreased ability to cope with pain; without restful sleep, a person is likely to feel more irritable and tired during the day. Poor sleep may be a symptom of poor sleeping habits (falling asleep on the couch, napping during the day, falling asleep to the TV), emotional difficulties (often coexisting with depression and anxiety) or pain during sleep. A contributing factor of sleep difficulties may require separate intervention.

Oral and lifestyle habit assessments are critical to treatment planning. In attempts to find anatomic bases for pain and to discover the "perfect" diagnosis, practitioners often miss the opportunity for common-sense interventions. If a patient reports that gum chewing aggravates jaw pain, for example, the treatment of choice is "no gum chewing." Even if an occlusal problem is simultaneously evident, treatment of the occlusion should not necessarily be the priority. Common-sense and "straightforward" treatments may be more helpful for many patients than complicated splint therapies, physical therapy, or psychological interventions. Common sense and good health care provider-patient relationships are major contributors to treatment success with patients.

Pain Management Skills. Pain management skill assessment involves gathering information about the role of the pain condition in the patient's life. This is especially important for patients with chronic pain. Regular complaining, secondary gain, or receipt of some overt or subtle "benefit" from talking about pain (e.g., avoidance of work, dependence on others to complete tasks, monetary gain), and strained interpersonal relationships may be seen in some chronic pain patients. When operative, these behaviors take on importance independent of the pain itself and often need to be addressed separately. In such patients, management must incorporate treatments for the pain, the emotion associated with the pain, and the dysfunctional lifestyles resulting from the pain and its presentation. These issues are discussed in more detail in the literature on chronic pain conditions.[7,8] The "pain patient" personality and "secondary gain" concerns are seen in only a small percentage of craniofacial pain patients but should be routinely evaluated. Often a simple question (e.g., "How has the pain affected your day-to-day living?" or "If I followed you around every day, how would I know that you had pain?") can yield a wealth of information about the role that pain is playing in a patient's life.

Stress Management Skills. Stress management skill assessment may be helpful in planning for treatment of craniomandibular disorders. "Stress," however loosely defined, may result in biochemical changes in the body that subsequently alter function. Similarly, biochemical changes may result in altered ability to cope and related perception of increased stress. The exact relationship between stress and orofacial pain is difficult to ascertain. To date, research does not support assumptions such as (1) bruxism is the result of stress, (2) stress causes patients to clench more, (3) stress causes people to cope inadequately, or (4) stress causes people to be less compliant. However, skills for coping with life's challenges may be affected by (or affect) the pain condition and its sequelae.

Many patients benefit from looking at stressors and coping strategies as influences on treatment outcome. Individuals expending significant amounts of energy to "cope" with the demands of their environment may have difficulty finding the time and energy necessary to make significant lifestyle changes, exercise consistently, or wear an occlusal appliance as requested. As with the findings for other "emotional" issues, the research does not support stress as a clear *etiologic* factor in orofacial pain conditions, although it may contribute to poor treatment outcome. An assessment of stress issues is helpful when discussing the timing of treatment or the benefit of additional stress management interventions to augment other TMD treatments.

Compliance with Self-Management. A review of likely compliance with prescribed care is extremely important in the prediction of treatment outcome. A history of poor compliance (e.g., poor follow-through with exercise programs, inability to wear splints as prescribed) is often not a positive indicator for treatment. Poor compliance with previous treatment is one of the best predictors of poor future compliance. When self-management is recommended in the treatment protocol, good compliance is even more crucial to treatment success.[8,9] Clinicians can use many techniques to better predict treatment adherence and to facilitate compliance, in turn significantly improving the likelihood of treatment success.[10]

General Physical Health. All patients should be screened for general health. Ongoing health conditions and treatments may interact unfavorably with treatment of the orofacial pain condition. A brief review of systems and general questions about patients' perception of their health (e.g., "Rate your physical health on a scale of 1 [good] to 10 [bad]; what would make it a 10?") can elicit much information for treatment planning.

Emotional Health. General emotional health can be screened in a manner similar to that for general health, with questions about previous contact with counselors, psychologists, or psychiatrists; use of medication for emotional issues; and again, a general question rating emotional health on a scale of 1 to 10. This type of question usually is not regarded as threatening and often can help patients gain personal insight. Direct questioning about depression, suicidal thinking, and anxiety is critical to a thorough screening.

Although the research does not support emotional difficulties as primary etiologic contributors, mood disorders and anxiety are common among chronic pain patients. Researchers and clinicians recognize the high prevalence of depression among chronic pain patients in particular, postulating that it often results from unrelenting or untreated pain.[11] These emotional issues must be addressed as part of the treatment package, or the physical pain may be reduced while the emotional pain persists.

Chemical dependency. Chemical dependency screenings are recommended for all acute and chronic health conditions. Dependency on either prescription or OTC drugs is common among pain patients. General practice physicians miss chemical dependency diagnoses more than 70% of the time.

Overuse or misuse of medication for pain management needs to be addressed before treatment begins, often coordinated with the patient's other medical practitioners. Patients can exhibit dependencies (either physical or psychological) on OTC medications (e.g., acetaminophen, ibuprofen, sleep medications), resulting in rebound symptoms. Recreational agents (e.g., alcohol, marijuana) may complicate treatment, and patients may use them to relax or reduce pain.

Specific questions about prescription and OTC medications include strength, amounts, time taken, and formulation; an answer such as "when the pain gets really bad" is not particularly informative. Chemical interactions and self-medication must be addressed as possible contributing factors to poor pain management.

Hypothesis of Pain. A patient's hypothesis about the etiology of the pain can be elicited by a specific question (e.g., "What do you believe is the reason you have pain?"). Often the answer will be vague (e.g., "It's related to clenching my teeth"), and occasionally it will be very specific. The health care provider should take this opportunity to begin educating the patient about the medical and/or dental hypothesis and basic physiology (e.g., muscle/joint function). Understanding a patient's conception of the pain condition is critical to treatment planning; it may be the most important part of the evaluation.

Patients may have some preferences for treatment; often they have heard or read facts about treatment that they believe will be particularly helpful. A thorough assessment, again with specific questions (e.g., "What do you think would be particularly helpful for you in addressing this pain?"), will yield information about these preferences.

Obstacles to Treatment. It is important to obtain information about obstacles that could interfere with effective treatment, including time, money, or competing health demands that will complicate compliance. When necessary, it may be better to defer treatment until later rather than risk frustrating both the patient and the health care provider with a lack of progress.

Assessment Instruments and Checklists

"Paper and pencil" checklists and inventories may assist practitioners in assessing psychosocial factors in patients with TMD. These include the Beck Depression Inventory (BDI), Minnesota Multiphasic Personality

Inventory II (MMPI-II), Millon Clinical Multiaxial Inventory (MCMI), Symptoms 90 Checklist, Mooney Problem Checklist, and Multidimensional Pain Inventory (MPI) (Box 21-1).

Generally, these instruments require at least an eighth-grade reading level, and some (e.g., MMPI, MCMI) require a specialist for scoring and interpreting test results. A partnership between the mental health community and the TMD practitioner will assist the dental practitioner in assessment and the development of a more complete treatment protocol and subsequent biopsychosocial therapies.

Beck Depression Inventory. The BDI is a test of 21 questions designed to produce a singular score related to depression. Scores are added, and the degree of depression is determined from the total score, ranging from severe to mild depression. The BDI is

---

BOX 21-1

Assessment Tests for Psychosocial Factors in Behavioral Management

Minnesota Multiphasic Personality Inventory
1982, University of Minnesota Press; distributed by National Computer Systems, PO Box 1416, Minneapolis, MN 55440

Millon Clinical Multiaxial Inventory
1987, National Computer Systems, PO Box 1416, Minneapolis, MN 55440

Beck Depression Inventory
1978, Center for Cognitive Therapy, Room 602, 133 S 36th St, Philadelphia, PA 19104

Mooney Problem Checklist
1978, The Psychological Corp, Harcourt Brace Jovanovich, New York

Symptoms 90 Checklist
1992, Clinical Psychometric Research, Towson, MD 21204

Multidimensional Pain Inventory
Turk DC, Rudy TE: Toward an empirically derived taxonomy of chronic pain patients: integration of psychological assessment data, *J Consult Clin Psychol* 56 (2):1-6, 1988.

particularly useful as a quick way to assess depression in patients, and several items are good predictors of suicidality.

Minnesota Multiphasic Personality Inventory. The MMPI-II is a psychological test designed to measure the presence of psychopathology in an individual by using three validity scales and 10 clinical scales. Scores are reported by profile from highest to lowest and include measures of depression, anxiety, and somatic focus, as may be found in TMD patients.

Millon Clinical Multiaxial Inventory. The MCMI is a brief instrument that provides a measure of 22 personality disorders and clinical syndromes for adults. The MCMI-II was specifically designed to coordinate with categories of personality disorders and clinical syndromes from the *Diagnostic and Statistical Manual of Mental Disorders* (in this case, DSM-III-R). The 22 clinical scales and three correction scales are divided into five categories to reflect more accurately the distinction between relatively enduring personality features and acute symptoms. The test also includes a validity index that is sensitive to careless, confused, or random responses.

Symptoms 90 Checklist. This self-reporting instrument consists of 90 items concerning common problems. The items are rated by the subject on a distress scale ranging from 0 (not distressful) to 4 (extremely distressful). The results are thought to reflect the patterns of the subject's psychological symptoms.

Mooney Problem Checklist. In this series of 288 possible statements or concerns, the individual is initially asked to underline items of consequence, then circle those of major importance. This provides insight into the various stresses in the patient's life.

Multidimensional Pain Inventory. The MPI is a set of empirically derived scales designed to assess appraisal of patients with chronic pain with regard to their pain severity, interference with social and familial activities, impact on their lives, current mood state (psychosocial factors), responses from significant others, and performance of common daily activities (behavioral factors).

From the list of contributing factors and possible concurrent emotional issues of psychopathology, a treatment protocol can be developed to address each concern.

Behavioral Treatments

Aside from occlusal treatments, the most common treatments for the orofacial pain patient involve behavior therapy for oral habits. Behavioral treatments are based on the learning theory that persistent behaviors can be unlearned. Most treatment approaches involve a *cognitive component* (to increase understanding of the importance of changing the behavior), an *emotional component* (to deal with any anxiety involved in the behavior change), and a *behavior change component* (habit reversal). Each patient will benefit differently from intervention in each area. A patient must gain greater insight regarding the consequences of the behavior (e.g., clenching results in significant muscle and joint strain) and the possible need to address anxiety resulting from making a change (e.g., learning to relax instead of tighten when experiencing pain). The greatest challenge, however, is the habit change itself. To change a behavior, a patient must have (1) the *motivation and commitment* to change the behavior, (2) a clear understanding of *alternate actions* to replace the behavior (e.g., relax the facial muscles instead of clench), and (3) a *regular routine* for engaging in (practicing) the correct behavior more often. Often the approach to behavior change is simply, "You need to stop clenching." It is more beneficial to set the goal of *increased muscle relaxation.* In this manner, patients can address several habits at the same time by replacing them with the incompatible behavior of relaxation.

Habit-reversal training is perhaps one of the best behavioral techniques for treatment of oral habits.[12] This technique involves a series of interventions to (1) increase an individual's awareness of a behavior such as clenching, (2) interrupt the chain of behaviors involved in the habit as soon as possible, (3) teach the patient a behavior incompatible with the maladaptive habit, and (4) eliminate any possible reinforcement for the habit. Good success has been reported with this approach,[13] which is straightforward, easy to orchestrate, and well received by patients.

A typical treatment program based on this approach involves instruction to patients in correct tongue and teeth position (tongue up, teeth apart, jaw muscles relaxed). After instruction, patients are told to self-monitor (to increase awareness and practice the new habit) on a regular schedule (e.g., put the tongue up, teeth apart, with jaw muscles relaxed). The new (incompatible) behavior is to be practiced frequently (e.g., every 20 to 30 minutes), increasing orofacial muscle relaxation and decreasing tooth contact activities. When the monitoring and correction are consistent, the habit can be changed effectively within a relatively short time. It does require a commitment to self-monitor and some guidance to make consistent use of reminders. Patients will soon realize that every minute the jaw is relaxed is a minute that the teeth cannot be clenched, the muscles cannot be held rigid, or gum cannot be chewed. The patient is reversing the maladaptive oral habit by replacing it with an incompatible behavior (relaxation). Patients rarely have difficulty with the first two phases of the behavior change; some will make the changes rapidly and without much guidance from the health care team. Others will have more trouble, using reminders inefficiently. Some guidance in this area is usually necessary and generally welcome.

The simple approach just outlined will not be effective with all patients. For some, lack of treatment success can be attributed to poor guidance from team members. For others it is a sign of poor motivation or commitment. Patients often want to change habits but want the change to be easy. They need to be told that the change will require effort and will take time. The health care provider is responsible for teaching good skills and educating the patient about the consequences of behavior. On occasion, however, a patient "catches herself biting her nails but does it anyway." Clinical expertise has little power when motivation is lacking, but motivational techniques may be helpful.[14] The patient can again be reminded of the importance of making the change. The health care provider can work to reduce the damage sustained by such behavior but should not expect miraculous treatment results.

Nocturnal Habits

Nocturnal habits such as bruxism present a unique treatment challenge.[15] To date, no treatment has proven superior to others in helping patients eliminate nighttime habits. The best approaches may involve (1) working with daytime habits (in the hope that some of the orofacial muscle relaxation will transfer to nocturnal activities), (2) use of occlusal devices to reduce the impact of the habits, and (3) consideration of presleep relaxation or biofeedback to facilitate nocturnal jaw relaxation. Currently, treatment applications are limited, and clinicians should be wary of claims about treatments or medications that will "cure" or eliminate nocturnal habits. However,

several treatments can be good augmentations, especially when combined with splint therapy.

Biofeedback

Biofeedback is a treatment based on both applied relaxation techniques and principles of learning. The premise behind biofeedback is that individuals can learn to change some physiologic activities when given information (feedback) about the activities. In the case of muscle activity, electromyography is used to monitor muscle activity, and patients are given feedback about the degree of tension or relaxation of the muscles. This information, coupled with training in relaxation, gives patients opportunities to reduce muscle tightness. Biofeedback has been used in patients with orofacial habits such as bruxism with equivocal but some positive results.[16] Many patients benefit from receiving concrete information about muscle activity and the means by which to change it. Biofeedback may be a good adjunct to occlusal splints and diurnal habit reversal in the treatment of daytime bruxism, particularly in patients who have not responded to other therapies.

Stress Management Techniques

Stress management techniques are often used with other treatments to address conditions involving chronic muscle tension or pain. No two people experience "stress" in the same way, however, and stress should not be viewed as a universal experience triggered by different external events. Each patient is equipped with a variety of adaptive mechanisms, strengthened or weakened by knowledge and experience. Each person deals with the same challenge differently as well, based on capabilities and understanding. Clinicians can help patients learn the skills of adaptation, balance, behavior change, and health management. This goal is much more important than that of "managing" stress. There is no simple or easy answer to the challenges of living and no ideal "stress management" technique, but a variety of techniques have proved helpful.

Stress management techniques must incorporate methods to help patients alter *cognitive patterns* that may be maladaptive, *emotional patterns* that may be disruptive, and *physical behaviors* that place strain on the body. Good stress management approaches involve all three areas. Cognitive and emotional attitudes may aggravate pain by influencing an individual's ability to tolerate symptoms. Although stress does not *cause* an individual to engage in maladaptive habits, it can distract a person from changing habits effectively.

Stress management and relaxation treatments are most often used in clinical settings as adjunctive treatments for pain management and for facial relaxation. Relaxation exercises and techniques to change thinking patterns can be effective treatment techniques. These strategies (1) increase physical, cognitive, and emotional relaxation; (2) increase the patient's self-confidence and sense of control; and (3) have no known negative side effects. The effect of relaxation exercises is global and is helpful when patients feel a desire to "unwind" generally. They can help improve general coping.

Lifestyle Counseling

Lifestyle counseling also can help patients change behaviors and attitudes that result in unhealthy lifestyles. Behaviors such as poor general exercise, poor nutritional intake, and excessive caffeine use can contribute in a significant way to increased muscle tension and joint strain. Interventions designed to help patients make changes in these areas are often time-consuming for both the patient and the health care provider. Many patients experiencing pain, however, are ready to make major changes and welcome the opportunity. Helping patients improve their quality of life is a major goal for health psychology and for public health worldwide.[17] It is not sufficient to change diet, for example, if the intervention does not reduce pain and improve the quality of a patient's life. Health care providers need to gear treatment toward health enhancement, particularly with patients experiencing chronic discomfort.

Pain management approaches generally involve cognitive, emotional, and physical interventions to help patients alter their perceptions of themselves as "pain patients."[18,19] These interventions may be short (e.g., instruction to return to work) or may be very complicated (e.g., family interventions to discuss pain behaviors and secondary gain issues with family members, discuss complications arising from litigation). Occasionally it will be necessary to coordinate treatment with chronic pain programs to help patients address complications and the chronic pain's impact on their lives with an interdisciplinary management team. This is extremely limited, however, because of limited availability and difficulty obtaining insurance coverage for this effective but costly approach.

Psychotherapy

A psychotherapeutic intervention may be helpful for orofacial pain patients. In these patients, personality issues must be treated as independent but related factors. Psychotherapy refers to individual or group sessions with a trained psychotherapist to help a patient make a major personality or life change. The change may be emotional, cognitive, and/or behavioral and is in a specified direction, such as a decrease in depression or an improvement in interpersonal relationships with family members. Goals for therapy are mutually determined by both patient and therapist and can be either short term (up to 10 sessions) or long term (more than 10 sessions). There are many different approaches to psychotherapy, and each therapy has its advantages. The "best fit" of therapist, patient, and therapeutic intervention is the best predictor of success.

Pharmacologic Treatments

Medications may also be helpful for many patients with emotional issues. A full mental health evaluation can help determine the appropriateness of psychotropic medication and psychotherapy. Psychopathology does not preclude the existence of a physical problem that requires treatment, however. It is important to coordinate efforts with the psychotherapist; the question generally involves timing (i.e., should orofacial pain treatment precede or follow psychotherapeutic intervention?). Some pharmacologic therapies are designed to decrease pain and address mood; these are familiar to the general practitioner and are discussed elsewhere.

Chronic pain patients have different needs than do acute pain patients, however, and medications should be used with extreme caution. When patients do not have other skills to use for pain reduction, they can become reliant on medications for maintaining their comfort. In addition, pain patients often sleep poorly (e.g., awakening with pain), and the health care practitioner is often tempted to treat the sleep issue as well. Pharmacologic treatments should be well designed. Most interventions should be short term and targeted at pain reduction.

Sleep medications and agents that allegedly reduce bruxism should be used with extreme caution, if at all. Generally these fall into the category of muscle relaxants. Their effects are nonspecific, and when positive results are reported, it is unclear whether the effects are from a reduction in muscle pain, a reduction in oral habits, general muscle relaxation, or sedation. Although they may be helpful in the short term, medications for treatment of oral habits currently cannot be recommended for long-term treatment.

Treatment Model and Options

Much has been written on the causes and management of TMD, as well as treatment modalities that best serve TMD patients.

Fig. 21-1 provides a working model to help the practitioner in treating TMD patients. On axis I the patient is differentiated by physical dysfunction, muscular hyperarousal, structural abnormalities, and internal derangement with intensity of pain. Patients reporting a positive or plus score generally acknowledge a lower intensity of pain and limited physical symptoms. Patients with a negative or minus score have increasing intensity of pain and physical symptoms.

On axis II the patient is differentiated by psychosocial factors. Positive or plus scores are characterized by good coping skills and by individuals who are functionally independent with low depression and low symptom endorsement. Negative or minus scores characterize persons who are identified as dysfunctional, disabled, or dependent, often with severe depression, and who have many symptoms associated with TMD.

More complex treatments for TMD will probably be needed for patients in categories II, III, and IV, with treatment emphasis on psychosocial factors only in categories III and IV. Patients in category IV are likely to present as difficult and will need a stronger, multidisciplinary approach, such as that found in pain centers that combine medical, psychological, physical, occupational, and speech therapies.[20]

Referral to a mental health professional for consultation and possible treatment can be difficult for the dental practitioner. Some patients resent the suggestion that any part of their pain problem is "in their head," "caused by stress," or representative of an "emotional problem." Often the referral involves a discussion of the contributing factors and a decision on the most appropriate treatment. Since factors such as oral habits and pain management are better addressed by those skilled in assisting patients with behavior changes, a good choice is a mental health provider with expertise in health issues (e.g.,

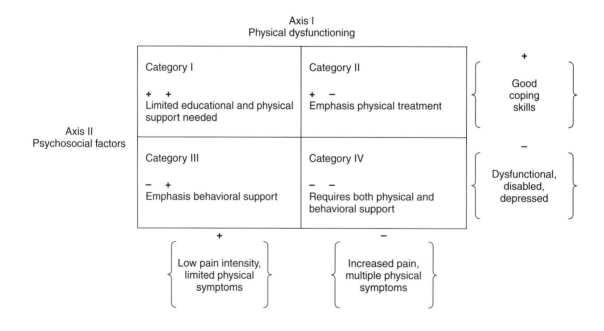

Fig. 21-1 Model for treatment of patients with temporomandibular disorders.

health psychologist). Often patients are relieved to have an opportunity to discuss issues with a trained professional. Many respond favorably to a question such as, "Have you thought about discussing some of these issues with a therapist?" or a statement such as, "I would like you to consider talking with a health psychologist or health educator about ways to reduce oral habits."

Patients often have opinions about what characteristics they would like in a therapist (e.g., female/male, location, orientation). The best gains in therapy generally occur when patient and therapist are well matched and when the goals are mutually designed by therapist and patient. Some of this matching can be done at the referral stage.

Therapeutic Recommendations

Working with patients who have pain can be very challenging, but it is extremely rewarding. Pain is experienced more than just physically,[21] and chronic pain often cannot be treated with physical intervention alone.[22] Every physical sensation is associated with an emotion (e.g., fear, sadness) and a cognitive experience (e.g., attempt to explain it). The emotional and cognitive components of the experience become more and more important as the pain lingers, and the best pain treatment programs are interdisciplinary. A health care provider working alone has fewer opportunities to effect change; working with other providers increases the likelihood of a positive treatment outcome. Each practitioner (dentist, physician, psychologist, physical therapist) will plan a treatment program designed to address the contributing factors. Together these plans will offer the most comprehensive program (Table 21-1).

Tailored, interdisciplinary approaches like these will succeed in treating the *whole patient,* not just the patient's pathophysiology. In this process, the most important member of the treatment team is the *patient.* The goals, desires, and priorities of the patient should always take precedence over the goals of the treatment team, even if this means deferment of treatment until mutual goals can be established. It is important that practitioners realize that the patient is the expert about his or her personal concerns. For this reason, the most important facet of treatment for TMD patients occurs before treatment begins, during a complete evaluation as contributing factors are listed and patient hypotheses and goals are discussed.

The treatment team must educate, collaborate with patients and other team members, and make treatment "user friendly." Treatments work best when individually tailored to patients' diagnoses and contributing factors and to their priorities and abilities. Therapies must address physical, cognitive, and emotional aspects of the patients' pain experience. With inclusion of these treatment priorities, TMD patients can invariably experience greater physical comfort and improved general health.

TABLE 21-1

Pain Symptoms with Treatment Options and Possible Providers

Symptoms	Treatment Options	Possible Providers
Oral habits	Habit reversal	Trained dentist
	Relaxation (adjunctive)	Health educator
	Biofeedback (adjunctive)	Psychotherapist
Unhealthy lifestyle	Lifestyle counseling	Any team member
"Stress"	Stress management	Psychotherapist
Poor coping	Pain management	All team members
	Pain program (inpatient or outpatient)	Pain specialist team
Chemical dependency (CD)	CD treatment	CD specialist
Emotional issues	Psychotherapy	Psychotherapist
	Medication	Physician
Poor compliance	Limit setting	Trained dentist
	Patient education	Psychotherapist

References

1. Marbach JJ: The temporomandibular pain dysfunction syndrome personality: fact or fiction? *J Oral Rehabil* 19(6):545-560, 1992.
2. Gatchel RJ, Gavonfale JP, Ellis E, et al: Major psychological disorders in acute and chronic TMD and initial examination, *J Am Dent Assoc* 127:1365, 1996.
3. List T, Dworkin S: Comparing TMD diagnoses and clinical findings at Swedish and U.S. TMD centers using research diagnostic criteria for temporomandibular disorder, *J Orofac Pain* 10:240-252, 1996.
4. McCreary CP et al: Predicting response to treatment for temporomandibular disorders, *J Craniomand Disord* 6(3): 161-169, 1992.
5. Fricton JR, Kroening RJ, Hathaway KM, editors: *TMJ and craniofacial pain: diagnosis and management,* St Louis, 1988, Ishiyaku EuroAmerica.
6. Lobbezoo F, Montplaisir JY, Lavigne GL: Bruxism: a factor associated with temporomandibular disorders and orofacial pain, *J Back Musculoskel Rehabil* 6:165-176, 1996.
7. Turk DC, Meichenbaum D, Genest M: *Pain and behavioral medicine: a cognitive-behavioral perspective,* New York, 1983, Guilford.
8. Turk DC, Rudy TE: Neglected topics in the treatment of chronic pain patients: relapse, noncompliance, and adherence enhancement, *Pain* 44(1):5-28, 1991.
9. Turk DC, Rudy TE: Toward an empirically derived taxonomy of chronic pain syndromes and definitions of pain terms, *Pain,* suppl 3, 1986.
10. Meichenbaum D, Turk DC: *Facilitating treatment adherence: a practitioner's guidebook,* New York, 1987, Plenum.
11. Haythornthwaite JA, Sieber WJ, Kerns RD: Depression and the chronic pain experience, *Pain* 46(2):177-184, 1991.
12. Azrin NJ, Nunn RG: Habit-reversal: a method of eliminating nervous habits and tics, *Behav Res Ther* 11(4):619-628, 1973.
13. Rosenbaum MS, Ayllon T: Treating bruxism with the habit-reversal technique, *Behav Res Ther* 19(1):87-96, 1981.
14. Prochaska JO, Norcross JC, DiClemente CC: *Changing for good,* New York, 1994, Morrow.
15. Hathaway KM: Bruxism: definition, measurement and treatment. In Fricton JR, Dubner R, editors: *Orofacial pain and temporomandibular disorders,* New York, 1995, Raven.
16. Lund JP, Widmer CF: Evaluation of the use of surface electromyography in the diagnosis, documentation, and treatment of dental patients, *J Craniomand Disord* 3(3):125-137, 1989.
17. Kaplan RM: Health outcome models for policy analysis, *Health Psychol* 8(6):123-135, 1989.
18. Turk DC: Psychological and behavioral assessment of patients with temporomandibular disorders: diagnostic and treatment implications, *Oral Surg* 53:65-71, 1997.
19. Gamsa A: The role of psychological factors in chronic pain. 1. A half century of study, *Pain* 57(1):5-15, 1994.
20. Hathaway KM: Behavioral and psychosocial management. In Pertes RA, Gross SG, editors: *Clinical management of temporomandibular disorders and orofacial pain,* Carol Stream, Ill, 1995, Quintessence.
21. Fernandez E, Turk DC: Sensory and affective components of pain: separation and synthesis, *Psychol Bull* 112(2):205-217, 1992.
22. Dworkin SF, LeResche L: Research diagnostic criteria for temporomandibular disorders: review, criteria, examination and specifications, critique, *J Craniomand Disord* 6:301-355, 1992.

CHAPTER 22

Diagnosis of Chronic Orofacial Pain

Yoshiki Imamura
Jeffrey P. Okeson

CHAPTER OUTLINE

Pain is one of the most common complaints of patients visiting a dental office. Most often the dental practitioner finds a cause for the pain, and proper treatment of this cause eliminates the pain. In some patients, however, the practitioner finds it difficult to identify the source of the pain, especially when referred pain is present. The dental structures are a common site of referred pain. Pain may be felt in the teeth or periodontal structures, but the origin of the pain can possibly be from another region. The practitioner must be aware of this type of pain, since toothache that results from referred pain will fail to respond to site-specific dental procedures. When referred pain continues after treatment of the tooth or periodontal structures, the patient can become discouraged and may pursue treatment with another dentist. The dental practitioner must be able to identify other sources of orofacial pain, beginning with knowledge of the various pain conditions that can occur in the orofacial structures.

In addition to the problems of identifying and treating the source of pain, therapeutic considerations can change when pain becomes chronic. The International Association for the Study of Pain (IASP) defines chronic pain as "pain that persists for a given length of time," as determined by common medical experiences. Two important factors that characterize chronic pain are time and psychological/environmental factors. Patients may complain of severe pain, but this pain may not be considered chronic pain unless it has been experienced for a length of time. For example, wound healing associated with pain rarely produces chronic pain. Chronic pain is associated with duration, continuity, and varying intensities, usually disturbing the individual's daily life activities. It is generally accepted that the pain experience becomes chronic if it has lasted longer than 6 months, although some individuals develop chronic pain behavior in less time.

This chapter reviews the various types of orofacial pain disorders that the dental practitioner must be able to recognize so that proper treatment can be selected. Common types of headache that can mimic orofacial pain are also described to aid in the differential diagnosis between dental conditions and conditions best referred to a neurologist, otolaryngologist, or other physician for evaluation and treatment.

Assessment of the Chronic Orofacial Pain Patient

Cranial Nerve Examination

The 12 cranial nerves supply sensory information to and motor impulses from the brain. Any gross problem relating to their function must be identified so abnormal conditions can be immediately and appropriately addressed. A cranial nerve examination does not need to be a complex evaluation. Any clinician who regularly evaluates pain problems can test the gross function of the cranial nerves to evaluate for any neuropathic disorders. Each nerve can be assessed by using simple evaluation procedures.

Olfactory Nerve (I). The first cranial nerve has sensory fibers originating in the mucous membrane of the nasal cavity and provides the sensation of smell. It may be tested by asking the patient to detect differences between odors, such as peppermint, vanilla, and chocolate. (It is helpful to have these available in the office for testing.) To determine if the patient's nose is obstructed, the patient exhales through the nares onto a mirror; fogging of the mirror from both nostrils denotes adequate airflow.

Optic Nerve (II). The second cranial nerve is also sensory and provides for sight through fibers originating in the retina. Sight is tested by having the patient cover one eye at a time and read a few sentences. The limits of the visual field are assessed by the examiner standing behind the patient and slowly bringing the fingers from behind and into view. The patient reports when the fingers first appear, normally with no variation between when they are seen on the right and on the left.

Oculomotor, Trochlear, and Abducens Nerves (III, IV, VI). The third, fourth, and sixth cranial nerves, supplying motor fibers to the extraocular muscles, are tested by having the patient follow the examiner's finger while making an X. Both eyes should move smoothly and similarly as they follow the finger. The pupils should be of equal size and rounded and should react to light by constricting. The accommodation reflex is tested by having the patient change focus from a distant to a near object. The pupils should constrict as the object (examiner's finger) approaches the patient's face. Both pupils should constrict not only to direct light but also to light directed in the other eye (consensual light reflex).

Trigeminal Nerve (V). The fifth cranial nerve is both sensory (from the face, scalp, nose, and mouth) and motor (to the muscles of mastication). Sensory input is tested by lightly stroking the face with a cotton tip bilaterally in three regions: forehead, cheek, and lower jaw. This provides a sense of the function of the ophthalmic, maxillary, and mandibular branches of the trigeminal nerve. The patient should describe similar sensations on each side. The trigeminal nerve also contains sensory fibers from the cornea. The corneal reflexes can be tested by observing the patient's blink response to light touch on the cornea with a sterile cotton pledget or tissue. Gross motor input is tested by having the patient clench while the examiner palpates both the masseter and the temporalis muscles. The muscles should contract equally and bilaterally.

Facial Nerve (VII). The seventh cranial nerve also is sensory and motor. The sensory component supplies taste sensations from the anterior portion of the tongue. Sensory function can be tested by asking the patient to distinguish between sugar and salt using just the tip of the tongue. The motor component, which innervates the muscles of facial expression, is tested by asking the patient to raise both eyebrows, smile, and show the lower teeth. During these movements, any bilateral differences are recorded.

Acoustic Nerve (VIII). Also called the *vestibulocochlear nerve,* the eighth cranial nerve supplies the senses of balance and hearing. The patient should be questioned regarding any recent changes in upright posture or in hearing, especially if associated with the problem that initiated the office visit. If there is a question regarding balance, the patient should walk heel to toe along a straight line. Gross hearing can be evaluated by rubbing a strand of hair between the first finger and thumb near the patient's ear and noting any difference between right and left sensitivities.

Glossopharyngeal and Vagus Nerves (IX, X). The ninth and tenth cranial nerves are tested together because they both supply fibers to the back of the throat. The patient is asked to say "ah," and the soft palate is observed for symmetric elevations. Touching

each side of the pharynx with a dental mirror or similar dull instrument tests the gag reflex.

Accessory Nerve (XI). The spinal accessory nerve supplies fibers to the trapezius and sternocleidomastoid muscles. Asking the patient to shrug the shoulders against resistance tests the motor function of the trapezius. The sternocleidomastoid is tested by having the patient look first to the right and then to the left against resistance. Note any differences in muscle strength.

Hypoglossal Nerve (XII). The twelfth cranial nerve supplies motor fibers to the tongue. The patient protrudes the tongue, and the examiner notes any uncontrolled or consistent lateral deviation. The strength of the tongue also can be evaluated by having the patient push laterally against a tongue blade.

Autonomic Nerve Examination. Evaluating the pupillary accommodation to light as part of the third cranial nerve examination also tests the parasympathetic functioning of the oculomotor nerve. The autonomic function of the facial and glossopharyngeal nerves is evaluated by the presence of lacrimation and salivation. The parasympathetic functioning of the vagus nerve can be evaluated by the carotid sinus reflex, which produces a reduction in heart rate in response to pressure on the internal carotid artery at the level of the cricoid cartilage. A deficit in cranial sympathetic functioning is recognized by the presence of *Horner's syndrome*, which presents with narrowing of the palpebral fissure, ptosis of the upper lid, elevation of the lower lid, constriction of the pupil, and facial anhydrosis.

Ear Evaluation

The ear is a common source of pain that needs to be evaluated to differentiate the pain requiring consultation with an otolaryngologist from the pain referred from other sites in the craniofacial region. The proximity of the ear to the temporomandibular joint and muscles of mastication, as well as to their common trigeminal innervation, frequently results in pain referral to the ear from these sites. A clinician who treats orofacial pain should become proficient at examining the ear for gross pathology. Hearing should be checked as described for the eighth cranial nerve examination. Infection of the external auditory meatus (otitis externa) can be identified by simply pushing inward on the tragus. If this causes pain, the patient may have an external ear infection and should be immediately referred to an otolaryngologist. An otoscope is necessary to visualize the tympanic membrane for inflammation, perforations, and fluid.

The practitioner's role is to identify the source of pain. When ear disease is suspected, the patient should be referred to an otolaryngologist for a more thorough evaluation and appropriate treatment. Normal findings from an otologic examination indicate further evaluation to find the true source of pain or dysfunction.

Somatosensory and Reflex Examination

Somatosensory Function. Applying tactile, thermal, and electric stimuli to examination areas permits assessment of somatosensory function. A brush is dragged gently from the intact area into the affected area to determine the border between these two areas. Moving stimuli may elicit abnormal sensations around the region a damaged nerve covers, such as allodynia and dysesthesia. A von Frey filament set consists of nylon filaments with varying diameters that produce increasing pressure when applied to the skin. Applying the fibers in ascending and descending movements reveals loss of sensation, either anesthesia or hypoesthesia. Thermal stimuli can be applied by hot or cold water or specific thermal-testing instruments. Hot water over 45° C usually produces pain sensation (a noxious stimulus). Low-frequency pulses (1 Hz) are adequate to assess the detective threshold of large-diameter (α-β) fibers, whereas short trains of high-frequency stimulation (100 Hz, 1 ms) are effective to observe pain at the detection threshold (allodynia).

The results of somatosensory testing are then used to classify deficits in normal sensation using the following terms, as defined by the IASP:

- *Anesthesia.* Complete loss of sensation. Patients cannot detect any stimuli.
- *Hypoesthesia.* Partial loss of sensation. Thresholds for nonnoxious stimuli are elevated in the affected area.
- *Hyperalgesia.* Increased sensitivity to noxious stimuli. Enhanced painful sensation to a noxious heat stimulus (over 45° C) is called *heat hyperalgesia* or *thermal hyperalgesia*. Patients with *mechanical hyperalgesia* respond to a mechanical

noxious stimulus, such as a pinprick, more strongly than normal subjects.
- *Allodynia.* Lowered pain thresholds to stimuli. *Heat (thermal) allodynia* shows an excessive response to a nonnoxious thermal stimulus under 43° C. *Mechanical allodynia* is defined as a painful sensation to a nonnoxious mechanical stimulus, such as a brush application.
- *Dysesthesia.* An unpleasant abnormal sensation, whether evoked or spontaneous. Special cases of dysesthesia include hyperalgesia and allodynia.
- *Paresthesia.* An abnormal sensation, whether spontaneous or evoked. This sensation is not described as unpleasant.

Superficial Reflexes. The *corneal reflex* is tested by closure of the eyelids in response to irritation of the cornea by touching with a sterile cotton applicator. It involves afferent impulses transmitted by the trigeminal nerve and efferent motor impulses via the facial nerve. The *palatal reflex* is involuntary swallowing in response to stimulation of the soft palate. It involves afferent impulses transmitted by the trigeminal and glossopharyngeal nerves and efferent motor impulses via the glossopharyngeal and vagus nerves. The *pharyngeal reflex*, or *gag reflex*, is contraction of the constrictor muscle of the pharynx, which is elicited by touching the posterior wall of the pharynx. It involves afferent impulses transmitted by the glossopharyngeal nerve and efferent motor impulses via the glossopharyngeal and vagus nerves.

Summary. Any abnormalities found during the cranial nerve examination should be viewed as important and should be assessed for their relationship to the pain condition. The purpose of this evaluation is to determine with certainty whether referral to a neurologist is essential and justified. When one or more of the following conditions are observed, immediate neurologic consultation is indicated:

- Areas of facial hypoesthesia
- Loss of normal corneal reflex
- Persistent muscular weakness
- Simultaneous involvement of otherwise unrelated nerve trunks

Eye Evaluation

The patient is questioned about vision and any recent changes, especially if associated with the reason for seeking treatment. As in the cranial nerve examination, simple techniques are sufficient for testing gross vision. With the left eye covered, the patient is asked to read a few sentences from a paper. The other eye is similarly examined. Any diplopia or blurriness of vision is noted, as well as whether this relates to the pain problem. Pain felt in or around the eyes is noted, as well as whether this affects reading. Reddening of the conjunctivae should be recorded, along with any tearing or swelling of the eyelids.

Differential Diagnosis of Orofacial Pain Disorders

Neuralgias

Neuralgia was originally used to describe a symptom, not a disorder. Characteristics common to all neuralgias are sudden, severe, brief, stabbing, recurrent pain (paroxysmal) in the distribution of the affected nerve.

Idiopathic Trigeminal Neuralgia (Tic Douloureux).

According to the IASP definition, trigeminal neuralgia is a sudden, usually unilateral, severe, brief, stabbing, recurrent pain felt in the distribution of one or more branches of the fifth cranial nerve.

Trigeminal nerve compression may be the primary cause of trigeminal neuralgia.[11] Vascular loops compressing or contracting the trigeminal nerve at the root entry zone are observed in more than 80% of these patients. The main vessel responsible is the superior cerebellar artery and in some patients the inferior cerebellar artery. With age, arteriosclerosis can make small vessels shift. Vascular anomaly, aneurysm, and bone architecture can also result in nerve compression.[26] Multiple sclerosis may also contribute to trigeminal neuralgia through segmental demyelination and microneuroma formation.

The paroxysmal pain attacks occur in one or more divisions of the trigeminal nerve, usually unilaterally.[44] Bilateral trigeminal neuralgia is rare. Pain is precipitated by light stimuli, such as talking, eating, shaving, washing the face, brushing the teeth, combing the hair, and putting on makeup. The incidence in females is almost twofold greater than with males. The age distribution of the first attack usually occurs in the 40s, with attacks peaking in the 50s. Right branches are affected more frequently

than left branches. Pain typically occurs according to the distribution of the second and the third branches, with the first branch rarely involved. Pain is always transient, lasting seconds (occasionally up to a few minutes). The intensity of pain is excruciating, and the characteristic of pain is expressed as lancinating, shooting, electrical, shocklike, and stabbing. Between episodes, sensations are essentially normal or slightly desensitized. No pain and numbness are observed in the affected area between ectopic paroxysmal pain periods. A short refractory period follows each of the pain attacks. An episode of pain attacks can last months, and a pain relief period can follow. Pain, however, usually rekindles months or years later.

Trigeminal neuralgia is diagnosed when pain satisfies the features of the IASP definition and can be excluded from symptomatic trigeminal neuralgia. Diagnosis of typical trigeminal neuralgia is, in a way, the denial of symptomatic trigeminal neuralgia and other conditions. Therefore pain is never accompanied by marked sensory abnormality or dysfunction of the cranial nerves. Trigeminal neuralgia may relate to an obvious cause, such as a lesion in cerebellopontine angle. In other patients, the etiology remains obscure. Recent magnetic resonance imaging (MRI) studies reveal improved lesion detection and may therefore assist in identifying possible tumors or multiple sclerosis.[56] Specific areas or points called *trigger zones* can initiate a pain attack with a light tactile stimulus. The trigger zone is often located in the lips and gingival tissues and is different from the allodynic area in neuropathy. Trigeminal neuralgia is not associated with anesthetic or marked hypoesthetic areas, whereas neuropathies often have both hypoesthetic and allodynic areas.

Trigeminal neuralgia responds well to certain anticonvulsant medications, such as carbamazepine (Tegretol), clonazepam (Klonopin), and baclofen (Lioresal), but not barbiturates. If an adequate dose of carbamazepine is administered without side effects (see Chapter 23), the neuralgic pain often can be completely relieved. If pain attacks are relieved by this medication and the patient has no neurologic abnormalities, the diagnosis is usually trigeminal neuralgia. Local anesthetic injected into the trigger zone often relieves the paroxysmal episodes. As this condition advances, however, patients gradually fail to respond to this pharmacologic management because of the change in the site of compression or the intensity of root compression.[42,54]

Glossopharyngeal Neuralgia. Glossopharyngeal neuralgia is a sudden, severe, brief, stabbing, recurrent pain in the distribution of the glossopharyngeal nerve. It occurs with very low frequency (0.7/100,000 for both genders), with peak of onset between ages 40 and 60, usually after 50. Left-sided involvement predominates in females. Bilateral involvement occurs in one fourth of the patients.[7]

Microvascular compression is a primary cause of glossopharyngeal neuralgia. The posterior inferior cerebellar artery is the most common vessel responsible. However, vascular decompression does not reveal the same success as with trigeminal neuralgia, indicating the possibility of other etiologies.[46] Invasion or compression by parapharyngeal and posterior fossa tumors, arteriovenous malformation, and choroid plexus are other etiologies of glossopharyngeal neuralgia.

Sudden, severe, brief pain can be elicited several times a day. The pain attacks are triggered by swallowing, yawning, light mechanical stimuli, and chemical stimuli. The trigger zone is usually located in the unilateral pharyngeal region, especially the tonsillar area. The excruciating, sharp, stabbing pain lasts seconds to minutes. The pain often radiates to the deep ear, neck, and angle of jaw. The pain attacks are rarely followed by syncope and clonicity.

The diagnosis of glossopharyngeal neuralgia is largely based on the clinical presentation. A magnetic resonance imaging (MRI) study may be useful, not only for vascular looping and compression, but also for obscure tumors. Infection and an elongated styloid process should be considered in the differential diagnosis. Carbamazepine and local anesthetic blocks are often helpful in the differential diagnosis.

Superior Laryngeal Neuralgia. Neuralgia of the superior laryngeal nerve is felt as sudden, brief, recurrent lancinating pain in the throat and laryngeal area. This pain can also be felt in the deep ear and angle of the jaw and is provoked by yawning, coughing, swallowing, and gargling. In some patients, symptoms resembling stimulation of the vagus nerve, such as salivation or hiccups, may be observed. Superior laryngeal neuralgia is more likely attributable to local lesions than intracranial lesions.

Differential diagnosis from glossopharyngeal neuralgia is often difficult because of similarity in clinical presentation. The trigger zone is often located in the larynx. Only a local anesthetic block of the superior laryngeal nerve is useful for the differ-

ential diagnosis. Tumors and infections should be investigated.

Neuralgia of Nervus Intermedius (Geniculate Neuralgia). Nervus intermedius is characterized by sudden, brief, severe pain felt directly in the ear. The pain may also present with a gradual onset and have a dull, persistent nature, with occasional sharp, stabbing pain. The trigger zone may be observed in the auditory canal. The etiology of nervus intermedius is unknown. Vascular compression is not observed on exploration for nervus intermedius neuralgia.

Ramsay Hunt syndrome has a similar presentation and should be differentially diagnosed (see later discussion). Vestibular and cochlear function should be assessed and auricular vesicles explored.

Tolosa-Hunt Syndrome. Tolosa-Hunt syndrome is characterized by severe unilateral stabbing pain around the orbit with ophthalmoplegia. Pain intensity may fluctuate and, unlike other neuralgias, may present with some constancy. Paresis of the eye muscles may be associated with this condition during early onset but usually subsides gradually within a few weeks to several months.[14]

The etiology of Tolosa-Hunt syndrome is unknown. A review of the literature suggests an unspecific inflammatory granulation tissue around the intracavernous portion of the carotid artery and on the dura mater near the cavernous sinus. Changes in orbital venography indicate venous vasculitis.

A history of relapsing and remitting painful ophthalmoplegia suggests the diagnosis of Tolosa-Hunt syndrome. Pain is experienced either as pressure behind the eye or as boring pain in the orbital region. The pain may fluctuate in intensity and increase when the eyes are strained. Pain may also increase when cold wind is blown against the face and with a change in weather. Tolosa-Hunt syndrome is often accompanied by a feeling of swelling in the affected region but not by nausea or vomiting. Steroids can dramatically ameliorate the symptoms, but conventional headache drugs provide little relief. Tenderness is observed when pressure is applied to the ipsilateral supraorbital foramen. Carotid arteriography may show stationary waves of this artery and narrowing of the intracavernous part of the internal carotid artery. Orbital venography may demonstrate occlusion of the supraorbital vein and the obstruction of the cavernous sinus. The pain is often relieved with steroid therapy within 48 to 72 hours.

Tolosa-Hunt syndrome should be differentiated from other causes of painful ophthalmoplegia, including tumors, aneurysms, collagen disease, specific infections, diabetes mellitus, paranasal mucocele, carotid cavernous fistula, and benign granulomas of unknown etiology.

Raeder's Syndrome. Raeder's syndrome is characterized by severe stabbing paroxysms in the first division of trigeminal nerve, with paralysis of the sympathetic nervous system (Horner's syndrome). Sympatholysis is usually not accompanied by sudomotor dysfunction. The most common clinical presentation is a middle-aged male who reports a severe, throbbing, supraorbital headache accompanied by ptosis and miosis. The headache is intermittently present for several weeks or months.[13]

Raeder's syndrome has two clinical presentations. The first type is related to a serious lesion in the middle cranial fossa, such as a neoplasm. The second type is related to benign conditions, such as unilateral vascular headache syndromes. Any lesion affecting the postganglionic oculosympathetic fibers distal to the bifurcation of the common carotid artery may cause Raeder's syndrome. Parasellar neoplasms often involve multiple cranial nerves; lesions of the internal carotid artery may elicit unilateral vascular headache syndromes.[21]

Raeder's syndrome can be distinguished from Horner's syndrome by observing facial sweating. The combination of MRI and magnetic resonance (MR) angiography is a reliable noninvasive tool to investigate the differential diagnosis of pericarotid syndrome and paratrigeminal lesions.

Neuropathic and Deafferentation Pain

Pain originating in a primary lesion or due to dysfunction of the nervous system is called *neuropathic pain*. Pain caused by loss of sensory input into the central nervous system (CNS) is called *deafferentation pain*. Deafferentation pain is observed in a completely denervated area. Neuroma formation and sprouting typically occur at sites of nerve transection or damage. These sites are extremely sensitive and result in hyperalgesia, allodynia, and dysesthesia. Neuroma formation and sprouting can cause spontaneous and ectopic discharges that can lead to a barrage of ascending impulses from injured primary afferent C fibers and surrounding fibers. This ongoing nociceptive input results in an increased state of excitability of the N-methyl-D-aspartate (NMDA) receptors for excitatory amino acids, with subsequent enhancement of neuronal discharge. Increased excitability of the NMDA receptors results in neurons becoming sensitive not only for nociceptive but also nonnociceptive stimuli. When this occurs, even nonnoxious stimuli can be processed as noxious by the CNS, a condition characterized as *central sensitization*. This pathology can be recognized when a peripheral conduction nerve block relieves pain from the injured nerve and from nerves innervating the surrounding tissues. In addition, sympathetic efferent and afferent nerve fibers play an important role in some neuropathic pain conditions (see Sympathetically Maintained Pain).

Neuritis Secondary to Herpes Zoster Infection. Acute herpetic neuralgia is characterized by severe constant pain with swelling, redness, and vesicles presenting in one or more branches of the trigeminal nerve. The patient may have paroxysmal stabbing pain in addition to the constant pain. *Acute herpetic neuralgia* is defined as pain that occurs during the first 30 days after rash onset.

Herpes zoster is caused by a recurrent infection of a nerve by the varicella-zoster virus (VZV). VZV remains latent in certain nerve ganglions after chickenpox has resolved. If the latent virus remains in the trigeminal and geniculate ganglion and the immune activity of the host declines, the infection can involve the trigeminal nerve branches and facial nerve branches, respectively.[2] Although most patients only recognize the dermal condition because the skin symptoms are the most prominent, the virus also affects nerves, vessels, bones, and other structures.[53] In postmortem studies, marked loss of myelin in peripheral nerves and sensory roots is found in all herpes zoster patients.

Trigeminal herpes zoster pain usually precedes dermal symptoms by a few days to a week, with sensory abnormality in moderate and severe cases.[15] Eruptions spontaneously heal within 3 weeks in patients with mild and moderate disease, possibly with pigmentation, but scars may remain in severe cases. The trigeminal nerve is involved in about 30% of all herpes zoster patients. The first division of trigeminal nerve is affected most frequently in all dermatomal divisions. Sixty percent of patients with trigeminal herpes zoster have vesicular eruptions in the first division. The second division follows in frequency, with the third division least affected.

Induration of lymph nodes and high fever is often observed. One of the most common complications in herpes zoster ophthalmicus is paropsis (20.5%), primarily from corneal opacity. In some patients with severe disease, corneal ulcer results in loss of vision in the affected eye, thus the importance of immediate referral to an ophthalmologist for evaluation if this diagnosis is a possibility. Ophthalmoplegia, meningoencephalitis, and hemiplegia are also rarely observed. Alveolar bone can be destroyed, and in severe cases, teeth can be lost in the second and third divisions.

Diagnosis can be revealed by laboratory examinations. Elevated antibody level of VZV should be observed for the diagnosis of trigeminal herpes zoster and Ramsay Hunt syndrome. The cerebrospinal fluid (CSF) titer of VZV elevates within 3 weeks from the onset. The antibody must be detected at least twice to confirm the diagnosis, immediately after the onset of herpes zoster and 2 to 3 weeks later. CSF titer should be increased at least eightfold. Some studies report that enzyme-linked assays are more useful to observe the changes of antibody for VZV for early detection of infection. Anti-VZV-IgM and anti-VZV-IgG antibodies increase within several days. Some patients with symptoms similar to trigeminal herpes zoster and Ramsay Hunt syndrome without vesicles can be infected by VZV, and proper diagnosis requires timely laboratory examinations.

Ramsay Hunt Syndrome. Ramsay Hunt syndrome is observed in 2% to 3% of patients with cranial herpes zoster and is characterized by severe constant pain felt in or around the ear and auricular vesicles. Ipsilateral peripheral facial palsy and vestibulocochlear symptoms may also be present. Typical patients with Ramsay Hunt syndrome will show the complete triad: vesicles in the auricle, ipsilateral peripheral facial palsy, and vestibulocochlear symptoms. Redness, swelling, and vesicles usually follow pain at the auricle, external auditory canal, postauricular region, occiput, or pharynx. Some patients have symptoms of trigeminal herpes zoster and Ramsay Hunt syndrome without eruptions. These conditions are called *zoster sine herpete.* Patients are often misdiagnosed.

Postherpetic Neuralgia. Postherpetic neuralgia (PHN) is characterized by burning, tearing pain with hyperalgesia, allodynia, and dysesthesia that lasts much longer than the clinical appearance of the vesi-cles associated with herpes zoster. The hyperalgesia and allodynia are more prominent outside the anesthetic skin area than inside. The diagnosis of PHN is assisted by a history of eruptions in the affected area and the presence of somatosensory abnormalities. Serum VZV antibody level is not helpful for diagnosis in chronic cases.

PHN is characterized by chronic pain with somatosensory abnormalities that persist in the affected trigeminal divisions after eruptions of acute trigeminal herpes zoster have healed. PHN is defined as pain that persists more than 4 months after the onset of rash. Approximately 12% of the patients with trigeminal herpes zoster complain of persistent pain, leading to the diagnosis of PHN. Risk factors become more problematic when the following conditions become more severe: (1) acute pain, (2) cutaneous manifestations, (3) sensory dysfunction in the affected dermatome, (4) humoral and cell-mediated immune responses, (5) painful prodrome, and (6) fever, during acute herpes zoster. The patient's age may also be a risk factor, with older patients at greater risk than younger patients.

Pathology of PHN centers on denervation of the affected nerve. Skin in severely denervated areas generally shows anesthesia. Atrophy of the dorsal horn and pathologic changes in sensory ganglion are found on the affected side, but not on the unaffected side. Central sensitization and neuroplasticity are believed to be important mechanisms contributing to PHN.

Neuritis Secondary to Trauma. Paroxysmal pain in the affected trigeminal divisions may follow trauma, surgery, and peripheral lesions. Persistent burning, throbbing, or dull pain may also be observed. Peripheral neuropathy (secondary trigeminal neuralgia) occurs with relative frequency after orthognathic surgery and fractures. Deafferentation and partial injury of peripheral nerves result in degeneration and regeneration.

Neuritis is commonly characterized as a burning pain. Hypoesthesia and dysesthesia are also commonly observed in the affected nerve division as are allodynia and hyperalgesia.

Complex Regional Pain Syndromes

A complex regional pain syndrome (CRPS) follows injury and has a predominance of abnormal findings exceeding the expected clinical course of the inciting event in both magnitude and duration and often resulting in significant impairment of motor function. CRPS consists of two types: type I, or reflex sympathetic dystrophy (RSD), and type II, or causalgia.[50] These two conditions are classified according to the presence and absence of direct peripheral nerve injury. RSD and causalgia were initially recognized to be observed only in extremities and not in the orofacial region. However, currently CRPS is not defined as being limited to the extremities.[24]

Type I: Reflex Sympathetic Dystrophy. RSD is a painful syndrome that develops after tissue damage. It is not limited to the distribution of a single peripheral nerve. Trauma is usually mild and not associated with significant nerve injury. This syndrome is associated at some point with edema, changes in skin blood flow, abnormal sudomotor activity, and sometimes atrophy of muscles and bones in the region of the pain.

RSD is clinically characterized by persistent burning pain with allodynia, hyperalgesia, and dysesthesia and usually occurs within 1 month after trauma. The pain is aggravated by jaw movement or skin/membrane stimulation. Pain intensity varies over time. Sympathetically maintained pain may be observed concomitantly (see later discussion). Skin temperature in the affected area usually elevates in an early stage, then declines. Abnormal sudomotor activity may exist, but the symptom does not necessarily match the vasomotor activity. Bone scans may indicate increased periarticular uptake in the affected area.

The IASP has proposed the following diagnostic criteria for CRPS type I:

1. Presence of an initiating noxious event or cause of immobilization
2. Continuing pain, allodynia, or hyperalgesia with pain disproportionate to the inciting event
3. Evidence at some time of edema, changes in skin blood flow, or abnormal sudomotor activity in the region of the pain
4. The diagnosis is excluded by the existence of conditions that would otherwise account for the degree of pain and dysfunction.

RSD in the head is described as lacking skin symptoms, which complicates the diagnosis. RSD occurs after mild tissue damage not necessarily directed to a nerve.

Type II: Causalgia. Causalgia is a painful syndrome that develops after partial injury of a nerve or one of its major branches. Spontaneous and evoked pains and skin symptoms similar to type I are present. Causalgia is characterized by continuous burning, throbbing, or aching pain. It is also often observed with allodynia, hyperalgesia, and dysesthesia in the affected area. Symptoms are not restricted to the distribution of the damaged nerve or branch. Tactile and thermal stimuli and movement of the affected area exacerbate the pain. Edema and hyperhydrosis or hypohydrosis are observed. Immobilization of the affected area may induce muscle atrophy and contracture.

The following criteria must be satisfied for the diagnosis of CRPS type II:

1. The presence of continuing pain, allodynia, or hyperalgesia after a nerve injury, not necessarily limited to the distribution of the damaged nerve
2. Evidence at some time of edema, changes in skin blood flow, or abnormal sudomotor activity in the region of the pain
3. The diagnosis is excluded by the existence of conditions that would otherwise account for the degree of pain and dysfunction.

Causalgia is diagnosed only when patients show changes in peripheral tissues, although symptoms resemble those in neuropathic pain conditions.

Sympathetically Maintained Pain

Sympathetically maintained pain (SMP) is described as a pain condition that is maintained, but not necessarily initiated, by sympathetic activity or regional noradrenergic action. Other painful disorders also have a sympathetic component. If pain depends strongly on sympathetic activity or noradrenergic action and sympatholysis relieves 70% of pain, by definition the pain has a 70% SMP component. The residual component of 30% pain is called *sympathetically independent pain* (SIP). This sympathetic component differs from patient to patient and at different times in a given patient. Continuous burning or aching pain is observed in the affected area in both states. In SMP, elevated vasomotor and sudomotor activities may be present but are not necessary for the diagnosis. The sympathetic component can change over time from being maintained as independent of sympathetic input, but the reverse does not occur.

SMP is diagnosed by sympathetic ganglion blocks and pharmacologic challenge with selective blockers. A stellate ganglion block and intravenous phentolamine relieves SMP. Pain that is not improved by these measures is diagnosed as sympathetically independent. Neuropathic pain and SMP also can be relieved by somatosensory nerve blocks. This evidence may confuse practitioners, especially when pain is located in the neck, because the local anesthetic used for a stellate ganglion block can spread to the cervical nerve roots. However, SMP of the head and face origin can be differentially diagnosed by use of a stellate ganglion block, as well as a cervical epidural block, which does not affect the trigeminal nerve.[9]

Temporomandibular Disorders

Temporomandibular disorders (TMD) is a collective term that describes a number of clinical complaints involving the muscles of mastication, temporomandibular joints (TMJ), and associated orofacial structures.[38] Previous terms include Costen syndrome, TMJ dysfunction, and craniomandibular disorders.[10] TMD is a major cause of nondental pain in the orofacial region and is considered a subclassification of musculoskeletal disorders. In many TMD patients the most common complaint is not the TMJ but rather the muscles of mastication.[12] Therefore the terms "TMJ dysfunction" and "TMJ disorder" are inappropriate for many of these complaints. For this reason, the American Dental Association adopted the more general term, *temporomandibular disorders.*[20]

Signs and symptoms associated with TMD are a common source of pain complaints in the head and orofacial structures.[29] These complaints can be associated with general joint problems and somatization.[30] The primary signs and symptoms associated with TMD originate from the masticatory structures and are associated with jaw function.[31] Pain during opening of the mouth or when chewing is common. Some individuals will even report difficulty speaking or singing. Patients often report pain in the preauricular areas, face, and temples. TMJ sounds are frequently described as clicking, popping, grating, or crepitus and can produce locking of the jaw during opening or closing.[16] Patients frequently report painful jaw muscles and occasionally a sudden change in their bite coincident with the onset of the painful condition.

The pain associated with most TMD is increased with jaw function. Since this is a condition of the musculoskeletal structures, function of these structures generally increases the pain.[28] When a patient's pain complaint is not influenced by jaw function, other sources of orofacial pain should be suspected.

TMD can be subdivided into two broad categories related to the primary source of pain and dysfunction: intracapsular (TMJ) disorders and masticatory muscle disorders.[18]

Temporomandibular Joint (Intracapsular) Disorders. The signs associated with functional disorders of TMJ are probably the most common findings on examination of a patient for masticatory dysfunction. Many of these signs do not produce painful symptoms, and therefore the patient may not seek treatment. When present, however, they generally fall into three broad categories: derangements of the condyle-disc complex, structural incompatibility of the articular surfaces, and inflammatory joint disorders. The first two categories have been collectively referred to as *disc-interference disorders.* Disc-interference disorder first described a category of functional disorders arising from problems with the condyle-disc complex. These conditions (1) are caused by a derangement or alteration of the disc's attachment to the condyle; (2) result from an incompatibility between the articular surfaces of the condyle, disc, and fossa; or (3) are present in anatomically normal structures extended beyond their physiologic range of movement. With time, inflammatory disorders may arise from a localized response of the TMJ tissues because of chronic or progressive degenerative changes.

The two major symptoms of functional TMJ problems are pain and dysfunction. Joint pain can arise from healthy joint structures that are mechanically overused during function or from structures that have become inflamed. Pain originating from healthy structures is felt as sharp, sudden, and intense pain that is closely associated with joint movement. When the joint is rested, the pain resolves quickly. The patient often reports the pain as being localized to the preauricular area. If the joint structures have become inflamed, the pain is reported as constant, even at rest, but accentuated by joint movement.

Dysfunction is common with functional TMJ disorders. Usually it presents as a disruption of the normal condyle-disc movement, with the production of joint sounds. The joint sounds may be a single event of short duration known as a *click.* If this is loud, it may be referred to as a *pop. Crepitation* is a long, rough, gravel-like sound described as grating and complicated. Dysfunction of TMJ may also present as catching sensations when the patient opens the mouth. Occasionally the jaw may lock. Dysfunction of TMJ is always directly related to jaw movement.

A single click during opening of the mouth is often associated with an anterior displaced disc, which is returned to a more normal position during the opening movement; this condition is known as *disc displacement with reduction*. Often, when the patient closes the mouth, a second click is felt, representing the disc's redisplacement to the anterior displaced position. For some patients the displacement of the disc progresses anteriorly, and the disc may not return to its normal relationship with the condyle during opening; this condition is known as *disc displacement without reduction*. Often the patient cannot fully open the mouth because the disc is blocking the translation of the condyle. For this reason, the condition is often referred to as a *closed lock*.

Masticatory Muscle Disorders. Functional disorders of masticatory muscles are probably the most common TMD complaint of patients seeking treatment in the dental office.[45] With regard to pain, these conditions are second only to odontalgia (i.e., tooth or periodontal pain) in terms of frequency. They are generally grouped in a large category known as masticatory muscle disorders.

The two major symptoms of masticatory muscle disorders are muscle pain and muscle dysfunction. *Muscle pain* felt in muscle tissue is termed *myalgia* and can range from slight tenderness to extreme discomfort. Myalgia usually arises from increased levels of muscular use.[34] The symptoms are often associated with a feeling of muscle fatigue and tightness. Patients often describe the location of the pain as broad, diffuse, and often bilateral. This complaint differs from the specific location reported in intracapsular disorders. Although its exact origin is unknown, some suggest that this muscle pain is related to vasoconstriction of the relevant nutrient arteries and the accumulation of metabolic waste products in the muscle tissues.[27] Within the ischemic area of the muscle, certain algogenic substances (e.g., bradykinins, prostaglandins) are released, causing muscle pain.[33,35] Muscle pain, however, is more complex than simple overuse and fatigue. In fact, muscle pain associated with TMD does not seem to be strongly correlated with increased activity (e.g., spasm). It is now appreciated that muscle pain can be greatly influenced by central mechanisms (see Chapter 2).

The severity of muscle pain is directly related to the functional activity of the muscle involved. If a patient does not report an increase in pain associated with jaw function, the disorder is not likely related to a masticatory muscle problem, and other diagnoses should be considered.

Muscle dysfunction is often associated with masticatory muscle disorders, usually seen as a decrease in the range of mandibular movement. When muscle tissues have been compromised by overuse, any contraction or stretching increases the pain.[41] Therefore to maintain comfort, the patient restricts movement within a range that does not increase pain levels. Clinically this is seen as an inability to open the mouth widely. The restriction may be at any degree of opening, depending on where discomfort is felt. In some myalgic disorders, the patient can slowly open wider, but the pain is still present and may even become worse.

Acute malocclusion refers to any sudden change in the occlusal position that has been created by a disorder. An acute malocclusion may result from a sudden change in the resting length of a muscle that controls jaw position. The patient describes a change in the occlusal contact of the teeth. The mandibular position and resultant alteration in occlusal relationships depend on the muscles involved. For example, with slight functional shortening of the inferior lateral pterygoid, disocclusion of the posterior teeth on the ipsilateral side will occur, with premature contact of the anterior teeth (especially the canines) on the contralateral side. With functional shortening of the elevator muscles (clinically a less detectable acute malocclusion), the patient will generally complain of an inability to occlude normally. Since an acute malocclusion is the *result* of the muscle disorder, not the cause, treatment should never be directed toward correcting the malocclusion.[49] Rather, treatment should be aimed at eliminating the muscle disorder.[47] When this condition is reduced, the occlusal condition will return to normal.

Carotidynia. Carotidynia is characterized by continuous aching or throbbing pain in the unilateral head, usually starting in the ipsilateral anterior neck. The etiology of carotidynia is unknown. Some cases have been associated with migraine, aneurysm, and long intraluminal clots with incomplete vessel obstruction of the internal carotid artery.[8]

Tenderness of the carotid artery, especially around the bifurcation, is the most common feature of carotidynia. Palpation may aggravate head and neck pain. In patients with headache, the pain complaint may resemble migraine. Autonomic symptoms are not observed, although symptoms associated with migraine, such as photophobia and nausea, may be present. Pain is precipitated by swallowing, coughing, and rotating or extending the neck.

Only a careful review of the history and physical examination can lead to the diagnosis of carotidynia. Laboratory studies may help exclude other causes. Migraine, giant cell arteritis, and glossopharyngeal neuralgia should be differentiated.

Sinusitis. Sinus pain may be confused with TMD associated with TMJ and masticatory musculature. Sinusitis is characterized by continuous aching or throbbing pain in the infraorbital, temporal, or frontal regions; the ear; or the upper molars and premolars; this results from inflammation of the sinuses. Pain is located unilaterally in the early stages but may extend bilaterally to involve both sinuses. Pain from inflammation is exacerbated when the mucosa is swollen and ostia of the sinuses are occluded.

Acute inflammation of sinuses may cause throbbing or wrenching headache, whereas chronic sinusitis usually causes dull or tender pain. The patient may have oppressive pain in the infraorbital region. Purulent discharge to the pharynx is a common finding. Rapid change of atmospheric pressure induced by diving and airplane travel usually aggravates the pain.

Sinusitis is readily diagnosed by purulent discharge from the sinus ostia and radiographic opacity in ipsilateral and bilateral sinuses. Laboratory examination may show changes associated with inflammation.

Oral Cavity Pain

Causes of pain in the oral cavity include inflammation of the dental pulp or periodontal tissue and trauma of hard and soft tissues. This section describes uncommon causes that are difficult to diagnose in usual dental practice.[39]

Atypical Facial Pains. Atypical facial pain in the oral cavity manifests as pain in the tongue, teeth, periodontal tissue, or in the whole mouth and has an uncertain etiology. *Glossodynia, atypical odontalgia,* and *burning mouth syndrome* are diagnosed only when more definitive diagnoses from all other possible causes have been ruled out. These syndromes occur more frequently in females over age 40.

Patients complain of a continuous, sore, throbbing or burning pain of moderate intensity in the tongue, teeth, or periodontal tissue or affecting the whole mouth. The pain may fluctuate, but precipitating factors are rarely found. Neither pathology nor a distinct

somatosensory abnormality can be observed at the location the patient complains of pain. Atypical facial pain most often occurs in the molar and premolar regions. Thermal and mechanical (oppression and percussion) tests for the teeth in the affected area are equivocal. These syndromes are considered to have a psychosomatic aspect and a relationship with menopause, although clinical investigation revealed no particular findings to personality evaluation in patients with atypical odontalgia.

The diagnoses of glossodynia, atypical odontalgia, and burning mouth syndrome should be given only after all other possible causes have been ruled out; misdiagnosis often involves neuropathic pain. History and somatosensory findings should be evaluated carefully.[40]

Cracked Tooth Syndrome. Pain may result from an *incomplete fracture* (cracked tooth) and a *complete fracture* (split tooth). A cracked tooth induces dental pulp sensitization and pulpitis, and deep pockets can give rise to severe periodontal pain. Cracked tooth syndrome is mostly seen in the molar and the premolar teeth, often associated with an intracoronal restoration; with no protection of the cusps from occlusal loading, a complete or partial fracture results. Vertical root fractures most frequently occur in endodontically treated posterior teeth in patients 45 to 60 years of age.[52] An incomplete fracture involving the dentinal layer of a vital posterior tooth may cause pain.[1] Caries, inappropriate cavity design, overloading of the tooth, atypical root canal anatomy, and external root resorption of the tooth may predispose the patient to cracked tooth syndrome.

Location of the dentinal crack is often difficult and must be guided by a precise history, thermal pulp testing, and inspection of the dentinal walls within the suspect tooth. The number, extent, and direction of the fracture lines may be ascertained readily using transillumination and magnification, which allow the clinician to distinguish between oblique and vertical cracks. Intraalveolar root fractures can be detected only by radiographs; detection can be increased by films taken from more than one angle. Radiolucent areas occur seven times more often in the region of the root fracture than in the periapical region.

Differential Diagnosis of Headache

Headache symptoms may mimic some types of chronic orofacial pain and may complicate the diagnosis and treatment of orofacial pain by the dental practitioner.[19] Interdisciplinary care is generally the optimal method for management of patients with orofacial pain and headache. The following descriptions can assist in the differential diagnosis of headaches with the exclusion of orofacial pain.[23]

Migraine

Migraine is usually unilateral, has a gradual onset, and is accompanied by photophobia, phonophobia, nausea, and vomiting. The intensity of the headache is moderate to severe. Migraine may be associated with sensory, motor, and mood disturbances and predominantly occurs in females.

The detailed etiology of migraine is still unknown. Two phases of intracranial vasomotor dysfunction during attacks have been reported in most migraine disorders.[37] In the initial phase, blood flow gradually decreases because of vasoconstriction in the involved hemisphere. Symptoms associated with the aura are related to cerebral ischemia. The headache is provoked by vasodilation in the later phase. The vessels responsible for the pain of migraine are innervated primarily by the trigeminal nerve, with some innervation from the glossopharyngeal and vagus nerves. Neurogenic inflammation may be a pathogenetic mechanism for migraine and cluster headache. Neurotransmitters from these nerves may play a role in the onset of migraine. Nociceptive chemical mediators, such as serotonin, histamine, bradykinin, leukotrienes, potassium, and prostaglandins, may have an important role as well. Plasma extravasation and ultrastructural changes, as well as increases in plasma calcitonin gene-related peptide (CGRP), are blocked by serotonin (5-HT) receptor agonists.

Migraine with Aura (Classic Migraine). Some migraine headaches are proceeded by a group of neurologic events or symptoms collectively called an *aura.* Migraine with aura is usually a unilateral pain condition but may be bilateral for some patients. The aura is typically felt before any pain experience and lasts 5 to 20 minutes. Shortly after the aura resolves, the headache begins and may last 1 hour to several days. During the aura, the patient may experience sensory abnormalities (hyperesthesia, paresthesia, dysesthesia) and motor defects (weakness, paralysis). Patients may experience abnormal sensations in the lips and the oral structures and may complain of speech difficulties. The aura may also be accompanied by visual abnormalities, such as zigzag flashing (*teichopsia*) or loss of visual field (*scotoma*).

The International Headache Society has proposed the following diagnostic criteria for a diagnosis of migraine with aura:

1. At least two attacks fulfilling characteristics in the second criterion
2. At least three of the following four characteristics:
   a. One or more fully reversible aura symptoms, indicating focal hemispheric or brainstem dysfunction
   b. At least one aura symptom developing gradually over more than 4 minutes, or two or more symptoms occurring in succession
   c. No aura symptom lasting more than 60 minutes. If more than one aura symptom is present, accepted duration is proportionally increased.
   d. Headache following aura, with a free interval of less than 60 minutes, but occasionally beginning before aura
3. At least one of the following:
   History, physical, and neurologic examinations do not suggest organic disorder.
   History, physical, and neurologic examinations do suggest organic disorder, but such disorder is ruled out by neuroimaging procedures or other laboratory investigations.

Migraine without Aura (Common Migraine) Migraine headaches with an aura are characterized by repetitive, unilateral, throbbing or pulsating pain attacks. Preceding aura is absent. Migraine without aura occurs twofold to threefold more frequently than migraine with aura. The duration of migraine without aura ranges from a few hours to 2 or 3 days, with an average duration of 6 to 8 hours. In some female migraine patients, a relationship exists between their menstrual cycle and precipitation of the migraine. The headache experience is the same for migraine patients with or without aura, and the diagnosis is based on the same criteria as described earlier.

Cluster Headache Syndrome

Cluster headache syndrome is divided into type types: cluster headache and chronic paroxysmal hemicrania. These disorders have similar features, but the gender predominance is different. The common features of these disorders are repetitive unilateral headache with autonomic symptoms and symptom-free intervals.

Cluster Headache. Cluster headache is characterized by episodes of severe, unilateral, throbbing pain in the frontal and temporal regions. Ipsilateral autonomic symptoms, such as Horner's syndrome, lacrimation, and nasal stuffiness, accompanies the episode. The incidence of cluster headache is 9.8 per 100,000 population, or approximately $\frac{1}{25}$ that of migraine. Cluster headache predominantly occurs in middle-aged males. The incidence in males is about fourfold greater than in females.[51]

Cluster headache is recognized as a neurovascular headache because it is aggravated by vasodilating substances and is improved by prophylactic drugs for migraine. However, the exact mechanism is still unknown. The episodes of cluster headache occur a few times in a day, often awaking the patient at night. Each episode lasts 1 to 3 hours, and a cluster of episodes is observed over 2 to 6 weeks. A pain-free interval between the clusters of headaches usually lasts 6 to 12 months.[5] Episodes can be precipitated by alcohol and other vasoactive agents. Associated autonomic symptoms during an attack are ptosis, miosis, conjunctival injection, nasal congestion, rhinorrhea, facial sweating, and lacrimation. Some patients feel nausea, but vomiting is rare. Referred pain to midface and teeth is often seen in cluster headache patients.

It is important to differentiate cluster headache from migraine and Raeder's syndrome. Pain associated with cluster headache is described as relatively short and occurs predominantly in males, whereas that of migraine is usually longer and occurs predominantly in females. The diagnostic characteristics differentiating cluster headache from Raeder's syndrome are the duration of an attack and intervening Horner's syndrome. Horner's syndrome ameliorates within an hour in cluster headache. The age at onset is usually younger in cluster headache patients than in those with Raeder's syndrome, but this difference is not always clear.

Chronic Paroxysmal Hemicrania. Chronic paroxysmal hemicrania is characterized by repetitive excruciating attacks of unilateral headache with autonomic symptoms. The pain attacks predominantly occur in females at both day and night. Unlike cluster headache, patients with chronic paroxysmal hemicrania report a few mild to moderate attacks per day after a severe headache period. In remitting cases a cluster of repetitive pain attacks is followed by a

pain-free period. Patients have diurnal and nocturnal attacks, and nocturnal attacks often disturb sleep. Pain is located around the ipsilateral orbit, forehead, and temple. Each attack usually lasts up to 30 minutes, significantly shorter than for cluster headache. Ptosis, conjunctival injection, lacrimation, nasal stuffiness, nasal discharge, and increased perspiration are often observed during an attack on the affected side of the face. Nausea and vomiting are not usually reported. Chronic paroxysmal hemicrania affects females four to six times more often than males.

Chronic paroxysmal hemicrania must be differentiated from cluster headache, migraine, and Raeder's syndrome. Indomethacin is a useful drug in the differential diagnosis; it relieves chronic paroxysmal hemicrania completely but generally not the other painful disorders.

Tension-Type Headache

Tension-type headache is characterized by mild to moderate recurring pain anywhere in the head or suboccipital area.[43] It is equally distributed in males and females. The quality of the headache is described as being constant, dull, aching, tightening, and pressure. Both muscle tension and psychologic tension can cause headache. Tension-type headache varies in pain intensity, duration, and frequency. This headache disorder is classified into two types, episodic and chronic, by its frequency and duration. *Episodic* tension-type headache is characterized by episodes that last from 30 minutes to a week. The diagnosis of *chronic* tension-type headache is used when the patient experiences the headache more than 15 days/ month (180 days/year).

Common features of both subtypes are the absence of nausea, vomiting, photophobia, and phonophobia. Tension-type headaches are rarely so debilitating as to disturb the patient's daily activities. Abnormal electromyographic findings are observed in pericranial muscles when the headache is caused by muscle tension. Psychosocial and behavioral factors contribute to this disorder, and patients are free from headache when they are away from these factors.

Tension-type headache is diagnosed by ruling out other headache disorders. Symptoms are sometimes similar to migraine without aura, but the intensity is less and the duration is more variable. The following clinical characteristics can help differentiate migraine from tension-type headache:

1. Tension-type headache is not exacerbated by routine physical activity.

2. Migraine is usually located unilaterally, whereas tension-type headache is more often bilateral.
3. The quality of migraine pain is described as pulsating, whereas pressure and tightness are more common in tension-type headache.

Sometimes it is difficult to differentiate tension-type headache from migraine. Some researchers regard these two headache disorders as having similar mechanisms with different presentations (Fig. 22-1).

Temporal Arteritis

Temporal arteritis is a vasculitis that predominantly affects large and medium-sized arteries. Intensity of headache varies from moderate to severe. Boring or throbbing pain is often reported in the unilateral temporal region. The pain is constant but sometimes paroxysmal. Patients with severe disease describe the pain quality as lancinating and sharp. Temporal arteritis is reported to occur in three to nine people per million per year. It predominantly occurs in females over 50 years old.

Temporal arteritis is probably caused by *giant cell arteritis,* a rheumatic disease.[48] The etiology is unknown. Fibrous tissue formation in the arterial wall results in blood supply deficiency. If giant cell arteritis occurs in shoulder and hip muscles first, it appears as *polymyalgia rheumatica.*

Headache, fever, fatigue, and tenderness of the temporal artery occur with the onset of temporal arteritis. Headache is usually located in the temple and forehead but is also reported in the occiput and maxilla. Some patients report symptoms seen in TMD, such as tenderness of masticatory muscles, TMJ pain, and occlusal dysfunction. However, occlusal dysfunction is

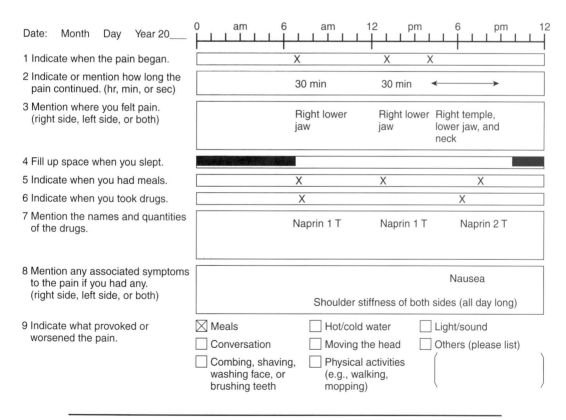

Fig. 22-1 Self-reporting pain diary provides useful information about patient's pain features. In most pain disorders, intensity and quality change day by day and point to point. To investigate pain frequency, duration, intensity, quality, and associated symptoms, practitioners use patients' pain diary and daily symptom report.

caused by ischemia in masticatory muscles (claudication of the jaw). Other symptoms from ischemia caused by giant cell arteritis may be seen. Visual impairment usually occurs in the early stages. Clinical manifestations include irreversible visual loss; lip, scalp, and tongue necrosis; carpal tunnel syndrome; stroke, angina pectoris, or myocardial infarction; hematuria; cough; and other CNS symptoms.

The clinical symptoms and laboratory findings may provide the diagnosis of temporal arteritis. Erythrocyte sedimentation rate and plasma fibrinogen are greatly elevated, and giant cells may be detected in the biopsy of the temporal artery. Corticosteroids improve pain and other symptoms, providing additional support for the diagnosis of temporal arteritis. Because of the risk of blindness with this condition, patients suspected to have this diagnosis should be referred immediately to an ophthalmologist for evaluation and interdisciplinary care.

SUMMARY

A correct diagnosis is essential for correct treatment. Detailed information is necessary to make a correct diagnosis.[32] Cues for the diagnosis are often hidden in the patient's history or examination, such as a pattern of pain onset and frequency or an associated symptom[3,4] (see Fig. 22-1). Even after diagnosis and initiation of treatment, it is important to assess the efficacy of treatment frequently and to reevaluate the diagnosis.[17]

Chronic pain research has advanced significantly in the last decade. Innovative theories of pain mechanisms, such as central sensitization and neuroplasticity, have been proposed and the effectiveness of newer treatments and drugs has been proved. Practitioners should understand the importance of a correct diagnosis and the treatment of acute pain in the prevention of chronic pain.

Bibliography

1. Bender IB, Freedland JB: Clinical considerations in the diagnosis and treatment of intra-alveolar root fractures, *J Am Dent Assoc* 107:595-600, 1983.
2. Bennett GJ: Hypotheses on the pathogenesis of herpes zoster-associated pain, *Ann Neurol* 35:S38-S41, 1994.
3. Beyer JE, Aradine CR: Patterns of pediatric pain intensity: a methodological investigation of a self-report scale, *Clin J Pain* 3:130-141, 1987.
4. Bieri D, Reeve RA, Champion GD, et al: The Faces Pain Scale for the self-assessment of the severity of pain experienced by children: development, initial validation, and preliminary investigation for ratio scale properties, *Pain* 41:139-150, 1990.
5. Bittar G, Graff-Radford SB: A retrospective study of patients with cluster headaches, *Oral Surg Oral Med Oral Pathol* 73:519-525, 1992.
6. Bonica JJ et al, editors: *The management of pain*, ed 2, Malvern, Pa, 1990, Lea & Febiger.
7. Bruyn GW: Glossopharyngeal neuralgia, *Cephalalgia* 3:143-157, 1983.
8. Cannon CR: Carotidynia: an unusual pain in the neck, *Otolaryngol Head Neck Surg* 110:387-390, 1994.
9. Chambers BR, Donnan GA, Riddell RJ, et al: Carotidynia: aetiology, diagnosis, and treatment, *Clin Exp Neurol* 17:113-123, 1981.
10. Costen JB: Syndrome of ear and sinus symptoms dependent upon functions of the temporomandibular joint, *Ann Otol Rhinol Laryngol* 3:1-4, 1934.
11. Dandy WE: Concerning the cause of trigeminal neuralgia, *Am J Surg* 24:447-455, 1934.
12. De Kanter RJ, Truin GJ, Burgersdijk RC, et al: Prevalence in the Dutch adult population and a meta-analysis of signs and symptoms of temporomandibular disorder, *J Dent Res* 72:1509-1518, 1993.
13. Desai BT, McHenry L Jr, Stanley JA: Raeder's syndrome, *Ann Ophthalmol* 7:1082-1084, 1975.
14. Dornan TL, Espir ML, Gale EA, et al: Remittent painful ophthalmoplegia: the Tolosa-Hunt syndrome? A report of seven cases and review of the literature, *J Neurol Neurosurg Psychiatry* 42:270-275, 1979.
15. Dworkin RH, Portemoy RK: Pain and its persistence in herpes zoster, *Pain* 67, 1996.
16. Eriksson L, Westesson PL, Rohlin M: Temporomandibular joint sounds in patients with disc displacement, *Int J Oral Surg* 14(5):428-436, 1985.
17. Fields HL, Liebeskind JC, editors: *Pharmacological approaches to the treatment of chronic pain: new concepts and critical issues*, Seattle, 1996, IASP Press.
18. Fricton JR, Kroening RJ, Hathaway KM, editors: *TMJ and craniofacial pain: diagnosis and management of pain*, St Louis, 1988, Ishiyaku EuroAmerica.
19. Graff-Radford SB: Headache problems that can present as toothache, *Dent Clin North Am* 35:155-170, 1991.
20. Griffiths RH: Report of the President's Conference on examination, diagnosis, and management of temporomandibular disorders, *J Am Dent Assoc* 106:75-77, 1983.
21. Grimson BS, Thompson HS: Raeder's syndrome: a clinical review, *Surv Ophthalmol* 24:199-210, 1980.
22. Harkins SW, Bush FM, Price DD, et al: Symptom report in orofacial pain patients: relation to chronic pain, experimental pain, illness behavior, and personality, *Clin J Pain* 7:102-113, 1991.
23. International Headache Society: Classification and diagnostic criteria for headache disorders, cranial neuralgias, and facial pain, *Cephalalgia* 7:1-96, 1988.

24. Janig W, Stanton-Hicks M, editors: *Reflex sympathetic dystrophy: a reappraisal,* Seattle, 1996, IASP Press.

25. Keele KD: A physician looks at pain. In Weisenberg M, editor: *Pain: clinical and experimental perspectives,* St Louis, 1975, Mosby.

26. Kerr F: Pathology of trigeminal neuralgia: light and electron microscopic observations, *J Neurosurg* 26(suppl):151-156, 1967.

27. Layzer RB: Muscle pain, cramps, and fatigue. In Engel AG, Franzini-Armstrong C, editors: *Myology,* New York, 1994, McGraw-Hill.

28. Lund JP, Widmer CG: Evaluation of the use of surface electromyography in the diagnosis, documentation, and treatment of dental patients, *J Craniomand Disord* 3(3):125-137, 1989.

29. Lund JP, Widmer CG, Feine JS: Validity of diagnostic and monitoring tests used for temporomandibular disorders, *J Dent Res* 74(4):1133-1143, 1995.

30. McCreary CP, Clark GT, Merril RL, et al: Psychological distress and diagnostic subgroups of temporomandibular disorder patients, *Pain* 44:29-34, 1991.

31. McNeill C, Danzig D, Farrar W, et al: Craniomandibular (TMJ) disorders: state of the art, *J Prosthet Dent* 44:434-437, 1980.

32. Melzack R, editor: *Pain measurement and assessment,* New York, 1983, Raven.

33. Mense S: Considerations concerning the neurobiological basis of muscle pain, *Can J Physiol Pharmacol* 69(5):610-616, 1991.

34. Mense S: Nociception from skeletal muscle in relation to clinical muscle pain, *Pain* 54(3):241-289, 1993.

35. Mense S, Meyer H: Bradykinin-induced sensitization of high-threshold muscle receptors with slowly conducting afferent fibers, *Pain* 1(suppl):S204, 1981.

36. Merskey H, Bogduk N, editors, Task Force on Taxonomy of the International Association for the Study of Pain: *Detailed descriptions of pain syndromes and classification of chronic pain, descriptions of chronic pain syndromes, and definitions of pain terms,* ed 2, Seattle, 1994, IASP Press.

37. Moskowitz MA: Basic mechanisms in vascular headache, *Neurol Clin* 8:801-815, 1990.

38. Okeson JP: *Management of temporomandibular disorders and occlusion,* ed 4, St Louis, 1997, Mosby.

39. Okeson JP: *Bell's orofacial pains,* ed 5, Chicago, 1995, Quintessence.

40. Okeson JP: *Orofacial pain: guidelines to assessment, diagnosis, and management,* ed 3, Chicago, 1996, Quintessence.

41. Paesani DA, Tallents RH, Murphy WC, et al: Reproducibility of rest activity of the anterior temporal and masseter muscles in asymptomatic and symptomatic temporomandibular subjects, *J Orofac Pain* 8:402-406, 1994.

42. Panagopoulos K, Chakraborty M, Deopujari CE, et al: Neurovascular decompression for cranial rhizopathies, *Br J Neurosurg* 1:235-241, 1987.

43. Rapoport AM: The diagnosis of migraine and tension-type headache, then and now, *Neurology* 42:11-15, 1992.

44. Rappaport ZH, Devor M: Trigeminal neuralgia: the role of self-sustaining discharge in the trigeminal ganglion, *Pain* 56:127-138, 1994.

45. Reid KI, Gracely RH, Dubner RA: The influence of time, facial side, and location on pain-pressure thresholds in chronic myogenous temporomandibular disorder, *J Orofac Pain* 8:258-265, 1994.

46. Resnick DK, Jannetta PJ, Bissonnette D, et al: Microvascular decompression for glossopharyngeal neuralgia, *Neurosurgery* 36:64-68, 1995.

47. Schiffman EL, Fricton JR, Haley DP, et al: The prevalence and treatment needs of subjects with temporomandibular disorders, *J Am Dent Assoc* 120(3):295-303, 1990.

48. Sherard RK, Coleridge ST: Giant-cell arteritis, *J Emerg Med* 4:293-299, 1986.

49. Shore NA: *Occlusal equilibration and temporomandibular joint dysfunction,* Philadelphia, 1959, JB Lippincott.

50. Stanton-Hicks M, Janig W, Hassenbusch S, et al: Reflex sympathetic dystrophy: changing concepts and taxonomy, *Pain* 63:127-133, 1995.

51. Swanson JW, Yanagihara T, Stang PE, et al: Incidence of cluster headaches: a population-based study in Olmsted County, Minnesota, *Neurology* 44:433-437, 1994.

52. Testori T, Badino M, Castagnola M: Vertical root fractures in endodontically treated teeth: a clinical survey of 36 cases, *J Endod* 19:87-91, 1993.

53. Tomita H, Tanaka M, Kukimoto N, et al: An ELISA study on varicella-zoster virus infection in acute peripheral facial palsy, *Acta Otolaryngol Suppl* 446:10-16, 1988.

54. Van Loveren H, Tew J Jr, Keller JT, et al: A 10-year experience in the treatment of trigeminal neuralgia: comparison of percutaneous stereotaxic rhizotomy and posterior fossa exploration, *J Neurosurg* 57:757-764, 1982.

55. Wall PD, Melzack R, editors: *Textbook of pain,* ed 3, New York, 1994, Churchill Livingstone.

56. Yang J, Simonson TM, Ruprecht A, et al: Magnetic resonance imaging used to assess patients with trigeminal neuralgia, *Oral Surg Oral Med Oral Pathol Oral Radiol Endod* 81:343-350, 1996.

CHAPTER 23

Pharmacologic Treatments for Temporomandibular Disorders and Other Orofacial Pain

LAUREN E. TA
JOHN K. NEUBERT
RAYMOND A. DIONNE

CHAPTER OUTLINE

Pharmacologic intervention in the management of chronic orofacial pain is usually considered adjunctive on the assumption that more definitive treatments will eventually correct the underlying pathophysiologic process. It is now recognized, however, that many putative dental and surgical therapies for temporomandibular disorders (TMDs) have not withstood scientific scrutiny for adequate efficacy and safety, which has led to the use of medications as the primary interventions for many of these disorders. Long-term palliative treatment of intractable pain through pharmacologic management may be the only option for some individuals when pain is poorly controlled after failed surgical interventions.

This chapter reviews the use of medications for TMDs and other forms of chronic orofacial pain in clinical situations where adequate evidence supports their efficacy and safety for this indication. Other drug classes are also described that may be considered based on their documented effectiveness for related chronic pain conditions.

Clinical Evaluation of Pharmacologic and Other Therapies

No generally accepted agreement exists on the etiology and pathophysiology of TMDs, the need for aggressive treatment, or the safety and efficacy of most current clinical treatments. Professional differences often result from a lack of appreciation for the differences between clinical observations, which may form the basis for therapeutic interventions, and the need to verify the safety and effectiveness of treatments in studies that control for factors that can mimic clinical success. Although these considerations apply to all areas of therapy, the management of chronic orofacial pain has a history of therapeutic misadventures, charismatic-based treatment philosophies, and a lack of scientific documentation for most clinical practices. The potential for significant morbidity and mortality with drug classes used for TMD mandates that their effectiveness be documented and outweigh safety concerns, especially when administered chronically.

In the natural history of therapeutic interventions for the management of pain, novel treatments that are first described on the basis of initial case reports, case series, or poorly controlled clinical trials usually appear to have therapeutic benefit, or the results would not be publicized. After evaluation of a putative therapy in well-controlled clinical trials, however, a number of alternative interpretations are possible. If several trials indicate that the treatment is effective and has minimum toxicity, it is considered a *validated* therapeutic practice, such as the use of nonsteroidal antiinflammatory drugs (NSAIDs) for the control of acute pain. If the treatment is found not to be effective or toxicity becomes evident, the drug is removed from the market, as occurred with zomepirac (Zomax) in the 1970s, or labeling restrictions are imposed, as with ketorolac (Toradol) more recently.

Most therapies that are used for chronic orofacial pain do not fall under the jurisdiction of the U.S. Food and Drug Administration (FDA) as either drugs or devices and are not subjected to rigorous examination before being used in humans. Other review processes, such as the U.S. Pharmacopeial Convention, use expert panels to review non-FDA-approved uses for marketed drugs but do not address devices or clinical practices. As a consequence, most drugs, devices, and therapeutic strategies used for chronic orofacial pain fall into the category of *invalidated* clinical practices. This does not imply that these treatment modalities do not have therapeutic value. Rather, they have not been subjected to well-controlled trials that allow the biomedical community to determine (1) if the modality is a validated clinical practice whose efficacy exceeds the potential for toxicity or (2) if the modality represents an irrational clinical practice that should not be continued. The hazard of using a seemingly effective therapy in humans without appropriate validation of safety is illustrated by the current plight of patients who received Proplast implants for the surgical treatment of TMD.[1]

Another factor that may affect the evaluation of treatment outcome to drug therapy for TMD is the fluctuating nature of chronic pain, which may undergo remissions and exacerbation independent of treatment.[2] The high psychological comorbidity described in this population may also influence the onset of symptoms, reporting of pain intensity or its affective component, and treatment response.[3] Many patients eventually improve even if an initial course of therapy is not successful or if they receive no treatment at all. Such responses may explain the high rates of success reported in case series and loosely controlled studies for many of the therapeutic modalities used for TMD.

Drug regimens and classes for the treatment of TMD range from short-term treatment with NSAIDs for joint pain and muscle relaxants for pain of muscular origin to chronic administration of antidepressants for diffuse pain. In general, claims of efficacy based on clinical observations are often superseded by equivocal findings of efficacy or belated recognition of adverse effects and toxicity with long-term administration. The principles of pain management for TMD rests on the same principles that apply to the use of all drugs: demonstrated efficacy for the indication, an acceptable incidence of adverse reactions for the condition being treated, and safety when used in large numbers of patients for prolonged periods.

Antiinflammatory Drugs

Nonsteroidal Antiinflammatory Drugs

NSAIDs comprise a heterogeneous group of drugs with diverse structures, similar therapeutic effects, good oral efficacy, and similar side effect profiles. They are better tolerated than opioid drugs by ambulatory patients, have less sedative side effects, and are not likely to produce dependence or result in tolerance. Conversely, the hazards of long-term administration of NSAIDs have been belatedly recognized as serious toxicity to the gastrointestinal (GI) tract and renal disease.

A comprehensive review of the primary literature reveals little scientific support that the daily use of NSAIDs offers benefit for chronic orofacial pain.[4] Standard texts and summaries of expert opinion often provide recommendations or extrapolate from chronic inflammatory conditions such as arthritis. The results of two placebo-controlled studies, however, suggest that NSAIDs are ineffective for chronic orofacial pain. The analgesic effects of ibuprofen, 2400 mg/day for 4 weeks, could not be separated from placebo in a group of patients with chronic orofacial myogenous pain.[5] A similar comparison of piroxicam, 20 mg daily for 12 days, to placebo for TMD pain also failed to demonstrate any therapeutic advantage for the NSAID.[6]

Both clinical and animal studies suggest that tolerance to NSAIDs can develop with repeated administration. The mean reduction in chronic lower back pain intensity after an initial dose of 1200 mg of ibuprofen was 23%.[7] After 2 weeks of 2400 mg/day of ibuprofen or placebo, the mean reduction in pain intensity for the last dose was fourfold lower in the drug group. The initial low level of response suggests that low back pain is not particularly sensitive to

ibuprofen and may partly explain the poor response seen for chronic musculoskeletal pain in the orofacial area. The development of tolerance over 2 weeks suggests a similar process for TMD pain, which could make the analgesic response negligible after 4 weeks. Tolerance to diflunisal with repeated administration has been demonstrated in animals without a reduction in the amount of drug in the blood over time after administration of the first dose versus a dose given after 3 days of diflunisal.[8] This suggests a functional change in the pharmacologic response rather than enhanced pharmacokinetic disposition, such that the same amount of drug elicits less analgesia.

The lack of clinical studies to support the efficacy of ibuprofen for TMD contrasts with the growing body of evidence on the potential serious toxic effects of NSAIDs when given chronically at high doses.[9] A short trial of an NSAID may be considered for patients with an inflammatory component to their pain complaint. A lack of therapeutic effect after a 7- to 10-day trial, however, or the development of any GI symptoms should prompt discontinuation of the NSAID. The development of selective cyclooxygenase-2 (COX-2) inhibitors may offer an alternative for use of antiinflammatory drugs in TMD pain without the risks of chronic administration of nonselective COX-1/COX-2 inhibitors. Table 23-1 compares the side effects and efficacy of nonselective NSAIDs and COX-2 selective NSAIDs.

Selective COX-2 Inhibitors

At standard therapeutic doses, conventional NSAIDs exert their analgesic and antiinflammatory effects through COX-2 inhibition. At the same time, however, NSAIDs also block COX-1, which in turn leads to diminished production of the prostaglandins that regulate homeostatic functions. As a sequence, these agents induce substantial platelet effects, along with the potential for renal and GI toxicity, which may interfere with clinical use. The discovery and characterization of the COX-2 isoform led to the hypothesis that selective inhibition of COX-2 would provide the potent antiinflammatory and analgesic effects of NSAIDs without influencing COX-1 and its important physiologic functions. Based on this hypothesis and encouraged by the significant morbidity and mortality associated with NSAIDs, there have been substantial efforts to develop specific inhibitors of the COX-2 isoform. Both isoforms of cyclooxygenase have the same molecular weight of 71,000 daltons.

TABLE 23-1

Comparison of Nonselective NSAIDs and COX-2 Selective NSAIDs

	Nonselective NSAIDs	COX-2 Selective NSAIDS
Side Effects		
Gastric ulcers, bleeding, perforation, obstruction	Uncommon*	Close to placebo†
Decreased platelet function	Common	None
Decreased renal function (reversible) in high-risk patients	Uncommon	Unknown
Pulmonary complications (bronchospasm in sensitive patients)	Uncommon	Unknown
Central nervous system effects	Rare*	Unknown
Efficacy		
Acute pain	Moderate*	Moderate‡
Pain in chronic osteoarthritis	Moderate*	Moderate
Pain in chronic rheumatoid arthritis	Moderate	Moderate§
Pain in acute migraine	Moderate*	Unknown
Pain in chronic spondylitis	Mild*	Unknown
Pain in acute gout	Strong*	Unknown
Approved for Children	Yes*	No

*Varies among individual NSAIDs.
†Longer follow-up required for patients using these drugs.
‡Indicated for rofecoxib only.
§Indicated for celecoxib only.

The major difference in the two enzymes resides in their substrate-binding pocket at the active sites, thus it has been possible to develop drugs that differ in their selectivity for inhibition of COX-1 and COX-2 in vitro.

COX-1 is primarily expressed constitutively in many tissues and produces arachidonic acid metabolites that regulate many physiologic functions under normal resting conditions, including GI mucosal protection, platelet aggregation, vascular homeostasis, and regulation of renal hemodynamics and electrolyte balance. In contrast, under basal conditions, COX-2 expression is limited to the brain[10] and kidney,[11] but it is greatly expressed in response to inflammatory and other physiologic stimuli and growth factors. COX-2 has been shown to be upregulated at sites of inflammation,[12,13] where it appears to mediate the production of arachidonic acid metabolites involved in pain and inflammatory diseases, such as osteoarthritis (OA) and rheumatoid arthritis (RA).[14,15] Furthermore, COX-2 may have an essential role in central pain mediation and is highly expressed in central nervous system (CNS) in response to peripheral stimuli[16,17] (Figs. 23-1 and 23-2).

More recent studies suggest that the original paradigm regarding the roles of COX-1 and COX-2 was overly simplistic. Findings from animal studies have demonstrated constitutive expression of COX-2 in the kidney, brain, ovary, uterus, cartilage, and bone.[10,18-22] Evidence also suggests that COX-1 can be induced by stressful stimuli, such as radiation injury to the intestine, and may play a protective role in

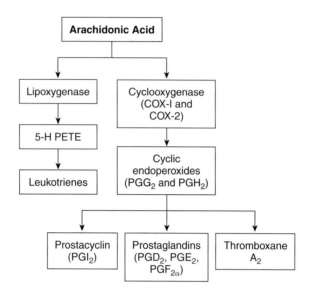

Fig. 23-1 Arachidonic acid pathway. *5-H PETE,* 5-Hydroperoxyeicosatetraenoic acid.

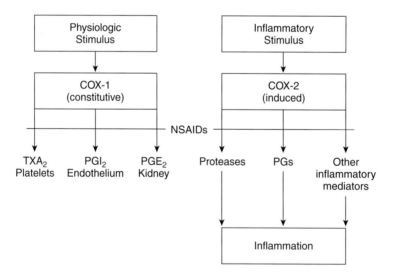

Fig. 23-2 Cyclooxygenase isoenzymes.

such circumstances.[23] Both COX-1 and COX-2 probably have more complex physiologic and pathophysiologic roles than originally thought.

The two currently available COX-2 inhibitors are considered to be highly selective for COX-2 suppression at the doses administered clinically, with minimal effects on COX-1 activity. Celecoxib (Celebrex), a sulfonamide, was the first family of COX-2 specific inhibitor approved by the FDA for RA and OA. Rofecoxib (Vioxx) was subsequently approved for osteoarthritis, acute pain in adults, and primary dysmenorrhea. It is a furanone, which allows patients with sulfonamide allergies to use rofecoxib safely.

Celecoxib. In recombinant enzyme assays, celecoxib has been reported to be 375-fold selective for COX-2.[24] Celecoxib at 600 mg twice daily (50% higher than the highest dose evaluated for efficacy in trials) has no effect on serum thromboxane or platelet function.[25] It is rapidly absorbed, with a peak plasma levels in about 3 hours. Celecoxib is metabolized and excreted primarily by the liver into bile, with a half-life of 11.2 hours.

Celecoxib has been extensively evaluated for the efficacy in OA and RA of the knees and hips, which should be comparable to the signs and symptoms of OA and RA in the temporomandibular joint (TMJ). Dosage ranges of 100 to 400 mg/day for OA and 200 to 800 mg/day for RA, established in phase II trials,[26] have been demonstrated efficacy in phase III trials.[27] Celecoxib at these dosages has been shown to have similar efficacy to naproxen (1000 mg/day) or diclofenac (150 mg/day) in the management of the symptoms of OA and RA. In a 12-week trial involving a large sample of patients with OA of the knee, significant pain relief and improvement in physical function were achieved with celecoxib (100 or 200 mg twice daily) and naproxen (500 mg twice daily).[28]

Upper GI complications, in the presence of a confirmed upper GI mucosal lesion, occur eightfold less frequently in patients receiving celecoxib than those receiving standard NSAIDs (naproxen, diclofenac, ibuprofen).[29] Furthermore, the incidence of endoscopic ulceration was consistently low with celecoxib and comparable to rates reported with placebo, but significantly higher with naproxen in a 12-week study.[27]

Rofecoxib. In recombinant enzyme assays, rofecoxib has been reported to be 1000-fold selective for COX-2.[30] When assessed by whole-blood assay ex vivo, rofecoxib was shown to have no effect on COX-1 by not interfering with thromboxane production at doses up to 1 g/day.[30] It is rapidly absorbed, with maximum plasma concentrations in 2 to 3 hours. Rofecoxib is metabolized in the liver and excreted primarily in the urine, with a half-life of approximately 17 hours. The specificity of rofecoxib for COX-2 versus COX-1 inhibition has also been demonstrated in a study with normal healthy volunteers. Rofecoxib is well tolerated up to a dose of 375 mg (10 times greater than the clinically recommended dose), retains COX-1/COX-2 selectivity at these doses, and had no effect on bleeding time.[31]

In OA studies using end points of pain relief, walking pain, and global assessments, rofecoxib showed clinical efficacy in doses of 12.5 or 25 mg/day and was as effective as ibuprofen (2400 mg daily over 6 weeks)[32] or diclofenac (100 mg daily over 6 to 12 months).[33] The rate of ulceration in endoscopic studies for patients receiving rofecoxib (25 or 50 mg/day) was compared with placebo over 12 weeks and ibuprofen (2400 mg/day) for 24 weeks.[34] Treatment with 25 or 50 mg daily was associated with a significantly lower percentage of patients with endoscopic gastroduodenal ulcers than treatment with 2400 mg of ibuprofen daily.

Adverse Effects. Based from the data presented to the FDA hearing for new drug applications, the occurrence of clinically significant perforations, gastric obstructions, and upper GI hemorrhages is significantly less with both celecoxib and rofecoxib compared to traditional NSAIDs (e.g., diclofenac, ibuprofen, diclofenac, naproxen) or close to the rate with placebo. However, the new COX-2 selective NSAIDs still produce some of the minor side effects attributed to the currently available NSAIDs, such as dyspepsia and diarrhea, but not to a major degree in clinical trials. Postmarketing surveillance studies will help to determine the significant difference of these effects of the COX-2 selective NSAIDs. The full extent of the antiinflammatory and analgesic actions and the side effect potential of celecoxib and rofecoxib can be fully recognized only with long-term use in the general population.

COX-2 inhibition has shown to delay mucosal healing in animals.[35] To establish clinical relevance, however, longer evaluation with general use in humans is needed. Caution should be taken in treating patients with prior history of GI mucosal problems, such as *Helicobacter pylori* infection, since it is unclear at present if COX-2 inhibitors are without toxicity.

Clinical studies are underway to address this issue. Bleeding and platelet aggregation studies for COX-2 inhibitors have shown negative effect. Since these are surrogate markers, however, it is difficult to determine the clinically significant bleeding episodes. No clinical trials have indicated that selective COX-2 inhibitors have any advantage over nonselective NSAIDs in terms of perioperative bleeding complications. A COX-1-sparing agent would seem to be a reasonable choice for an NSAID in the perioperative setting (Box 23-1).

Corticosteroids

Corticosteroids have been injected directly into the TMJ and applied topically in an attempt to reduce the pain and dysfunction associated with TMDs. Few controlled studies of intraarticular injection have been reported, with wide-ranging results including demonstration of efficacy, no difference in comparison to placebo, and deleterious effects in the absence of therapeutic benefit.

The iontophoretic administration of steroids is also recommended based on clinical observations. It is hypothesized that iontophoresis will result in higher drug levels at the site of injury or pain, in this case the TMJ, by applying an electrical current to ionized drug solutions. One study compared iontophoresis with dexamethasone in a lidocaine vehicle to saline placebo for TMD after three drug administration sessions over 5 days and with 7 and 14 days of follow-up.[36] Both groups of subjects (active drug and placebo) showed improvement over the course of therapy and continued to report less pain and improved range of motion at the 7- and 14-day follow-ups. These data illustrate the dichotomy that often exists between clinical observations and the results of controlled clinical trial. If one compared the pain and dysfunction reported before treatment and at the follow-up appointments, it would appear logical to conclude that the improvement was the result of the treatment being evaluated, in this case the iontophoretic application of a steroid to the TMJ. Evaluation of the active drug in the presence of a placebo-controlled clinical trial leads to the opposite conclusion, that the drug has no detectable therapeutic effect. Alternative explanations include cyclic fluctuations in symptomatology over time and patient expectations of improvement from receiving medications applied by a novel method in a therapeutic environment.

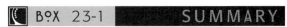

BOX 23-1   **SUMMARY**

Nonsteroidal Antiinflammatory Drugs in Treatment of Orofacial Pain

No well-controlled clinical trials have provided evidence that NSAIDs have a therapeutic effect in patients with temporomandibular disorders.

If an NSAID is prescribed for chronic orofacial pain, it should be discontinued if there is a lack of therapeutic effect or development of GI symptoms.

Selective COX-2 inhibitors provide pain relief and antiinflammatory effects for chronic conditions such as rheumatoid arthritis and osteoarthritis without the significant morbidity associated with chronic NSAID administration. They may also be useful for TMD.

Centrally Acting Drugs

Benzodiazepines

Drugs of the benzodiazepine class are frequently administered to patients with chronic pain, often for prolonged periods, despite long-standing concern about their potential for abuse and dependence, and the possibility of initiating or exacerbating depression in patients with chronic pain. Although the efficacy of benzodiazepines for chronic pain is not generally recognized, several studies have demonstrated therapeutic effects for musculoskeletal pain.

A study evaluating *diazepam*, ibuprofen, and the combination in patients with chronic orofacial pain of myogenic origin demonstrated a significant decrease in pain in the diazepam and diazepam plus ibuprofen groups compared with placebo, indicating that the pain relief was attributable to diazepam.[5] Administration of *clonazepam* to patients with chronic myofascial pain in the orofacial region was also demonstrated to be superior to placebo in a double-blind 30-day trial.[37] No cases of dependence or withdrawal symptoms were noted on discontinuation of the drug in either of these studies. A larger study of patients with fibromyalgia receiving *alprazolam*, ibuprofen, or the combination reported improvement in patients rating of disease severity and tenderness on palpation after 6 weeks.[38] The dose of alprazolam (0.5 to 3.0 mg/day) was well tolerated in patients completing 24 weeks of therapy; many patients tapered their daily dosage, contrary to a pattern of drug abuse. Data from these three studies support benzodiazepine-mediated relief of symptoms in chronic orofacial pain of myogenic origin.

A nonsystematic review of the long-term use of benzodiazepines for chronic pain concluded that benzodiazepines are effective for some musculoskeletal symptoms.[39] However, the antidepressant effects attributable to triazolo-benzodiazepines, such as alprazolam, may be artifactual because of overlaps in diagnostic criteria used for depression and anxiety disorders and because of the sedative effects on rating scales used to assess depression. Conversely, high doses of benzodiazepines may produce reversible side effects that are mistakenly interpreted as depression.

The scientific literature does not provide unequivocal support either for the use of benzodiazepines on the basis of their efficacy or for their condemnation because of potential toxicity. Patients whose pain appears to be of musculoskeletal origin may benefit from a 2- to 4-week course. Benzodiazepines should not be prescribed in large amounts that would permit dose escalation without professional supervision. A lack of treatment response or the onset of sedative side effects or depressive symptoms should prompt a dose reduction or drug discontinuation. If difficulties in sleep onset or duration are the primary complaint, consideration should be given to the use of a hypnotic benzodiazepine to minimize drug effects during the day. Patients who present with depressive symptoms should be further evaluated by a psychiatrist to rule out depression or other mood disorders. Antidepressant therapy, if indicated, should be pursued rather than prescribing a benzodiazepine with putative antidepressant properties.

Therapy with a benzodiazepine should not be extended beyond a few weeks. When a therapeutic course of a benzodiazepine and conservative therapy do not produce a therapeutic response, patients should be reevaluated rather than "managed" with long-term benzodiazepine treatment.

Muscle Relaxants

Drugs that are thought to reduce skeletal muscle tone are often administered to patients with chronic orofacial pain to help alleviate the increased muscle activity attributed to certain TMD subtypes. Muscle relaxants are thought to decrease muscle tone without impairment in motor function by acting centrally to depress polysynaptic reflexes. Other drugs with sedative properties also depress polysynaptic reflexes, making it difficult to differentiate between drugs that may be centrally acting muscle relaxants versus nonspecific sedatives that also produce muscle relaxation. Benzodiazepines (e.g., diazepam) are used in TMD partly on the basis of putative muscle relaxant properties, but they only decrease muscle tone at doses that produce unacceptable levels of CNS depression.

A critical review of *carisoprodol* and related propandiols concluded that they are better than placebo for acute musculoskeletal disorders but less effective for chronic conditions.[40] A possible exception to this generalization is *cyclobenzaprine* (Flexeril), which is effective in some chronic musculoskeletal disorders. Cyclobenzaprine is superior to placebo for pain in cervical and lumbar regions associated with skeletal muscle spasms and reduces electromyographic signs of muscle spasm.[41,42] Although cyclobenzaprine has not been directly assessed for TMDs, these findings suggest its efficacy for muscle relaxation in the orofacial region.

A discrepancy appears to exist between common clinical use of skeletal muscle relaxants and the results of controlled clinical trials evaluating their efficacy compared with placebo. It is also not clear whether they are specific for muscle relaxation or produce CNS depression, thereby reducing muscle tone. Little evidence exists for their efficacy in chronic orofacial pain of myogenic origin, and it has not been demonstrated that muscle relaxants provide additive effect with exercises or splint therapy aimed at muscle relaxation. Given this modest scientific support, use of muscle relaxants for decreasing muscle tone in patients with TMD should probably be limited to a brief trial in conjunction with physical therapy modalities.

Opioids

Administration of opioids for nonmalignant pain is controversial but may be considered for certain orofacial pain conditions, especially if other more conservative options have failed or if more surgery is likely to result in iatrogenic injury. Both open-label and double-blind studies demonstrate that oral opioids such as codeine and morphine result in significant analgesia, with no signs of respiratory depression but with an increased incidence of adverse events compared with placebo or an NSAID. Although patients with head and neck pain were included in these studies, no direct evaluation was made of long-term administration of opioids for TMD patients.

Most concern over the chronic use of opioids relates to the potential for "addiction," the maladaptive behaviors associated with illicit drug seeking. This term implies the development of physical dependence and tolerance requiring continued opioid use with increasing doses. Physical dependence or the development of tolerance in a therapeutic context does not necessarily equate with addictive behavior, and drug seeking is not necessary if the drug is medically available. Similarly, cycles of intoxication and withdrawal should not occur with sustained-release formulations.

The other major concern with prescribing opioids is the surveillance and additional record keeping required in some states. The long-term use of opioids in clinical practice was assessed in a survey of randomly selected physicians ($n = 1912$).[43,44] The results of this survey indicate that prescription of opioid for long-term administration is widespread for the treatment of nonmalignant chronic pain in medical practice. Surprisingly, physicians in states that require multiple copies of prescription forms indicated a greater frequency of opioid prescriptions, which suggests that drug regulations and surveillance are not barriers to the use of opioids in clinical practice.

Given the serious adverse effects associated with NSAIDs when given chronically and the absence of effective therapies for certain orofacial pain conditions, the use of opioids should be considered when more conservative measures have failed. Sustained-release formulations should minimize cyclic fluctuations in pain associated with standard-release formulations with short duration of action. The chronic use of opioids for patients with TMD requires careful patient selection to rule out drug-seeking behavior or other personality disorders, careful monitoring to individualize dose and minimize side effects and dose escalation, and careful attention to regulatory procedures.

Antidepressants

Antidepressant drugs have been used for more than 30 years for the management of pain from a wide variety of conditions, including orofacial pain. Three independent reviews of controlled studies of the use of antidepressants for pain management indicate that the analgesic effects are largely independent of antidepressant activity.[45,46] The analgesic effects can be differentiated from placebo, are seen at doses lower than those usually effective in depression, and can occur in patients who are not depressed. In studies of patients with nondental chronic pain, primarily those with diabetes and postherpetic neuropathy, drugs that inhibit reuptake of both serotonin and norepinephrine, such as amitriptyline, are more efficacious than drugs that are selective for either neurotransmitter.[47,48]

Evidence that antidepressants produce analgesia independent of the alleviation of depression comes from studies with low doses of amitriptyline in patients with chronic pain. A low dose of amitriptyline (mean dose, 24 mg) was as effective for chronic orofacial pain as a higher dose (mean, 129 mg) in the range of the usual daily antidepressant dose (75 to 150 mg).[49] A daily dose of 25 mg of amitriptyline for 3 weeks was superior to placebo in a variety of patients with chronic nonmalignant pain.[50] A dose-response comparison of 25, 50, and 75 mg of amitriptyline demonstrated increased analgesia with increasing dose, improved sleep with the 75-mg dose, but a significantly higher incidence of adverse effects at the 75-mg dose.[51] Another study also reported analgesia with 75 mg of amitriptyline and improved sleep over 6 weeks.[52] If antidepressants produced therapeutic effects solely through alleviation of depression, the doses used in these studies would be similar to those needed for depression.

The biomedical literature,[44-52] the United States Pharmacopeia Drug Information (USPDI),[53] and the National Institutes of Health Technology Assessment Conference Statement[54] support the clinical use of antidepressants for treatment of neuropathic pain, for chronic nonmalignant pain when other treatments have failed, or if depression accompanies the pain. Tricyclic antidepressants with both serotonergic and noradrenergic effects (e.g., amitriptyline, doxepin) appear to be most effective. Lower dosages (25 to 75 mg) should be used initially for undepressed patients. Antidepressant doses are reserved for depressed patients and are best prescribed in consultation with a clinician experienced in the diagnosis and treatment of psychiatric illness. Sedative-antidepressants may be useful when patients have sleeping problems and may help to reduce the dose of other hypnotic drugs.

The dose of antidepressant will usually be limited by anticholinergic side effects (e.g., dry mouth, constipation, blurred vision, urinary retention) and should be adjusted in response to individual variation in analgesic response and side effects. Cardiovascular effects range from postural hypotension to serious ventricular arrhythmias, especially in patients with preexisting heart disease; medical consultation or parallel management is advisable in patients at risk.

Drugs for Neuropathic Pain

A wide spectrum of drug classes have been used for the treatment of neuropathic disorders. Anticonvulsant medications have been reported to provide effective treatments for many orofacial pain disorders (e.g., trigeminal neuralgia) and related pain disorders (e.g., migraine). Additionally, the use of N-methyl-D-aspartate (NMDA) receptor antagonists may provide a new line of therapy for orofacial pain. Although most of these drug classes are used in the treatment of other neuropathic disorders, their use in the treatment of orofacial pain has not been systematically evaluated, and no evidence is available on their use in the treatment of early-onset TMD pain. As TMD pain persists, however, CNS changes may occur (central plasticity), making use of these medications a therapeutic option.

Carbamazepine. Pharmacologic treatment of trigeminal neuralgia has remained relatively unchanged for the past 10 years. Carbamazepine (Tegretol) remains the treatment of choice and is diagnostic for this disorder.[55,56] Although efficacious in most patients, carbamazepine has some rare, potentially life-threatening side effects (aplastic anemia, hepatic effects) that warrant careful monitoring of these patients. It is necessary to obtain baseline blood tests to evaluate hepatic and renal function and blood cell counts before initiating carbamazepine therapy.

Baclofen and Phenytoin. Other common medications used for the treatment of trigeminal neuralgia are baclofen (Lioresal) and phenytoin (Dilantin). Baclofen, a gamma-aminobutyric acid (GABA) agonist, can be considered an alternative first-line drug in patients with preexisting hematologic abnormalities or when frequent blood monitoring is unavailable or impractical.[57] Phenytoin has been used as a second-line medication in refractory cases or in patients who cannot tolerate carbamazepine or baclofen.

Gabapentin. Gabapentin represents a new generation of drug originally developed as an antiepileptic agent but also studied as an analgesic for chronic conditions. Although structurally similar to the inhibitory neurotransmitter GABA, the mechanism of action for pain inhibition is still unknown. The use of gabapentin for a variety of disorders, including epilepsy, movement disorders, migraine prophylaxis, and chronic pain, suggests a nonspecific mechanism. Benefits of gabapentin include low toxicity, favorable side effect profile, and good patient tolerance compared with other anticonvulsants (e.g., carbamazepine).[58] These attributes make gabapentin a suitable candidate for management of chronic pain disorders such as trigeminal neuralgia.

Numerous placebo-controlled, double-blind studies demonstrate the effectiveness of gabapentin on pain reduction and quality of life for patients with postherpetic neuralgia and diabetic neuropathies.[59,60] Only a limited number of studies have evaluated the use of gabapentin for the treatment of trigeminal neuralgia (Table 23-2). None, however, can be considered a prospective, double-blind, or placebo-controlled study, so the true therapeutic value of gabapentin is uncertain. Gabapentin may be considered as a single treatment agent for patients with trigeminal neuralgia who cannot tolerate the untoward effects of the first-line medications (carbamazepine, baclofen) and as an adjuvant agent for use with these drugs.

NMDA Receptor Antagonists. Extensive animal data and more limited results of clinical trials suggest that drugs blocking the effects of excitatory amino acids at the NMDA receptor interfere with the development and maintenance of central hyperalgesia.[61,62] In a double-blind, placebo-controlled crossover study comparing the effects of dextromethorphan in patients with either postherpetic neuralgia or diabetic neuropathy, dextromethorphan significantly reduced pain in the diabetic neuropathy group but not the postherpetic neuralgia group, compared with placebo.[63] Although several studies have demonstrated the effectiveness of NMDA receptor antagonists in the reduction and treatment of chronic pain,[64-66] their use is limited primarily because of the intolerability of their side effects, including sedation, dizziness, dissociative effects, nausea, and visual disturbances.[67] NMDA receptor antagonists may be useful when

TABLE 23-2

Studies on Gabapentin Treatment for Trigeminal Neuralgia (TGN) and Multiple Sclerosis (MS)

Study	Type	n	Population	Dose (mg/day)	Results
Sist et al (1997)	Case report	2 TGN	Unable to tolerate other medications	900-2400	Reduction of pain from severe (8-10/10) to mild (0-1/10)
Merren (1998)	Prospective, open label, not placebo controlled	5 TGN 2 MS-TGN	Patients from private neurology practice	600-2400	Excellent improvement for TGN patients; no to mild improvement for MS-TGN patients
Solaro et al (1998)	Prospective, open label, not placebo controlled	6 MS-TGN	Patients from neurologic center	600-1200	5 of 6 subjects had complete pain remission
Khan	Prospective, open label, not placebo controlled	7 MS-TGN	Previous drug treatment failure	900-2400	6 of 7 subjects had complete pain remission; 5 were taking other medications
Solaro et al (2000)	Prospective, open label, not placebo controlled	11 MS-TGN	Combination of carbamazepine + gabapentin *or* lamotrigine + gabapentin	300-1200	Dose reduction of other anticonvulsants; decrease in pain report
Eckhardt et al (2000)	Randomized, placebo-controlled, double-blind	12 normal subjects	Comparison of gabapentin/ morphine vs gabapentin/ placebo vs morphine/placebo vs placebo/placebo	600	Significant increase in pain tolerance with gabapentin/ morphine group to other groups

combined with opioids, since there appears to be a synergistic effect in reducing pain and a decrease in the development of tolerance to the opioid.[68-70] This strategy may be useful in patients who did not respond to TMJ surgery and whose only treatment options are limited to use of high doses of opioids.

Despite the scientific literature supporting the use of anticonvulsants for the treatment of pain, most studies do not provide well-controlled clinical data to support anticonvulsants for treatment of TMD, which are primarily arthritic and muscular in origin. It is increasingly recognized, however, that secondary central changes occur as these conditions become chronic. Central activation and changes may follow a focal TMJ injury and contribute to the long-lasting symptoms reported by these patients.[71] Acute inflammation of the TMJ in animal models produces central activation of immediate early genes, including *c-fos*, and can provide a pathway for development of chronic pain.[72] TMD patients may experience a spreading, lancinating, or burning pain associated with a neuropathic component. These patients should not be classified simply as TMD patients; rather, they fall in the broader classification of patients with orofacial pain. In patients who develop these secondary changes, appropriate use of an anticonvulsant or NMDA antagonist may be beneficial, as outlined earlier.

Therapeutic Recommendations

Review of the drug classes most often used for TMD and other chronic orofacial pain reveals few data on which to base therapy. Given the potential for serious toxicity that can accompany long-term administration of drugs that are safe enough to be marketed without a prescription (e.g., NSAIDs), some drug classes may be associated with risks to the patient without therapeutic benefits. A need exists for well-controlled studies of drugs for TMD and related orofacial pain in the relevant patient population, for a duration of administration that approximates their use clinically, with appropriate indices of therapeutic efficacy and toxicity, and with groups that control for cyclic fluctuations in symptoms. In the interim, clinicians should consider the use of many drug classes for TMD as invalidated clinical practices and limit treatment to short trials subject to some evidence of clinical efficacy and with careful attention to potential adverse events.

The decision to use a traditional NSAID or one of the newer selective COX-2 inhibitors is first predicated on whether *any* NSAID is appropriate therapy. In a patient with a high risk for gastropathy, COX-2 selective NSAIDs provide a useful alternative to combination therapy with a gastroprotective drug and a nonselective NSAID. When treating inflammation associated with TMD, the NSAIDs and selective COX-2 inhibitors should be considered based on proven efficacy in the oral surgery model and for both RA and OA. A short trial of celecoxib or rofecoxib may be considered for patients with TMJ synovitis, capsulitis, or acute flare of TMJ osteoarthritis. Whether a nonselective NSAID or a COX-2 selective inhibitor is prescribed, close monitoring is important to ensure patient safety.

Pain primarily of musculoskeletal origin is best managed by physical medicine procedures (see Chapter 24), possibly with a short trial of a muscle relaxant or benzodiazepine. As with many other chronic pain conditions, low doses (10 to 75 mg/day) of tricyclic antidepressants may be considered for patients with musculoskeletal pain, particularly those who are mildly depressed or have sleep disturbances. In these patients it becomes necessary to consult with the appropriate physician to comanage the patient's needs.

The use of antidepressants and anticonvulsants provides effective treatments for many orofacial pain disorders, including various neuropathies (e.g., diabetic, trigeminal), muscle disorders (e.g., myofascial pain, fibromyalgia), and related pain disorders (e.g., migraine). Use of NMDA receptor antagonists also may provide a new line of pharmacotherapy or adjuvant therapy for orofacial pain patients. Although most of these drug classes are routinely used in the treatment of neuropathic disorders, their use in the treatment of TMD has not been systematically evaluated, and no evidence is available on the treatment of early-onset TMD pain.

The decision to treat complex orofacial neuropathic pain patient depends on the clinician's knowledge, training, experience, and comfort with diagnosing and managing these patients. The clinician can treat with medication or make a referral to the appropriate specialist, either a dentist with advanced training in orofacial pain or a neurologist. In either case it is important to recognize signs and symptoms that require immediate evaluation and referral, including presentation of new, unusual, systemic, and unresolved or worsening symptoms. The clinician must also consider that many medications (e.g., carbamazepine) require careful management and monitoring through the course of treatment. The choice of medications is based on presenting symptoms, the patient's history, systemic conditions, and general logistical considerations. These are merely guidelines, since each patient's treatment response may vary, and the clinical presentation of TMD must be assessed individually.

For patients in whom other therapeutic modalities have failed or a specific treatment is not readily apparent, such as those with failed TMJ implants or multiple surgeries, a trial with an opioid should be considered. Although concerns for the development of tolerance and dependence need to be considered, opioids may represent a more favorable therapeutic ratio than risk of iatrogenic injury from further surgery or experimentation with nonvalidated or irrational clinical practices.

References

1. Ta LE, Phero JC, Pillemer SR, et al: Evaluation of patients with TMJ implants, Submitted for publication.
2. Magnusson T, Egermark-Eriksson I, Carlson GE: Five-year longitudinal study of signs and symptoms of mandibular dysfunction in adolescents, *J Craniomandibular Pract* 4:338-353, 1986.
3. Speculand B, Goss AN, Hughes A, et al: Temporomandibular joint dysfunction: pain and illness behavior, *Pain* 17:139-150, 1983.

4. Antczak-Bouckoms A: Reaction paper to chapters 12 and 13. In Sessle BJ, Bryant P, Dionne RA, editors: *Temporomandibular disorders and related pain conditions,* Seattle, 1995, IASP Press.

5. Singer EJ, Dionne RA: A controlled evaluation of diazepam and ibuprofen for chronic orofacial muscle pain, *J Orofac Pain* 11:139-146, 1997.

6. Gordon SM, Montgomery MT, Jones D: Comparative efficacy of piroxicam versus placebo for temporomandibular pain (abstract), *J Dent Res* 69:218, 1990.

7. Walker JS, Lockton AI, Nguyen TV, et al: Analgesic effect of ibuprofen after single and multiple doses in chronic spinal pain patients, *Analgesia* 2:93-101, 1996.

8. Walker JS, Levy G: Effect of multiple dosing on the analgesic actions of diflunisal in rats, *Life Sci* 46:737-742, 1990.

9. Rainsford KD: Review of published clinical trial data on the adverse reactions from ibuprofen and paracetamol/ acetaminophen at OTC dosages. In Rainsford KD, Powanda MD, editors: *Safety and efficacy of non-prescription (OTC) analgesics and NSAIDs,* London, 1999, Kluwer Academic Publishers.

10. Yamagata K, Andreasson KI, et al: Expression of a mitogen-inducible cyclooxygenase in brain neurons: regulation by synaptic activity and glucocorticoids, *Neuron* 11(2):371-386, 1993.

11. Komhoff MH, Grone HL, et al: Localization of cyclooxygenase-1 and -2 in adult and fetal human kidney: implication for renal function, *Am J Physiol* 272(4, pt 2):F460-F468, 1997.

12. Masferrer JL, Zweifel BS, et al: Selective inhibition of inducible cyclooxygenase 2 in vivo is antiinflammatory and nonulcerogenic, *Proc Natl Acad Sci USA* 91(8):3228-3232, 1994.

13. Seibert K, Zhang Y, et al: Pharmacological and biochemical demonstration of the role of cyclooxygenase 2 in inflammation and pain, *Proc Natl Acad Sci USA* 91(25):12013-12017, 1994.

14. Crofford LJ: Expression and regulation of cyclooxygenase-2 in synovial tissues of arthritic patients. In Bazan N, Botting J, Vane J, editors: *New targets in inflammation: inhibitors of COX-2 or adhesion molecules,* New York, 1996, Kluwer/ Harvey.

15. Kang RY, Freire-Moar J, et al: Expression of cyclooxygenase-2 in human and an animal model of rheumatoid arthritis, *Br J Rheumatol* 35(8):711-718, 1996.

16. Laird JM, Herrero JF, et al: Analgesic activity of the novel COX-2 preferring NSAID, meloxicam, in mono-arthritic rats: central and peripheral components, *Inflamm Res* 46(6):203-210, 1997.

17. Taniguchi Y, Yokoyama K, et al: Inhibition of brain cyclo-oxygenase-2 activity and the antipyretic action of nimesulide, *Eur J Pharmacol* 330(2-3):221-229, 1997.

18. Zhang M, Wang JL, et al: Cyclooxygenase-2 in rat nephron development, *Am J Physiol* 273(6, pt 2):F994-F1002, 1997.

19. Kaufmann WE, Worley PF, et al: COX-2, a synaptically induced enzyme, is expressed by excitatory neurons at post-synaptic sites in rat cerebral cortex, *Proc Natl Acad Sci USA* 93(6):2317-2321, 1996.

20. Lim HB, Paria BC, et al: Multiple female reproductive failures in cyclooxygenase 2-deficient mice, *Cell* 91(2):197-208, 1997.

21. Chakraborty I, Das SK et al: Developmental expression of the cyclo-oxygenase-1 and cyclo-oxygenase-2 genes in the peri-implantation mouse uterus and their differential regulation by the blastocyst and ovarian steroids, *J Mol Endocrinol* 16(2):107-22, 1996.

22. Kawaguchi HC, Pilbeam CC, et al: The role of prostaglandins in the regulation of bone metabolism, *Clin Orthop* 313:36-46, 1995.

23. Cohn SM, Schloeman S, et al: Crypt stem cell survival in the mouse intestinal epithelium is regulated by prostaglandins synthesized through cyclooxygenase-1, *J Clin Invest* 99(6):1367-1379, 1997.

24. Lipsky PE, Isakson PC: Outcome of specific COX-2 inhibition in rheumatoid arthritis, *J Rheumatol* 24(suppl 49):9-14, 1997.

25. Leese PT, Hubbard RC, et al: Effects of celecoxib, a novel cyclooxygenase-2 inhibitor, on platelet function in healthy adults: a randomized, controlled trial, *J Clin Pharmacol* 40(2):124-132, 2000.

26. Simon LS, Lanza FL, et al: Preliminary study of the safety and efficacy of SC-58635, a novel cyclooxygenase 2 inhibitor: efficacy and safety in two placebo-controlled trials in osteoarthritis and rheumatoid arthritis, and studies of gastrointestinal and platelet effects, *Arthritis Rheum* 41(9):1591-1602, 1998.

27. Simon LS, Weaver AL, Graham DL, et al: Anti-inflammatory and upper gastrointestinal effects of celecoxib in rheumatoid arthritis: a randomized controlled trial, *JAMA* 282(20):1921-1928, 1999.

28. Bensen WG, Fiechtner JJ, et al: Treatment of osteoarthritis with celecoxib, a cyclooxygenase-2 inhibitor: a randomized controlled trial, *Mayo Clin Proc* 74(11):1095-1105, 1999.

29. Goldstein JL, Silverstein FE, et al: Reduced risk of upper gastrointestinal ulcer complications with celecoxib, a novel COX-2 inhibitor, *Am J Gastroenterol* 95(7):1681-1690, 2000.

30. Chan CC, Boyce S, et al: Rofecoxib: pharmacological and biochemical profiles, *J Pharmacol Exp Ther* 290(2):551-560, 1999.

31. Depre ME, Ehrich E, et al: Pharmacokinetics, COX-2 specificity, and tolerability of supratherapeutic doses of rofecoxib in humans, *Eur J Clin Pharmacol* 56(2):167-174, 2000.

32. Day R, Morrison B, et al: A randomized trial of the efficacy and tolerability of the COX-2 inhibitor rofecoxib vs ibuprofen in patients with osteoarthritis, Rofecoxib/ Ibuprofen Comparator Study Group, *Arch Intern Med* 160(12):1781-1787, 2000.

33. Cannon GW, Caldwell JR, et al: Rofecoxib: results of a one-year, randomized, clinical trial in patients with osteoarthritis of the knee and hip, Rofecoxib Phase III Protocol 035 Study Group, *Arthritis Rheum* 43(5):978-987, 2000.

34. Hawkey CL et al: Comparison of the effect of rofecoxib (a cyclooxygenase 2 inhibitor), ibuprofen, and placebo on the gastroduodenal mucosa of patients with osteoarthritis, *Arthritis Rheum* 43(2):370-377, 2000.

35. Schmassmann A: Mechanisms of ulcer healing and effects of nonsteroidal anti-inflammatory drugs, *Am J Med* 104(3A): 43S-51S, 79S-80S, 1998.

36. Reid KI, Dionne RA, Sicard-Rosenbaum L, et al: Evaluation of iontophoretically applied dexamethasone for painful pathologic temporomandibular joints, *Oral Surg Oral Med Oral Pathol* 77:605-609, 1994.

37. Harkins S, Linford J, Cohen J, et al: Administration of clonazepam in the treatment of TMD and associated myofascial pain: a double-blind pilot study, *J Craniom Disord* 5:179-186, 1991.

38. Russell IJ, Fletcher EM, Michalek JE, et al: Treatment of primary fibrositis/fibromyalgia syndrome with ibuprofen and alprazolam, *Arthritis Rheum* 34:552-560, 1991.

39. Dellemijn PJ, Fields HL: Do benzodiazepines have a role in chronic pain management? *Pain* 57:137-152, 1994.

40. Elenbaas JK: Centrally acting oral skeletal muscle muscle relaxants, *Am J Hosp Pharm* 37:1313-23, 1980.

41. Brown BR, Womble J: Cyclobenzaprine in intractable pain syndromes with muscle spasm, *JAMA* 240:1151-1152, 1978.

42. Basmajiam JV: Cyclobenzaprine hydrochloride effect on skeletal muscle spasm in the lumbar region and neck: two double-blind controlled clinical and laboratory studies, *Arch Phys Med Rehabil* 59:58-63, 1978.

43. Turk DC, Brody MC, Okifuji EA: Physicians' attitudes and practices regarding the long-term prescribing of opioids for non-cancer pain, *Pain* 59:201-208, 1994.

44. Magni G: The use of antidepressants in the treatment of chronic pain, *Drugs* 42:730-738, 1991.

45. Egbunike IG, Chaffee BJ: Antidepressants in the management of chronic pain syndromes, *Pharmacotherapy* 10:262-270, 1990.

46. Onghena P, Van Houdenhove B: Antidepressant-induced analgesia in chronic nonmalignant pain: a metanalysis of 39 placebo-controlled studies, *Pain* 42:205-219, 1992.

47. Max MB, Culnane M, Schafer SC, et al: Amitriptyline relieves diabetic neuropathy pain in patients with normal or depressed mood, *Neurology* 37:589-596, 1987.

48. Max MB, Gilron I: Antidepressants, muscle relaxants, and NMDA receptor antagonists. In Loeser JD, editor, *Bonica's The Management of Pain*, ed 3, Philadephia, 2000, Lippincott-Williams & Wilkins.

49. Sharav Y, Singer E, Schmidt E, et al: The analgesic effect of amitriptyline on chronic facial pain, *Pain* 31:199-209, 1987.

50. McQuay HJ, Carroll D, Glynn CJ: Low dose amitrptyline in the treatment of chronic pain, *Anaesthesia* 47:646-652, 1992.

51. McQuay HJ, Carroll D, Glynn CJ: Dose-response for analgesic effect of amitriptyline in chronic pain, *Anaesthesia* 48:281-285, 1993.

52. Zitman FG, Linssen ACG, Edelbroek PM: Low dose amitriptyline in chronic pain: the gain is modest, *Pain* 42:35-42, 1990.

53. US Pharmacopeial Convention: *Tricyclic antidepressants*, Micromedex, 2000, Englewood, Colorado.

54. National Institutes of Health Technology Assessment Conference Statement: Management of temporomandibular disorders, *J Am Dent Assoc* 127:1595-1603, 1996.

55. Fields HL: Treatment of trigeminal neuralgia [editorial comment], *N Engl J Med* 334:1125-1126, 1996.

56. Sweet WH: The treatment of trigeminal neuralgia (tic douloureux), *N Engl J Med,* 315:174-177, 1996.

57. Fromm GH: Baclofen as an adjuvant analgesic, *J Pain Symptom Manage* 9:500-509, 1994.

58. Magnus L: Nonepileptic uses of gabapentin, *Epilepsia* 40:S66-74, 1999.

59. Backonja M, Beydoun A, Edwards KR, et al: Gabapentin for the symptomatic treatment of painful neuropathy in patients with diabetes mellitus: a randomized controlled trial [see comments], *JAMA* 280:1831-1836, 1998.

60. Rowbotham M, Harden N, Stacey B, et al: Gabapentin for the treatment of postherpetic neuralgia: a randomized controlled trial [see comments], *JAMA* 280:1837-1842, 1998.

61. Mao J, Price DD, Hayes RL, et al: Intrathecal treatment with dextrorphan or ketamine potently reduces pain-related behaviors in a rat model of peripheral mononeuropathy, *Brain Res* 605:164-168, 1993.

62. Tal M, Bennett GJ: Dextrorphan relieves neuropathic heat-evoked hyperalgesia in the rat, *Neurosci Lett* 151:107-110, 1993.

63. Nelson KA, Park KM, Robinovitz E, et al: High-dose oral dextromethorphan versus placebo in painful diabetic neuropathy and postherpetic neuralgia, *Neurology* 48:1212-1218, 1997.

64. Backonja M, Arndt G, Gombar KA, et al: Response of chronic neuropathic pain syndromes to ketamine: a preliminary study [published erratum appears in *Pain* 58(3): 433, 1994], *Pain* 56:51-57, 1994.

65. Felsby S, Nielsen J, Arendt-Nielsen L, et al: NMDA receptor blockade in chronic neuropathic pain: a comparison of ketamine and magnesium chloride, *Pain* 64:283-291, 1996.

66. McQuay HJ, Carroll D, Jadad AR, et al: Dextromethorphan for the treatment of neuropathic pain: a double-blind randomised controlled crossover trial with integral n-of-1 design, *Pain* 59:127-133, 1994.

67. Hewitt DJ: The use of NMDA-receptor antagonists in the treatment of chronic pain, *Clin J Pain* 16:S73-79, 2000.

68. Advokat C, Rhein FQ: Potentiation of morphine-induced antinociception in acute spinal rats by the NMDA antagonist dextrorphan, *Brain Res* 699:157-160, 1995.

69. Katz NP: MorphiDex (MS:DM) double-blind, multiple-dose studies in chronic pain patients, *J Pain Symptom Manage* 19:S37-41, 2000.

70. Trujillo KA, Akil H: Inhibition of opiate tolerance by noncompetitive N-methyl-D-aspartate receptor antagonists, *Brain Res* 633:178-188, 1994.

71. Bereiter DA, Bereiter DF: Morphine and NMDA receptor antagonism reduce c-fos expression in spinal trigeminal nucleus produced by acute injury to the TMJ region, *Pain* 85:65-77, 2000.

72. Bereiter DA, Benetti AP: Excitatory amino release within spinal trigeminal nucleus after mustard oil injection into the temporomandibular joint region of the rat, *Pain* 67:451-459, 1996.

Physical Medicine for Masticatory Pain and Dysfunction

GLENN T. CLARK

CHAPTER OUTLINE

When a patient exhibits pain or dysfunction of the masticatory musculature and temporomandibular joints (TMJs), this is globally described as a *temporomandibular disorder* (TMD). The myriad of problems that can cause TMDs are generally categorized into four subgroups: disc derangements, arthritic disease, muscle disorders, and uncommon presentations[1-4] (Tables 24-1 to 24-4). Even though these subgroups have clear and distinctly different mechanisms, all are treated with some form of physical medicine in addition to the pharmacologic and surgical therapies indicated. Because many patients do not want or cannot tolerate medications, or because they have a less severe problem, physical medicine methods are often first-line treatments. Physical medicine modalities can also be used to supplement pharmacologic therapies and closed-joint or open-joint surgical interventions as well. For example, acute joint hypomobility may be caused by masticatory muscle dysfunction (e.g., trismus) or disc derangement (e.g., displacement without reduction). For both disorders, treatment will involve stretching of the jaw to increase opening.

This chapter defines the scope of physical medicine treatments and provides available evidence in assessing their efficacy for TMDs.

The broad categories of physical medicine methods used for treating TMDs are (1) general instruction about limited function and rest/exercise, (2) mobilization and manipulation for hypomobile jaw muscles and TMJ locking problems, (3) active physical therapy modalities for arthromyogenous disorders of the jaw, (4) muscle injections (including trigger points) for arthromyogenous jaw disorders, (5) counterstimulation methods for chronic orofacial pain symptoms, (6) orthotic devices (occlusal appliances) used to modify oral habits and bruxism, and (7) injectable agents for joint lubrication, patient mobilization, and pain relief.

General Instructions about Limited Function and Rest/Exercise

Depending on the nature of the TMD, different self-directed treatments can be used. Such instruction or "advice" is given for TMJ clicking, recurrent open locking of the jaw, myalgia and trismus disorder of the jaw, and joint pain due to inflammation and arthritic disease of the TMJ.

Temporomandibular Joint Clicking

Education about the need to avoid this frictional event during function is essential to reducing the likelihood of progression of a painless click to a painful click with dysfunction. This approach is called *avoidance therapy* and involves three components. First, show the patient how limiting the degree of jaw opening and protrusion generally stops translation and TMJ clicking. This is best done with a plastic model of jaw joint. Second, inform the patient that chewing on same side of the click usually helps avoid it. Provide some gum so the patient can test (under your observation) this assertion. Third, educate the

TABLE 24-1

Disorders of the Masticatory Muscles

Disorder	Primary Signs	Alternative Terms
Myalgia	Pain	Myofascial pain, fibrositis, fibromyalgia
Myositis	Swelling	Muscle effusion, muscle edema
Trismus/myospasm	Limited opening	Bracing, splinting, protective guarding

TABLE 24-2

Derangements of the Temporomandibular Joint

Disorder	Primary Signs	Alternative Terms
D/C incoordination	Joint noise	Clicking, disc displacement with reduction
D/C restriction	Cannot open	Disc displacement without reduction, closed locking
Dislocation	Cannot close	Condyle displacement
Open locking	Cannot close	Open condyle jamming, TMJ subluxation
Partial open locking	Cannot close	Posterior disc displacement

D/C, Disc-condyle.

TABLE 24-3

Arthritic Disease of the Temporomandibular Joint

Disorder	Primary Signs	Alternative Terms
Arthralgia/arthritis	Pain	Capsulitis, synovitis
Osteoarthritis	Pain/noises	Degenerative joint disease
Polyarthritis	Pain/noises	Various types

TABLE 24-4

Uncommon Disorders of the Temporomandibular Joint

Disorder	Primary Signs	Alternative Terms
Growth disorders	Facial asymmetry	Hyperplasias and hypoplasias, hypertrophy and atrophy
Mobility disorders	Either limited or excessive jaw motion	Contracture, ankylosis, hypermobility, and extracapsular restrictions
Motor disorders	Involuntary movement or contraction	Myospasm, dyskinesias, dystonias, tics, tremors, myoclonus, bruxism

patient that a diet change to small bites and soft food will be necessary to avoid the click. Strict avoidance of all clicking and all gum chewing is required. The patient must understand that this approach will not stop clicking, only reduce the number of times the disc is jammed between the condyle and eminence, thus reducing wear and tear of these tissues.

In 1959, Schwartz[5] first advocated this type of avoidance approach to help reduce TMJ clicking. Unfortunately, the efficacy of this approach is not established by randomized controlled trials (RCTs). A prospective case-series study on adults applied strict avoidance of the persistent click and reported that this method was ineffective at eliminating clicking phenomena in the jaw joints.[6] In contrast, another study used a much younger patient population with recent-onset TMJ clicking. The authors evaluated the effect of jaw hinge exercises on clicking and reported that this exercise helped eliminate the click.[7] The degree to which spontaneous remission occurred in the latter report is not known. This avoidance approach seems empirically logical and may be a reasonable treatment alternative for a patient with a persistent TMJ click. Results of most longitudinal observational studies suggest that most clicking patterns do not change in prevalence for a given population but rather "come and go" in individuals.[8,9] Data suggests that only a few patients with "joint noises" will ever develop a serious TMJ locking or degenerative joint disease.

Open Locking

After the patient's lock is reduced and joint imaging has demonstrated that the joint is not deformed or arthritic, the simplest treatment approach is to suggest that the patient practice avoiding all forms of wide-open mouth movement. This generally involves instructing the patient to flex the head forward when yawning and to avoid eating foods that require wide mouth opening. A final avoidance strategy is to instruct the patient to use a rubber bite block between the teeth during dental treatment. With a bite block the patient can use the jaw closers to hold the jaw open and therefore stabilize the joint and better avoid overstretching.

Myalgia and Trismus

If the patient has masticatory muscle pain with or without trismus, and if the pain seems to be caused by repeated parafunctional behaviors (e.g., clench-

ing, facial tension habits, nocturnal bruxism), the TMD is managed with a series of tongue and jaw posture exercises. These exercises involve two primary methods. In the *"n" position exercise* the patient holds the jaw and tongue for a count of 10 in the position achieved when saying the letter "n." The patient is instructed to perform this exercise hourly each day (or 12 times a day). The goal is to put and hold the jaw in the most relaxed jaw position where the teeth are apart and the lips not touching.

Once the patient's initial pain symptoms are reduced, the *jaw coordination exercise* involves instructing the patient (using mirror feedback) to move the jaw carefully along a border pathway to a maximum lateral position. Once achieved, this position is held for 3 seconds; the patient then retraces the motion back into ICP. This is done three times to the right and the left and is also done hourly (or 12 times a day). This exercise tests the patient's ability to selectively activate some jaw muscles but not others.

The third exercise is instruction in proper *upper body mechanics.* This involves training the patient how to keep the head, neck, and shoulders in an upright, "non-slumped-forward" posture. The primary motion needed to do the exercise is to pull both hands back over the top of the shoulders while keeping the elbows close to the side of the chest. Then the patient pulls the chin back, extending the neck fully. Both exercises and postural instruction are provided on how to correct postural defects of the head-neck-shoulder complex.

Patients who have stiffness and reduced pain-free motions of the jaw and/or the neck are shown how to effectively stretch out stiff and shortened cervical and jaw muscles. For the patient who has a trismus diagnosis (confirmed by a reduced active opening, which can substantially increase with passive stretching), a series of home-based exercises for neck and jaw stretching must be developed. Correctly used, these gentle-to-moderate stretching exercises will be helpful in remobilizing the jaw and neck and keeping the patient aware of orofacial habits. It is always advisable to follow these exercises with 20 minutes of heat therapy (hot towels, moist heating pad) applied to the sorest muscles. Heat helps to reduce pain and stiffness by relaxing aching muscles and increasing circulation to the area.

Although these methods have been described in many textbooks and review articles,[10-14] no RCTs have been performed to compare the effectiveness of these exercises versus a no-treatment approach for acute-onset masticatory myalgia and myositis.

Despite this, these methods are often prescribed to provide symptomatic treatment for acute muscle pain problems because they are both logical and common-sense approaches to self-applied therapy.

Joint Pain

When the TMJ is inflamed and tender, initial therapies include (1) jaw rest, (2) soft-food diet, and (3) nonsteroidal antiinflammatory drugs (NSAIDs).[15,16] In addition, the patient should conduct joint hinge-motion exercises but avoid a wide range of opening motions to prevent further injury to a fragile joint.[17-19] The hinge-motion exercise is not traumatic because it involves a short-arc opening and closing of the jaw without translation. The movement is performed 10 times and should be done hourly each day during the treatment period. The primary purpose of this exercise is to disrupt jaw tension and clenching patterns and to pump synovial fluid into the joint spaces over the articular surfaces.

When the joint has undergone substantial arthrotic remodeling change, and when moderate-to-extensive crepitation is evident with motion, the patient is usually placed on a limited-function program. At a minimum the program includes (1) periodic recall for monitoring of further joint and occlusal changes; (2) continued hinge-motion exercises and, if strong bruxism or clenching is present or an unstable occlusion exists, use of an occlusal appliance at night to provide a stable bite during nocturnal clenching episodes; (3) pain-modulating medications; (4) thorough explanation of necessary dietary limitations; and (6) discussion of long-term occlusal effects of progressive joint remodeling and adaptation.

The hinge-motion exercise and limited-function protocol are both reasonable and logical, but no RCTs have tested the validity or efficacy of these methods relative to other approaches. Nonpharmacologic physical medicine procedures have not been reported to reverse or stop any polyarthritic joint disease process. Patients with intraarticular osseous changes often avoid movement of the involved joint.

Mobilization and Manipulation for Hypomobility and Jaw Locking

The manual therapy selected depends on the TMD category. Manual therapy is used for jaw muscle tightness caused by acute trismus, sustained (nonreducing) open locking of the jaw, acute closed

locking of the jaw, chronic contracture of the jaw, and immediate postsurgical passive motion devices.

Trismus and Splinting

Because a trismus must be considered as one explanation for the loss of active mouth-opening ability, a diagnostic procedure called the *passive stretch test* is the first step in treatment. The passive stretch test is performed by either spraying the masseter and temporalis muscles with a vapocoolant spray (fluormethane) or rubbing the jaw muscles with ice. The induced cutaneous chilling helps transiently block the protective muscle-guarding response, which prevents opening. In the second step the examiner stretches the jaw opening by applying a mild-to-moderate force (approximately 1 kg of pressure) between the maxillary and mandibular teeth with the fingers. If a muscular-induced limitation is present, jaw opening will increase to a normal distance; this result implies a diagnosis of trismus. For patients who demonstrate increased movement, other treatment procedures are recommended, as discussed next.

Trismus and splinting of the masticatory muscles result in a decreased range of voluntary jaw opening.[20] Limited mandibular movements may also result from nonmuscular causes. For this discussion, however, decreased range of mandibular movement is assumed to be a protective reflex induced during opening in which jaw-opening muscles are inhibited and jaw-closing muscles are excited.

A common physical medicine approach for patients with complaints of trismus is application of ice or vapocoolant spray to the skin over the painful muscle, followed by stretching of the involved muscles.[21-23] Except as a diagnostic test, this approach is not typically recommended for acute (less than 5 days) trismus caused by a recent injury or trauma. If the patient's condition is caused by acute psychological distress, this etiology must be addressed by a psychologist.[24] In most patients, acute traumatic trismus and hysterical trismus are self-limiting and resolve in 7 to 14 days as the injury heals or the emotional crisis passes.

Posttraumatic trismus is usually easily recognized since the patient is fully aware of the injury and its acute onset. Any unresolved trismus can produce a chronic restriction of movement, which is caused by long-term shortening of the unmoving muscle and joint tissues. Occasionally, trismus is caused by a strong emotional reaction, such as that seen in catatonia. *Hysterical trismus* usually is not treated by physical medicine but rather with behavioral and pharmacologic methods (see later discussion).

Advocates of vapocoolant spray and stretch procedures claim that stretching helps alleviate chronic myofascial pain and dysfunction by desensitizing the *trigger point* in the muscle.[25] Although the mechanism is not known, the clinical effectiveness of this procedure has been accepted due to clinical success. The application of spray and stretch procedures in cases without muscle shortening is not logical. In fact, vigorous overstretching can produce muscle microtearing and is potentially damaging. Trismus is usually a symptom secondary to regional pain. Treatment of trismus without appropriate management of the underlying pathology is not likely to be efficacious.

Open Locking

If a patient presents with a jaw that is locked open, the clinician should first manipulate the jaw to close the opening. Patients who recently had a problem with jaw closing should first have a thorough history and examination, then tomographic imaging of the jaw. If the jaw is currently locked and no panoramic film has been taken recently, or if a traumatic event induced the locking, this film of the jaw should be taken before proceeding. If no new film is needed, or if the film shows no osseous abnormality, the clinician should attempt the manual manipulation.

Depending on how long the jaw has been locked, manipulation of the jaw can usually be performed without adjunctive medications (antispasmodics). Assuming the mandible is locking in a wide-open position, manipulation involves holding the mandible with both hands, placing the thumb on the back molars of the lower jaw and the fingers under the mandible on each side. The manipulation is performed by pushing down on the mandible with the thumbs while pulling up on the mandible with the fingers in an attempt to pull the condyle down and then back so that it can then move posterior to the TMJ eminence.

If manual manipulation alone is not possible, the next step is to sedate the patient with a short-acting benzodiazepine, administered orally (if the patient can swallow) or intravenously (if the patient cannot swallow). Once reasonable sedation is achieved, the manipulation is usually much easier to perform.

Closed Locking

For the patients who do not show a substantial increase of motion, the potential diagnosis of an acute TMJ restriction caused by an intracapsular disorder becomes the working diagnosis. Although the reported success of manual reduction varies widely, typically less than half of all patients have a return of normal mobility. One study reported that manual manipulation was successful in 26 of 30 patients.[26] Arthrographic imaging, however, showed a normal disc position after manipulation in only a few patients. These reports are all case-series descriptions; no RCTs have been performed comparing manipulation to two other treatments, arthroscopy or arthrocentesis. Many authors who reported success also described a postmanipulation protocol involving the insertion of a mandibular repositioning appliance. They assume that the clicking and locking would recur if no appliance is used.[27,28] Whether the appliance is necessary after manipulation has never been addressed by an RCT. Frequent use of such a protocol might suggest that the results of manipulation are short term.

Stretching of Contractures

For patients with severe contracture who are not candidates for releasing surgeries of the jaw, a jaw muscle-stretching program should be implemented. This process employs an external-force jaw-opening device applied to the teeth in an attempt to stretch the jaw muscles. At present, no studies have evaluated these methods, but conventional wisdom and experience suggest that they are not highly effective.

Passive Motion Devices

Any joint must be mobilized as soon as possible after surgery, such as through a continuous motion device. One study evaluated the efficacy of continuous passive motion (CPM) in TMJ meniscectomy patients.[29] Chewing movement was analyzed before surgery and 6 months after surgery in 31 patients with CPM and 26 patients without CPM. Chewing in patients receiving CPM was closer to the normal range than for patients in the non-CPM group.

Active Physical Therapy for Arthromyogenous Jaw Disorders

Depending on the nature of the TMD, different physical therapy modalities are used to assist patients. This section describes acute pain relief therapy approaches for arthromyogenous disorders of the jaw and rehabilitation-oriented physical therapy.

Acute Pain Relief

As the first component of the physical medicine program, physical therapy is often recommended for patients with muscle and joint pain disorders who have had no relief from a home-based therapy program. This therapy can be performed by either a dentist trained in physical medicine or an experienced physical therapist. Therapy is usually divided into two phases. Methods include ice packs, heat packs, ultrasound, massage, and soft tissue laser therapy. The therapist usually provides these modalities at a 30- to 45-minute visit two times per week for 2 to 5 weeks. The specifics of the actual therapy for ultrasound and soft tissue laser vary according to the specifics of the device.

The first modality used for joint pain is usually a small ice pack, which can be applied to the involved joint several times a day for 20 minutes. For those patients with secondary muscle pain and stiffness, it is also advisable to use movement exercises, such as hinge-motion exercise for the jaw and head and neck range of motion exercises, followed by heat packs applied to the sorest muscles. The combination of heat, ice, and exercise under the specific direction of a trained physical therapist is a common treatment intervention for patients with severe arthritis.

One RCT evaluated the efficacy of physical therapy in the treatment of patients with rheumatoid arthritis (RA).[30] This study did not focus on TMJ arthritis but is still applicable. Physicians referred their patients for physical therapy (PT). Participants were randomized to either an experimental group (EG) or a wait list control group (CG). The intervention was a standardized program of education and exercise consisting of at least four PT visits over 6 weeks. Assessments of morning stiffness, grip strength, and tender joint count were collected at 6 weeks from 127 of 150 eligible and randomized participants. Results showed a mean change (improvement) of 13.5% in the EG and 5.8% in the CG, representing a 7.7% difference. Since a PT intervention does nothing to neutralize the RA disease itself, disease status measures did not change with treatment, except for duration of morning stiffness. The authors concluded that patients were better at managing their disease and had less morning stiffness.

Heat, cold heat, or cold can provide temporary relief of stiffness. Heat helps relax aching muscles and relieve joint pain and soreness, and cold helps numb the area. For example, a hot shower will help limber up the body before exercise, and an ice pack applied to an injured joint will constrict blood vessels and reduce swelling.

When the myalgia disorder is recalcitrant to treatment and therefore considered chronic, other methods are traditionally prescribed, such as topical pain-relieving and inflammation-reducing modalities (e.g., ultrasound, ice/heat pack applications to injured site) that increase regional arterial perfusion. Although no specific evidence exists for the masticatory muscles, physical therapists have proved these methods to be clinically effective in treating other body parts.[31-33]

Most authors accept the conservative use of cold for an acute traumatic injury and even for more resistant subacute problems. The question remains whether thermal agents are appropriate and efficacious for chronic myalgia problems. In a comparative study on ultrasound versus electrical stimulation and jaw exercises for a TMD patient group with chronic muscle pain, all treatments were partially helpful, but with no significant difference in treatment results.[34]

Rehabilitation

Once acute pain relief has been achieved, an exercise-based program may include jaw posture ("n" position) exercises (see earlier discussion), jaw coordination exercises, jaw stretch and spray procedures, head and neck posture exercises, neck-stretching range of motion exercises, and cardiovascular-based exercises (usually at a gym or exercise facility). To jaw posture exercises the therapist will add *jaw coordination exercises,* or careful movement of the jaw along a border pathway to the right and back to ICP and left and back to ICP. This exercise tests the patient's ability to activate jaw muscles selectively. The *stretching exercises* are usually best done with a vapocoolant spray or ice rubbed over the skin overlying a tight painful muscle for about 15 seconds. After applying the ice or spray, stretching of the jaw or neck muscle is performed.

Additional therapy options in the rehabilitation phase includes soft tissue mobilization and manipulation and training the patient how to keep their head, neck, and shoulders in a upright, nonslumped posture. Exercises and postural instruction focus on how to correct postural defects of the head and neck and stretch out stiff and shortened cervical muscles. Finally, toward the end of the rehabilitation program, a cardiovascular exercise program is implemented to keep the patient active and well exercised. In general, the acute physical treatment program is limited to six to ten visits, and the rehabilitation program involves an additional 5 to 6 weeks of treatment.

Postural awareness and *range of motion exercises* are typically used when, on evaluation, the myalgia symptoms appear to be related to mandibular muscle parafunction. No RCT data have demonstrated that these exercises are more effective than a no-treatment approach for myalgia and myositis in the masticatory muscles. These statements also apply to *deep tissue massage* and *stretching techniques,* which are used to relax chronically contracted muscles, stretch related tissue, alter motor patterns, and increase the patient's postural awareness.

Muscle Injections for Arthromyogenous Jaw Disorders

Again, depending on the nature of the muscle dysfunction, different physical medicine methods are used to help patients. These treatments include local anesthetic and other medication injections into trigger points, steroid muscle injections for myositis and tendinitis, and paralyzing injections using botulinum toxin into chronically contracted or hypertrophied jaw muscles.

Trigger Point Injections

The injection of a local anesthetic agent is another common technique used for chronic myogenous pain conditions. Usually, 1.0% procaine hydrochloride without epinephrine is injected into the identified tender areas or trigger points in the muscle. The injection is typically performed using a 1-ml tuberculin syringe with a 27-gauge needle. The anesthetic solution should be injected into the most tender area of the muscle, followed by strong stretching of the stiff muscle. Extremely tender muscle may require dexamethasone added to the anesthetic solution. Other physical therapy modalities, such as prolonged application of ice packs, heat packs, and electrical or ultrasonic stimulation to the tender muscles, may also be recommended.

The efficacy of local anesthetic injections into tender areas or muscle trigger points for regional myalgia and myositis has not been substantiated with RCT-based research. However, numerous case reports have described how anesthetic blocking of the tender areas in an involved muscle has helped a patient.[35-37]

Steroid Injections for Myositis and Tendinitis

If prolonged trismus develops after muscle injection, reevaluation of the original diagnosis is appropriate. These patients may develop prolonged trismus from ongoing microtrauma and jaw muscle parafunctions or an unusual healing process.

Counterstimulation for Chronic Orofacial Pain

Counterstimulation therapies include acupuncture for generalized chronic orofacial pain and transcutaneous nerve stimulation (either with electrical or laser-light irradiation) for local neuropathic pain affecting a nerve branch or division.

Acupuncture

The most common form of strong counterstimulation is acupuncture treatment, which has been shown to be a strong therapeutic intervention for chronic muscle pain problems. The acupuncture is usually applied by a clinician trained in the method and will involve local needling in sore sites plus several distant but strong neurologic sites in the region. As with the trigger point injections, strong stretching of the stiff muscle after the injection is recommended. To the traditional acupuncture stimulation with manual manipulation of the needles, the therapist may add 30 minutes of low-frequency electrical stimulation (2 to 3 Hz) by clipping the stimulator directly to the inserted needle. After 8 to 10 visits, therapy is reevaluated. RCTs have compared acupuncture to occlusal appliances for the treatment of TMD problems.[38,39] Both methods have generally resulted in a substantial improvement in chronic muscle pain symptoms immediately after the treatment period and at 1 year. These data are encouraging and hold promise for acupuncture as a therapeutic method of managing local myalgia and myositis in the masticatory system.

Transcutaneous Electrical Nerve Stimulation

Some patients are unable to have needles or prefer noninvasive forms of counterstimulation. In transcutaneous electrical nerve stimulation (TENS), electrodes are placed directly on the skin. As with acupuncture, TENS involves local stimulation of sore sites plus distant but strong neurologic sites in the region, followed by strong stretching of the stiff muscle. Therapy is reevaluated after 8 to 10 visits. The efficacy of TENS procedures has been challenged. Several controlled trials indicate they have no greater benefit than a placebo therapy program.[40-42]

Laser Irradiation of Pain Sites

Other transcutaneous therapies, such as ultrasound, cold lasers, and low-frequency electrical pulsing devices for muscle stimulation, also generally have no RCT data to prove their efficacy. *Soft (cold) lasers* have been investigated as a tool for wound healing and muscle pain relief. The cold laser usually causes no pain and is aseptic, nonthermal, and noninjurious to tissues. The proposed empiric biostimulatory effects include accelerated collagen synthesis, increased vascularity of healing tissue, and decreased pain.[43] Most studies of cold laser therapy have been on chronic musculoskeletal, rheumatologic, and neurologic pain conditions.[44-49] The results have been mixed, and most studies lacked proper research design. The work on laser irradiation of musculoskeletal trigger points as a substitute for direct local anesthetic injections is interesting, but additional work is needed. A decrease in trigger point pain has been reported after irradiation in a sample of patients with neck and lower back pain.[50,51] Two case studies have been published in which cold laser treatment was used on persistent TMJ pain.[52,53] After laser treatment, pain and crepitation decreased, and range of motion increased; however, the studies lacked controls, blinding, and adequate sample sizes.

Orthotic Devices (Occlusal Appliances) for Orofacial Habits and Motor Disorders

Occlusal appliances are used for TMJ derangement symptoms (e.g., clicking), arthromyalgia secondary to clenching and bruxism behaviors, acute tooth pain symptoms caused by clenching behaviors, stabilization of an occlusion, and management of occlusal dysesthesia.

Temporomandibular Joint Clicking and Other Derangement Symptoms

In the treatment of TMJ clicking, a discussion of open surgical manipulation (e.g., discal plication, discoplasty) and closed surgical manipulation (e.g.,

arthroscopic lavage, arthroscopically assisted discal plication) is beyond the scope of this chapter. TMJ clicking is the most resistant symptom to treatment.[54] Some studies have reported improvement of other symptoms (e.g., pain) with a stabilization appliance, but few of the subjects exhibited diminished clicking.[55-57] In subjects with TMJ clicking randomly assigned to one of two treatments (repositioning versus stabilization appliances), those using the stabilization appliance had no change in joint clicking.[58] Another study compared the outcome of 55 patients who had disc displacement (both with and without reduction) with 342 others who had TMD and no disc displacement.[59] All patients underwent conventional treatment (physical therapy and stabilization appliances). After 1 year, 69% of disc displacement subjects and 74% of other TMD patients improved.

Repositioning appliances have also been used extensively to treat clicking since they were first described in 1971 as a therapy for TMJ disc displacement.[60] Another report describes 25 patients prospectively followed with a repositioning appliance for TMJ clicking for 1 to 2 years.[61] Ten of 20 patients (50%) still had clicking at follow-up. Within the same group, 70% had improvement in pain symptoms. Similar results were reported in 1988 for clicking reduction (39%) and improvement in other symptoms (39%) at 19 months of follow-up.[62] Two additional studies had similar results, with greater improvement in symptoms (e.g., pain) other than clicking at follow-up.[63,64] A large study reported that only 36% of 241 repositioning cases followed for 3 years maintained the absence of clicking.[65] The authors suggested the repositioning device was less effective on late-opening than early-opening clicks.

In contrast to these multiple studies, only one study compared patients who received repositioning appliances ($n = 10$) with patients who received stabilization appliances ($n = 10$).[66] The authors claimed that after 90 days of treatment, clicking was gone in 80% of the repositioned group and in none of the stabilization appliance group. In fact, two cases became locked in the stabilization appliance group during treatment. The authors further reported that pain symptoms improved in 60% of the repositioned group and in none of the stabilization appliance group.

Another study also compared repositioning to other techniques.[58] The authors randomly assigned 72 subjects to a stabilization splint, a repositioning appliance, or a wait list condition. At 1 year, clicking was present in all the patients with a stabilization appliance and in 81% of the wait list group. The repositioning appliance stopped clicking in 22 of 24 patients, but clicking returned in 18 patients after the repositioning appliance was discontinued. One patient's jaw became locked. The authors recommended permanent repositioning of the jaw for long-lasting effect and subsequently conducted such a study.[67] They reported that the permanently repositioned group had a continued clicking cessation, but not the other two groups. A third study reported 3-year results for 15 patients with TMJ clicking after exchanging the removable repositioning appliance for cemented posterior tooth onlays.[68] Thirteen patients were click free after treatment, and 82% had normal disc position (two had anterior disc position).

Arthromyalgia Secondary to Clenching and Bruxism

Oral orthotic devices, best known as *occlusal appliances,* are used for myalgia and arthralgia as a physical medicine treatment if clenching is strongly evident or if the patient has a unstable bite (e.g., missing teeth, uneven occlusion). This approach is also helpful for the patient who has tender, painful, or inflamed muscles; sore teeth; or joint pain due to bruxism.

Typically the preferred appliance is a full-arch, hard acrylic device designed to cover one entire arch (maxillary or mandibular). This appliance has a flat occlusal surface, which is adjusted to have several teeth make contact in a habitual, comfortable, jaw closure position. When first delivered, this appliance is adjusted to an unstrained habitual closure. The appliance is worn for the first 5 weeks 24 hours a day (except eating) and is readjusted at least twice during this period. After the symptoms decrease, the patient should decrease use of the device after 6 to 8 weeks. It may be used for many years if the patient has clear evidence of nocturnal bruxism.

The purpose of the appliance is not to find a new therapeutic jaw position, but to serve as a behavioral feedback device that makes the patient conscious of any oral parafunction. The patient must therefore be instructed not to bring the teeth together on the appliance while it is worn. After relief of symptoms the patient should reduce the amount of daytime wear of the appliance. Continued use of the appliance at night is indicated only if there is evidence of ongoing

wear of its occlusal surface, indicating a strong clenching or bruxism habit.

Joint Pain

Two studies reported improvement of joint pain with stabilization appliance use.[57,69] In contrast, another study reported no effect of appliances on joint pain at follow-up.[70]

Myalgia

Myalgia is generally considered to be a function of local tissue inflammation and vascular alterations in the muscle and pain referred from other sources. The pathophysiologic changes in the muscle tissue are not established. Occlusal splints have been used for many years to treat this condition under the assumption that masticatory muscle parafunction was contributing to the pain production.[71-75] Two studies evaluated the relationship among nocturnal muscle parafunction, myogenous pain symptoms, and stabilization appliances.[76,77] Of the myofascial pain dysfunction patients, 52% ($n = 25$) had significantly reduced nocturnal muscle activity levels, and 80% experienced overall improvement in pain symptoms when full-arch stabilization splints were used. Patients with more severe symptoms were less likely to be helped with occlusal appliances as a sole treatment modality. Other studies have also demonstrated a good correlation between occlusal appliance therapy and reduction of bruxism[78] and relief of masticatory muscle pain.[54] Another study reported decreased myalgia symptoms in 71% of patients wearing stabilization appliances.[57]

Except for studies using electromyography to measure masseter function directly, most prior studies did not assess whether muscle pain patients had parafunctional behaviors or were strictly exhibiting muscle pain that might be described as *myofascial* in character (i.e., spontaneous onset, daytime occurrence, stress component in fluctuation). This distinction might be important because occlusal appliances could work differently on these two patterns of muscle pain. Patients who have parafunction-aggravated myalgia might be more likely to respond to stabilization appliances.

An RCT of 100 subjects evaluated the efficacy of stabilization appliances versus biofeedback, exercises, no treatment, and auditory feedback at night (triggered by tooth clenching).[79] The stabilizing appliance and the auditory feedback significantly interfered with bruxism. Unfortunately, the authors did not report or evaluate muscle pain levels in these subjects. Another RCT on the efficacy of stabilization appliances for the specific management of myofascial pain patients found no remarkable efficacy for stabilization appliances compared with two placebo-controlled conditions.[80] These data suggest that the primary mechanism for the reported efficacy of the stabilization appliance (especially in myofascial patients without strong oral parafunction) is nonspecific and likely to be more behavioral in its treatment action. The stabilization appliance does appear to be a strong behavior-modifying device.[81] An RCT based study reported that the occlusal appliance approach was as effective as a biofeedback/stress management program for pain reduction in TMD patients. When combined, the two therapies (appliances and biofeedback) were more effective than either one alone.

For spontaneous onset of chronic myofascial pain, the stabilization appliance might best be conceptualized as a behavior modification device. The stabilization appliance is a moderately powerful treatment for modifying parafunctional activities in the jaw. In myalgia patients without a strong parafunctional origin for symptoms, appliances are comparable to both acupuncture treatment and most other behavioral therapies. Further, if a credible pseudotherapy is used in a clinical trial on pain of musculoskeletal origin, stabilization appliances are not routinely shown to be superior to other treatments. When either stabilization appliances or behavioral therapies for TMD are compared to a no-treatment or wait list program, patients typically report that these treatments are very helpful, whereas the no-treatment program has a weak effect.

Trismus and Splinting

Anecdotally, appliances are used successfully to treat trismus, probably because they alter parafunctional behaviors. Unfortunately, there is no specific research on the effect of splints on trismus.

Dyskinesia and Motor Incoordination

Studies on motor coordination suggest that occlusal appliances improve motor skills in patients who exhibit reduced coordination but are not helpful (except as protective devices) in patients with a true involuntary motor abnormality.[82-84]

Arthritis

When TMJ arthritic changes are severe, joint inflammation may destroy condyles. These condylar effects alter the occlusion, producing either a unilateral bite opening or, if the destruction is bilateral, an anterior open bite. Alternatively, some patients with severe arthritis have an unstable occlusion for unrelated reasons. In either group, a well-balanced occlusal appliance may provide the patient with a stable occlusal contact pattern during sleep, when they will clench or grind their teeth with force. Patients with low levels of jaw function may tolerate this malocclusion without complaint, but a splint clearly helps bite instability in others. Eventually, occlusal therapy (orthodontics, prosthetics, occlusal adjustments) may be required to provide a reasonably stable posterior occlusion. Definitive occlusal evaluation during the acute phase of joint inflammation should be avoided, however, because the intracapsular swelling may cause a dramatic acute change, which will return to normal after the joint inflammation subsides.

Injectable Agents for Joint Lubrication, Patient Mobilization, and Pain Relief

Depending on the nature of the TMJ derangement, a variety of agents are used to improve joint function and assist patients. These treatment include infusion of saline into a closed-locking patient to assist with mobilization, infusion of hyaluronate into an arthritic or clicking joint to reduce joint friction and promote healing, and infusion of steroids into the acutely inflamed joint to reduce pain and inflammation (see earlier discussion).

Saline

Arthrocentesis using saline infusion to increase joint mobility was first described in the late 1980s and early 1990s, specifically to treat an acute closed-locking condition.[85-87] All three studies reported success rates comparable to those for arthroscopy (greater than 80%). The major flaw of these studies is that none involved an RCT comparing arthrocentesis to arthroscopy or manual manipulation. Finally, even if no attempt is made to mobilize a locked joint, patients will eventually experience a near-full restoration of jaw mobility and a substantial decrease in painful symptoms.[55,88-90] This improvement is generally slower than after an arthroscopic surgical or arthrocentesis procedure. Regardless of the method, the amount of pain and lost mobility in these chronically locked joints is usually minimal after 6 to 12 months. Signs of crepitation and arthrotic remodeling are present in some untreated closed-locking patients. It is not known whether these signs are less likely to occur after successful arthroscopy or arthrocentesis.

Hyaluronate

Joint surface lubrication using a sodium hyaluronate (hyaluronic acid, HA) is another physical medicine technique. Data from other joints (knee) undergoing HA infusion suggest that a high-molecular-weight hyaluronate has the potential to be a conservative, safe, efficacious, and essentially hazard-free adjunctive "lubricating" agent to reduce joint friction and promote healing of intracapsular disorders.[91-94] In a multisite RCT, injections of HA were moderately efficacious for the management of painful symptoms associated with TMJ clicking, but the clicking did not disappear.[95] The HA infusion procedure is limited because HA is not yet approved by the U.S. Food and Drug Administration (FDA) for intraarticular use in humans.

Expected Outcomes

In most studies a physical medicine method has produced a positive response in approximately 75% of patients with masticatory pain or dysfunction. The definition of a "positive response" is not always clear, however, and may mean "no further treatment sought," "a satisfied patient," or "a substantial reduction of the jaw pain complaint." Regardless of the measurement, most studies report that three of four patients have a good result. It is not known whether the 25% of patients who do not respond have been inaccurately diagnosed or ineffectively and perhaps inappropriately treated. The percentage of patients who state that they require further treatment varies between 14% and 34%.[96-101]

These data are not unexpected, since many of these patients' clinical problems are not "cured," but instead "managed" by a physical medicine program. For example, jaw pain secondary to a strong bruxism or tooth-clenching habit or a generalized stress reaction might be managed in the acute phase by a physical medicine program, but the behavior often continues, as do the pain and dysfunction symptoms, although in a less aggravated state. This observation also applies to jaw pain and dysfunction secondary to arthritis or disc derangement of the TMJ. Therefore the clinician must expect some limited or negative outcomes for all treatment approaches.

Therapeutic Recommendations

Before summarizing the previous information into a set of recommendations to help clinicians select logical treatment methods and to help researchers establish the future agenda of investigations needed to advance the discipline, the following perspective must be considered. First, the typical problems seen in TMD patients are not usually disabling or extremely long-lasting. Even when TMD symptoms are prolonged for more than 6 months, they are not disabling and usually do not interfere substantially with the patient's work or social life (except eating). *Irreversible* therapy, however, may cause iatrogenic damage, and therefore conservative treatments with reasonable efficacy should be selected and advocated. Second, a conceptual framework for organizing and understanding the available treatments is helpful. The most common method of treatment for TMDs includes a combination of techniques derived from a physical medicine model (e.g., physical therapy and physical medicine procedures applied at home or in the office, including dental occlusal appliances) and a behavioral medicine model (e.g., counseling, biofeedback, stress management, relaxation training). These two models are generally considered *reversible* treatments, with low morbidity and high efficacy.

Because some conditions affecting the TMJ substantially interfere with function, two additional, minimally invasive models of care are also often used: the pharmacologic model (e.g., NSAIDs, antidepressants, antispasmodics, steroid injections) and the closed-joint surgical manipulation model (e.g., arthrocentesis, arthroscopy). Both these latter models have greater potential risks than physical medicine and behavioral models. If selected for the appropriate patient and used in the proper situation, however, these minimally invasive approaches should have low morbidity and good efficacy. Finally, in all areas of medicine, it is assumed that if a correct and specific diagnosis is made, appropriate and logical treatment will follow. Unfortunately, diagnosis is difficult and choice of therapy often complicated. Treatments are selected based on numerous factors, including cost, risk/benefit ratio, prior experience, degree of invasiveness, patient's confidence in the care provider, and clinician's judgment on the optimal treatment for the patient.

Temporomandibular Clicking

The sparse research and clinical observation data indicate that the clicking TMJ is not cured by the use of avoidance and exercise therapy. This approach may be viable in slowing the progression of a dysfunctional clicking joint, but there is no experimental verification. Open discoplasty, arthroscopic lavage, and discal plication methods have been advocated for painful TMJ click but have not been reviewed for efficacy. Data suggest that the stabilization appliance has poor efficacy for management of TMJ clicking. For repositioning appliances the short-term (1 year or less) data suggest that these appliances can modify and perhaps eliminate some TMJ clicking problems. The long-term data are less convincing, however, and the cost of reconstructing a permanently repositioned occlusion, whether surgically, orthodontically, or prosthetically, is substantial and irreversible. This approach does not seem warranted except in rare cases.

Studies on the efficacy of repositioning for TMJ clicking had several design problems. Few studies used random assignment, and none were "double-blind" evaluation studies. There are no good methods of measuring clicking over time in the natural environment. All prior data are based on patients' self-reporting or a laboratory-based measurement of clicking. Laboratory-based assessments are useful, but the problem's frequency in the patient's day-to-day routine is more relevant than the click's loudness in the laboratory. The development of portable devices to measure long-term TMJ noise would be beneficial in future studies of TMJ clicking.

Criteria for selecting patients who "require" permanent repositioning are not clear and need to be refined and tested. Until well-designed research compares the treatments described in this chapter for TMJ clicking to newer, minimally invasive methods, such as hyaluronate infusion into the joint, no definitive prediction can be made regarding which treatment is the most efficacious or has the lowest morbidity and the best longevity. Further, the entire phenomenon of TMJ clicking requires investigation to determine if early painless clicks are more likely to progress and become painful dysfunctional clicks, which in turn will induce prolonged interference in jaw movement.

Temporomandibular Locking

Since the mid-1970s the patient with acute-onset loss of TMJ motion has been managed with methods that directly invade or manipulate the joint. From about 1978 to 1988, open-surgical TMJ disc repositioning was widely performed. This procedure was described as a method for treating closed-locking problems.[102,103] Since the advent of arthroscopic surgery in 1986, the closed-locking problem has been managed with this less invasive method. Whether manual manipulation, arthrocentesis, or arthroscopic lavage or lysis is the best way to manage these cases has not been established. Until more research compares these treatment methods, no prediction can be made regarding which treatment is the most efficacious and has the lowest morbidity and the best longevity.

A clear problem with all prior research is that the method of measuring passive jaw opening is not standardized. Methodologic research on this issue needs to be performed. Maximum passive opening is the interincisal distance achieved by stretching the patient's jaw open with the examiner's fingers. The resulting value is partially dependent on the level of force applied by the examiner. Additional information about the natural course of an untreated closed-locking condition also is needed because some cases will resolve fully without invasive therapy, whereas others progress to a rapid degeneration of the articular surfaces. The anatomic and functional status of the disc itself or of the intracapsular fluid constituents might be important variables in such prognostic prediction. At present, decisions about treatment for individual cases should be based on both the patient's history and at least 2 weeks of continued pain and disability from the closed-locking condition even after appropriate, noninvasive pharmacologic and physical medicine therapy has been attempted. Therapy with the lowest morbidity should be used first.

Joint Pain

Few well-designed clinical outcome research studies have been conducted that specifically evaluate the efficacy of individual physical medicine techniques to relieve TMJ pain beyond a brief therapeutic period. RCTs have compared corticosteroid and sodium hyaluronate infusions for TMJ pain management associated with TMJ arthritis. Clinical case reports and therapeutic logic generally support the claim that the rest/soft-diet/NSAID approach is helpful for acute trauma-induced joint pain, but its efficacy in chronic TMJ pain is not proven. Chronic TMJ pain appears to respond only weakly to the stabilization appliance. Better scientific research is needed to evaluate its efficacy for this condition. Clearly, comparative studies are needed to determine the relative effectiveness of treatment approaches: physical medicine versus pharmacology versus surgery.

TMJ pain rarely occurs as an isolated problem, and secondary myogenous symptoms are usually present. Identifying the etiology of the problem is essential, since treatment will provide only transient relief if the etiology is ongoing (e.g., systemic arthritic disorder). More reliable and valid methods (e.g., joint fluid markers of inflammation) are needed to assess and quantify joint pain versus adjacent muscle pain.

Temporomandibular Polyarthritis

The efficacy of physical medicine procedures for symptomatic management of the TMJ with a polyarthritic disease process has not been well studied. Nevertheless, these procedures are widely used for other body joints. Physical medicine procedures, especially the postural awareness and range of motion exercises, probably can reduce secondary arthritic symptoms. Patient education on how to reduce the strain on an arthritic joint may be the critical factor. No published scientific evidence indicates that nonpharmacologic physical medicine, including occlusal appliances, can reverse or stop the bony erosive process of substantial polyarthritic disease. Intraarticular steroid injections have been widely accepted as the standard approach for an isolated inflamed joint; the relative efficacy of other pharmacologic agents for TMJ arthritis is beyond the discussion in this chapter. Separate literature is not available on the efficacy of occlusal appliances for managing polyarthritic pain symptoms. Stabilization appliances might be more beneficial in the patient with substantial polyarthritic destruction of the TMJ than in the TMJ pain patient without arthritic change. The former patient often has a disturbed dental occlusion (e.g., open bite), and the stabilization appliance theoretically supports the occlusion.

Myalgia and Myositis

Common modalities for muscle pain include exercise, stretching, and thermal agents, but their individual efficacy for myogenous jaw pain has received limited study. The more invasive modalities, such as trigger point injections, acupuncture, TENS, muscle stimulation, and cold lasers, have not been fully tested for efficacy. The most reasonable data on physical medicine modalities for treatment of chronic jaw muscle pain involve acupuncture. If a credible pseudo-acupuncture treatment were tested in an RCT, however, these findings might weaken. Additional testing of acupuncture versus a control condition and other myalgic management methods seems warranted. Comparative studies of various physical medicine methods of treating musculoskeletal pain in other anatomic areas have not consistently rated one method better than other methods. Further, tests comparing traditional physical medicine procedures with behavioral medicine methods (e.g., biofeedback, stress management) find similar efficacy, suggesting a strong behavioral component in most physical medicine methods or a strong physical component in behavioral methods.

Until the therapeutic effectiveness of one approach or modality can be well correlated with a specific clinical, etiologic-based diagnosis, the physical medicine modalities selected for the treatment of chronic myalgia will continue to be based solely on the clinician's best judgment and experience. Use of occlusal appliances for masticatory muscle pain is likely to be comparably effective as any other approach. No physical medicine methods (e.g., occlusal appliances) have been shown to be superior to a credible pseudotherapy control condition.

Trismus and Splinting

Most clinicians recognize the potential of physical medicine modalities to interrupt a significant masticatory muscle trismus response of extracapsular origin. Unfortunately, no clear experimental evidence has documented the use of various physical medicine modalities, including occlusal appliances, for trismus.

Dyskinesia and Motor Incoordination

The literature does not support the effectiveness of any physical medicine procedures in the management of involuntary motor disorders, except as a purely palliative measure. Exercise methods involving movement feedback can help mild masticatory muscle incoordination problems if they are learned behaviors.

Additional research must be performed that compares the various treatment methods for masticatory muscle pain, trismus, and movement incoordination problems. Available data suggest that occlusal appliances have a strong beneficial effect on jaw muscle incoordination.

References

1. McNeill C, editor: *Temporomandibular disorders: guidelines for classification, assessment, and management,* American Academy of Orofacial Pain, Chicago, 1993, Quintessence.
2. Clark GT: Diagnosis and treatment of painful temporomandibular disorders, *Dent Clin North Am* 31:645-674, 1987.
3. Clark GT, Seligman DA, Solberg WK, et al: Guidelines for the examination and diagnosis of temporomandibular disorders, *J Craniomandib Disord Fac Oral Pain* 3:7-14, 1989.
4. McNeill C, Mohl ND, Rugh JD, et al: Temporomandibular disorders: diagnosis, management, education, and research, *J Am Dent Assoc* 120:253-261, 1990.
5. Schwartz L: Disorders of the temporomandibular joint, Philadelphia, 1959, Saunders.
6. Messenger K, Barghi N: The effect of function and rest on the amplitude of the TMJ click, *J Oral Rehabil* 14:261-266, 1987.
7. Au AR, Klineberg IJ: Isokinetic exercise management of temporomandibular joint clicking in young adults, *J Prosthet Dent* 70:33-39, 1993.
8. Lundh H, Westesson P, Kopp S: A three-year follow-up of patients with reciprocal temporomandibular joint clicking, *Oral Surg Oral Med Oral Pathol* 63:530-533, 1987.
9. Greene CS, Turner C, Laskin DM: Long term outcome of TMJ clicking in 100 MPD patients, *J Dent Res* 61:218, 1982.
10. Clark GT: The diagnosis and treatment of painful temporomandibular disorders. In Curro F, editor: *Dental Clinics of North America,* Philadelphia, 1987, WB Saunders.
11. Clark G, Seligman D, Solberg W, et al: Guidelines for the treatment of temporomandibular disorders, *J Craniomand Disord Fac Oral Pain* 4:80-88, 1990.
12. Yavelow I, Forster I, Wininger M: Mandibular relearning, *Oral Surg* 36:632-641, 1973.
13. Friedman MH, Weisberg J: Joint play movements of the temporomandibular joint: clinical considerations, *Arch Phys Med Rehabil* 65:413-417, 1984.
14. Bush FM: Physical therapy for mandibular movement–jaw pain, *J Dent Res* 63:172, 1984.
15. Okeson JP: *Management of temporomandibular joint disorders and occlusion,* St Louis, 1989, Mosby.
16. Kraus S: Physical therapy management of temporomandibular joint dysfunction. In Kraus S, editor: *TMJ disorders: management of the craniomandibular complex,* New York, 1988, Churchill Livingstone.
17. Maitland J: *Peripheral manipulation,* ed 2, London, 1979, Butterworth.
18. Wyke B: Articular neurology and manipulative therapy. In *Aspects of manipulative therapy,* ed 2, London, 1975, Churchill Livingstone.
19. Carstensen B: Indications and contraindications of manual therapy for temporomandibular joint dysfunction. In Grieve G, editor: *Modern manual therapy,* New York, 1986, Churchill Livingstone.
20. Tveteras K, Kristensen S: The etiology and pathogenesis of trismus, *Clin Otolaryngol* 11:383-387, 1986.
21. Schultz LW: Report of ten years of treating hypermobility of the temporomandibular joint, *J Oral Surg* 5:202-207, 1947.
22. Schwartz L: Ethyl chloride treatment of limited painful mandibular movement, *J Am Dent Assoc* 48:497-507, 1954.
23. Burgess J, Sommess E, Truelove E, et al: Effects of ice, sketch, and reflex inhibition on TMD, *J Dent Res* 65:307, 1986.
24. Salmon TN, Tracy NH, Hiatt NR: Hysterical trismus (conversion reaction): report of a case, *Oral Surg* 34:187-191, 1972.
25. Travell J: Myofascial trigger points: clinical view. In Bonica J, Albe-Fessard P, editors: *Advances in pain research and therapy,* vol 1, New York, 1976, Raven.
26. Segami N, Murakami K, Iizuka T: Arthrographic evaluation of disk position following mandibular manipulation technique for internal derangement with closed lock of the temporomandibular joint, *J Craniomand Disord Fac Oral Pain* 4:99-108, 1990.
27. McCarty W: Diagnosis and treatment of internal derangements of the articular disc and mandibular condyle. In Solberg WK, Clark GT, editors: *Temporomandibular joint problems,* Chicago, 1980, Quintessence.
28. Friedman MH, Anstendig HS, Weisberg J: Treatment of disc dysfunction, *J Clin Orthodont* 16:408-411, 1982.
29. Kuwahara T, Bessette RW, Maruyama T, et al: Effect of continuous passive motion on the results of TMJ meniscectomy. I. Comparisons of chewing movement, *J Craniomaxillofac Surg* 14(3):190-199, 1996.
30. Bell MJ, Lineker SC, Wilkins AL, et al: A randomized controlled trial to evaluate the efficacy of community based physical therapy in the treatment of people with rheumatoid arthritis, *J Rheumatol* 25(2):231-237, 1998.
31. Cordray YM, Krusen EM: Use of hydrocollator packs in the treatment of neck and shoulder pains, *Arch Phys Med Rehabil* 40:105-108, 1959.
32. Fountain FP, Gersten JW: Decrease in muscle spasm produced by ultrasound, hot packs, and infrared radiation, *Arch Phys Med Rehabil* 41:293-298, 1960.

33. Keene J: Ligament and muscle-tendon unit injuries. In Gould J, Davies G, editors: *Orthopedic and sports physical therapy*, St Louis, 1985, Mosby.

34. Eisen R, Kaufman A, Greene C: Evaluation of physical therapy for MPD syndrome patients, *J Dent Res* 63:344, 1984.

35. Toller P: Non-surgical treatment of dysfunctions of the temporo-mandibular joint, *Oral Sci Rev* 7:70-85, 1976.

36. Bell WH: Nonsurgical management of the pain-dysfunction syndrome, *J Am Dent Assoc* 79:161-170, 1969.

37. Bonica JJ: Management of myofascial pain syndrome in general practice, *JAMA* 164:732-738, 1957.

38. List T, Helkimo M, Anderson S, et al: Acupuncture and occlusal splint therapy in the treatment of craniomandibular disorders. I. A comparative study, *Swed Dent J* 12:125-141, 1992.

39. Johansson A, Wenneberg B, Wagersten C, et al: Acupuncture in treatment of facial mandibular pain, *Acta Odontol Scand* 49:153-158, 1991.

40. Block SL, Laskin DM: The effectiveness of transcutaneous nerve stimulation (TNS) in the treatment of unilateral MPD syndrome, *J Dent Res* 59(special issue A): 519, 1980.

41. Graff-Radford SB, Reeves JL, Baker RL, et al: Effects of transcutaneous electrical nerve stimulation on myofascial pain and trigger point sensitivity, *Pain* 37:1-5, 1989.

42. Deyo RA, Walsh NE, Martin DC, et al: A controlled trial of transcutaneous electrical nerve stimulation (TENS) and exercise for chronic low back pain, *N Engl J Med* 322:1627-1634, 1990.

43. Seitz LM, Kleinkort JA: Low-power laser: its applications in physical therapy. In Michlovitz SL, Wolf SL, editors: *Thermal agents in rehabilitation*, Philadelphia, 1986, FA Davis.

44. Snyder-Mackler L, Bork CE: Effect of helium-neon laser irradiation on peripheral sensory nerve latency, *Phys Ther* 68:223-225, 1988.

45. Strang R, Moseley H, Carmichael A: Soft lasers: have they a place in dentistry? *Br Dent J* 165:221-225, 1988.

46. Zakariasen K, Dederich D: Lasers in dentistry: "Star Wars" dreaming or a future reality? *Can Dent Assoc J* 54:27-30, 1988.

47. Kleinkort JA, Foley R: Laser acupuncture: its use in physical therapy, *Am J Acupunct* 12:51-56, 1984.

48. Walker J: Relief from chronic pain from low-power laser irradiation, *Neurosci Lett* 43:339-344, 1983.

49. Goldman JA, Chiapella J, Casey H, et al: Laser therapy of rheumatoid arthritis, *Lasers Surg Med* 1:93-101, 1980.

50. Olavi A, Pekka R, Pertti K, et al: Effects of the infrared laser therapy at treated and non-treated trigger points, *Acupunct Electro-Ther Res* 14:9-14, 1989.

51. Snyder-Mackler L, Barry A, Perkins A, et al: Effects of helium-neon laser irradiation on skin resistance and pain in patients with trigger points in the neck and back, *Phys Ther* 69:336-341, 1989.

52. Hansson TL: Infrared laser in the treatment of craniomandibular arthrogenous pain, *J Prosthet Dent* 61:614-617, 1985.

53. Palano D, Martelli M, Avi R, et al: A clinic statistical investigation of laser effect in the treatment of pain and dysfunction of the temporomandibular joint (TMJ), *Med Laser Rep* 2:21-29, 1985.

54. Greene CS, Laskin DM: Splint therapy for the myofascial pain-dysfunction (MPD) syndrome: a comparative study, *J Am Dent Assoc* 84:624-628, 1972.

55. Mejersjo C, Carlsson GE: Long term results of treatment for temporomandibular joint pain-dysfunction, *J Prosthet Dent* 49:809-815, 1983.

56. Goharian RK, Neff PA: Effect of occlusal retainers on temporomandibular joint and facial pain, *J Prosthet Dent* 44:206-208, 1980.

57. Agerberg G, Carlsson GE: Late results of treatment of functional disorders of the masticatory system: a follow-up by questionnaire, *J Oral Rehabil* 1:309-316, 1974.

58. Lundh H, Westesson P, Kopp S, et al: Anterior repositioning splint in the treatment of temporomandibular joints with reciprocal clicking: comparison with a flat occlusal splint and an untreated control group, *Oral Surg Oral Med Oral Pathol* 60:131-136, 1985.

59. Helkimo E, Westling L: History, clinical findings, and outcome of treatment of patients with anterior disk displacement, *J Craniomand Pract* 5:269-276, 1987.

60. Farrar WB: Diagnosis and treatment of anterior dislocation of the articular disc, *J Dent* 41:348-351, 1971.

61. Clark GT: Treatment of jaw clicking with temporomandibular repositioning: an analysis of 25 cases, *J Craniomand Pract* 2:263-270, 1984.

62. Clark GT, Lanham F, Flack VF: Treatment outcome for consecutive TMJ clinic patients, *J Craniomand Disord* 2:87-95, 1988.

63. Okeson JP: Long-term treatment of disk-interference disorders of the temporomandibular joint with anterior repositioning occlusal splints, *J Prosthet Dent* 60:611-616, 1988.

64. Le Bell Y, Kirveskari P: Treatment of reciprocal clicking of the temporomandibular joint using a mandibular repositioning splint and occlusal adjustment, *Proc Finn Dent Soc* 81:251-255, 1985.

65. Moloney F, Howard JA: Internal derangements of the temporomandibular joint: anterior repositioning splint therapy, *Aust Dent J* 31:30-39, 1986.

66. Anderson GC, Schulte JK, Goodkind RJ: Comparative study of two treatment methods for internal derangement of the temporomandibular joint, *J Prosthet Dent* 53:392-397, 1985.

67. Lundh H, Westesson P, Jisander S, et al: Disk-repositioning onlays in the treatment of temporomandibular joint with disk displacement: comparison with a flat occlusal splint and with no treatment, *Oral Surg Oral Med Oral Pathol* 66:155-162, 1988.

68. Lundh H, Westesson P: Long-term follow-up after occlusal treatment to correct abnormal temporomandibular joint disk position, *Oral Surg Oral Med Oral Pathol* 67:2-10, 1989.

69. Carraro JJ, Caffesse RG: Effect of occlusal splints on TMJ symptomatology, *J Prosthet Dent* 40:563-566, 1978.

70. Magnusson T, Carlsson GE: Treatment of patients with functional disturbances in the masticatory system: a survey of 80 consecutive patients, *Swed Dent J* 4:145-153, 1980.

71. Hamada T, Kotani H, Kawazoe Y, et al: Effect of occlusal splints on the EMG activity of masseter and temporal muscles in bruxism with clinical symptoms, *J Oral Rehabil* 9:119-123, 1982.

72. Rugh JD: Muscle activity studies of MPD in the natural environment, *J Dent Res* 61(S-24):175, 1982.

73. Kawazoe Y, Kotani H, Hamada T, et al: Effect of occlusal splints on the electromyographic activities of masseter muscles during maximum clenching in patients with myofascial pain-dysfunction syndrome, *J Prosthet Dent* 43:578-580, 1980.

74. Carlsson GE, Ingervall B, Kocak G: Effect of increasing vertical dimension on the masticatory system in subjects with natural teeth, *J Prosthet Dent* 41:284-289, 1979.

75. Fuchs P: The muscular activity of the chewing apparatus during night sleep, *J Oral Rehabil* 2:35-48, 1975.

76. Clark GT, Beemsterboer PL, Solberg WK, et al: Nocturnal electromyographic evaluation of myofascial pain dysfunction in patients undergoing splint therapy, *J Am Dent Assoc* 99:607-611, 1979.

77. Clark GT, Beemsterboer PL, Rugh JD: Nocturnal masseter muscle activity and the symptoms of masticatory dysfunction, *J Oral Rehabil* 8:279-286, 1981.

78. Solberg WK, Clark GT, Rugh JD: Nocturnal electromyographic evaluation of bruxing patients undergoing short-term splint therapy, *J Oral Rehabil* 2:215-223, 1975.

79. Pierce CJ, Gale EN: A comparison of different treatments for nocturnal bruxism, *J Dent Res* 67:597-601, 1988.

80. Dao TT, Lavigne GJ, Charbonneau A, et al: The efficacy of oral splints in the treatment of myofascial pain of the jaw muscles: a controlled clinical trial, *Pain* 56:85-94, 1994.

81. Turk DC, Zaki HS, Rudy TE: Effect of intraoral appliance and biofeedback/stress management alone and in combination in treating pain and depression in patients with temporomandibular disorders, *J Prosthet Dent* 70:158-164, 1993.

82. McCall WD, Bailey JO, Ash MM: A quantitative measure of mandibular joint dysfunction: phase plane modelling of jaw movement in man, *Arch Oral Biol* 21:685-689, 1976.

83. Beard CC, Clayton JA: Effect of occlusal splint therapy on TMJ dysfunction, *J Prosthet Dent* 44:324-335, 1980.

84. Monteiro AA, Clark GT: Mandibular movement feedback versus occlusal appliances in the treatment of masticatory muscle dysfunction, *J Craniomand Disord Fac Oral Pain* 2:41-47, 1988.

85. Murakami K, Matsuki M, Iizuka T, et al: Recapturing of persistent anteriorly displaced disc by mandibular manipulation after pumping and hydraulic pressure to the upper joint cavity of the temporomandibular joint, *J Craniomand Pract* 5:17-24, 1987.

86. Ross JB: The intracapsular therapeutic modalities in conjunction with arthrography: case reports, *J Craniomand Disord Fac Oral Pain* 3:35-43, 1989.

87. Nitzan DW, Dolwick MF, Martinez GA: Temporomandibular joint arthrocentesis: a simplified treatment for severe, limited mouth opening, *J Oral Maxillofac Surg* 49: 1163-1167, 1991.

88. Rasmussen OC: Description of population and progress of symptoms in a longitudinal study of temporomandibular joint arthropathy, *Scand J Dent Res* 89:196-213, 1981.

89. McNeill C: Nonsurgical management of internal derangements. In Helms CA, Katzberg RW, Dolwick MF, editors: 1985, Radiology Research and Education Foundation.

90. Carlsson GE: Long-term effects of treatment of craniomandibular disorders, *J Craniomand Pract* 3:337-342, 1985.

91. Rydell N, Balazs EA: Effect of intra-articular injection of hyaluronic acid on the clinical symptoms of osteoarthritis and on granulation tissue formation, *Clin Orthop* 80:25-32, 1971.

92. Peyron JG, Balazs EA: Preliminary clinical assessment of Na-hyaluronate injection into human arthritic joints, *Pathol Biol* 22:731-736, 1974.

93. Namiki O, Toyoshima M, Morisaki N: Therapeutic effect of intra-articular injection of high molecular weight hyaluronic acid on osteoarthritis of the knee, *Int J Clin Pharmacol Ther Toxicol* 20:501-507, 1982.

94. Ruth DT, Swites BJ: Comparison of the effectiveness of intra-articular hyaluronic acid and conventional therapy for the treatment of naturally occurring arthritic conditions in horses, *Equine Pract* 7:25, 1985.

95. Bertolami CN, Gay T, Clark GT, et al: Use of sodium hyaluronate in treating temporomandibular disorders, *J Oral Maxillofac Surg* 51:232-242, 1993.

96. Greene CS, Laskin DM: Long-term evaluation of treatment for myofascial pain-dysfunction syndrome: a comparative analysis, *J Am Dent Assoc* 107:235-238, 1983.

97. Wedel A, Carlsson GE: Factors influencing the outcome of treatment in patients referred to a temporomandibular joint clinic, *J Prosthet Dent* 54:420-426, 1985.

98. Salter MW, Brooke RI, Merskey H: Temporomandibular pain and dysfunction syndrome: the relationship of clinical and psychological data to outcome, *J Behav Med* 9:97-109, 1986.

99. Clark GT, Lanham F, Flack F: Treatment outcome results for consecutive TMJ clinic patients, *J Craniomand Disord Fac Oral Pain* 2:87-95, 1988.

100. Okeson JP: Long-term treatment of disk-interference disorders of the temporomandibular joint with anterior repositioning occlusal splints, *J Prosthet Dent* 60:611-616, 1988.

101. Agerberg G, Carlsson GE: Late results of treatment of functional disorders of the masticatory system: a follow-up by questionnaire, *J Oral Rehabil* 1:309-316, 1974.

102. Wilkes CH: Arthrography of the temporomandibular joint in patients with the TMJ pain-dysfunction syndrome, *Minn Med* 61(11):645-652, 1978.

103. Wilkes CH: Structural and functional alterations of the temporomandibular joint, *Northwest Dent* 57(5):287-294, 1978.

Treatment of Stomatitis and Oropharyngeal Pain in the Oncology Patient

JANE M. FALL-DICKSON

The American Cancer Society estimated that 1,268,000 new cases of cancer would be diagnosed in 2001 and that 553,400 Americans would die from cancer.[1] Aggressive therapies, including chemoradiotherapy, high-dose chemotherapy followed by bone marrow or peripheral blood stem cell transplantation (BMT), and hyperfractionation of radiation therapy, are increasingly used to improve cure rates.[2] Although these treatment strategies may lead to increased survival, they also may increase the incidence of potentially life-threatening toxicities. Specifically, the use of growth factors to speed recovery time of the hematopoietic system has converted nonhematologic, cancer treatment-related side effects to major dose- and treatment-limiting complications, including stomatitis.

Stomatitis and Cancer Treatment

Stomatitis is an inflammation of the mucous membranes of the oral cavity, which may range from redness to ulceration, secondary to intensive chemotherapy and radiation therapy.[3] The clinical significance of stomatitis and acute oral pain was highlighted during the National Institutes of Health (NIH) Consensus Conference on Oral Complications of Cancer Therapies, Diagnosis, Prevention, and Treatment.[4] The consensus was that research should be directed toward interventions for stomatitis as a treatment-related complication. The management of stomatitis-related acute oral pain has also been recognized as clinically significant through inclusion within the Clinical Practice Guideline for the Management of Cancer Pain commissioned by the U.S. Agency for Health Care Policy and Research.[5]

Oncology patients who develop stomatitis often experience a cascade of related negative sequelae,[6] with one complication exacerbating another.[7-9] Stomatitis may alter oral comfort and lead to loss of taste.[10] Acute stomatitis-related oropharyngeal pain often leads to altered voice and difficulty speaking, limiting the patient's communication ability, and to dysphagia and related difficulty drinking and eating.[8,9,11] Patients experiencing difficulty drinking and eating may have compromised hydration and nutritional status, necessitating the use of total parenteral nutrition (TPN).[12] These negative sequelae have great potential to decrease the patient's quality of life during and after treatment.

The clinical literature strongly supports a central tenant of oncology treatment: each chemotherapeutic drug or modality should be administered on the basis of its optimal dose and schedule.[13] Violation of this central tenant may lead to less than optimal treatment outcomes. For example, a 20-year retrospective analysis of patients with node-positive breast cancer who received adjuvant cyclophosphamide, methotrexate, and 5-fluorouracil showed that patients who received less than 65% of the planned dose experienced significant reductions in both relapse-free survival (30%) and overall survival (25%).[14] Stomatitis impacts survival as a dose- and rate-limiting toxicity in selected chemotherapy and radiation treatment plans. Also, stomatitis may be so severe that patients themselves choose to discontinue chemotherapy.[15]

Patients with stomatitis also have an increased risk for local and systemic infections. Neutropenic patients with stomatitis have a four times greater relative risk of septicemia compared with patients without stomatitis.[16] Stomatitis also has considerable economic impact. For example, patients undergoing BMTs for hematologic malignancies who develop stomatitis have a length of hospital stay 5 days longer than this population without stomatitis.[17] This increased length of stay translated into additional charges of $22,500 per patient, based on an average daily hospitalization rate for this population of $4500.[18] Higher hospitalization charges of $42,749 have also been reported for BMT patients with evidence of ulcerative stomatitis compared with those without such evidence.[19]

Epidemiology

The frequency and severity of stomatitis vary and are influenced by numerous risk factors (Box 25-1). In contrast to these reports, however, Driezen[20] stated that there is no age or gender disposition to the development of stomatitis. Periodontal disease with chronic infection may be synergistic with stomatitis, and ulcerative lesions often spread with surface necrosis. Drug metabolism also affects the severity of stomatitis; patients who cannot adequately metabolize or excrete certain chemotherapeutic agents experience an increased incidence of stomatitis.[6] Risk factors related to chemotherapy and radiation treatment are described in the following sections.

Chemotherapy

Approximately 40% of oncology patients who receive chemotherapy develop some degree of stomatitis,[21] and about 50% of these patients with stomatitis develop severe, painful lesions requiring treatment modification or TPN.[18] Oncology patient populations at high risk for stomatitis are those who receive continuous infusion therapy for breast and colon cancer (5-fluorouracil and leucovorin) and who are treated with high-dose chemotherapy before BMT.

In general, more than 60% of high-risk BMT patients experience stomatitis.[9,22] Incidence rates of 97% ($n = 30$),[23] 89% ($n = 47$),[9] and 75% ($n = 59$)[22] have been reported in mixed samples of autologous and allogeneic BMT patients. In a series of breast cancer patients undergoing autologous BMT, 100% of patients ($n = 32$) experienced some degree of stomatitis.[24] Incidence rates of ulcerative stomatitis of 78% ($n = 59$),[22] 49% ($n = 47$),[9] and 36% ($n = 32$)[24] have been demonstrated in BMT populations.

The duration and time pattern of stomatitis over the course of treatment has been described in BMT populations. Kolbinson et al.[8] reported that in patients receiving allogeneic and other BMT ($n = 23$) the onset of oral cavity changes began on BMT day 0 (day of bone marrow or peripheral stem cell reinfusion), with a sharp increase seen from BMT day +1 to BMT day +11. Although oral scores decreased after BMT day +14, they remained above baseline. Most oral cavity change occurred from BMT day +7 to BMT day +14, as supported by a mixed allogeneic and autologous ($n = 47$) BMT sample in whom stomatitis began on average at BMT day +3, lasted 9.5 days, and resolved by BMT day +12.[9] In a mixed sample of allogeneic and autologous BMT patients

($n = 188$), 120 of whom also had received total body irradiation, the Oral Mucositis Index scores increased on BMT days 0 to +2, peaked on BMT days +6 to +16, and then decreased.[25] Scores remained greater than baseline after BMT day +38. Oral assessment scores from BMT patients treated with chemoradiation were consistently higher and showed slower recovery times.

Radiation Therapy

More than 90% of patients receiving experimental therapies (e.g., combined chemotherapy and radiation therapy) experience severe stomatitis.[26] Stomatitis is virtually universal if radiation therapy includes the oropharyngeal region.[2] Stomatitis is a dose- and rate-limiting toxicity of radiation therapy for head and neck cancer.[2] Although hyperfractionated radiotherapy and chemotherapy may improve survival, this treatment is frequently limited by the severity of stomatitis.

Pathogenesis

Stomatitis is a complex oral complication of cancer treatment resulting from toxicities, tissue damage, and inflammation (Fig. 25-1). The primary event is cell damage. Secondary influences include indirect toxicities, which lead to neutropenia, reactivation of latent virus, and opportunistic infections. Salivary gland dysfunction secondary to dehydration and direct effects of therapy on gland function may also alter the local mucosal defenses.

Sonis[18] proposed a mechanism for stomatitis development and healing to correlate clinical and laboratory findings and present a comprehensive picture of this complex biologic process. The four phases of the model are (1) inflammatory/vascular, (2) epithelial, (3) ulcerative/bacterial, and (4) healing (Box 25-2). Each phase is interdependent and results from cytokine-mediated actions, direct effects of chemotherapeutic drugs on the epithelium, oral bacterial flora, and the patient's bone marrow status. Observations in models of graft-versus-host disease have demonstrated that injury to host tissue from radiation and chemotherapy may cause cytokine release from the epithelium and connective tissue.[27]

The well-documented, relatively acute *inflammatory/vascular phase* occurs shortly after radiation therapy or chemotherapy administration.[18] Cytokines are released from epithelial tissue, including tumor

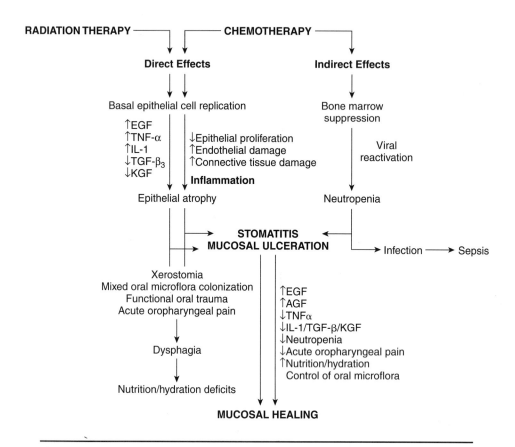

Fig. 25-1 Multifactorial etiology of stomatitis. *EGF,* Epidermal growth factor; *TNF-α,* tumor necrosis factor alpha; *IL-1,* interleukin-1; *TGF-β₃,* transforming growth factor beta-3; *KGF,* keratinocyte growth factor; *AGF,* angiogenic growth factor. (Modified from Loeser JD, Butler SH, Chapman CR, Turk DC, editors: *Bonica's management of pain,* ed 3, Philadelphia, 2001, Lippincott/ Williams & Wilkins; and Sonis ST: *Oral Oncol* 43:39-43, 1998.)

BⓞX 25-2

Four Phases of Stomatitis Development and Resolution

1. *Inflammatory/vascular:* shortly after radiation therapy or chemotherapy administration
2. *Epithelial:* 4 to 5 days after chemotherapy administration
3. *Ulcerative/bacterial:* about 1 week after chemotherapy; generally with maximum neutropenia
4. *Healing:* by BMT day +15 in more than 90% of BMT patients; with neutrophil recovery

From Sonis ST: *Oral Oncol* 43:39-43, 1998.

necrosis factor alpha (TNF-α), which leads to tissue damage; interleukin-1 (IL-1), which incites the inflammatory response and increases subepithelial vascularity and has the potential to increase levels of chemotherapy delivered locally to the oral cavity; and perhaps also IL-6.

The *epithelial phase* is associated with reduced epithelial renewal and atrophy and typically begins 4 to 5 days after chemotherapy administration. Stomatitis begins approximately 5 days after bone marrow infusion. The cell cycle S-phase-specific agents, including methotrexate, 5-fluorouracil, and cytarabine, are most efficient in this phase and are targeted at deoxyribonucleic acid (DNA) synthesis. The dividing cells of the oral basal epithelium are affected, and therefore children are three times more likely than adults to develop stomatitis because of children's higher proliferating fraction of basal cells. Epidermal growth factor (EGF) in animals pretreated with 5-flurouracil greatly increased the incidence of stomatitis through the increased rate of basal cell proliferation. Taking basal cells out of cell cycle with transforming growth factor beta-3 (TGF-β_3) appears to be protective, as does modification of apoptotic cell death.

The *ulcerative/bacterial phase* is the most biologically complex stage, beginning about 1 week after chemotherapy and generally coincident with maximum neutropenia[18] (Fig. 25-2). This stage is probably not related to specific classes of agents. Localized areas of full-thickness erosions are often covered by a fibrinous pseudomembrane. Bacterial colonization of mucosal ulceration leads to local secondary infection, and the mucosal ulceration is a portal of entry for microorganisms, which may lead to sepsis. Endotoxin flows into submucosal tissue, which reacts with tissue-borne mononuclear cells, leading to the release of IL-1 and tumor necrosis factor (TNF) and production of nitric oxide, which may lead to local mucosal injury. Radiation therapy and chemotherapy are likely to amplify and prolong the release of cytokines, exacerbating tissue response. The atrophy and ulceration are likely to be exacerbated by functional trauma.

This third stage is most symptomatic for the patient, accompanied by acute oropharyngeal pain and leading to dysphagia, nutritional deficits, and communication difficulties. Transcription factors may modify genetic expression of cytokines and enzymes critical in tissue damage. There may be a role for transcription factors (e.g., NF-kappa B) in the rate increase of rate gene transcription and thereby the rate of messenger ribonucleic acid (mRNA) and protein production.[18] Although the environmental modification of transcription factor expression has been described, the impact of chemotherapy has yet to be investigated.[18] Future research may elucidate the variance in patient response to chemotherapy.

The *healing phase* is affected by any factor that impacts negatively on wound healing. Resolution of stomatitis occurs in more than 90% of BMT patients by BMT day +15, when the white blood cells (WBCs) recover. This phase is associated with renewal of epithelial proliferation and differentiation, normalization of peripheral WBCs, reestablishment of local microbial flora, and decrease in acute oropharyngeal pain.

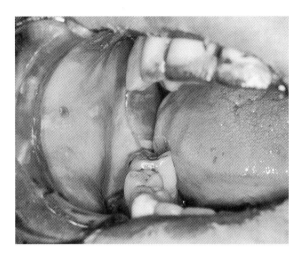

Fig. 25-2 Ulcerative stomatitis in a 44-year-old male after allogeneic BMT for acute lymphocytic leukemia. (Courtesy Dr. Vidya Sankar.)

Stomatitis and Acute Oropharyngeal Pain

Pain is an extremely complex subjective experience composed of multiple dimensions and affected by both physiologic and psychological variables.[28] Stomatitis is the principal etiology of most pain experienced during the 3-week post-BMT period[29] and is a major source of morbidity for BMT patients, often described as the "most unforgettable ordeal" of BMT.[30] High incidence rates of stomatitis-induced acute oral pain of 86% ($n = 47$)[9] and 89% ($n = 100$)[31] have been found in mixed samples of allogeneic and autologous BMT patients. A 47% incidence of stomatitis-related acute oral pain both at rest and with swallowing was observed in a sample of 32 breast cancer patients undergoing autologous BMT.[24]

The multiple dimensions of stomatitis-related acute oropharyngeal pain include physiologic, sensory, affective, behavioral, cognitive, and sociocultural. The sensory receptors of the oropharynx are innervated by the trigeminal (cranial nerve V), facial (VII), glossopharyngeal (IX), and the vagus (X) nerves.[32] The predominantly free nerve-ending receptors of the pharyngeal epithelium contribute to both the sensation of pain and the discriminative ability for hot and cold liquids.[32] Any degree of stomatitis can lead to pain.[33] McGuire et al.[9] reported that (1) oral pain in autologous and allogeneic BMT patients may be detected before stomatitis is clinically evident, (2) intensity of pain is not directly related to the extent of mucosal injury, and (3) some patients experience limited or no pain after BMT. In contrast to these findings, Kolbinson et al.[8] reported in a sample of patients treated with either allogeneic or other BMT treatment, oral pain increased from BMT days +4 to +21, with BMT days +4 to +14 having the highest pain scores. Overall pain ratings paralleled the trend for oral tissue and salivary changes during the 2 weeks after BMT.

The *sensory dimension* of stomatitis-related acute oropharyngeal pain refers to its location, intensity, duration, and quality, as well as the interrelationships among these components.[34] Assessment of these components of the pain experience is necessary before and during treatment of stomatitis to ensure adequate pain control. Breast cancer patients undergoing BMT has been shown to differentiate pain in six oropharyngeal locations: lips (upper and lower), buccal mucosa (right and left), tongue, and throat.[24]

Stomatitis-related oral pain is continuous and is exacerbated by normal activities of daily living, such as oral care, swallowing, and sleeping.[9] The intensity of this oral pain associated with general mucosal inflammation and breakdown ranges from mild discomfort to severe and debilitating pain requiring high-dose opioid analgesics.[25] Patients treated with high-dose chemotherapy and BMT and those receiving standard-dose chemotherapy report similar oral sensations, with oral discomfort perceived as dryness and mild burning, progressing to a raw and painful mouth.[5,35] Duration of stomatitis-related acute oral pain follows the acute pain taxonomy of the International Association for the Study of Pain (IASP),[36] which covers several orders of magnitude of less than 3 months.[9,36,37] Breast cancer patients undergoing BMT can clearly differentiate sensory pain components from affective pain components, with the sensory component of pain most frequently described as sore, aching, and dull and the affective component as annoying, troublesome, and nagging.[24]

Oral infections may increase stomatitis-related acute oral pain. Allogeneic and autologous BMT patients may experience severe oral pain or esophageal infection in the first 20 days after transplantation.[38] Stomatitis may be more severe in the presence of oral infection, particularly *herpes simplex virus* (HSV).[8,39,40] Immunocompromised cancer patients with HSV infections exhibit atypical biologic behavior compared

with their immunocompromised counterparts.[41] These patients develop larger, more tissue-destructive lesions and experience greater resulting pain than noncancer patients. The immunocompromised patients unable to overcome the invasion may develop localized infections of the oral mucosa, which may lead to systemic, life-threatening complications, such as esophagitis, necrotizing and hemorrhagic ulcers, and septicemia.[42]

The *affective dimension* of the acute oral pain experience refers to emotional responses to pain, which may be exhibited as anxiety, depression, mood changes, anger, and irritability, or conversely as anticipation of relief.[34] Patients have attached special biologic, emotional, and psychological meaning to pains in the face, head, mouth, and throat.[43] Nociceptive transmitting neurons at all segmental levels of the spinal cord project to the medial and lateral hypothalamus, as well as to several telencephalic regions.[44] These projections provide the neurophysiologic link between tissue injury, such as stomatitis, and the hypothalamic response. Extensive research has documented a positive relationship between pain, anxiety, and depression.[45-47]

The *behavioral dimension* of pain is related to communication, interpersonal interaction, and physical behaviors that demonstrate the presence and perhaps the severity of pain, and development of behaviors to manage pain.[9] The acute oral pain related to stomatitis may change the patient's communication patterns by preventing talking for days.[48] Behaviors used by cancer patients to relieve pain include medications and sleep,[49] relaxation and guided imagery, hypnosis, biofeedback, and distraction.[50]

The *cognitive dimension* of pain refers to influences on the patient's thought processes and self-image and the personal meaning of the pain.[34] Cognitive coping strategies, such as distraction, reinterpretation of the pain as another sensation, and ignoring the pain, have been used successfully by cancer patients to relieve pain.[37] The individual's attitudes, knowledge, and beliefs about pain and its treatment are important to assess before treatment begins.

The *sociocultural dimension* includes demographic characteristics, cultural background, personal family and work roles, family factors, and caregiver perspectives.[34] Research reports conflicting results regarding the association between age and pain perception[51,52] and intraethnic differences in the perception of pain.[53,54] The attitudes, knowledge, and beliefs of the patient's caregiver have become vital to the management of treatment-related oral pain in the home setting because caregivers are assuming increasing responsibility for pain management after the patient is discharged from the hospital.

Management

The optimal treatments for stomatitis and related acute oropharyngeal pain have not been established. Prevention and management strategies for stomatitis and related negative sequelae have been comprehensively reviewed[2,55,56] and include antimicrobial, antiinflammatory, and topical approaches. Limitations of previous research studies include use of small sample sizes and single clinical sites, lack of description of standardized oral assessment procedures, use of stomatitis measurement tools without reported validity and reliability, and lack of adequate description of methodology to allow study replication.

Pretreatment oral/dental stabilization is necessary to (1) eliminate sites of oral infection and trauma, (2) provide adequate cleaning, and (3) encourage appropriate oral hygiene. Challenges to pretreatment evaluation and stabilization include timing of therapy, knowledge base of the dental team regarding potential complications of cancer therapies, and patient compliance with oral hygiene and treatment plans.

Antimicrobial approaches include systemic administration of antimicrobial agents, such as antibiotics, antivirals (e.g., acyclovir, ganciclovir), and the antifungal agent fluconazole. *Acyclovir* prophylaxis is accepted treatment for BMT patients who are HSV and cytomegalovirus (CMV) seropositive. However, no correlation was found between severity of stomatitis and serologic status of HSV or CMV patients.[57] *Ganciclovir* has been found to be effective in suppressing CMV infection in patients with leukemia undergoing allogeneic BMT.[58] A randomized controlled clinical trial comparing *fluconazole* to placebo in BMT patients demonstrated that fluconazole prevented systemic fungal infections (7% fluconazole vs. 18% placebo) and significantly reduced the incidence of mucosal infection and oropharyngeal colonization by *Candida albicans*.[59] Epstein et al.[60] evaluated fluconazole versus prophylaxis in patients with leukemia treated with BMT and found reduced oropharyngeal colonization by *C. albicans*.

Donnelly et al.[61] demonstrated the importance of minimizing stomatitis through the combined use of intravenous clindamycin, 900 mg three times a day (tid), and ceftazidime, 2 g tid, in the initial manage-

ment of fever in allogeneic BMT patients. Bacteremia caused by *Viridans streptococci* was seen in 70% of patients during the maximum observed stomatitis. Culture results were positive 1 day before the onset of fever in one third of the patients. Mucosal ulceration predisposes the patient to systemic infection by oral flora, and therefore stomatitis attenuation is clearly important.

Antiinflammatory approaches include the use of topical agents such as prostaglandins and corticosteroids. Dinoprostone (Prostin E2, 0.5 mg/tablet) or placebo was tested for stomatitis prophylaxis in a sample of BMT patients.[62] The incidence, severity, and duration of stomatitis were similar for both groups. In the dinoprostone group, however, the stomatitis was more severe and the incidence of HSV infection higher.

Topical approaches have had varying results. Topical antimicrobial agents include chlorhexidine and antimicrobial lozenges. Use of *chlorhexidine*, a bisbiguanide compound and antiplaque agent with strong antimicrobial activity,[63] has demonstrated conflicting results. In hospitalized patients receiving BMT and radiation therapy, chlorhexidine appears to be beneficial in reducing stomatitis,[64-67] with a tendency toward reduced oral colonization of *Candida* species.[65] Confounding factors in these studies of chlorhexidine include the effects of oral hygiene and rinses on plaque levels, gingival inflammation, and caries risk; although not primary end points in the studies, these are logical factors to include in selected clinical trials. In contrast to these findings, results from a double-blind, placebo-controlled, randomized clinical trial (RCT) with ambulatory (non-BMT) chemotherapy patients ($n = 222$), who were treated with a 0.12% chlorhexidine or sterile water oral rinse and a nurse-initiated oral hygiene teaching program, demonstrated no statistically significant difference between the two treatment arms in regard to incidence, days to onset, and severity of stomatitis.[68] These researchers did acknowledge that chlorhexidine is effective in reducing stomatitis in a hospitalized chemotherapy population. *Antimicrobial lozenges* containing polymyxin, tobramycin, and amphotericin B have been shown to prevent ulcerative stomatitis in head and neck radiation therapy patients, perhaps because of reduction in gram-negative bacteria.

Studies regarding the use of *sucralfate* suspension are inconclusive. Although less severe stomatitis has been reported with the use of sucralfate,[69-71] in a randomized prospective trial of sucralfate prophylaxis in radiation therapy patients receiving high daily fractions, no difference in stomatitis was observed.[72] Less oral pain was noted early in the radiation therapy time course in the sucralfate group.

Biologic response modifiers include granulocyte-macrophage colony-stimulating factor (GM-CSF), granulocyte colony-stimulating factor (G-CSF), EGF, and TGF. The effects of these growth factors and cytokines (e.g., IL-11) in the development and severity of stomatitis have been evaluated using the animal cheek pouch model in Syrian golden hamsters. Results have demonstrated increased severity of mucosal damage in animals that received 5-fluorouracil and EGF[73] and decreased incidence, severity, and duration of stomatitis; decreased weight loss; and increased survival in animals that received TGF-β after chemotherapy.[74] In a randomized trial comparing IL-11 to placebo, a dose-dependent, statistically significant decrease in stomatitis ($p < 0.05$), increased survival (survival 85% IL-11 vs. 46% placebo), and less weight loss in the IL-11 group were found.[75]

GM-CSF has been tested in patients receiving a wide variety of treatment modalities. Head and neck squamous cell carcinoma patients ($n = 20$) treated with GM-CSF, cisplatin, 5-fluorouracil, and leucovorin demonstrated decreased incidence, duration, and severity of stomatitis.[76] Seventy-nine percent of head and neck cancer patients ($n = 14$) treated with radiation therapy and GM-CSF experienced decreased severity of stomatitis.[77] In contrast to these findings, Gordon[78] reported no effect on stomatitis severity in a pediatric oncology patient sample ($n = 26$) treated with hematopoietic stem cell transplantation and GM-CSF, although stomatitis duration was decreased. No difference in stomatitis was seen in a sample of BMT patients treated with G-CSF after BMT in a multicenter controlled study. Patients treated with G-CSF did have accelerated neutrophil recovery and decreased length of hospital stay.

Feber[79] compared saline to hydrogen peroxide oral rinses in a sample of patients receiving radiotherapy to more than 50% of the oral cavity ($n = 40$). No significant differences were seen in stomatitis between the two groups, and oral sensitivity was greater in the peroxide group. Tretinoin cream used from BMT day -7 until BMT day +21 was found to reduce stomatitis severity and decrease the number of patients who required systemic analgesics in a small sample of BMT recipients ($n = 6$).[80] Clinicians frequently recommend the use of oral mucosal coating agents (e.g., Milk of Magnesia, Amphojel liquid)

for stomatitis treatment. However, these agents have not been tested in the large RCT setting.

High-dose opioids are used to alleviate severe oropharyngeal pain associated with stomatitis and are often administered by patient-controlled analgesia pumps. Another approach has been the use of *capsaicin*, the active ingredient found in chili peppers.[81] Capsaicin was tested in a phase I study using a sample of chemotherapy and radiation therapy patients ($n = 11$).[82] The capsaicin was delivered in a taffy candy vehicle, which the subjects were instructed to let dissolve in their mouths. Partial and temporary pain reduction was reported in 11 patients with stomatitis. A double blind, placebo-controlled study is continuing to test the efficacy of capsaicin for pain control.[55]

Other strategies have included low-energy lasers, vitamin supplements, and anticholinergic agents (xerogenergic agents). *Azelastine* (2 mg daily, versus control) was tested in a sample of oral carcinoma patients who received chemoradiotherapy ($n = 63$).[83] Azelastine may suppress cytokine release from lymphocytes. Mild stomatitis ($n = 21$) and ulceration and severe pain ($n = 16$) were experienced by the treatment group. Mild reaction ($n = 5$) and severe stomatitis ($n = 21$) were observed in the control group. *Cryotherapy*, the use of ice chips or ice popsicles, has been shown to reduce stomatitis significantly in patients receiving 5-fluorouracil or melphalan treatment when these chemotherapy agents are given over short periods. Sucking on ice pops from 5 minutes before to 30 minutes after drug exposure may decrease stomatitis through a vasoconstrictive mechanism.

A meta-analysis of RCTs on prophylaxis for radiation-induced stomatitis in head and neck cancer patients ($n = 15$) revealed that narrow-spectrum antibiotic lozenges may be effective when stomatitis is assessed by clinicians.[26] When patient self-reporting was used to evaluate the stomatitis-related symptoms, however, none of the interventions appeared to be beneficial, and chlorhexidine was poorly tolerated. The analysis revealed that methodologic limitations were present in many studies.

Many treatment strategies for stomatitis and related oropharyngeal pain have been recommended but often have not been tested sufficiently in RCTs. Conflicting study results may be related to mixed diagnosis and treatment samples; inappropriate stomatitis assessment tools, which are unable to capture wide variations in oral cavity changes; and inappropriate timing and dose of interventions. Published research methodology should include the name of the research instrument used, items and scale, scoring, validity and reliability, and use in other samples to demonstrate appropriate choice of tool and therefore valid results.

Assessment Instruments

Historically, there have been several different approaches to the assessment and evaluation of the oral complications related to cancer chemotherapy. Oral cavity assessment tools have used two general approaches to date: (1) assigning a grade to the stomatitis observed in separate anatomic locations in the oral cavity and (2) staging the stomatitis holistically, including both the clinical observations and the functional status.[3] Each investigator or clinician must decide which assessment method and tool are most appropriate based on the purpose of the study.[84] Frequent assessment of stomatitis is necessary to capture changing clinical signs and symptoms over the treatment course.[5]

This section presents the instrument development rationale, psychometrics, and clinical utility for three widely used stomatitis assessment tools.

Oral Assessment Guide

The Oral Assessment Guide (OAG) was developed as a concise clinical tool to assess oral cavity complications in patients receiving stomatogenic cancer therapy.[85] The guide consists of eight assessment categories (voice, swallow, lips, tongue, saliva, mucous membranes, gingiva, teeth/dentures), each rated on three levels of descriptors: *1*, normal findings; *2*, mild alterations; and *3*, definitely compromised. Each category is a subscale, and an overall oral assessment score is obtained by summing the subscale scores, with a possible score range of 8 to 24. The OAG takes approximately 5 minutes to complete.

Content-related validity evidence for the OAG was obtained through a review of the nursing and dental literature and evaluation by an expert panel of dentists. The expert panel validated the eight separate categories of the OAG and the rating scale of 1 to 3. The appropriateness of the tool was tested through a pilot study using a sample of 20 sequential BMT patients with a variety of diagnoses and treatment protocols. Staff nurses used the OAG to make oral assessments after the nurse researchers outlined a protocol for assessment frequency. The pilot study for the OAG demonstrated construct validity evidence, support for the tool's clinical utility, and a high level of trained nurse-nurse interrater reliability ($r = .912$).[85]

Two limitations of the OAG are the combination of the functional performance ratings (voice, swallowing, oral hygiene) with the objective examiner-rater evaluations and unequal scoring for oral cavity areas.[25] The OAG has been used frequently to assess the effect of oral care protocols,[86,87] to compare methods on the nature and prevalence of oral mucositis,[84] and to determine incidence and severity of stomatitis in BMT patients in descriptive research studies.[24,31]

World Health Organization Index

The World Health Organization (WHO) index, which gives a simple, overall rating of stomatitis, has often been used as a general comparison index to other assessment scales.[3,88] The tool is scaled as follows: *grade 0*, no change; *grade 1*, soreness, erythema; *grade 2*, erythema and ulcers, solid diet tolerated; *grade 3*, ulcers, liquid diet only; and *grade 4*, alimentation not possible. Limitations include the lack of reliability or validity data for this guide, inability to capture the variety of oral changes that occur with cancer treatment, and inadequate assessment of the functional status of the patient.

Oral Mucositis Index

The Oral Mucositis Index (OMI) was derived from the Oral Mucositis Rating Scale (OMRS). The OMRS was developed as a research tool to measure comprehensively a broad range of cancer therapy–associated oral tissue changes, and as an index for assessing BMT-related stomatitis appropriate for use in patient care and research.[25]

The OMRS was constructed through the selection of clinical descriptors of oral mucosal changes related to BMT. The OMRS divides the oral cavity into seven distinct anatomic areas: (1) lips, (2) labial mucosa, (3) buccal mucosa, (4) tongue, (5) floor of mouth, (6) palate, and (7) attached gingiva. Each site is further divided into upper and lower (lips and labial mucosa); right and left (buccal mucosa); dorsal, ventral, and lateral (tongue); and hard and soft (palate). Descriptive categories include atrophy, pseudomembrane, erythema, hyperkeratosis, lichenoid, ulceration, and edema. Erythema, atrophy, hyperkeratosis, lichenoid, and edema are rated on the following scale: 0, normal/no change; 1, mild; 2, moderate; and 3, severe change. Ulceration and pseudomembrane are rated on scores based on estimated surface area involved: 0, none; 1, up to 1 cm^2; 2, from 1 cm^2 to 2 cm^2; and 3, 2 cm^2 or greater. The item pool consists of 91 items for 13 areas of the mouth that are assessed for several types of changes. The score is obtained by summing the scores of all items on the OMRS to yield a total possible score ranging from 0 to 273.

The psychometric analysis of the OMI was performed using a sample of 188 BMT patients (96 males, 92 females) ranging in age from 18 to 58 years, with a mean of 36 years.[25] Diagnostic categories in the sample included chronic myelogenous leukemia (38.8%), lymphoma (13.8%), acute myelogenous leukemia (9.0%), and other (17.6%). One hundred fifty-one (80%) patients received allogeneic transplants, and 37 received autologous transplants. No significant differences were found between the two groups regarding type of conditioning regimen. The ethnic composition of the sample was primarily Caucasian (94.4%), with African-American, Hispanic, and Asian ethnicity represented.

Construct validity evidence was collected based on a total item pool screening to exclude items that had little or no variance for three of the four assessment time periods corresponding to BMT days +3 to +16.[25] Although variance was too low for pseudomembrane and ulceration to satisfy psychometric criteria, these clinically significant variables were retained to define appropriately the range of mucosal damage seen with mucositis. A final set of 34 items was included in the OMI: 11 atrophy items (upper and lower lips; upper and lower labial mucosa; right and left buccal mucosa; dorsal, lateral, and ventral tongue; floor of mouth; soft palate); 11 pseudomembrane items (upper and lower lips; upper and lower labial mucosa; right and left buccal mucosa; dorsal, lateral, and ventral tongue; floor of mouth; soft palate); 10 erythema items (upper and lower lips; upper and lower labial mucosa; right and left buccal mucosa; dorsal, lateral, and ventral tongue; floor of mouth); and two edema items (right and left buccal mucosa).[25] The OMI has a total range of 0 to 102.

The reliability of the OMI was estimated using internal consistency and test-retest reliability statistics.

The internal consistency indices (Cronbach's alpha and Guttman split-half coefficients) ranged from 0.84 to 0.93, which indicate that the items related highly to each other. Correlations between OMI scores decreased as the time between scores increased, which is consistent with the clinical evidence that the extent and type of stomatitis are most consistent when assessments are performed closely to each other in time.[25]

Construct validity evidence of the OMI was gathered by comparing self-reported assessments of mouth pain (collected independently as part of another study) with the OMI matched by day post-BMT. Although the magnitude of Pearson product-moment correlation coefficients between the OMI and subjective reports of oral pain was low to moderate (0.33 to 0.67), they were statistically significant ($p < 0.0001$).[25] The OMI scores were also examined for two patient groups who were expected to differ in degree of stomatitis. Results confirmed the hypothesis that patients conditioned with both radiation and chemotherapy would have higher levels of stomatitis than those conditioned with only chemotherapy ($p < 0.05$). Patients who received chemoradiation therapy scored consistently higher and recovered more slowly, as measured by the OMI scores.

Recently, researchers have suggested the use of a downsized 20-item version of the OMI because numerous difficulties have been found with the original 34-item version,[89] including the following:

1. The atrophy parameter is difficult to measure reliably in the absence of histopathologic confirmation.
2. Use of all 34 items increases the probability of significant missing data because of patient difficulty in tolerating the oral examination.
3. Some of the parameters in the 34 items (e.g., atrophy in 11 anatomic locations, edema in right and left buccal mucosa) are less relevant to the acute oral pain experience.

The 20-item OMI was validated through a process of consensual judgment by an expert panel of leading BMT oral complications specialists in the United States. This 20-item version of the OMI has a possible score range of 0 to 60.

McGuire et al[90] tested the psychometrics of the 20-item OMI through a methodologic instrument evaluation design with repeated measures that was embedded in a larger intervention study. The convenience sample consisted of 133 patients who received allogenic or autologous BMT in a university-affiliated medical center. Patients were primarily Caucasian, with 43% men and 57% women, and the most common diagnoses were breast cancer, chronic myelogenous leukemia, and non-Hodgkin's lymphoma. Internal consistency reliability was demonstrated through Cronbach's alpha coefficients across time points that ranged from 0.90 to 0.96 for OMI total, 0.92 to 0.95 for erythema, and 0.71 to 0.90 for ulceration. Test-retest reliability was documented by significant positive correlations ($p < 0.001$) between each time point for OMI score ($r = 0.53$ to 0.86), erythema ($r = 0.53$ to 0.79), and ulceration ($r = 0.39$ to 0.83). Interrater reliability coefficients of 0.80 or greater were obtained for 17 of the 20 items when rated independently by three examiners at several time points during the study.

Construct-related evidence was demonstrated through positive correlations (most significant at $p < 0.01$) across time points between higher (worse) scores from the Brief Pain Inventory. Mean OMI total scores consistently discriminated ($p < 0.001$) between autologous BMT and allogeneic BMT patients at all time points. Criterion-related evidence was demonstrated through positive correlation of the OMI total scores ($r = 0.40$ to 0.62, $p < 0.01$), with summed mucous membrane and tongue items from the OAG scores across time. McGuire et al.[90] concluded that the 20-item OMI performed well in the BMT population, with the caveat that investigators need to acquire training and experience with the tool and the companion grading rules, which address the rating of stomatitis exhibiting more than one grade of change.

OMI Template. The OMI Template (Searle) is used with the OMI as a visual aid for scoring of erythema values of "normal," "mild," "moderate," and "severe," as well as scoring of the ulcer/pseudomembrane size in centimeter values. The template is a thin, white, laminated card measuring approximately 8 by 4½ inches. The erythema scale is located on the front side and consists of four rectangular strips, with ranges of the color red corresponding to "normal" coloration for mucous membranes, "mild" erythema, "moderate" erythema, and "severe" erythema. The back side of the template contains the ulcer/pseudomembrane scale and has square, circular, and rectangular figures corresponding to the surface area of grade 2 (≥ 1 cm^2 but < 2 cm^2) and

grade 3 (≥ 2 cm^2). Grade 2 figures are used as a reference to assess for grade 1 ulcer and pseudomembrane surface area.

Content validity for the shades of red corresponding to the values of "normal," "mild," "moderate," and "severe" was established through a collaborative effort among Peterson (University of Connecticut Health Center), Schubert (Fred Hutchinson Cancer Research Center), and a graphics designer.[91] The color scheme for erythema was reviewed, and the range of red within each category was selected based on Kodachrome slide sets and the oral medicine experts' experience with oral mucosa scoring.

Therapeutic Recommendations

Treatment for stomatitis and related oropharyngeal pain needs to be based on an understanding of the etiology of this condition and treatment results reported in the scientific literature. In general, the only standard forms of care are pretreatment oral/dental stabilization, saline mouthwashes, and pain management.[92] Prevention or attenuation of stomatitis begins with pretreatment oral/dental stabilization, which should be timed to allow healing before cancer treatment begins. This pretreatment requires collaboration among dental staff, cancer treatment team, and patient. Written instructions should be provided to the patient regarding self-care measures to prepare the oral cavity for the effects of cancer treatment. The dental progress notes should include specific risk factors for cancer therapy–related oral complications.

The treatment of stomatitis and related acute oropharyngeal pain begins with appropriate assessment of this cancer treatment–related oral inflammatory process and related symptoms. Use of reliable stomatitis and pain assessment tools with demonstrated clinical utility in the population assessed is critical to the assessment process. Stomatitis and related acute oropharyngeal pain should be assessed at least once each shift during active treatment and throughout the predicted time course of stomatitis and acute oral pain. More frequent pain assessments may be necessary during titration of opioid continuous infusions and during periods of uncontrolled pain. Assessment results need to be recorded and available to the health care team. Treatment recommendations should be made based on the outcomes of these assessments.

Meticulous oral hygiene must be maintained throughout the cancer treatment process. Numerous health care institution-based oral care policies and procedures exist for oncology patients during treatment and periods of treatment-related neutropenia and thrombocytopenia. The outcome of any oral care practice standard should be a clean, trauma-free, moist oral cavity, which is maintained in a physiologic environment conducive to healing. Institutional variability exists regarding these oral care protocols for patients treated with BMT, standard-dose therapy, and radiation therapy, and these practice standards should be evidence based.[93]

Hospital-based pharmacies typically formulate and dispense topical mixtures containing an analgesic, an antiinflammatory agent, and a coating agent as an oral comfort measure for oncology patients undergoing treatment. For example, one such topical formulation recommended for use at a large clinical research center contains lidocaine, viscous 2% (40 ml); diphenhydramine, 12.5 mg/5ml (40 ml); and Maalox, 10 mg (40 ml), every 3 to 4 hours as needed. Testing these various topical formulations through RCTs would promote evidence-based practice regarding these treatment recommendations.

Cryotherapy to induce vasoconstriction should be considered for patients who will be receiving 5-fluorouracil or melphalan over short infusion times. Lozenges containing amphotericin B, polymyxin, and tobramycin are useful in alleviating stomatitis associated with radiation therapy.

The increased use of the ambulatory setting for the delivery of cancer treatment has necessitated increased use of patient self-care activities and also the involvement of patient caregivers for pain management. Swisher, Scheidler, and Kennedy[94] described a mucositis pain management algorithm to enhance the transition from inpatient to ambulatory care for BMT patients. A key component of this successful program was the BMT patient self-reporting of oral pain to the multidisciplinary team.

Research Directions

Current research and clinical opportunities related to oral mucosal toxicities such as stomatitis and the related symptomatology of acute oral pain are significant and constantly evolving. Research directions regarding treatment of stomatitis and related oropharyngeal pain derive logically both from gaps in the scientific knowledge regarding the pathogenesis of this condition and from clinical research applications of the new scientific discoveries regarding the molecular genetic mechanisms of inflammation, pain, tissue injury, and repair. General research directions have the potential to advance the science of cancer treatment–related oral toxicities (Box 25-3).

Cooperative stomatitis clinical research groups, such as the Mucositis Study Group[95] and the Multinational Association for Supportive Care in Cancer/International Society for Oral Oncology, have demonstrated the excellent outcomes possible utilizing a targeted, multidisciplinary approach to this research. Pharmaceutical companies are also key players in the search for useful treatments for stomatitis. For example, the drug *repifermin* as a systemic formulation is currently being tested in phase IIa clinical trials for the prevention of stomatitis in the BMT setting.[96] Repifermin, also known as keratinocyte growth factor 2, promotes the growth and repair of epithelial cells in the mucosal tissues that line the mouth, throat, and other organs.

Key questions for inclusion in research programs on stomatitis and related oropharyngeal pain prevention and management include the following:

1. What are the roles of cytokines in the development of stomatitis?

BOX 25-3

Research Directions for Stomatitis and Related Oropharyngeal Pain

Characterize prognostic factors for the development of stomatitis and acute oropharyngeal pain.

Use randomized controlled clinical trials to test the effectiveness of pharmacologic and nonpharmacologic interventions to prevent or attenuate stomatitis and related oropharyngeal pain.

Establish optimal dose and timing of pharmacologic interventions for stomatitis.

Evaluate the contribution of oral microbial flora to stomatitis and oropharyngeal pain.

Establish valid and reliable measurement instruments for stomatitis appropriate for use in clinical research and/or clinical practice.

Establish valid and reliable measurement instruments for the multiple dimensions of stomatitis-related oropharyngeal pain.

2. Which patients are most at risk to develop stomatitis? Why?
3. What is the optimal stomatitis treatment for various oncology therapy populations?
4. What are optimal dosing schedules for stomatitis treatments?
5. Which patients are at risk to develop stomatitis-related acute oral pain?
6. Is there a genetic component of this acute oral pain?
7. What is the relationship among oral infection, stomatitis, and stomatitis-related acute oral pain?
8. What constitute reliable and valid research and clinical measurement tools for stomatitis and related acute oral pain?

Research also must explore the phenomenon of stomatitis-related acute oral pain itself, including patient and treatment factors that affect the perception of pain and response to pain.[97] Future research should focus on the interrelationships among the multiple dimensions for stomatitis-related acute oral pain in oncology patients, as well as the effectiveness of prophylactic and therapeutic interventions for this acute oral pain at rest and with swallowing.

SUMMARY

Stomatitis is a biologically complex oral condition experienced by many oncology patients that often leads to a cascade of negative sequelae, critical treatment alterations or cessation, and decreased quality of life. Oncology treatment protocols continue to examine the affect of dose-intensive treatments on clinical and survival outcomes. These vital outcomes are compromised when dose reduction or treatment cessation is necessary because of treatment-related stomatitis. Despite numerous recommendations for prevention and treatment of this oral condition, these interventions need to be evaluated in RCT settings using valid and reliable stomatitis assessment tools to both advance the science of oral toxicities and improve patient care.

References

1. Greenlee RT, Hill-Harmon MB, Murray T, et al: Cancer statistics, *CA Cancer J Clin* 51(1):15-37, 2001.
2. Epstein JB, Schubert MM: Oral mucositis in cancer patients. In Loeser JD, Butler SH, Chapman CR, Turk DC, editors: *Bonica's management of pain*, ed 3, Philadelphia, 2001, Lippincott/Williams & Wilkins.
3. Hyland S: Assessing the oral cavity. In Frank-Stromborg M, Olsen SJ, editors: *Instruments for clinical health-care research*, London, 1997, Jones and Bartlett.
4. National Institutes of Health Consensus Development Panel: Consensus statement: oral complications of cancer therapies, *Natl Cancer Inst Monogr* 9:3-8, 1989.
5. Jacox A, Carr DB, Payne R, et al: Mucositis. In *Management of cancer pain*, Clinical Practice Guideline No 9, AHCPR Pub No 94-0592, Agency for Health Care Policy and Research, Rockville, Md, 1994, US Department of Health and Human Services, Public Health Service.
6. Daeffler RJ: Mucous membranes. In Johnson BL, Gross J, editors: *Handbook of oncology nursing*, New York, 1985, Wiley.
7. Ford R, Ballard B: Acute complications after bone marrow transplantation, *Semin Oncol Nurs* 49:15-24, 1988.
8. Kolbinson DA, Schubert MM, Flournoy N, et al: Early oral changes following bone marrow transplantation, *Oral Surg Oral Med Oral Pathol* 66:130-138, 1988.
9. McGuire DB, Altomonte V, Peterson DE, et al: Patterns of mucositis and pain in patients receiving preparative chemotherapy, *Oncol Nurs Forum* 20:1493-1502, 1993.
10. Wujcik D: Current research in side effects of high-dose chemotherapy, *Semin Oncol Nurs* 8:102-112, 1992.
11. Barasch A, Peterson D, Tanzer JM, et al: Helium-neon laser effects on conditioning-induced oral mucositis in bone marrow transplantation patients, *Cancer* 76:2550-2556, 1995.
12. Wingard JR, Niehaus CS, Peterson DE, et al: Oral mucositis after bone marrow transplantation, *Oral Surg Oral Med Oral Pathol* 72:419-424, 1991.
13. Gillespie TW: Chemotherapy dose and dose intensity: analyzing data to guide therapeutic decision, *Oncol Nurs Forum* 28:5-10, 2001.
14. Bonadonna G, Valagussa P, Moliterni A, et al: Adjuvant cyclophosphamide, methotrexate, and fluorouracil in node-positive breast cancer: the results of 20 years of follow-up, *N Engl J Med* 332:901-906, 1995.
15. Fox PC: *Consensus Development Conference on Oral Complications of Cancer Therapies: Diagnosis, Prevention, and Treatment*, Bethesda, Md, 1990, National Cancer Institute.
16. Eting LS, Bodey GP, Keefe BH: Septicemia and shock syndrome due to viridans streptococci: a case-control study of predisposing factors, *Clin Infect Dis* 14:1201-1207, 1992.
17. Reuscher TJ, Sodeifi A, Scricani SJ, et al: The impact of mucositis on α-hemolytic streptococcal infection in patients undergoing autologous bone marrow transplantation for hematologic malignancies, *Cancer* 82:2275-2281, 1998.
18. Sonis ST: Mucositis as a biological process: a new hypothesis for the development of chemotherapy-induced stomatoxicity, *Oral Oncol* 43:39-43, 1998.
19. Sonis ST, Oster G, Fuchs H, et al: Oral mucositis and the clinical and economic outcomes of hematopoietic stem-cell transplantation, *J Clin Oncol* 19:2201-2205, 2001.
20. Driezen S: Description and incidence of oral complications, *Natl Cancer Inst Monogr* 9:11-15, 1990.

21. Sonis ST: Oral complications of cancer therapy. In DeVita VT, Hellman S, Rosenberg SA, editors: *Cancer: principles and practice of oncology,* ed 4, Philadelphia, 1993, Lippincott.

22. Woo S-B, Sonis ST, Monopoli MM, et al: A longitudinal study of oral ulcerative mucositis in bone marrow transplant recipients, *Cancer* 72:1612-1617, 1993.

23. Seto BG, Kim M, Wolinsky L, et al: Oral mucositis in patients undergoing bone marrow transplantation, *Oral Surg Oral Med Oral Pathol* 60:493-497, 1985.

24. Fall-Dickson JM: Stomatitis-related acute oral pain experience of breast cancer autotransplant patient, Unpublished dissertation data, 2000.

25. Schubert MM, Williams BE, Lloyd ME, et al: Clinical scale for the rating of oral mucosal changes associated with bone marrow transplantation, *Cancer* 69:2469-2477, 1992.

26. Sutherland SE, Browman GP: Prophylaxis of oral mucositis in irradiated head-and-neck cancer patients: a proposed classification scheme of interventions and meta-analysis of randomized controlled trials, *Int J Radiat Oncol Biol Phys* 49:917-930, 2001.

27. Antin JH, Ferrara JL: Cytokine dysregulation and acute graft-versus-host-disease, *Blood* 80:2964-2968, 1992.

28. Coyle N, Foley KM: Alterations in comfort: pain. In Baird SB, McCorkle R, Grant M, editors: *Cancer nursing: a comprehensive textbook,* Philadelphia, 1991, Saunders.

29. Syrjala KL, Chapko ME: Evidence for a biopsychosocial model of cancer treatment pain, *Pain* 61:69-79, 1995.

30. Eisen D, Essell J, Brown ER: Oral cavity complications of bone marrow transplantation, *Semin Cutan Med Surg* 16:265-272, 1997.

31. Waterman MR, Wool A, Brown J: The incidence and severity of stomatitis and oral pain in bone marrow transplant patients, *Oncol Nurs Forum* 20:325, 1993.

32. Capra NF: Mechanisms of oral sensation, *Dysphagia* 10:235-247, 1995.

33. Burke MB, Wilkes GM, Berg D, et al: Potential toxicities and nursing management. In *Cancer chemotherapy: a nursing process approach,* Boston, 1991, Jones and Bartlett.

34. National Institute of Nursing Research Priority Expert Panel on Symptom Management: Acute Pain: *The nature of pain: a conceptual perspective,* Bethesda, Md, 1994, US Department of Health and Human Services.

35. Lin EM, Tiernery DK, Stadtmauer EA: Autologous bone marrow transplantation: a review of the principles and complications, *Cancer Nurs* 16:204-213, 1993.

36. International Association for the Study of Pain, Subcommittee on Taxonomy: Pain terms: a current list with definition and notes on usage, *Pain* 6:249-252, 1979 (updated 1982, 1986).

37. Gaston-Johannson F, Franco T, Zimmerman L: Pain and psychological distress in patients undergoing autologous bone marrow transplantation, *Oncol Nurs Forum* 19:441-448, 1992.

38. Scott DA, Schimpff SC: Prevention of infection in cancer patients. In Klastersky J, Schimpff SC, Senn H-J, editors: *Handbook of supportive care in cancer,* New York, 1995, Marcel Dekker.

39. Redding SW: Role of herpes simplex virus reactivation in chemotherapy-induced oral mucositis, *Natl Cancer Inst Monogr* 9:103-105, 1990.

40. Woo S-B, Lee SF-K: Oral recrudescent herpes simplex virus infection, *Oral Surg Oral Med Oral Pathol Oral Radiol Oral Endod* 83:239-243, 1997.

41. Poland J: Prevention and treatment of oral complications in the cancer patient, *Oncology* 5:45-50, 1991.

42. Ezzone S, Jolly E, Replongle K, et al: Survey of oral hygiene regimens among bone marrow transplant centers, *Oncol Nurs Forum* 20:1375-1381, 1993.

43. Sessle BJ: Neural mechanisms of oral and facial pain, *Otolaryngol Clin North Am* 22:1059-1072, 1989.

44. Chapman CR: The affective dimension of pain. A model of pain and the brain: from nociception to cognition. In Bromm B, Desmedt JE, editors: *Advances in pain research and theory,* New York, 1995, Raven.

45. Gaston-Johansson F, Fall-Dickson JM, Bakos AB, et al: Fatigue, pain, and depression in pre-autotransplant breast cancer patients, *Cancer Pract* 7:240-247, 1999.

46. Massie MJ, Holland JC: The cancer patients with pain: psychiatric complications and their management, *J Pain Symptom Manage* 7:99-109, 1992.

47. Spiegel D, Sands S, Koopman C: Pain and depression in patients with cancer, *Cancer* 74:2570-2578, 1994.

48. Shuster GF, Steeves RH, Onega L, et al: Coping patterns among bone marrow transplant patients: a hermeneutical inquiry, *Cancer Nurs* 19:290-297, 1996.

49. Wilkie D, Lovejoy N, Dodd M, et al: Cancer pain control behaviors: description and correlation with pain intensity, *Oncol Nurs Forum* 15:723-731, 1998.

50. Whipple B: Methods of pain control: review of research and literature, *Image J Nurs Scholar* 19:142-146, 1987.

51. Ferrell BA, Ferrell BR: The experience of pain and quality of life in elderly patients, *Gerontology* 28:76A, 1988.

52. McMillan S: The relationship between age and intensity of cancer-related symptoms, *Oncol Nurs Forum* 16:237-241, 1989.

53. Greenwald HP: Interethnic differences in pain perception, *Pain* 44:157-163, 1991.

54. Cleeland CS, Ladinsky JL, Serlin RC: Multidimensional measurement of cancer pain: comparisons of US and Vietnamese patients, *J Pain Symptom Manage* 3:23-27, 1988.

55. Berger AM, Kilroy TJ: Oral complications. In DeVita VT, Hellman S, Rosenberg S, editors: *Principles and practice of oncology,* ed 6, Philadelphia, 2001, Lippincott.

56. Iwamoto RR: Alterations in oral status. In McCorkle R, Grant M, Frank-Stromborg M, et al, editors: *Cancer nursing: a comprehensive textbook,* ed 2, Philadelphia, 1996, Saunders.

57. Epstein JB, Ransier A, Sherlock CH: Acyclovir prophylaxis of oral herpes virus during bone marrow transplantation, *Oral Oncol Eur J Cancer* 32(B):158-162, 1996.

58. Goodrich JM, Bowden RA, Fisher L, et al: Ganciclovir prophylaxis to prevent cytomegalovirus disease after allogeneic marrow transplant, *Ann Intern Med* 118:173-178, 1993.

59. Slavin MA, Osborne B, Adams R, et al: Efficacy and safety of fluconazole prophylaxis for fungal infections after marrow transplantation: a prospective, randomized, double-blind study, *J Infect Dis* 171:1545-1552, 1995.

60. Epstein JB, Ransier A, Lunn R, et al: Prophylaxis of candidiasis in patients with leukemia and bone marrow transplants, *Oral Surg Oral Med Oral Pathol Oral Radiol Endod* 81:291-296, 1993.

61. Donnelly JP, Muus P, Horrevorts AM: Failure of clindamycin to influence the course of severe oromucositis associated with streptococcal bacteraemia in allogeneic bone marrow transplant recipients, *Scand J Infect Dis* 25:43-40, 1993.

62. Labor B, Mrsic M, Pavletic Z, et al: Prostaglandin E2 for prophylaxis of oral mucositis following BMT, *Bone Marrow Transplant* 11:379-382, 1993.

63. Davies A: The mode of action of chlorhexidine, *J Periodont Res* 8(suppl 12):68-75, 1973.

64. Verdi CJ: Cancer therapy and oral mucositis: an appraisal of drug prophylaxis, *Drug Safety* 9:185-195, 1993.

65. Epstein JB, Vickais L, Spinelli J, et al: Efficacy of chlorhexidine and nystatin rinses in prevention of oral complications in leukemia and bone marrow transplantation, *Oral Surg Oral Med Oral Pathol* 73:682-689, 1992.

66. Ferretti GA, Raybould TP, Brown AT, et al: Chlorhexidine prophylaxis for chemotherapy- and radiation-induced stomatitis: a randomized double-blind trial, *Oral Surg Oral Med Oral Pathol* 69:331-338, 1990.

67. Rutkauskas JS, Davis JW: Effects of chlorhexidine during immunosuppressive chemotherapy: a preliminary report, *Oral Surg Oral Med Oral Pathol* 76:441-448, 1993.

68. Dodd MJ, Larson PJ, Dibble SL, et al: Randomized clinical trial of chlorhexidine versus placebo for prevention of oral mucositis in patients receiving chemotherapy, *Oncol Nurs Forum* 23:921-927, 1996.

69. Adams S, Toth B, Dudley BS: Evaluation of sucralfate as a compounded oral suspension for the treatment of stomatitis, *Clin Pharmacol Ther* 2:178, 1985.

70. Pfeiffer P, Hansen O, Madsen EL, et al: A prospective pilot study on the effect of sucralfate mouth-swishing in reducing stomatitis during radiotherapy of the oral cavity, *Acta Oncol* 29:471-473, 1990.

71. Shenep JL, Kalwinsky K, Hutson DK: Efficacy of oral sucralfate suspension in prevention and treatment of chemotherapy-induced stomatitis, *J Pediatr* 113:758-763, 1988.

72. Epstein JB, Wong FL: The efficacy of sucralfate suspension in the prevention of oral mucositis due to radiation therapy, *Int J Radiat Oncol Phys* 28:693-698, 1994.

73. Sonis ST, Costa JW, Evitts SM, et al: Effect of epidermal growth factor on ulcerative mucositis in hamsters that receive cancer chemotherapy, *Oral Surg Oral Med Oral Pathol* 74:749-755, 1992.

74. Sonis ST, Lindquist IL, Van Vugt A, et al: Prevention of chemotherapy-induced ulcerative mucositis by transforming growth factor β3, *Cancer Res* 54:1135-1138, 1994.

75. Sonis S, Muska A, O'Brien J, et al: Alteration in the frequency, severity, and duration of chemotherapy-mucositis in hamsters by interleukin-11, *Eur J Cancer Oral Oncol* 31B:261-266, 1995.

76. Chi K-H, Chen C-H, Chan W-K, et al: Effect of granulocyte-macrophage colony-stimulating factor on oral mucositis in head and neck cancer patients after cis-platinum, fluorouracil and leucovorin chemotherapy, *J Clin Oncol* 13:2620-2628, 1995.

77. Masucci G: New clinical applications of granulocyte-macrophage colony-stimulating factor, *Med Oncol* 13:149-154, 1996.

78. Gordon B, Spadinger A, Hodges E, et al: Effect of granulocyte-macrophage colony-stimulating factor on oral mucositis after hematopoietic stem-cell transplantation, *J Clin Oncol* 12:1917-1922, 1994.

79. Feber T: Management of mucositis in oral irradiation, *Clin Oncol R Coll Radiol* 8:106-111, 1996.

80. Cohen G, Elad S, Or R, et al: The use of tretinoin as oral mucositis prophylaxis in bone marrow transplantation patients: a preliminary study, *Oral Dis* 3:243-246, 1997.

81. Berger AM, Bartoshuk LM, Duffy VB, et al: Capsaicin for the treatment of oral mucositis pain: PPO updates, *Princ Pract Oncol* 9:1-11, 1995.

82. Berger A, Henderson M, Nadoolman W, et al: Oral capsaicin provides temporary relief for oral mucositis pain secondary to chemotherapy/radiation therapy, *J Pain Symptom Manage* 10:243-248, 1995.

83. Osaki T, Ueta E, Yoneda K, et al: Prophylaxis of oral mucositis associated with chemoradiotherapy for oral carcinoma by azelastine hydrochloride (Azelastine) with other antioxidants, *Head Neck* 16:331-339, 1994.

84. Dodd MJ, Facione NC, Dibble SL, et al: Comparison of methods to determine the prevalence and nature of oral mucositis, *Cancer Pract* 4:312-317, 1996.

85. Eilers J, Berger AM, Petersen MC: Development, testing, and application of the Oral Assessment Guide, *Oncol Nurs Forum* 15:325-330, 1988.

86. Graham KM, Pecoraro DA, Venture M, et al: Reducing the incidence of stomatitis using a quality assessment and improvement approach, *Cancer Nurs* 16(suppl):117-122, 1993.

87. Kenny SA: Effect of two oral protocols on the incidence of stomatitis in hematology patients, Cancer Nurs 13:345-353, 1990.

88. World Health Organization: *Handbook for reporting results of cancer treatment*, Geneva, 1979, WHO.

89. Peterson DE, McGuire DB: Personal communication, 1998.

90. McGuire DB, Peterson DE, Miller S, et al: The 20-item oral mucositis index: reliability and validity in bone marrow and stem cell transplant patients. Paper presented at Fifth National Conference on Cancer Nursing Research, Newport Beach, Calif, 1999.

91. Peterson DE: Personal communication, 1999.

92. Biron P, Sebban C, Gourmet R, et al: Research controversies in management of oral mucositis, *Support Care Cancer* 8:68-71, 2000.
93. Peterson DE: Research advances in oral mucositis, *Curr Opin Oncol* 11:261-266, 1999.
94. Swisher ME, Scheidler VR, Kennedy MJ: A mucositis pain management algorithm: a creative strategy to enhance the transition to ambulatory care, *Oncol Nurs Forum* 25:309, 1998.
95. Sonis ST, Eilers JP, Epstein JB: Mucositis Study Group: validation of a new scoring system for the assessment of clinical trial research of oral mucositis induced by radiation or chemotherapy, *Cancer* 85:2103-2113, 1999.
96. Brzostowski M: From genomics to drugs, *Res Dev Direct* April 2001, pp 34-44.
97. Spross JA, McGuire DB, Schmitt R: Oncology Nursing Society position paper on cancer pain. Part II, *Oncol Nurs Forum* 17:751-760, 1990.

INDEX